ANNUAL REVIEW OF
PUBLIC HEALTH

EDITORIAL COMMITTEE (1992)

EDWARD L. BAKER
MARSHALL H. BECKER
JONATHAN E. FIELDING
WILLIAM H. FOEGE
JOYCE C. LASHOF
LESTER B. LAVE
PAUL E. LEAVERTON
GILBERT S. OMENN

Responsible for the organization of Volume 13
(Editorial Committee, 1990)

EDWARD L. BAKER
JONATHAN E. FIELDING
WILLIAM H. FOEGE
LAWRENCE W. GREEN
JOYCE C. LASHOF
LESTER B. LAVE
GILBERT S. OMENN
RICHARD D. REMMINGTON
LESTER BRESLOW (GUEST)

Production Editor   BONNIE MEYERS
Subject Indexer   SUZANNE COPENHAGEN

ANNUAL REVIEW OF PUBLIC HEALTH

VOLUME 13, 1992

GILBERT S. OMENN, *Editor*
University of Washington

JONATHAN E. FIELDING, *Associate Editor*
University of California at Los Angeles

LESTER B. LAVE, *Associate Editor*
Carnegie Mellon University

ANNUAL REVIEWS INC.   4139 EL CAMINO WAY   P.O. BOX 10139   PALO ALTO, CALIFORNIA 94303-0897

ANNUAL REVIEWS INC.
Palo Alto, California, USA

International Standard Serial Number: 0164–7525
International Standard Book Number: 0–8243–2713-6

Annual Review and publication titles are registered trademarks of Annual Reviews Inc.

⊗ The paper used in this publication meets the minimum requirements of
American National Standard for Information Sciences—Permanence of Paper
for Printed Library Materials, ANZI Z39.48-1984.

Annual Reviews Inc. and the Editors of its publications assume no responsibility for the
statements expressed by the contributors to this *Review*.

Typesetting by Kachina Typesetting Inc., Tempe, Arizona; John Olson, President;
Janis Hoffman, Typesetting Coordinator; and by the Annual Reviews Inc. Editorial Staff

PRINTED AND BOUND IN THE UNITED STATES OF AMERICA

PREFACE

The 1992 *Annual Review of Public Health* continues to meet the important need, increasingly recognized, to bridge academic public health and preventive medicine with public health practice and clinical preventive services.

We see growing attention to prevention and to a population-based orientation to health, health care needs, and costs among health care professionals and among health policy analysts and policymakers. We believe that the *Annual Review of Public Health* fuels this movement with essential substantive material.

We are working with a committee and the staff of the American College of Preventive Medicine to help them utilize the articles in the *Annual Review of Public Health* in their Continuing Education and Self-Assessment program. We believe that these volumes can be similarly used by public health schools and their constituent departments and by public health practitioners and their organizations.

In organizing the text, we have experimented this year with grouping the articles by heading. We have long organized the cumulative table of contents under Age and Disease Specific, Behavioral Aspects of Health, Environmental Health, Epidemiology/Biostatistics, and Health Services. The task is complicated by the fact that certain topics and certain articles deliberately combine public health areas, such as epidemiology and health services, or epidemiology and environmental health. This year, we have added the heading of Public Health Practice to give greater visibility to our commitment to bridging academia and practice, and to stimulate suggestions of topics and authors from a broadened array of sources, especially our readers. We welcome your comments.

Despite increased attention to developing country topics and more invitations to authors from other countries, we have not used the heading International Health. These articles cut across the headings, and a separate heading would be confusing. Also, we believe that many, if not most, of our articles have international relevance. Do look through the cumulative table of contents at the end of this text and "browse" beyond your own specialty field.

THE EDITORIAL COMMITTEE

Annual Review of Public Health
Volume 13, 1992

CONTENTS

EPIDEMIOLOGY AND BIOSTATISTICS

HIV Infection and AIDS in Children, *Thomas C. Quinn, Andrea
Ruff, and John Modlin*   1

Selected Methodological Issues in Evaluating Community-Based
Health Promotion and Disease Prevention Programs, *T. D.
Koepsell, E. H. Wagner, A. C. Cheadle, D. L. Patrick, D.
C. Martin, P. H. Diehr, E. B. Perrin, A. R. Kristal, C. H.
Allan-Andrilla, and L. J. Dey*   31

Public Health Assessment in the 1990s, *Michael A. Stoto*   59

The Hantaviruses, Etiologic Agents of Hemorrhagic Fever with
Renal Syndrome: A Possible Cause of Hypertension and
Chronic Renal Disease in the United States, *J. W. LeDuc, J.
E. Childs, and G. E. Glass*   79

How Much Physical Activity Is Good for Health?, *S. N. Blair,
H. W. Kohl, N. F. Gordon, and R. S. Paffenbarger, Jr.*   99

ENVIRONMENTAL AND OCCUPATIONAL HEALTH

The Health Effects of Low-Level Ionizing Radiation, *Arthur C.
Upton, Roy E. Shore, and Naomi H. Harley*   127

Occupational Health Concerns of Firefighting, *Tee L. Guidotti
and Veronica M. Clough*   151

Biological Interactions and Potential Health Effects of
Extremely-Low-Frequency Magnetic Fields from Power Lines
and Other Common Sources, *T. S. Tenforde*   173

Worksite Drug Testing, *Diana Chapman Walsh, Lynn Elinson,
and Lawrence Gostin*   197

PUBLIC HEALTH PRACTICE

Global Immunization, *R. Kim-Farley and the Expanded
Programme on Immunization Team*   223

Polio Eradication from the Western Hemisphere, *Ciro A. de
Quadros, Jon K. Andrus, Jean-Marc Olive, Carlyle Guerra
de Macedo, and Donald A. Henderson*   239

Health Issues for College Students, *Kevin Patrick, Ted W.
Grace, and Chris Y. Lovato*   253

viii   CONTENTS   *(Continued)*

Mortality of American Indian and Alaska Native Infants, *Everett R. Rhoades, George Brenneman, Jerry Lyle, and Aaron Handler*   269

The Public Health Practice of Tobacco Control: Lessons Learned and Directions for the States in the 1990s, *Thomas E. Novotny, Rosemary A. Romano, Ronald M. Davis, and Sherry L. Mills*   287

BEHAVIORAL ASPECTS OF HEALTH

Depression: Current Understanding and Changing Trends, *Myrna M. Weissman and Gerald L. Klerman*   319

Social Marketing: Its Place in Public Health, *Jack C. Ling, Barbara A. K. Franklin, Janis F. Lindsteadt, and Susan A. N. Gearon*   341

HEALTH SERVICES

Unnecessary Surgery, *Lucian L. Leape*   363

Causes of Low Preschool Immunization Coverage in the United States, *Felicity T. Cutts, Walter A. Orenstein, and Roger H. Bernier*   385

Access and Cost Implications of State Limitations on Medicaid Reimbursement for Pharmaceuticals, *Stuart O. Schweitzer and S. Renee Shiota*   399

SYMPOSIUM ON SELECTED CLINICAL SYNDROMES ASSOCIATED WITH AGING

Introduction, *Gilbert S. Omenn*   411

Acute Confusional States in Older Adults and the Role of Polypharmacy, *Ronald B. Stewart and William E. Hale*   415

Cognitive Impairment: Dementia and Alzheimer's Disease, *Eric B. Larson, Walter A. Kukull, and Robert L. Katzman*   431

Effects of Physical Activity on Health Status in Older Adults I: Observational Studies, *Edward H. Wagner, Andrea Z. LaCroix, David M. Buchner, and Eric B. Larson*   451

Effects of Physical Activity on Health Status in Older Adults II: Intervention Studies, *David M. Buchner, Shirley A. A. Beresford, Eric B. Larson, Andrea Z. LaCroix, and Edward H. Wagner*   469

Falls Among Older Persons: A Public Health Perspective, *Richard W. Sattin*   489

Nonfall Injuries in Older Adults, *Marsha E. Wolf and Frederick P. Rivara*   509

INDEXES

Subject Index   529

Cumulative Index of Contributing Authors, Volumes 1–13   539

Cumulative Index of Chapter Titles, Volumes 1–13   543

SOME RELATED ARTICLES IN OTHER *ANNUAL REVIEWS*

From the *Annual Review of Genetics*, Volume 25 (1991):

Transcription Activation by Estrogen and Progesterone Receptors, Hinrich
Gronemeyer
Genetic Risk Assessment, Udo H. Ehling
*Molecular and Genetic Insights into T Cell Antigen Receptor Structure and Func-
tion*, Arthur Weiss
Genetic Mechanisms for Adapting to a Changing Environment, Dennis A. Powers,
Tod Lauerman, Douglas Crawford, and Leonard DiMichele

From the *Annual Review of Medicine*, Volume 43 (1992):

*Therapeutic Approaches to Hemoglobin Switching in Treatment of Hemoglobino-
pathies*, Arthur W. Nienhuis and G. Stamatoyannopoulos
Immunologic Aspects of Schistosomiasis, André Capron and Jean-Paul Dessaint
Acute Progressive Epstein-Barr Virus Infections, Stephen E. Straus
Complications of Lyme Borreliosis, W. Donald Cooke and Raymond J. Dattwyler
The Resurgence of Measles in the United States, 1989–1990, William L. Atkinson,
Walter A. Orenstein, and Saul Krugman
A Putative Role of Hypercholesterolemia in Progressive Glomerular Injury,
Jonathan R. Diamond and Morris J. Karnovsky
Kidney Preservation ex vivo for Transplantation, Joseph V. Bonventre and Joel M.
Weinberg
Prospects for the Prevention of Breast Cancer, I. S. Fentiman
Suicide: Risk Factors and Prevention in Medical Practice, Randall D. Buzan and
Michael P. Weissberg
Risks and Benefits of Estrogen Replacement, Elizabeth Barrett-Connor
Chlamydia pneumoniae, *strain TWAR Pneumonia*, J. Thomas Grayston

From the *Annual Review of Nutrition*, Volume 12 (1992):

The Physiological Effect of Dietary Fiber: An Update, Martin A. Eastwood
Serum Cholesterol and Cancer Risk: An Epidemiologic Perspective, Stephen B.
Kritchevsky and David Kritchevsky
The Eosinophilia-Myalgia Syndrome and Tryptophan, Edward A. Belongia, Arthur
N. Mayeno, and Michael T. Osterholm
*Dietary Carotenes, Vitamin C, and Vitamin E as Protective Antioxidants in Human
Cancers*, Tim Byers and Geraldine Perry
The Influence of Maternal Nutrition on Lactation, Kathleen Maher Rasmussen

From the *Annual Review of Psychology,* Volume 43 (1992):

Behavioral Decision Research: A Constructive Processing Perspective, John W. Payne, James R. Bettman, and Eric J. Johnson
Negotiation and Mediation, Peter J. Carnevale and Dean G. Pruitt
Psychological Dimensions of Global Environmental Change, Paul C. Stern

From the *Annual Review of Sociology,* Volume 18 (1992):

Models for Sample Selection Bias, Christopher Winship and Robert D. Mare
Two Approaches to Social Structure: Exchange Theory and Network Analysis, K. S. Cook and J. M. Whitmeyer
Medicalization and Social Control, Peter Conrad
Social Science Research and Contemporary Studies of Homelessness, Anne B. Shlay and Peter H. Rossi
Stress Theory and Research, Carol S. Aneshensel
Changing Fertility Patterns and Fertility Policies in the Third World, Geoffrey McNicoll
Population Aging and Social Policy, Peter Uhlenberg

ANNUAL REVIEWS INC. is a nonprofit scientific publisher established to promote the advancement of the sciences. Beginning in 1932 with the *Annual Review of Biochemistry*, the Company has pursued as its principal function the publication of high quality, reasonably priced *Annual Review* volumes. The volumes are organized by Editors and Editorial Committees who invite qualified authors to contribute critical articles reviewing significant developments within each major discipline. The Editor-in-Chief invites those interested in serving as future Editorial Committee members to communicate directly with him. Annual Reviews Inc. is administered by a Board of Directors, whose members serve without compensation.

For the convenience of readers, a detachable order form/envelope is bound into the back of this volume.

Annu. Rev. Publ. Health. 1992. 13:1–30

HIV INFECTION AND AIDS IN CHILDREN[1]

Thomas C. Quinn, Andrea Ruff, and John Modlin

Departments of Medicine and Pediatrics, The Johns Hopkins School of Medicine; Department of International Health, The Johns Hopkins School of Public Health and Hygiene; Laboratory of Immunoregulation, National Institute of Allergy and Infectious Diseases, Baltimore, Maryland 21205

KEY WORDS: pediatrics, diagnosis, therapy, epidemiology

INTRODUCTION

As of January 1990, the World Health Organization (WHO) estimates that 8–10 million persons are infected with human immunodeficiency virus (HIV) worldwide. Approximately 3 million women, mostly of reproductive age, and more than 500,000 infants and children are infected (35). Eighty percent of these infected women and children reside in sub-Saharan Africa, where the estimated prevalence of HIV infection is 2500/100,000 women aged 15–49 (34). In some African cities, HIV prevalence rates of up to 30% have been documented (114, 142). As heterosexual transmission of HIV increases in other areas of the world, the numbers of infected women and, consequently, their children also increase (124). In Latin America, an estimated 200,000 women are infected, with a prevalence of 200/100,000 women aged 15–49 years (34). There is a rapid increase in HIV infection among drug users and prostitutes in some Asian countries (36). In the United States, women comprise 10% of the 171,865 adult cases of AIDS reported to the Centers for Disease Control as of May 1, 1991 (23). In 1991, AIDS was the fifth leading cause of premature death in women aged 15–49; in New York City, AIDS was the leading cause of death for women aged 20–40 (31, 38).

---

[1]The US Government has the right to retain a nonexclusive royalty-free license in and to any copyright covering this paper.

1

The World Health Organization estimates that the HIV pandemic will kill 3 million or more women and 2.7 million children worldwide during the 1990s (34, 37). AIDS will become the leading cause of death for women aged 15–49 in major cities throughout the Americas, western Europe, and sub-Saharan Africa, with infant and child mortality rates as much as 30% greater than previously projected. In addition, it is estimated that up to 5.5 million children under 15 will be orphaned because of the premature death of their HIV-infected mothers and fathers from AIDS (34, 130).

EPIDEMIOLOGY OF HIV IN WOMEN AND INFANTS

Because more than 90% of HIV-infected children acquired their infection perinatally, the incidence of HIV infection in infants and children is dependent upon the prevalence of HIV infection in women of reproductive age, the fertility rate of these women, and the risk of perinatal transmission. Because the latter two factors appear to be highly variable among women in different populations, the overall rate of perinatal infection is difficult to predict. The following section discusses the prevalence of HIV infection in women, the associated risk factors for HIV acquisition in women, and how these variables influence perinatal transmission of HIV. Acquisition of HIV through contaminated blood or blood products also remains a risk in many parts of the world; therefore, we also present data regarding this additional mode of transmission.

AIDS Surveillance

Globally, there has been a marked increase in the number of female AIDS cases. In sub-Saharan Africa and some parts of the Caribbean, the male-to-female ratio for AIDS cases is 1:1, primarily as a result of heterosexual transmission (69, 126, 135, 136). In developed countries, such as those in North America and Europe, the number of AIDS cases diagnosed in women is still fewer than male cases; however, the number is increasing at a faster rate each year because of intravenous (IV) drug use and heterosexual transmission. For example, in the US, the number of AIDS cases diagnosed in women aged 18–44 increased 29% from 1988 to 1989, as compared with an increase of 18% in men in the same age group (21). In 1991, 48% of female AIDS cases acknowledged IV drug use; 35% acknowledged heterosexual contact with an individual at risk for HIV; 7% had a history of receipt of blood transfusion; and 11% were listed as other or undetermined (23), including individuals who may have acquired HIV infection within health care settings, whose mode of exposure is unknown, and who may still be under investigation, have died, were lost to follow-up, or refused interview.

In the US, more than 3000 children have been reported to the Centers for

Disease Control (CDC) with AIDS: 88% acquired it from birth to a mother known to be at risk for HIV infection, 5% from a blood transfusion contaminated with HIV infection, 4% from factor 9 concentrates, and 4% from an undetermined source. In most other countries, more than 90% of children with AIDS acquired their infection from birth to an infected mother. In countries with evidence of heterosexual transmission and a male-to-female ratio approximating one, infants and children with AIDS may comprise as much as 20% of the total number of AIDS cases reported in national surveillance (136, 138). The demographic characteristics of AIDS cases in women and in children with perinatally acquired infection primarily reflect the characteristics of groups at risk for infection, especially IV drug users. In the US, 59% of perinatally acquired AIDS cases are among black children and 26% are in Hispanic children; their cumulative AIDS incidence rates are 21 and 13 times, respectively, the incidence rates in white children (25, 29). In parts of New York and New Jersey, most IV drug users in treatment are black or Hispanic and live in poor inner city communities, where the prevalence of HIV infection among these drug users is nearly 50% (28, 44, 45). Fifteen metropolitan areas, mostly along the East Coast, which include only 18% of the US pediatric population, account for 70% of the perinatal cases (25).

Although the greatest number of pediatric AIDS cases occurs in the first year of life, the relative impact of AIDS as the cause of death has been most striking in the 1–4 year age group: By 1990, AIDS was the leading cause of death among Hispanic children, and the second leading cause among black children in the US.

Increasing AIDS-related adult mortality in Africa, as recently documented (43), is creating a large and growing number of children under age 15 whose mothers have died of AIDS. During the 1990s, AIDS will kill 1.5–2.9 million women of reproductive age in Central Africa, thus producing 3.1–5.5 million AIDS orphans (130), 6–11% of the population under 15. In these countries, where 20% of mothers are HIV-infected, childhood mortality under five years of age will rise from 100/1000 live births to 136/1000, thereby negating or reversing the gains of childhood survival achieved in the past few decades. Similar large numbers of orphans are predicted in the Caribbean and several urban centers of the US. Many of these children will be driven to prostitution for survival, thus enhancing further transmission of HIV in adolescents. They are joining those now referred to by the United Nations Children's Fund as "children in extremely difficult circumstances," which includes children endangered by armed conflict and other disasters, those exploited by child labor, street children, and children who are victims of abuse and neglect (71, 130). Although the phenomenon of AIDS orphans is also affecting Western cities like New York, the predominance of heterosexual transmission and absolute number of parents infected with HIV make this problem considerably greater in Africa (34). As a result, national and international government and nongovernment service providers in Africa need to recognize this potential impact of HIV infection on children, expand AIDS prevention efforts, and develop policies and programs to address children's AIDS-related needs.

HIV Prevalence in Women

Because AIDS case reporting is variable and subject to a variety of problems, such as underreporting and difficulties with case definition, seroprevalence studies better reflect the real magnitude of HIV infection. Knowledge of the general prevalence and possible incidence of HIV infections is essential to monitor the epidemiologic patterns and scope of the HIV pandemic (35). Estimates of the number of future cases of HIV-related disease, including AIDS, will be dependent upon the number of persons currently infected with HIV. However, seroprevalence data must also be interpreted with caution, because of the differences in methods in the populations surveyed. Local or regional findings regarding HIV seroprevalence cannot be generalized to the national level, and the extraordinary cultural diversity of many countries should limit any unwarranted extrapolations from small, more intensely studied groups to large populations.

A variety of seroprevalence studies have attempted to estimate the frequency of HIV infection in women of reproductive age (Table 1). Female applicants for US military service are routinely tested and have shown a fairly stable seroprevalence rate nationally of 0.06%, although rates are much higher in certain inner cities of the Northeast: approximately 0.5% in northern New Jersey, New York City, and San Juan, Puerto Rico (27, 32, 42, 114). Seroprevalence rates in black and Hispanic female military applicants are eight and four times higher, respectively, than those among white applicants. Seroprevalence among first-time female blood donors is approximately 0.01%. Blinded antenatal screening and surveys of women delivering babies have also documented variable rates in different cities (114). However, several of these studies have shown that many seropositive women do not acknowledge or know they have risk factors for infection. For instance, among women delivering babies at a New York City hospital (92) and at the Johns Hopkins Hospital in Baltimore (4, 5), between one third and one half of the seropositive women had no reported risk for HIV infection. In other words, they were likely infected through heterosexual contact with a partner they did not recognize to be infected or at increased risk. Similar studies in sexually transmitted disease (STD) clinics have documented increasing rates among women who may have been infected through heterosexual contact with a partner of unknown risk. In the CDC blinded HIV surveys, seroprevalence of HIV in more than 100,000 women attending STD clinics was 2.2% (21). Median seroprevalence rates by clinic type for women attending prenatal, family planning, and drug-treatment clinics were 0.9%, 0.5%, and 3.7%, respectively (21). In 1988, a national survey of 2 million childbearing women per year was initiated in 44 states, the District of Columbia, and Puerto Rico to measure the prevalence of HIV infection among women delivering infants over time. These data will be useful in developing, targeting, and evaluating appropriate education and prevention programs. Thus far, the highest sero-prevalence rates have been in New York (0.58%, with 1.25% in New York City and 0.16% upstate), the District of Columbia (0.55%), New Jersey (0.49%), and Florida (0.49); most states have overall rates under 0.1%. The estimated national rate was 0.15%, which corresponds to 5500–6000 HIV-infected women delivering liveborn infants in 1989. If 30% is the rate of perinatal transmission, 1600–1800 of these children were infected as a result of maternal infection in 1989. This number is three times the number of children reported with perinatally acquired AIDS in 1989, which suggests that the future number of pediatric cases will be even higher. Rates of 1–4% have been documented in blacks and Hispanic childbearing women in these sur-veys, which clearly reflect the impact of HIV infection in minority pop-ulations.

In developing countries, antenatal surveys for HIV among apparently healthy women of childbearing age reveals that a surprisingly large proportion of those women living in urban areas in some countries have high rates of HIV infection. For example, in Port-au-Prince, Haiti, the rate of HIV infection in pregnant women rose from 8% to more than 10% between 1982 and 1988 (14). In African cities, seroprevalence rates of 5–30% have been documented among women who attend antenatal clinics (17, 59, 67, 90, 95, 105, 126, 137, 142, 143). Rates of HIV infection have risen from 0% in 1980 to 3% in

Table 1 Seroprevalence of HIV-1 infection in antenatal women

Location	Number tested	Rate
Rwanda	900	30.3%
Uganda	497	24.3%
Rwanda	3891	23.1%
Burundi	1255	17.5%
Zambia	1954	11.6%
Kenya	2400	7.1%
Zaire	1491	6.0%
New York	276,609	0.66%
Massachusetts	30,708	0.26%
United States	>2 million	0.15%
London	114,515	0.15%
Italy	23,491	0.024%
Sweden	130,508	0.013%

1988 in Nairobi (126, 127), and from 0.2% in 1970 to 8% in 1986 in Kinshasa, Zaire (142).

Heterosexual Transmission

Sexual behavior, exposure to an HIV-infected individual, and a history of STDs appear to be the major risk factors for HIV infection in both men and women. In some developing countries, urban prostitutes, who have a high infection rate (18–86%), played a prominent role in the initial dissemination of HIV in many parts of the world (39, 88, 126–128, 135, 148, 156). However, even among African prostitutes, the presence of STDs appears to be strongly associated with HIV transmission (122). In Nairobi, a prospective study of 124 HIV seronegative African prostitutes documented HIV seroconversion in 83 (67%) (128). Oral contraceptive use, genital ulcers, and *Chlamydia trachomatis* cervical infection were each independently associated with increased risk of HIV infection. Condom use reduced the risk of HIV infection. Of seroconverting women, 60% experienced one or more episodes of genital ulcers in the period before seroconversion, compared with 45% of HIV seronegative women. This relationship became stronger when the number of ulcer episodes was adjusted for length of follow-up. The mean number of annual ulcer episodes was 1.32 ± 0.55 in seroconverting women, compared with 0.48 ± 0.21 in seronegative women ($p < 0.02$).

The importance of STDs as cofactors was further emphasized among sexual couples in general population surveys. In studies in Rwanda (156) and Kinshasa (125), seropositivity was strongly associated with history of STDs in both men and women. More recently, several US studies have found that a positive serologic test for syphilis (133, 134) and seropositivity to herpes simplex virus type II (31), which is the predominant cause of genital herpes, were strongly associated with HIV infection among women with or without a history of IV drug use. Therefore, STDs appear to be intricately linked to HIV epidemiology and represent one of the major explanations for the heterosexual epidemic in central equatorial Africa, and for the increasing number of heterosexual cases in the US. These findings argue strongly for inclusion of STD control in AIDS prevention programs. The development of programs with an integrated approach to inducing behavioral change, promoting condom use, and controlling STDs would reduce the infectiousness of HIV transmitters (43) and the susceptibility of HIV-exposed persons (122). Limiting the transmission of HIV infection among women of reproductive age would obviously have the same impact on preventing perinatal transmission of HIV to infants.

Parenteral Transmission

In the US, 9% of children acquired HIV infection by receipt of HIV-contaminated blood transfusions or blood components, such as factor 8 and 9 concentrates for hemophilia. Fortunately, with HIV screening of all blood donations, this mode of transmission has dramatically decreased. In contrast, recent outbreaks of HIV infection in children in the Soviet Union, Romania, and in many developing countries in Africa and Latin America emphasize the risk of nosocomial transmission and the continued need for blood screening and sterilization of medical equipment. For example, among hospitalized children less than 24 months old in Zaire, five (31%) of 16 seropositive infants born to seronegative mothers had been transfused, compared with 15 (7%) of 220 seronegative children in the same age group (100). Also, 147 (14.1%) of 1046 pediatric patients in Kinshasa, Zaire, had a history of blood transfusion. Of these pediatric patients, 40 (3.8%) were HIV seropositive, and there was a strong dose-response association between blood transfusion and HIV seropositivity (58).

HIV INFECTION AND PREGNANCY

Studies in Zaire, Zambia, Uganda, Kenya, Haiti, and Malawi have shown highest rates of adverse pregnancy outcomes, such as spontaneous abortion, stillbirth, prematurity, low birth weight, and neonatal mortality in seropositive women compared with seronegative controls (17, 59, 67, 90, 95, 105, 143). However, the findings have not been consistent and appear to be related to the severity of maternal HIV disease. In Haiti, children born to HIV seropositive mothers were significantly more likely to be premature, of low birth weight, and malnourished at three and six months of age than were infants born to HIV negative women (62). In Nairobi (17), the mean birth weight of singleton neonates of HIV positive women was significantly lower than that of controls (3090 vs. 3220 g, p = 0.005), and birth weight was < 2500 g in 9% of cases and 3% of controls [odds ratio (OR) 3.0, p. = 0.007]. Among neonates of HIV seropositive women, birth weight was less than 2500 g in 17% if mothers were symptomatic and 6% if mothers were asymptomatic (OR 3.4, p = 0.08). In Malawi, the seroprevalence for HIV infection in 461 consecutive pregnant women was 17.6% (104). The estimated annual incidence of HIV seroconversion in urban pregnant women was 3–4% per annum between 1985 and 1987, and 7–13% between 1987 and 1989. HIV infection was significantly associated with a positive syphilis serology and correlated with history of STDs, although it was not statistically significant. A history of spontaneous abortion was also associated with reactive syphilis serology, HIV infection, and history of STDs; in a logistic regression analysis, HIV infection remained the only significant variable.

Predicting HIV infection in pregnant women without serologic testing has been extremely difficult, even in high prevalence areas. Obstetrical history may be a better predictor of HIV infection in women of childbearing age than socioeconomic and sexual history parameters, with a strong association between intrauterine fetal death and maternal HIV infection in case-controlled studies performed in Nairobi (152) and in Kigali, Rwanda. The rates of prematurity, low birth weight, congenital malformations, and neonatal mortality and socioeconomic statistics were comparable in the two groups (95). However, infants of HIV positive mothers were a mean birth weight of 130 g lower than the infants of HIV negative mothers (p<0.01).

Because HIV infection in women may be associated with behavioral attributes, such as alcohol consumption, smoking, illicit drug use, or coinfection with such STDs as syphilis or bacterial vaginosis, which may also lead to low birth weight or premature birth, it is important to control for these potentially confounding factors. In the European prospective studies (10, 51), lower birth weight was not related to HIV infection in the child, but to maternal IV drug use during pregnancy. It is not possible to ascertain whether the adverse pregnancy outcomes reported are the direct consequence of maternal infection or caused by fetal infection (110). In other European and US studies, HIV infection has not been associated with adverse pregnancy outcomes (80, 147). In a study of 39 seropositive and 58 seronegative pregnant women enrolled in a methadone program in New York, there were no differences in the frequency of spontaneous or elective abortions, ectopic pregnancies, preterm delivery, stillbirth, low birth weight, or antenatal, intrapartum or perinatal complications (147). In Germany, Lutz et al (99) reported no difference in pregnancy complications or proportion of low birth weight children in HIV positive women with severe lymphocyte depletion.

Investigators have also suggested that pregnancy may accelerate the course of HIV infection, but in more recent prospective studies, in which pregnant and nonpregnant infected IV drug users were compared, there was no difference in the progression of HIV disease over a three-year period (9, 153). The appearance of p24 antigen during pregnancy was transient and not an indicator of disease progression (9). Further information is needed, especially for symptomatic women and those without IV drug use.

VERTICAL TRANSMISSION OF HIV

Like other vertically transmitted viral diseases, HIV infection occurs in only a portion of children born to HIV infected women. The observed rate of vertical transmission has varied widely among prospective studies conducted in the United States, Europe, Africa, and Haiti (Table 2) (3, 10, 50, 55, 62, 74, 76, 108, 143). Not only have rates varied considerably among different locations, but longitudinal studies conducted by the same investigators in the same populations have, in general, reported declining vertical transmission rates over time (50, 51).

The reasons for the wide geographic and temporal variation in reported

Table 2   Vertical HIV transmission rates in selected locations

Location	Number	Rate	Reference
Zaire	92	39%	143
France	117	35%	108
Italy	89	33%	76
Miami, Florida	82	30%	74
New York City	55	29%	62
Haiti	230	25%	55
New Haven, Connecticut	59	24%	50
Western Europe	372	13%	10
Edinburgh, Scotland	28	7%	3

vertical transmission rates are not known. The wide confidence limits surrounding the means in those studies with small numbers may account for some of the differences, as may the different case definitions and other methodologic variations. Some investigators believe that the observed decline in vertical transmission rates in some locations over time may reflect the increasing efficiency of detecting asymptomatically infected pregnant women via obstetrical screening programs. Furthermore, the duration of the HIV epidemic undoubtedly differs from one location to the next. If women with more advanced HIV disease are more likely to transmit infection to their newborns (vide infra), then higher transmission rates in some locations may reflect a longer duration of the HIV epidemic among women of child bearing age.

Factors that May Affect the Risk of Transmission

MATERNAL FACTORS   One of the most important determinants of newborn HIV infection may be the stage of maternal infection. To date, this has been difficult to assess in our domestic maternal population, because about 80% of HIV infected pregnant women followed in US studies have been asymptomatic (60). However, reports from France and central Africa indicate a much higher rate of transmission of HIV from women with advanced symptoms than among women who are asymptomatic or have only mild symptoms of HIV infection (13, 143, 157). Two of these studies (13, 157) found a marked increase in risk of newborn infection when maternal CD4+ cell counts are less than $150/mm^3$. Individuals with advanced HIV infection and low CD4+ cell counts are more likely to have higher concentrations of virus in blood and other tissues (41, 68). Not surprisingly, several markers for progressive maternal HIV infection correlate with an increased risk of perinatal infection, including p24 antigenemia (13), HIV viremia (13), and serum IgA concentration (75).

Older women also appear more likely to have HIV-infected infants than younger women (75). The potential influence of other STDs, particularly those that cause genital ulceration, is currently under investigation. To date, there is little information on whether rates of vertical transmission vary among women with different risk factors for HIV infection.

GESTATIONAL AGE   Investigators at the National Institute of Child Health and Development and a consortium of New York City hospitals have reported that infants delivered before 37 weeks' gestation have a 60% risk of infection, compared with an infection rate of 22% for term infants (74). However, Hutto and colleagues (74) subsequently reported no increased relative risk of infection for premature infants in a cohort of 82 cases prospectively studied in Miami. Clearly, conclusions regarding the influence of premature delivery on risk of newborn infection must wait the results of additional studies.

MATERNAL ANTI-HIV ANTIBODY   Since 1989, several groups of investigators have suggested that maternal antibody to the HIV viral envelope protein gp120 protects the newborn from infection (46, 55, 141). Two of these groups reported that the protective maternal antibodies are directed against epitopes on, or adjacent to, the immunodominant V3 loop, which is the principal neutralizing domain of the gp 120 protein (46, 141). If these intriguing observations are confirmed by others, then it may be possible to predict which pregnancies are likely to produce an infected infant, and vertical transmission might be prevented by immunomodulation. However, Goldstein et al (56) have reported that the presence of maternal HIV neutralizing antibody did not affect the rate of transmission. Experienced clinical scientists are reserving judgment until more complete data are available. Unfortunately, a wider discussion of this topic exceeds the scope of this review.

Mechanisms of Vertical HIV Transmission

Interest has focused on three possible routes by which HIV is transmitted from a pregnant woman to her fetus or newborn infant: intrauterine (or transplacental) transmission, intrapartum transmission, and postpartum transmission via breast feeding. The strength and nature of the evidence supporting each of these mechanisms varies, and there are no data to indicate the relative contribution of each potential route of transmission.

INTRAUTERINE TRANSMISSION   There is little doubt that at least some infants are infected in utero early in gestation. HIV has been recovered in cell culture from the tissues of fetuses aborted between 12 and 20 weeks' gestation (47, 81, 83, 149). The virus has also been detected by in situ cDNA hybridization in the peripheral blood mononuclear cells of a one-day-old infant (65), and by polymerase chain reaction (PCR) in several infants within a few days of birth (93, 163).

Because not all infants of HIV infected pregnant women become infected, considerable attention has been paid to the role of the human placenta in either facilitating or inhibiting viral passage from the maternal circulation to the fetal circulation. The placenta contains several cell types that may support HIV replication. The HIV cell membrane receptor protein, CD4, has been identified on the surface of trophoblast cells and on stromal macrophages from both first trimester and term normal human placentas (2, 56, 103). Maury et al (103) have reported that monoclonal antibodies also identify CD4 antigen on endothelial cells of villous capillaries.

Studies of term placentas from HIV seropositive pregnancies have produced contradictory data. Chandwani and colleagues (33) found HIV p24 antigen within rare trophoblast cells in only two of 41 placentas of HIV seropositive women, but observed no staining within villous macrophages. In contrast, other investigators have noted HIV p24 antigen to be predominantly within villous stromal macrophages (78, 102). In the only reported study of preterm placental tissue from HIV seropositive pregnancies, Lewis and colleagues (97) identified HIV gp41 antigen by immunoperoxidase staining and HIV DNA by in situ hybridization in trophoblast cells and within chorionic macrophages of placental tissue obtained at eight weeks' gestation.

The numerous macrophages (Hofbauer cells) distributed throughout the villous stroma in the human placenta are capable phagocytes (161), can be activated by gamma interferon (162), and produce interleukin-1 (52). Many of these placental macrophages express membrane CD4 antigen throughout pregnancy (56). The role that these cells play in vertical transmission is not known. In some model systems, the placental macrophage is associated with protection of the fetus from viral infection (106). In human HIV infection, the macrophage may protect the fetus, may serve as the mechanism by which the placental barrier is breached, or both.

INTRAPARTUM TRANSMISSION   The role of intrapartum (i.e. during labor or delivery) transmission of HIV is less settled. The majority of infants of HIV seropositive women escape infection in utero. It is entirely plausible, if not likely, that some of these infants are infected at the time of delivery as a result of contact with maternal blood or genital tract secretions. Documenting intrapartum transmission is difficult, however. The best evidence, albeit indirect, comes from observations that some HIV infected infants test negative at birth or during the first few weeks of life, by sensitive and specific assays, such as HIV culture (54, 85), PCR (140), and anti-HIV serum IgA testing (159).

If the intrapartum route proves to be an important mechanism for vertically acquired HIV infection, it is possible that the postnatal natural history of HIV infection will be different for infants infected perinatally, compared with infants infected in utero. In fact, survival curves for infected infants appear to have a bimodal distribution (145). There are also implications for possible prevention of vertical HIV transmission or altering the course of intrapartum acquired infection, i.e. an antiviral agent, such as zidovudine or dideoxyinosine, or HIV immune globulin administered to either the mother or the infant in the perinatal period could prevent neonatal HIV infection, just as intrapartum hepatitis B infection can be prevented (30).

A large clinical trial of zidovudine administration to HIV-infected pregnant women and their newborn infants has been initiated by the AIDS Clinical Trials Group to test this hypothesis. In this multicenter, randomized trial, pregnant HIV-infected women receive either zidovudine or placebo beginning as early as 14 weeks' gestation, and their newborn infants receive the same preparation as their mothers for six weeks after delivery. Although phase I trials in both pregnant women and newborn infants have produced preliminary evidence of zidovudine safety in these populations, side effects will also be closely monitored during the efficacy trial.

POSTNATAL TRANSMISSION   There are several reported cases of postnatal HIV infection of infants who appear to have acquired HIV infection via breast feeding from their postnatally infected mothers (115). HIV has been isolated from the breast milk of healthy seropositive women (154). Furthermore, a prospective French study suggests an increased risk of infection among infants of seropositive women; however, the number of infants at risk was small (10). In contrast, several large studies have not demonstrated an increased risk among children born to HIV seropositive mothers who breast feed their infants (N. Halsey 1991, personal communication; 63, 100, 107, 150). The level of infectivity of breast milk has yet to be established. As noted above, one group reports the successful culture of HIV from cell-free extracts of breast milk (154), but other investigators have repeatedly failed in their attempts to culture virus from breast milk samples obtained from seropositive mothers. With the exception of breast feeding, it is unlikely that infants are at risk of HIV infection from postnatal maternal exposure.

CLINICAL PRESENTATION

The incubation period, or the time between infection and development of AIDS, varies considerably among perinatally infected infants. The vast majority of HIV-infected infants are asymptomatic at the time of birth. Although some HIV infected children may remain minimally symptomatic for several years, the median age at AIDS diagnosis is 12 months (114).

Because relatively few large pediatric cohorts have been prospectively followed, the spectrum of HIV manifestations in children is still being defined (50, 145). Early signs and symptoms, such as generalized lymphadenopathy, hepatosplenomegaly, and failure to thrive, are relatively nonspecific. As in adults, progression of HIV infection typically involves multiple organ systems.

HIV is a neutrotropic virus, and some degree of neurologic dysfunction develops in the majority of infected infants and children (17). Static encephalopathy, detected in approximately 25% of HIV-1 infected children, is manifested by nonprogressive cognitive and motor deficits of varying severity (6, 17). Children may also demonstrate a steady decline in language and motor and adaptive skills, which is consistent with a progressive encephalopathy. Computed tomographic examinations typically demonstrate cerebral atrophy, increased ventricular size, calcification of the basal ganglia, and decreased attenuation in the white matter. The majority of neurologic abnormalities in HIV-infected children appear to be caused by direct effects of the virus itself. Although central nervous system lymphomas and opportunistic infections are not infrequent among adult patients with AIDS, they are relatively rare among pediatric patients (17).

Acute or chronic pulmonary disease develops in approximately 80% of HIV-infected children (40, 145, 158). Acute pulmonary disease, which is generally due to bacterial, viral, or *Pneumocystis carinii* infections, is discussed below. Chronic pulmonary disease involving a spectrum of lymphoid lesions is common among HIV-infected children. Focal lymphocytic infiltration is seen in some children, whereas the diffuse lymphocytic infiltration of alveolar septae characteristic of lymphoid interstitial pneumonitis (LIP) develops in others. Although LIP rarely develops in HIV-infected adults, it has been reported in approximately 40% of children with perinatally acquired HIV infection (40).

In HIV-infected children over one year of age, LIP generally presents as an asymptomatic pulmonary infiltration. Clinical symptoms, including cough, tachypnea, wheezing, and hypoxemia, develop gradually. Chest radiographs show persistent or progressive bilateral diffuse reticulonodular infiltrates unresponsive to antimicrobial therapy. Although the combination of an indolent clinical course and typical radiographic findings in an older child may be highly suggestive of LIP, the definitive diagnosis can only be made by biopsy.

HIV-infected children may have abnormalities of numerous other organ systems. Cardiac abnormalities, detected by echocardiography in 62–93% of infected children, include pericardial effusion, dilated cardiomyopathy, and left and right ventricular dysfunction (84, 98). Electrocardiographic abnormalities include ventricular hypertrophy, nonspecific ST-T changes, prolonged QT interval, and arrhythmias. The etiology of the cardiac abnormalities has not been determined; several'factors, including infection by HIV and other pathogens and immunologic or nutritional abnormalities, may be involved (84). The clinical manifestations of cardiovascular disease may be difficult to interpret in the setting of multisystem disease, and early signs of myocardial dysfunction may be erroneously attributed to infection.

Gastrointestinal dysfunction is common and may involve any region of the digestive tract. Diarrhea and failure to thrive appear to be the most prevalent clinical findings in the pediatric population (48, 124). Enteric parasites, such as cryptosporidium and *Giardia lamblia,* bacteria, such as Salmonella, Shigella, and *Mycobacterium avium intracellulare,* and viruses, such as cytomegalovirus, have all been detected. Noninfectious causes of gastrointestinal symptoms include carbohydrate, protein, and fat malabsorption (124).

Nephropathy has been detected in 29% of perinatally infected children (119). Renal manifestations include nephrotic syndrome, acute nephritic syndrome, renal tubular dysfunction, and acute renal failure (144).

Hematologic abnormalities include normochromic normocytic anemia, granulocytopenia, and thrombocytopenia (19). Lymphopenia, frequently observed in HIV-infected adults, occurs far less often in infected children. Malignancies also appear to occur less frequently in HIV-infected children; however, as children receiving antiretroviral therapy survive for longer periods, the risk of malignancy may increase.

Both infectious and noninfectious skin disorders are very common among HIV-infected children (132). Thrush, monilial diaper rash, and atopic dermatitis tend to be more severe and and refractory to therapy in HIV-infected children. Other common diseases may present with unusual lesions, organisms, or clinical course. Chronic varicella-zoster infection with atypical lesions may require biopsy or culture to establish the diagnosis (82, 116). Seborrheic dermatitis and Kaposi's sarcoma, both frequently detected in HIV-infected adults, are much less common among infected children (132).

Abnormalities of the immune system characterize HIV infections. Early in the disease, most children with perinatally acquired HIV demonstrate B-cell dysfunction, with relative sparing of T-cell function (8, 118, 151). This presentation, which differs from that in HIV-infected adults and older children, is probably due to acquisition of HIV during the development of the immune system. Among the initial manifestations of B-cell dysfunction is elevation of one or all immunoglobulins; hypergammaglobulinemia may be one of the first indicators that a child has acquired HIV infection perinatally. Despite the high levels of immunoglobulins, HIV-infected children demonstrate significant deficiencies in their ability to mount appropriate antibody responses to specific antigens (8, 12). B-cell dysfunction may also result in increased production of autoantibodies, which may mediate some of the renal, cardiac, and hematologic abnormalities found with HIV infection. T-cell abnormalities may be less pronounced than those in adults; children are less likely to have lymphopenia or profound T helper cell (CD4) depletion. However, because normal newborns and young infants have a striking lymphocytosis, CD4 numbers in HIV-infected children, which appear normal by adult standards, may represent significant depletion. As discussed below, recommendations regarding prophylaxis for *Pneumocystis carinii* pneumonia (PCP) have recently been revised, considering these age-related differences.

A variety of infections are likely to develop in HIV-infected children during the course of their disease. The timing of HIV infection to some extent influences the types of other infections acquired by the host. HIV appears to interfere with antibody responses to antigens encountered after acquisition of HIV. The lymphocytes of children who acquire HIV infection perinatally will not have been primed to large numbers of antigens before infection with HIV. This immunologic naivete, combined with HIV-induced suppression of the humoral immune system, significantly increases the susceptibility of these children to bacterial infections (7, 12, 121). Of bacterial diseases, HIV-infected children are most likely to have bacteremia and sepsis, pneumonia, gastroenteritis, urinary tract infections, sinusitis, and recurrent otitis media. Bacteremia is most often due to *Streptococcus pneumoniae,* followed by *Haemophilus influenzae* type B, enterococcus, group B *Streptococcus* and *Salmonella,* and other gram negative enteric species (7, 86, 121). Bacteremia due to *Staphlococcus aureus* and *Staphlococcus epidermidis,* generally associated with catheter or wound infections, has also been reported. Pulmonary pathogens include *S. pneumoniae, Pseudomonas aeruginosa, S. aureus, Klebsiella pneumoniae,* and *H. influenzae,* and less commonly *Salmonella, Nocardia, Listeria,* and *Legionella* (121).

Opportunistic infections due to pathogens associated with defects in cell-mediated immunity also develop in HIV-infected children (64). *Pneumocystis carinii* pneumonia develops in approximately 50% of children with AIDS (70). Although PCP in adults is due to reactivation of a previously acquired infection, it more likely represents a primary infection in infants and children. The risk of pneumocystis appears to be age-related; children less than one year old are much more likely to have PCP than are older children (91, 139, 145). In many young infants, PCP is the first manifestation of HIV infection. Although numerous studies have documented an association between low CD4 cell numbers and PCP in HIV-infected adults, the CD4 count is not a reliable predictor of pneumocystis infection in children (22, 70, 145). Clinically, PCP is characterized by tachypnea, dyspnea, cough, and fever associated with hypoxemia. The onset of PCP is generally acute with a fairly rapid progression, particularly in infants; however, a more insidious presentation has also been observed. The chest radiographic typically shows bilateral diffuse interstitial infiltrates without hilar lymphadenopathy, although a variety of other findings have been described.

Mycobacteria are common opportunistic pathogens in HIV-infected individuals. The number of tuberculosis cases is increasing with the AIDS epidemic (66). Although the majority of cases have been reported in adults, it is likely that tuberculosis due to both greater exposure and immune dysfunction will increasingly develop in HIV-infected children. Disseminated infection with *M. avium-intracellulare* complex (MAC) organisms is frequently detected in HIV-infected adults and children (49, 72). Multiple organ involvement and persistent bacteremia are typically present.

Fungal infections are also significant causes of morbidity and mortality in HIV-infected children. Mucocutaneous candidiasis with oropharyngeal and esophageal involvement is by far the most common fungal infection; surprisingly, disseminated candidiasis rarely occurs in patients with AIDS. Other fungi, such as *Cryptococcus neoformans,* which frequently cause systemic infections in HIV-infected adults, are unusual in children. The most common opportunistic viral pathogens in HIV-infected children are herpes simplex virus, varicella-zoster virus, and cytomegalovirus.

Laboratory Diagnosis of HIV Infection in Infants

Early diagnosis of perinatally acquired HIV infection is needed to identify infants that might benefit from early antiviral therapy and prophylactic treatment for opportunistic infections, and to determine the timing of transmission from mother to infant. Early diagnosis would aid parents and other caretakers of these children who want to know the status of HIV infection in their children as soon as possible. Furthermore, natural history data suggest that the time scale for disease progression in children is compressed compared with adults. From a cohort of 172 perinatally infected infants, 25% of the cohort died by two years of age (145). *Pneumocystis carinii* pneumonia occurred in over 10% of the median age of five months and was associated with a median survival of one month. Thus, for some infants the window of opportunity for intervention between laboratory diagnosis and the development of symptoms is narrow.

Diagnosis of HIV infection in infants during the first year of life is, however, problematic. The clinical manifestations of HIV infection in children are varied and nonspecific, including chronic pneumonitis, failure to thrive, hepatosplenomegaly, thrombocytopenia, and chronic diarrhea. Diagnosis of HIV infection is more difficult in infants because the current testing for evidence of infection depends on serologic confirmation of the presence of IgG antibody to specific viral proteins of HIV. However, all infants passively acquire maternal IgG antibodies in utero, which can persist for 15 months (51, 79). Serum tests for IgG antibody, therefore, do not differentiate between infant and maternal antibody; thus, a positive IgG HIV antibody test in an infant only indicates exposure. Consequently, in children less than 15 months, documentation of HIV infection requires a more thorough investigation of the immune system with CD4 lymphocyte determination, exclusion of congenital immunodeficiency, and identification of viral components (such as p24 HIV antigen), HIV culture, or PCR. Alternative tests in the process of evaluation include assays for neonatal IgM and IgA and in vitro assays to determine the ability of neonatal peripheral blood mononuclear cells to secrete HIV-specific IgG antibody (155).

The current gold standard for establishing HIV infection in neonates is recovery of the virus from the infant by culture. Although this is a highly specific assay, its sensitivity varies and may be as low as 50% in HIV-infected infants during their first few weeks of life because of the low viral load (89). Culture has limited use as a diagnostic test for HIV. Cultures typically take 7–28 days or more to complete and require special biosafety precautions to prevent exposure to laboratory personnel. Cultures are costly, labor intensive, and not practical for resource-poor settings. The sensitivity of virus culture for detecting HIV infection also varies among laboratories and during the course of illness.

DNA amplification by PCR offers several advantages over culture. Because PCR detects the presence of the virus, rather than antibody to the virus, it avoids the problem of persistent maternal antibody (73). Polymerase chain reaction requires a small amount of blood and can be performed within 24 hours. Although sensitivity appears to be improved compared with culture, it is also limited during the early neonatal period. For example, in a study of infants later defined as being HIV-infected, only eight of 20 had detectable proviral sequences by PCR in the neonatal period within the first week of life (140). Of the 11 infants who had CDC-defined AIDS in the first 18 months, seven were positive for PCR in the neonatal period, compared with one of nine other infants who have other HIV-related clinical signs and symptoms, thus suggesting a prognostic role for PCR. All 22 HIV-infected infants tested in the postnatal period were PCR positive; of these, 20 were PCR positive by six months of age. Some infected infants test negative in the neonatal period, possibly because of infection during late gestation or in the intrapartum period, and their level of virus is below detectable levels for the test.

The specificity of the assay in this particular study was excellent (140). None of 93 infants who had lost maternal antibody and remained antibody negative were repeatedly PCR positive. Three of 93 infants tested PCR positive on one occasion; however, subsequent PCR testings were negative, and these children remained clinically well. As with culture, there are several limitations with this assay besides its low sensitivity in the neonatal period. Currently, the test is not completely standardized, and different laboratories report varying sensitivities and specificities with known samples. Finally, PCR is not widely available in a diagnostic format and still may be impractical for developing countries. However, it is hoped that soon the technology will be inexpensively exportable to the developing world. Paterlini et al (120) detected HIV DNA sequences in 20 (64%) of 31 babies born to seropositive mothers in Kinshasa. Clearly, this high rate needs confirmation and may represent falsely high rates because of contamination, a particular problem in developing countries.

Serologic assays, which are less expensive and better standardized, offer yet another alternative to early diagnosis. Because IgM and IgA antibodies do not cross the placenta, assays for the measurement of these antibodies to HIV have been developed. IgM assays have lacked sensitivity and specificity because of cross reaction with rheumatoid factor and the transient nature of IgM antibodies (160). However, the sensitivity of IgA detection increases by removal of IgG, which competes for antigen-binding sites. In a preliminary study, Weiblen et al (159) demonstrated IgA antibodies in 12 of 18 samples from HIV-infected infants aged six to 12 months, five of 10 of infants aged three to five months, and two of 13 of infants under three months. More promising results were recently reported in another study, in which IgA antibody was detected in eight of nine infected infants by 12 weeks of age (101).

Another serologic assay is the p24 antigen assay. Available HIV antigen detection kits fail to detect serum p24 antigen in the presence of high titers of HIV-specific antibodies. Studies of infants born to HIV-infected mothers have found very few infants to be antigen-positive early in the course of infection because of the presence of excess maternal antibody (15). As maternal IgG antibody declines, infant p24 antigen may be transiently measurable, although some of this may be bound by infant IgG antibody, which increases in titer with age.

Other techniques for perinatal diagnosis include the in vitro antibody production assay (IVAP) (117) and the ELISPOT (94), which detect the presence of antibody-producing B-lymphocytes, not the antibody itself, thus avoiding the problem of persistent maternal antibody. Preliminary data indicate that the IVAP test and ELISPOT, although sensitive, were neither specific nor predictive for HIV infection during the first few months of life. These data, like many of the other assays, confirm the difficulty with early diagnosis during the first few months of life, but reliability of the assays appears to improve after three to six months of age.

Clinical Diagnosis

The Centers for Disease Control has developed a definition and classification system of HIV infection in children less than 13 years of age (31). However, in developing countries, limited diagnostic capabilities have precluded routine use of the CDC criteria. In these areas, diagnosis relies upon the provisional pediatric clinical case definition of AIDS developed by WHO (164). Although the WHO case definition appears to be fairly specific, it lacks sensitivity and positive predictive value (137). HIV-infected children who die acutely with an overwhelming infection may be missed by this case definition, which emphasizes chronic signs and symptoms. In addition, the broad spectrum of disease associated with HIV in children, and the overlap with other common diseases in developing countries, hinders the diagnosis of AIDS based solely on clinical criteria. Thus, in countries with limited diagnostic resources, establishing the diagnosis and determining the natural history of HIV infection will continue to be a significant problem.

CLINICAL MANAGEMENT

Clinical management of an HIV-infected child should include both specific antiviral therapy and aggressive diagnosis and treatment of associated infectious and noninfectious conditions. Several therapeutic agents with activity against HIV, including the dideoxynucleosides, azidothymidine (zidovudine, AZT), dideoxycytidine (ddC), and dideoxyinosine (ddI), are being evaluated in both pediatric and adult patients. By inhibiting reverse transcriptase, these drugs interfere with HIV replication. In a recently completed phase II study, children receiving zidovudine showed an improvement in weight gain and cognitive function; their serum and cerebrospinal fluid p24 antigen levels declined, and their CD4 cell counts transiently improved (104). Studies currently underway include one in which two doses of zidovudine are being compared in less symptomatic children and one involving the coadministration of IVIG or placebo. Smaller studies, which use ddI, ddC, or soluble CD4, are also being conducted.

Zidovudine is currently the only agent approved for use in children. The standard dose is 180 mg/square meter given every six hours. The most common toxicity is bone marrow suppression with anemia and, less often, neutropenia, both of which generally respond to dose reduction or temporary discontinuation of the medication (104). Children who cannot tolerate zidovudine or who have progressive disease while on therapy can be considered for trials that use other antiretroviral agents.

Opportunistic and other serious infections are a major cause of morbidity and mortality among HIV-infected children. Therefore, early detection and treatment of these infections is critical. It is important to remember that common childhood pathogens are also likely to be problems in HIV-infected children; however, the diagnosis and management of these diseases may be complicated by an atypical presentation or progression. An HIV-infected child who has an acute febrile illness should be aggressively evaluated to determine the site of infection and potential etiologic agent. Because infections may rapidly progress and the social situation is often not optimal, the decision to observe a febrile HIV-infected child at home should be made with caution.

The presentation of an HIV-infected child with fever, cough, and dyspnea should prompt consideration of PCP, as well as other pulmonary infections. Differentiation of PCP from other infections of LIP by radiograph may be very difficult, and definitive diagnosis requires demonstration of *P. carinii* in specimens generally obtained by bronchoscopy or open lung biopsy. Tissue specimens are particularly useful to determine the presence of concurrent infections with cytomegalovirus or other organisms. Induced sputum, often used to establish the diagnosis of PCP in adults, cannot reliably be obtained in very young children. Because untreated PCP is associated with high mortality rates, therapy should be started quickly; it can be started presumptively in very ill children or in situations in which the diagnostic workup is likely to be delayed. The therapy of choice is intravenous trimethoprim-sulfamethoxazole; although associated with a relatively high incidence of adverse effects in adults with AIDS, fewer data regarding toxicity in pediatric patients are available (57). Patients who fail to respond clinically after five to seven days of therapy or who cannot tolerate trimethoprim-sulfamethoxazole should be treated with pentamidine isethionate. Although both drugs are equally efficacious, pentamidine is associated with a higher incidence of serious adverse effects. Therapy of PCP is generally continued for two to three weeks; the high rate of recurrence in HIV-infected patients indicates the need for subsequent prophylaxis.

The use of corticosteroids should be considered as adjunctive therapy. Studies of adults with AIDS have indicated that the early use of steroids reduces the risk of respiratory failure and improves survival (15, 53). Although no data are yet available regarding the use of corticosteroids in HIV-infected children, many centers are now using them in children with moderate to severe PCP.

The high mortality rates associated with PCP among HIV-infected infants and children warrant aggressive use of chemoprophylaxis. In children with perinatally acquired HIV infection, the risk of PCP is greatest during the first year of life; therefore, prophylaxis often needs to be instituted before a definitive diagnosis of HIV infection has been established. The Working Group on PCP Prophylaxis in Children recently issued guidelines for initiation of PCP prophylaxis for HIV-infected children (22). Trimethoprim-sulfamethoxazole, administered three times per week, is the recommended regimen. Although few data are available regarding efficacy in children, aerosolized pentamidine can be used for PCP prophylaxis in children aged five years or older (22). Intravenous pentamidine or dapsone are also being used prophylactically in some children.

The management of other opportunistic infections is problematic. The diagnosis of MAC infection is generally established by blood mycobacterial culture or histopathology of biopsy specimens. Although numerous drug regimens have been examined, no effective therapy for MAC infections is currently available; new drugs with increased in vitro activity against MAC are now being examined in adults and children. Oral candidiasis can be diagnosed clinically, whereas the definitive diagnosis of esophageal candidiasis requires culture and histopathology of specimens obtained at endoscopy. Nystatin or clotrimazole are often adequate treatment for oropharyngeal candidiasis, whereas esophageal candidiasis requires the use of ketoconazole, or less often, amphotericin B. The diagnosis of cytomegalovirus (CMV) infections, other than retinitis, generally requires histopathologic evidence of invasive disease and isolation of the virus. Ganciclovir, an analogue of acyclovir, has been used in small numbers of HIV-infected children with severe CMV-related disease (18). There are no data currently available regarding use of other therapeutic agents, such as foscarnet, high dose acyclovir, CMV hyperimmuneglobulin, or interferon, in HIV-infected children.

The management of other HIV-related noninfectious conditions is largely supportive. Initial management of an asymptomatic child with LIP should include aggressive therapy of intercurrent pulmonary infections; appropriate use of influenza, pneumococcal, and *Haemophilus influenzae* vaccines; and close monitoring for progression of LIP. Children with significant hypoxemia may require supplemental oxygen. Several investigators have advocated the use of a 4–12 week course of prednisone in children with PaO_2 less than 65 mmHg (40, 113).

Other organ systems should be carefully evaluated in HIV-infected children. These children should undergo routine cardiovascular screening with electrocardiography and echocardiography at six-month intervals. Patients with significant gastrointestinal dysfunction may become malnourished and rapidly deteriorate clinically; therefore, reversible causes of gastrointestinal disease, such as infectious diarrhea, should be aggressively sought, and nutritional support should be implemented early in the course of HIV infection. Renal function should be monitored, urinary tract infections should be promptly treated, and potentially nephrotoxic drugs should be used cautiously. If drug toxicity, acute tubular necrosis, or other potentially reversible conditions precipitate acute renal failure in a child who otherwise has a reasonable prognosis for short-term survival, acute dialysis should be considered (144). Decisions regarding dialysis for irreversible renal failure are made on an individual basis, depending on the patient's overall state of health.

Although several immunomodulating agents are under investigation in HIV-infected adults, relatively few options are available to the pediatric patient. A recently completed multicenter placebo-controlled IVIG trial concluded that monthly IVIG prolonged the time free from serious bacterial infections in children with symptomatic HIV infection and CD4 cell counts greater than 200 (109). These data have led the American Academy of Pediatrics to recommend that pediatricians consider the use of IVIG for their patients.

Prognosis

Infants with perinatally acquired HIV infection progress clinically and immunologically much more quickly than adults (114, 145). Available data suggest that children who have AIDS or become symptomatic during the first year of life have median survival times of 6.7 months and 24.8 months, respectively (139, 145). Children who have LIP appear to have a more favorable prognosis than do children who have opportunistic infections. Although the use of zidovudine may somewhat improve their prospects of survival, the overall prognosis for HIV-infected children remains bleak.

PREVENTION

As the numbers of HIV-infected women continue to increase in this and other countries, the specter of perinatal HIV infection also increases. HIV, which has emerged as the ninth leading cause of death in infants aged one to four years in the United States, has already had a significant impact on infant survival (146). The accelerated course of the disease in children and the inadequacy of available therapeutic modalities make prevention of infection a priority. Preventive efforts include two approaches: prevention of transmission to the infant and prevention of infection in women of childbearing age.

A multicenter study has recently evaluated the safety, tolerance, and pharmacokinetics of zidovudine administered to 30 infants born to HIV seropositive women. Infants less than 30 days old demonstrated increased clearance of zidovudine, and overall the drug was well tolerated (131). The next step, a trial designed to determine whether maternal infant transmission can be prevented with zidovudine, is being undertaken in several medical centers under the auspices of the AIDS Clinical Trials Group. This study assumes that a significant portion of HIV transmission occurs around the time of delivery and that the use of zidovudine can interrupt such transmission. HIV seropositive pregnant women will be randomized to receive either zidovudine or placebo during pregnancy and through delivery; infants will be treated for six weeks and then followed for 18 months. Data from this trial will not be available for several years. Additional trials with other therapeutic agents are being considered.

Women in the United States are now becoming infected with HIV primarily through heterosexual transmission or through intravenous drug use. Because attempts to diminish high risk sexual activity or drug use have often been ineffective, prevention of transmission has been very difficult. Increasing numbers of obstetricians are recognizing their obligation to educate, counsel, and screen their patients; however, their ability to alter high risk behavior effectively is limited. Intense educational efforts must be undertaken in this country; unfortunately, the populations at highest risk are also the most difficult to reach. There is now increasing recognition of the urgency to educate adolescents, in an attempt to modulate high risk behaviors traditionally undertaken during adolescence. The difficulties inherent in changing high risk behavior of any population should not dissuade public health practitioners. The reality of the AIDS epidemic, with its increasing toll on children, should provide sufficient motivation for the development, implementation, and careful evaluation of intervention strategies.

Literature Cited

1. Amadori, A., De Rossi, A., Giaquinto, C., Faulkner-Valle, G., Zacchello, F., Chieco-Binachi, L. 1988. In vitro production of HIV-specific antibody in children at risk of AIDS. *Lancet* 1:852–54

2. Amirhessami-Aghili, N., Spector, S. A. 1990. Human immunodeficiency virus (HIV) infection of human placenta. *Pediatr. Res.* 27(2):165A

3. Andiman, W. A., Simpson, B. J., Olson, B., Dember, L., Silva, T. J. 1990. Rate of transmission of human immunodeficiency virus type 1 infection from mother to child and short-term outcome of infection. *Am. J. Dis. Child.* 144:758–66

4. Barbacci, M., Dalabetta, G. A., Repke, J. T., Talbot, B. L., Polk, B. F., et al. 1990. Human immunodeficiency virus infection in women attending an inner-city obstetrics clinics: ineffectiveness of targeted screening. *Sex. Transm. Dis.* 17:122–26

5. Barbacci, M., Repke, J. T., Chaisson, R. E. 1991. Routine prenatal screening for HIV infection. *Lancet* 337:709–11

6. Belman, A. L. 1990. AIDS and pediatric neurology. *Neurol. Clin.* 8:571–603

7. Bernstein, L. J., Krieger, B. Z., Novick, B., Sicklick, M. J., Rubinstein, A. 1985. Bacterial infection in the acquired immunodeficiency syndrome of children. *Pediatr. Infect. Dis.* 4:472–75

8. Bernstein, L. J., Ochs, H. D., Wedgewood, R. J., Rubinstein, A. 1985. Defective humoral immunity in pediatric acquired immune deficiency syndrome. *J. Pediatr.* 107:352–57

9. Berrebi, A., Puel, J., Tricoire, J., Herne, P., Pontonnier, G. 1989. Influence of gestation in HIV infection. Presented at *Les Implications du SIDA pour la Mere et l'Enfant, Symp.* (Abstr. E1), Paris

10. Blanche, S., Rouzioux, C., Guihard-Moscato, M.-L., Veber, F., Mayaux, M. J., et al. 1989. A prospective study of infants born to women seropositive for human immunodeficiency virus type 1. *N. Engl. J. Med.* 320:1643–48

11. Borkowsky, W., Krasinski, K., Paul, D., Holzman, R., Moore, T., et al. 1989. Human immunodeficiency virus type 1 antigenemia in children. *J. Pediatr.* 114:940–45

12. Borkowsky, W., Steele, C. J., Grubman, S., Moore, T., LaRussa, P., et al. 1987. Antibody responses to bacterial toxoids in children infected with the human immunodeficiency virus. *J. Pediatr.* 110:563–66

13. Boue, F., Pons, J. C., Keros, L., Chambrin, V., Papiernik, E. 1990. *Risk for HIV 1 Perinatal Transmission Varies with the Mother's Stage of HIV Infec-*

tion. Presented at the 6th Int. Conf. on AIDS, San Francisco

14. Boulos, R., Halsey, N., Holt, E., Brutus, J. R., Quinn, T. C., et al. 1990. HIV-1 in Haitian Women 1982–1988. *J. Acquired Immune Defic. Syndr.* 3:721–28

15. Bozzette, S. A., Sattler, F. R., Chiu, J., Wu, A. W., Gluckstein, D., et al. 1990. A controlled trial of early adjunctive treatment with corticosteroids for *Pneumocystis carinii* pneumonia in the acquired immunodeficiency syndrome. *N. Engl. J. Med.* 323:1451–57

16. Braddick, M. R., Kreiss, J. K., Embree, J. E., Datta, P., Ndinya-Achola, J. O., et al. 1990. Impact of maternal HIV infection on obstetrical and early neonatal outcome. *AIDS* 4(10):1001–5

17. Brouwers, P., Belman, A. L., Epstein, L. G. 1990. Central nervous system involvement: manifestations and evaluation. See Ref. 127a, pp. 318–35

18. Bryson, Y., Arvin, A. 1990. Herpes group virus infections in HIV-1-infected infants, children, and adolescents. See Ref. 127a, pp. 245–65

19. Butler, K. 1990. Hematologic manifestations of HIV infection. See Ref. 127a, pp. 318–35

20. Cannon, R. O., Hook, E. W., Nahmias, A. J., Lee, F. K., Glasser, D. 1988. Association of herpes simplex virus type 2 with HIV infection in heterosexual patients attending sexually transmitted disease clinics. *Fourth Int. Conf. AIDS,* Stockholm

21. Cent. Dis. Control. 1991. Characteristics of, and HIV infection among women served by publicly funded HIV counseling and testing services-United States, 1989–1990. *Morbid. Mortal. Wkly. Rep.* 40:195–203

22. Cent. Dis. Control. 1991. Guidelines for prophylaxis against *Pneumocystis carinii* pneumonia for children infected with human immunodeficiency virus. *Morbid. Mortal.Wkly. Rep.* 40:1–13

23. Cent. Dis. Control. 1991. *HIV/AIDS Surveillance Rep.* May:1–18

24. Cent. Dis. Control. 1991. Mortality attributable to HIV infection/AIDS—United States, 1981–1990. *Morbid. Mortal. Wkly. Rep.* 40:41–44

25. Cent. Dis. Control. 1990. AIDS and the human immunodeficiency virus infection in the United States: 1989 Update. *Morbid. Mortal. Wkly. Rep.* 39:81–86

26. Cent. Dis. Control. 1990. AIDS in women-US *Morbid. Mortal. Wkly. Rep.* 39:845–46

27. Cent. Dis. Control. 1990. Estimates of HIV prevalence and projected AIDS cases: summary of a workshop, October 31–November 1, 1989. *Morbid. Mortal. Wkly. Rep.* 39:1–31

28. Cent. Dis. Control. 1989. Update: Acquired immunodeficiency syndrome associated with intravenous-drug use—United States, 1988. *Morbid. Mortal. Wkly. Rep.* 38:165–70

29. Cent. Dis. Control. 1989. Update: Heterosexual transmission of AIDS and HIV infection—U.S. *Morbid. Mortal. Wkly. Rep.* 38:423–34

30. Cent. Dis. Control. 1988. Prevention of perinatal transmission of hepatitis B virus: prenatal screening of all pregnant women for hepatitis B surface antigen. *Morbid. Mortal. Wkly. Rep.* 37:341–51

31. Cent. Dis. Control. 1987. Classification system for human immunodeficiency virus (HIV) infection in children under 13 years of age. *Morbid. Mortal. Wkly. Rep.* 36:225–35

32. Cent. Dis. Control. 1987. Human immunodeficiency virus infection in the United States; a review of current knowledge. *Morbid. Mortal. Wkly. Rep.* 36:1–48

33. Chandwani, S., Greco, M. A., Mittal, K., Antoine, C., Krasinski, K. 1991. Pathology and human immunodeficiency virus expression in placentas of seropositive women. *J. Infect. Dis.* 163:134–38

34. Chin, J. 1990. Current and future dimensions of the HIV/AIDS pandemic in women and children. *Lancet* 336:221–24

35. Chin, J. 1990. Global estimates of AIDS cases and HIV infection. *AIDS* 4:S277–83

36. Chin, J. 1990. Public health surveillance of AIDS and HIV infections. *WHO Bull.* 68:529–36

37. Chin, J., Sato, P. A., Mann, J. M. 1990. Projections of HIV infections and AIDS cases to the year 2000. *WHO Bull.* 68:1–11

38. Chu, S. Y., Buehler, J. W., Berkelman, R. L. 1990. Impact of the human immunodeficiency virus epidemic on mortality in women of reproductive age, United States. *J. Am. Med. Assoc.* 264:225–29

39. Clumek, N., Robert-Guroff, M., Van de Perre, P., Jennings, A., Sibomana, J. 1985. Seroepidemiological studies of HTLV-III antibody prevalence among selected groups of heterosexual Africans. *J. Am. Med. Assoc.* 254:2599–2602

40. Connor, E. M., Marquis, J., Oleske, J. M. 1990. Lymphoid interstitial pneumonitis. See Ref. 127a, pp. 318–35

41. Coombs, R. W., Collier, A. C., Allain, J.-P., Nikora, B., Leuther, M. 1989. Plasma viremia in human immunodeficiency virus infection. *N. Engl. J. Med.* 321:1626–31

42. Data for applicants tested Oct. 1985–Sept. 1989, provided by US Dep. Defense

43. DeCock, K. M., Barrere, B., Diaby, L., Lafontaine, M. F., Gnaore, E., et al. 1990. AIDS—the leading cause of adult death in the West African city of Abidjan, Ivory Coast. *Science* 249:793–96

44. Des Jarlais, D. C., Friedman, S. R., Novick, D. M., Sotheran, J. L., Thomas, P. 1989. HIV-1 infection among intravenous drug users in Manhattan, New York. *J. Am. Med. Assoc.* 261: 1008–12

45. Des Jarlais, D. C., Friedman, S. R., Stoneburner, R. L. 1988. HIV infection and intravenous drug use: critical issues in transmission dynamics, infection, outcome and prevention. *Rev. Infect. Dis.* 10:151–58

46. Devash, Y., Calvelli, T. A., Wood, D. G., Reagan, K. J., Rubinstein, A. 1990. Vertical transmission of human immunodeficiency virus is correlated with the absence of high-affinity/avidity maternal antibodies to the gp120 principal neutralizing domain. *Proc. Natl. Acad. Sci. USA* 87:3445–49

47. Di Maria, H., Courpotin, C., Rouzioux, C., Cohen, D., Rio, D. 1986. Transplacental transmission of human immunodeficiency virus. *Lancet* 2:215–16

48. Doyle, M. G., Pickering, L. K. 1990. Gastrointestinal infections in children with AIDS. *Semin. Pediatr. Infect. Dis.* 1:64–72

49. Ellner, J. J., Goldberger, M. J., Parenti, D. M. 1991. Mycobacterium avium infection and AIDS: a therapeutic dilemma in rapid evolution. *J. Infect. Dis.* 163: 1326–35

50. Eur. Collaborative Study. 1991. Children born to women with HIV-1 infection: natural history and risk of transmission. *Lancet* 337:253–60

51. Eur. Collaborative Study. 1988. Mother-to-child transmission of HIV infection. *Lancet* 332:1039–42

52. Flynn, A., Finke, J. H., Loftus, M. A. 1985. Comparison of interleukin 1 production by adherent cells and tissue pieces from human placenta. *Immunopharmacology* 9:19–26

53. Gagnon, S., Boota, A. M., Fischl, M. A., Baier, H., Kirksey, O. W., et al. 1990. Corticosteroids as adjunctive therapy for severe *Pneumocystis carinii*

pneumonia in the acquire immunodeficiency syndrome. A double-blind, placebo-controlled trial. *N. Engl. J. Med.* 323:1444–50

54. Gillespie, S., Miles, S., Deveikis, A., Church, J., Diagne, A. 1991. *Plasma Viremia and Virologic Markers of HIV Infection in Children.* Presented to Soc. Pediatr. Res., New Orleans, 29:172A

55. Goedert, J. J., Mendez, H., Drummond, J. E., Robert-Guroff, M., Minkoff, H. L. 1989. Mother-to-infant transmission of human immunodeficiency virus type 1: association with prematurity or low anti-gp120. *Lancet* 2:1351–54

56. Goldstein, J., Braverman, M., Salafia, C., Buckley, P. 1988. The phenotype of human placental macrophages and its variation with age. *Am. J. Pathol.* 133: 648–59

57. Gordon, F. M., Simon, G. L., Wofsy, C. B., Mills, J. 1984. Adverse reactions to trimethoprim-sulfamethoxazole in patients with the acquired immune deficiency syndrome. *Ann. Intern. Med.* 100:495–99

58. Greenberg, A. E., Nguyen-Dinh, P., Mann, J. M., Kabote, N., Colebunders, R. L. 1988. The association between malaria, blood transfusion, and HIV seropositivity in a pediatric population in Kinshasa, Zaire. *J. Am. Med. Assoc.* 259:545–49

59. Guay, L., Mmiro, F., Ndugwa, C., Kataha, P., Mugisha, K. 1990. *Perinatal Outcome in HIV-Infected Women in Uganda.* Presented at the 6th Int. Conf. on AIDS. Th.C.42(Abstr.)

60. Guinan, M. E., Hardy, A. 1987. Epidemiology of AIDS in women in the United States: 1981 through 1986. *J. Am. Med. Assoc.* 257:2039–42

61. Gwinn, M., Pappaioanou, M., George, J. R., Hannon, W. H., Wasser, S. C. 1991. Prevalence of HIV infection in childbearing women in the United States. Surveillance using newborn blood samples. *J. Am. Med. Assoc.* 265:1704–8

62. Halsey, N. A., Boulos, R., Holt, E., Ruff, A., Brutus, J. R. 1990. Maternal-infant HIV-1 infection in Haiti: impact on childhood mortality and malnutrition. *J. Am. Med. Assoc.* 264:2088–92

63. Halsey, N. A., Tafari, N. 1988. *Round Table: Breast Feeding, Vaccination, and Child Care in Developing Countries.* Discussion at 4th Int. AIDS Conf., Stockholm

64. Hanson, I. C., Kaplan, S. L. 1990. Opportunistic infections. *Semin. Pediatr. Infect. Dis.* 1:31–39

65. Harnish, D. G., Hammerberg, O., Wal-

ker, I. R., Rosenthal, K. L. 1987. Early detection of HIV infection in a newborn. *N. Engl. J. Med.* 316:272–73

66. Harries, A. D. 1990. Tuberculosis and human immunodeficiency virus infection in developing countries. *Lancet* 335:387–90

67. Hira, S. K., Kamanga, J., Bhat, G. J., Mwale, C., Tembo, G. 1989. Perinatal transmission of HIV-1 in Zambia. *Br. Med. J.* 299:1250–52

68. Ho, D. D., Moudgil, T., Alam, M. 1989. Quantitation of human immunodeficiency virus infection. *N. Engl. J. Med.* 321:1621–25

69. Holmes, K. K., Karon, J. M., Kreiss, J. K. 1990. The increasing frequency of heterosexually acquired AIDS in the United States. *Am. J. Public Health* 80:858–62

70. Hughes, W. T., Kennedy, W., Dugdale, M., Land, M. A., Stein, D. S., et al. 1990. Prevention of *Pneumocystis carinii* pneumonitis in AIDS patients with weekly dapsone. (Letter). *Lancet* 336:1066

71. Hunter, S. S. 1990. Orphans as a window on the AIDS epidemic in Sub-Saharan Africa: initial results and implications of a study of Uganda. *Soc. Sci. Med.* 31:681–90

72. Husson, R. N. 1990. Mycobacterial infection. See Ref. 127a, pp. 209–24

73. Husson, R. N., Comeau, A. M., Hoff, R. 1990. Diagnosis of human immunodeficiency virus infection in infants and children. *Pediatr. Res.* 86:1–10

74. Hutto, C., Parks, W., Lai, S., Mastrucci, M. T., Mitchell, C. 1991. A hospital-based prospective study of perinatal infection with human immunodeficiency virus type 1. *J. Pediatr.* 118:347–53

75. Hutto, C., Scott, G., Mitchell, C., Parks, W. 1989. *Maternal Risk Factors for Perinatal Transmission to human immunodeficiency Virus-1 (HIV-1).* Presented to 5th Int. Conf. on AIDS, Montreal

76. Italian Multicent. Study. 1988. Epidemiology, clinical features, and prognostic factors of paediatric HIV infection. *Lancet* 2:1043–46

77. Jacobson, M. A. 1988. Mycobacterila diseases. Tuberculosis and mycobacterium avium complex. *Infect. Dis. Clin. North Am.* 2:465–74

78. Jimenez, E., Backe, E., Unger, M., Vogel, M., Schafer, A. 1990. Immunohistochemical marker profiles of placentae of HIV-exposed pregnancies.

Presented to 6th Int. AIDS Conf., San Francisco

79. Johnson, J. P., Nair, P., Hines, S. E., Selden, S. W., Alger, L. 1989. Natural history and serologic diagnosis of infants born to human immunodeficiency virus-infected women. *Am. J. Dis. Child.* 143:1147–53

80. Johnstone, F. D., MacCallum, L., Brettle, R., Inglis, J. M., Peutherer, J. F. 1988. Does infection with HIV affect the outcome of pregnancy? *Br. Med. J.* 296:467

81. Jovaisas, E., Koch, M. A., Schafer, A., Stauber, M., Löwenthal, D. 1985. LAV/HTLV-III in 20-week fetus. (Letter). *Lancet* 2:1129

82. Jura, E., Chadwick, E. G., Josephs, S. H., Steinberg, S. P., Vogev, R. 1989. Varicella-zoster virus infections in children infected with human immunodeficiency virus. *Pediatr. Infect. Dis. J.* 8:586–90

83. Kashkin, J. M., Shliozberg, J., Lyman, W. D., Calvelli, T. A., Steinhauer, E. 1988. Detection of human immunodeficiency virus (HIV) in human fetal tissues. *Pediatr. Res.* 23(2):355A

84. Kavanaugh-McHugh, A., Ruff, A. J., Rowe, S. A., Herskowitz, A., Modlin, J. F. 1990. Cardiovascular manifestations. See Ref. 127a, pp. 318–35

85. Kesson, A., Miles, S., Daigne, A., Chen, I., Frenkl, L. 1990. Diagnosis of perinatally acquired HIV infection. Presented to 6th AIDS Conf., San Francisco

86. Krasinski, K., Borkowsky, W., Bonk, S., Lawrence, R., Chandwani, S. 1988. Bacterial infections in human immunodeficiency virus infected children. *Pediatr. Infect. Dis. J.* 7:323–28

87. Kreiss, J. K., Coombs, R., Plummer, F. A., Holmes, K. K., Nikora, B. 1989. Isolation of human immunodeficiency virus from genital ulcers in Nairobi prostitutes. *J. Infect. Dis.* 160:380–84

88. Kreiss, J. K., Koech, D., Plummer, F. A., Holmes, K. K., Lightfoote, M. 1986. AIDS virus infection in Nairobi prostitutes. Spread of the epidemic to East Africa. *N. Engl. J. Med.* 314:414–18

89. Krivine, A., Yakudima, A., LeMay, M., Pena-Cruz, V., Huang, A. S. 1990. A comparative study of virus isolation, polymerase chain reaction, and antigen detection in children of mothers infected with human immunodeficiency virus. *J. Pediatr.* 116:372–76

90. Lallemant, M., Lallemant-Le-Coeur, S., Cheynier, D., Nzingoula, S., Jourdain, G. 1989. Mother-to-child trans-

mission of HIV-1 and infant survival in Brazzaville, Congo. *AIDS* 3:643–46

91. Lampert, R., Milberg, J., O'Donnell, R., Kristal, A., Thomas, P. 1986. Life table analysis of children with acquired immunodeficiency syndrome. *Pediatr. Infect. Dis. J.* 5:374–75

92. Landesman, S., Minkoff, H., Holman, S., McCalla, S., Sijn, O. 1987. Serosurvey of human immunodeficiency virus infection in parturients. *J. Am. Med. Assoc.* 258:2701–3

93. Laure, F., Courgnaud, V., Rouzioux, C., Blanche, S., Veber, F. 1988. Detection of HIV1 DNA in infants and children by means of the polymerase chain reaction. *Lancet* 2:538–41

94. Lee, F. K., Nahmias, A. J., Lowery, S., Nesheim, S., Reef, S. 1989. ELISPOT: a new approach to studying the dynamics of virus-immune system interaction for diagnosis and monitoring of HIV infection. *AIDS Res. Hum. Retroviruses* 5:517–23

95. Lepage, P., Dabis, F., Hitimana, D.-G., Msellati, P., Van Goethem, C. 1991. Perinatal transmission of HIV-1: lack of impact of maternal HIV infection on characteristics of livebirths and on neonatal mortality in Kigali, Rwanda. *AIDS* 5:295–300

96. Lepage, P., Van de Perre, P. 1988. Nosocomial transmission of HIV in Africa: what tribute is paid to contaminated blood transfusion and medication injection. *Infect. Control Hosp. Epidemiol.* 9:200–3

97. Lewis, S. H., Reynolds-Kohler, C., Fox, H. E., Nelson, J. A. 1990. HIV-1 in trophoblastic and villous Hofbauer cells, and haematological precursors in eight-week fetuses. *Lancet* 335:565–68

98. Lipshultz, S. E., Chanock, S., Sanders, S. P., Colan, S. D., Perez-Atayde, A., McIntosh, K. 1989. Cardiovascular manifestations of human immunodeficiency virus in infants and children. *Am. J. Cardiol.* 63:1489–97

99. Lutz, R., Hiller, K., Stauber, M., Wintergerst, U., Notheis, G., Belohradsky, B. H. 1990. Effect of lymphocyte depletion during pregnancy on clinical complications, birth weight and HIV-infection of the newborn. *6th Int. Conf. on AIDS, Final Program and Abstr.* 2:189 (Abstr. F. B. 447)

100. Mann, J. M., Francis, H., Davachi, F., Baudoux, P., Quinn, T. C. 1986. Risk factors for human immunodeficiency virus seropositivity among children 1 to 24 months old in Kinshasa, Zaire. *Lancet* 2:654–57

101. Martin, N. L., Levy, J. A., Legg, H., Weintrub, P. S., Cowan, M. J., Wara, D. W. 1990. Detection of infection with human immunodeficiency virus (HIV) type 1 in infants by an anti-HIV immunoglobin A assay using recombinant proteins. *J. Pediatr.* 118:354–58

102. Mattern, C. F. T., Murray, K., Jensen, A., Pang, J., Farzadegan, H., et al. 1991. *Pediatrics.* In press

103. Maury, W., Potts, B. J., Rabson, A. B. 1989. HIV-1 infection of first-trimester and term human placental tissue: a possible mode of maternal-fetal transmission. *J. Infect. Dis.* 160:583–88

104. McKinney, R. E., Maha, M. A., Connor, E. M., Feinberg, J., Scott, G. B., et al. 1991. A multicenter trial of oral zidovudine in children with advanced human immunodeficiency virus disease. *N. Engl. J. Med.* 324:1018–25

105. Miotti, P. G., Dallabetta, G., Ndovi, E., Liomba, G., Saah, A. J., et al. 1990. HIV-1 and pregnant women: associated factors, prevalence, estimate of incidence and role of fetal wastage in Central Africa. *AIDS* 4:733–36

106. Modlin, J. F., Bowman, M. 1987. Perinatal transmission of coxackie B3 virus in mice. *J. Infect. Dis.* 156:21–25

107. Mok, J. Q., Giaquinto, C., De Rossi, A., Groschworner, I., Ades, A. E., Peckham, C. S. 1987. Infants born to mothers seropositive for human immunodeficiency virus. *Lancet* 1:1164–68

108. Mok, J. Y. Q., Hague, R. A., Yap, P. L., Hargreaves, F. D., Inglis, J. M., et al. 1989. Vertical transmission of HIV: a prospective study. *Arch. Dis. Child.* 64:1140–45

109. Natl. Inst. Child Health Hum. Dev. Intravenous Immunoglobulin Study Group. 1991. Intravenous immune globulin for the prevention of bacterial infections in children with symptomatic human immunodeficiency virus infection. *N. Engl. J. Med.* 325:73–80

110. Newell, M. L., Peckham, C. S., LePage, P. 1990. HIV-1 infection in pregnancy: implications for women and children. *AIDS* 4(Suppl. 1):S111–18

111. Nguyen Dinh, P., Greenberg, A. E., Mann, J. M., Kabote, N., Francis, H. 1987. Absence of association between *Plasmodium falciparum* malaria and HIV infection in children in Kinshasa, Zaire. *Bull. WHO* 65:607–11

112. Nzilambi, N., Colebunders, R. L.,

Mann, J. M., Francis, H., Nseka, K., 1987. HIV blood screening in Africa: are there no alternatives? *3rd Int. Conf. on AIDS.* (Abstr.)

113. Oleske, J. M., Connor, E. M., Grabenau, M., Minnefor, A. B. 1988. Treatment of HIV infected infants and children. *Ann. Pediatr.* 17:332–39

114. Oxtoby, M. J. 1990. Perinatally acquired human immunodeficiency virus infection. *Pediatr. Infect. Dis. J.* 9:609–19

115. Oxtoby, M. J. 1988. Human immunodeficiency virus and other viruses in human milk: placing the issues in broader perspective. *Pediatr. Infect. Dis. J.* 7:825–35

116. Pahwa, S., Biron, K., Lim, W., Swenson, P., Kaplan, M. H., et al. 1988. Continuous varicella-zoster infection associated with acyclovir resistance in a child with AIDS. *J. Am. Med. Assoc.* 260:2879–82

117. Pahwa, S., Chirmule, N., Leombruno, C., Lim, W., Harper, R., et al. 1989. In vitro synthesis of human immunodeficiency virus-specific antibodies in peripheral blood lymphocytes of infants. *Proc. Natl. Acad. Sci. USA* 86:7532–36

118. Pahwa, S., Fikrig, S., Menez, R., Pahwa, R. 1986. Pediatric acquired immunodeficiency syndrome: Demonstration of B lymphocyte defects in vitro. *Diagn. Immunol.* 4:24–30

119. Pardo, V., Meneses, R., Ossa, L., Jaffe, D. J., Strauss, J., et al. 1987. AIDS related glomerulonephropathy; occurrence in specific risk groups. *Kidney* 31:1167–73

120. Paterlini, P., Lallemant-Le Coeur, S., Lallemant, M., Mpele, P., Dazza, M. C., et al. 1990. Polymerase chain reaction for studies of mother to child transmission of HIV1 in Africa. *J. Med. Virol.* 30:53–57

121. Pelton, S. I., Kelin, J. O. 1990. Bacterial diseases in infants and children with infections due to human immunodeficiency virus. See Ref. 127a, pp. 199–208

122. Pepin, J., Plummer, F. A., Brunham, R. C., Piot, P., Cameron, D. W., et al. 1989. The interaction of HIV infection and other sexually transmitted diseases: an opportunity for intervention. *AIDS* 3:3–9

123. Peters, B., Francis, N., Boylston, A. W., Harris, J. R. W., Pinching, A. J. 1989. Investigation of HIV positive patients with gastrointestinal symptomatology. *5th Int. Conf. on AIDS*, Montreal

124. Pickering, L. K., Cleary, K. R. 1990. Problems of the digestive tract. See Ref. 127a, pp. 318–35

125. Piot, P., Kreiss, J. K., Ndinya-Achola, J. O., Ngugi, E., Plummer, F. A. 1988. Heterosexual transmission of HIV. *AIDS* 2:1–10

126. Piot, P., Plummer, F. A., Mhalu, J. L., Chin, F. S., Mann, J. M. 1988. AIDS: an international perspective. *Science* 239:573–79

127. Piot, P., Plummer, F. A., Rey, M. A., Ngugi, E. N., Rouzioux, C. 1987. Retrospective seroepidemiology of AIDS virus infection in Nairobi populations. *J. Infect. Dis.* 155:1108–12

127a. Pizzo, P. A., Wilfert, C. M., eds. 1990. *Pediatric AIDS: The Challenge of HIV Infection in Infants, Children, and Adolescents.* Baltimore: Williams & Wilkins

128. Plummer, F. A., Simonsen, J. N., Cameron, D. W., Ndinya-Achola, J. O., Kreiss, J. K. 1991. Cofactors in male-female sexual transmission of human immunodeficiency virus type 1. *J. Infect. Dis.* 163:233–39

129. Plummer, F. A., Wainberg, M. A., Plourde, P., Jessamine, P., D'Costa, L. J. 1990. Detection of human immunodeficiency virus type 1 (HIV-1) in genital ulcer exudate of HIV-1 infected man by culture and gene amplification (letter). *J. Infect. Dis.* 161:810–11

130. Preble, E. A. 1990. Impact of HIV/AIDS on African children. *Soc. Sci. Med.* 31:671–80

131. Prober, C. G., Gershon, A. A. 1990. Medical management of newborn infants born to seropositive mothers. See Ref. 127a, pp. 516–30

132. Prose, N. S. 1990. Skin disorders. See Ref. 127a, pp. 373–83

133. Quinn, T. C., Cannon, R. O., Glasser, D., Groseclose, S., Brathwaite, W. S. 1990. The association of syphilis with risk of human immunodeficiency virus infection in patients attending sexually transmitted diseases clinics. *Arch. Intern. Med.* 150:1297–1302

134. Quinn, T. C., Glasser, D., Cannon, R. O., Matuszak, D. L., Dunning, R. W. 1988. Human immunodeficiency virus infection among patients attending clinics for sexually transmitted diseases. *N. Engl. J. Med.* 318:197–203

135. Quinn, T. C., Mann, J. M., Curran, J. W., Piot, P. 1986. AIDS in Africa: an epidemiologic paradigm. *Science* 234:955–63

136. Quinn, T. C., Narain, J. P., Zacarias, F.

R. K. 1990. AIDS in the Americas: a public health priority for the region. *AIDS* 4:709–24

137. Quinn, T. C., Ruff, A., Halsey, N. 1990. Special considerations for developing nations. See Ref. 127a, pp. 714–44

138. Quinn, T. C., Zacarias, F. R. K., St. John, R. K. 1989. HIV and HTLV-1 infection in the Americas: A regional perspective. *Medicine* 68:189–209

139. Rogers, M. F. 1985. AIDS in children: a review of the clinical, epidemiologic and public health aspects. *Pediatr. Infect. Dis.* 4:230–36

140. Rogers, M. F., Ou, C. Y., Rayfield, M., Thomas, P. A., Schoenbaum, E. E. 1989. Use of polymerase chain reaction for early detection of proviral sequences of human immunodeficiency virus in infants born to seropositive mothers. *N. Engl. J. Med.* 320:1649–54

141. Rossi, P., Moschese, V., Broliden, P. A., Fundaró, C., Quinti, I., et al. 1989. Presence of maternal antibodies to human immunodeficiency virus 1 envelope glycoprotein gp120 epitopes correlates with the uninfected status of children born to seropositive mothers. *Proc. Natl. Acad. Sci. USA* 86:8055–58

142. Ryder, R. W., Hassig, S. E. 1988. The epidemiology of perinatal transmission of HIV. *AIDS* 2:S83–89

143. Ryder, R. W., Nsa, W., Hassig, S. E., Behets, F., Rayfield, M. 1989. Perinatal transmission of the human immunodeficiency virus type 1 to infants of seropositive women in Zaire. *N. Engl. J. Med.* 320:1637–42

144. Salcedo, J. R., Connor, E. M., Oleske, J. M. 1990. Renal complications. See Ref. 127a, pp. 318–35

145. Scott, G. B., Hutto, C., Makuch, R. W., Mastrucci, M. T., O'Connor, T. 1989. Survival in children with perinatally aquired human immunodeficiency virus type 1 infection. *N. Engl. J. Med.* 321:1791–96

146. Secretary's Work Group on Pediatr. HIV Infect. and Dis. 1988. A. Novello, Chairm. Dep. Health and Hum. Serv. Washington, DC: US GPO

147. Selwyn, P. A., Schoenbaum, E. E., Davenny, K., Robertson, V. J., Feingold, A. R. 1989. Prospective study of human immunodeficiency virus infection and pregnancy outcomes in intravenous drug users. *J. Am. Med. Assoc.* 261:1289–94

148. Simonsen, J. N., Plummer, F. A., Ngugi, E. N., Black, C., Kreiss, J. K. 1990. HIV infection among lower socioeconomic strata prostitues in Nairobi. *AIDS* 4:139–44

149. Sprecher, S., Soumenkoff, G., Puissant, F., Degueldre, M. 1986. Vertical transmission of HIV in 15-week fetus. *Lancet* 2:288–89

150. Stanback, M., Pape, J. W., Verdier, R., Jean, S., Johnson, W. D. Jr. 1988. Breastfeeding and HIV transmission in Haitian children. *Proc. 4th Int. Conf. on AIDS,* Stockholm

151. Stiehm, E. R., Wara, D. W. 1990. Immunology of HIV. See Ref. 127a, pp. 95–112

152. Temmerman, M., Kiragu, D., Farah, A., Plummer, F. A., Wamioia, I. A., et al. 1990. HIV infection and pregnancy outcome. *5th Int. Conf. on AIDS in Africa.* (Abstr. WOC5)

153. Terragna, A., Anselmo, M., Camera, M., Canessa, A., Mazzarello, G., Melica, F. 1989. Influence of pregnancy on disease progression in 31 HIV infected patients. Presented at *Les implications du SIDA pour la Mere et l'Enfant, Symp.* (Abstr. E2), Paris

154. Thiry, L., Sprecher-Goldberger, S., Jonckheer, T., Levy, J. 1985. Isolation of AIDS virus from cell-free breast milk of three healthy virus carriers. *Lancet* 1:881–92

155. Tudor-Williams, G. 1991. Early diagnosis of vertically acquired HIV-1 infection. *AIDS* 5:103–5

156. Van de Peere, P., Clumeck, N., Carael, M., Nzabihimana, E., Robert-Guroff, M. 1985. Female prostitutes: a risk group for infection with human T-cell lymphotropic virus type-III. *Lancet* 2: 524–27

157. Van de Perre, P., Simonon, A., Hitimana, D. G., Msellati, P., Dabis, F. 1990. *Mother to Child Transmission of HIV: First Immunologic and Serologic Features from an Ongoing Cohort Study in Kigali, Rwanda.* Presented to 6th Int. Conf. on AIDS, San Francisco

158. Vernon, D. D., Holzman, B. H., Lewis, P., Scott, G. B., Birriel, J. A. 1988. Respiratory failure in children with acquired immunodeficiency syndrome and acquired immunodeficiency syndrome related complex. *Pediatrics* 82:223–29

159. Weiblen, B. J., Lee, F. K., Cooper, E. R., Landesman, S. H., McIntosh, K. 1990. Early diagnosis of HIV infection in infants by detection of IgA antibodies. *Lancet* 335:988–90

160. Weiblen, B. J., Schumacher, R. T., Hoff, R. 1990. Detection of IgM and IgA HIV antibodies after removal of IgG

with recombinant protein G. *J. Immunol. Methods* 126:199–204

161. Wilson, C. B., Haas, J. E., Weaver, W. M. 1983. Isolation, purification and characteristics of mononuclear phagocytes from human placentas. *J. Immunol. Methods* 56:305–17

162. Wilson, C. B., Westall, J. 1985. Activation of neonatal and adult human macrophages by alpha, beta, and gamma interferons. *Infect. Immun.* 49:351–56

163. Wolinksy, S., Mack, D., Yogev, R., Herst, C., Sninsky, J. 1988. Direct detection of HIV infection in pediatric patients and their mothers by the polymerase chain reaction (PCR). *Proc. of the 4th Int. Conf. on AIDS*, Stockholm

164. World Health Organization. 1986. Acquired immunodeficiency syndrome (AIDS). *Wkly. Epidemiol. Rec.* 61:69–73

Annu. Rev. Publ. Health 1992. 13:31–57

SELECTED METHODOLOGICAL ISSUES IN EVALUATING COMMUNITY-BASED HEALTH PROMOTION AND DISEASE PREVENTION PROGRAMS

T. D. Koepsell[1], E. H. Wagner[2], A. C. Cheadle, D. L. Patrick, D. C. Martin, P. H. Diehr, and E. B. Perrin

Departments of Health Services, Epidemiology, and Biostatistics, University of Washington, Seattle, Washington 98195

A. R. Kristal[3], C. H. Allan-Andrilla, L. J. Dey

Cancer Prevention Research Unit, Fred Hutchinson Cancer Research Center, Seattle, Washington 98104

KEY WORDS: evaluation methods

INTRODUCTION

An important recent trend in health promotion and disease prevention has been the increasing number and scope of community-based interventions. These programs are aimed at entire populations, which are usually geographically defined, and they attempt to change health behavior and disease risk

[1]address correspondence to T. D. Koepsell, Departments of Health Services and Epidemiology, SC-37, University of Washington, Seattle, WA 98195

[2]also at Center for Health Studies, Group Health Cooperative of Puget Sound, Seattle, WA 98101

[3]also at Departments of Epidemiology and Health Services, University of Washington, Seattle, WA 98195

31

0163-7525/92/0501-0000$02.00

through mass media campaigns, activation of existing community organizations, or changes in the physical or sociocultural environment. Several large programs of this kind have been mounted for cardiovascular disease prevention (30, 33, 44, 56, 71), as reviewed by Shea & Basch (79, 80), and the approach is increasingly being applied to other disease areas and populations (3, 34, 67, 89, 92). As investment in community-based programs has grown, so has the importance of evaluating their effectiveness, as evidenced in part by the recent publications of Green & Lewis (38) and Bracht (6). In this review, we focus on a selection of methodological issues that assume special importance in evaluating community-based programs, but receive little coverage in standard texts on program evaluation. These issues include:

1. Specification of the theoretical model. The design of an intervention is usually based on some theory of program action. An important early step in program evaluation is to make this theoretical model explicit: What are the key intervention components, and what are the causal mechanisms by which they are expected to work? An explicit model is needed to guide evaluation design decisions, to help identify the specific shortcomings of a program found to be ineffective, or to facilitate dissemination of an effective one. The task can be complex for community-level interventions aimed at individual-level health behavior because of the need for a multilevel conceptualization.

2. Communities as units of allocation. Because interventions aim at entire communities, an evaluation design with concurrent controls will likely involve assignment of communities en bloc to intervention and control groups. This feature has important implications for both planning study size and data analysis.

3. Allocation of a small number of communities. Cost and feasibility considerations usually limit the intervention and evaluation to a small number of communities, thus complicating the task of achieving comparable study groups.

4. Longitudinal versus repeated cross-sectional samples. Community surveys may be needed to measure change in certain key outcomes. These surveys can be conducted by either following a panel of individuals in each community over time or drawing a fresh cross-sectional sample in each community at each time point. Both approaches have unique strengths and drawbacks.

5. Validity of self-reported health characteristics. Particularly because of the highly public nature of the intervention and the inability to blind participants to their treatment group membership, the validity of self-reported data on health behavior can be a concern.

6. Measures of community environment. Assessing features of the community environment can help test the underlying causal model, detect early

program effects, and avoid excessive reliance on self-reported behavior change.

We now discuss each of these six issues in turn.

SPECIFICATION OF THE THEORETICAL MODEL

The randomized controlled trial has become a widely accepted paradigm for evaluating the effect of health interventions, against which nonexperimental methods are judged and often found wanting. The design and the size of most randomized trials are usually driven by a primary research question, which typically concerns the effect of an intervention on final outcomes. Unfortunately, this focus on final outcomes may result in overlooking the need to characterize both the intervention itself and the causal mechanisms by which it is supposed to work. Interventions then become "black boxes" whose overall effects may be detectable, but whose contents are obscure. Careful specification of the intervention and its presumed mechanism of action is an important step in designing an appropriate evaluation.

What are black box interventions? Lipsey (57) describes them as "situations for which inputs and outputs can be observed, but the connecting processes are not readily visible." The black box then contains the causal sequence between inputs (e.g. receipt of grant funds and formation of a community coalition) and outputs (e.g. cessation of cigarette smoking). For simpler interventions, such as an immunization program, opening the black box, albeit desirable, may not be as essential to interpreting the evaluation results, replicating effective interventions, or tinkering with ineffective ones. For such interventions as community-based prevention efforts, the contents of the black box are much more complex, and their obscurity is a serious deterrent to understanding and progress.

A key reason to open black boxes is to improve interventions. With this in mind, an approach to process evaluation based on theoretical considerations has emerged in the evaluation literature (13, 14). At the heart of the approach is the notion of treatment theory, which describes how program inputs translate into outputs. An optimal treatment theory is specific enough to guide evaluation design and analysis, yet general enough to illuminate the field. The more critical need, however, is for specific applicability to the intervention under study and to the context in which it will be implemented. This need has led Lipsey (57) to label such intervention theories as "small theories of treatment." Large theories, such as diffusion theory or exchange theory, might guide the elaboration of treatment theory, but can be too abstract and general to guide evaluation design.

A useful treatment theory provides a model to show how the program will produce its postulated effects. At minimum, it must include key inputs (e.g. formation of a new community coalition) and outputs (e.g. avoidance of substance use by adolescents), and the sequence of events of processes connecting them. For community-based prevention programs, these events or processes must delineate a believable scenario by which the mobilization of community organizations and programs can motivate and assist individual citizens to change their behaviors. A useful small theory of treatment would describe how grant funds, program specifications, technical assistance, and other inputs translate into effective community structures that can produce and disseminate intervention components with a chance of success.

A critical aspect of useful treatment theory and process evaluation, in general, is the specification of key steps in program implementation (75). For most community-based health programs, major concerns include the functionality of the community coalition or board, the scientific quality of intervention components as actually delivered, and the exposure of community residents to those interventions.

Treatment Theory and Evaluative Design

A good treatment theory can greatly enhance the design, analysis, and interpretation of an evaluation (5, 57). From a study design perspective, there is almost no limit to what can be measured in a community-based program. Important events and processes may occur in the community environment or among community organizations, political leaders, health care providers, or individual members of the target population. Choosing the variables to measure requires some means of distinguishing that which is essential for determining program success or failure from the rest. Program theory provides a blueprint for measurement because, by definition, it specifies the critical steps on the path from input to output.

For example, Figure 1 shows the "small theory" of treatment that guides the evaluation of the Henry J. Kaiser Family Foundation's Community Health Promotion Grants Program (89). The conceptual basis for the model (27, 39, 40), based in social learning theory (a "large theory") (2), emphasizes modifying community norms and inducing changes in the physical, regulatory, and socioeconomic environments to make them more supportive of healthful behaviors and behavior change. To accomplish this, the model posits that projects must first activate their communities by developing a broadly based consensus among leading community organizations to address a health problem, coordinate planning, share resources, and engender broad citizen involvement. The "activated community" reaches individual citizens through high quality intervention components that change norms toward approval of healthful behaviors and disapproval of unhealthful ones (e.g. in media messages), change environments to encourage healthful behaviors and discourage

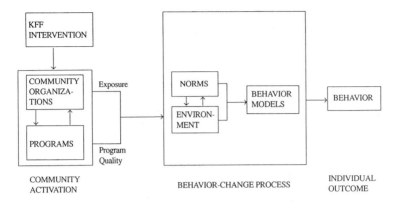

Figure 1 Intervention model.

unhealthful ones (e.g. worksite smoking policies), and provide more models of individuals who have adopted healthful norms and behaviors.

Measurements in this evaluation were then selected to correspond to the major components of the treatment theory. A survey of leaders of key community organizations provides data to assess the extent to which community organizations were collaborating and generating intervention activities. Surveys of restaurants and grocery stores and reviews of legislative activity monitor environmental changes, whereas surveys of adult and adolescent residents furnish information about exposure to interventions, norms, behavioral models, as well as behaviors.

Treatment Theory and Data Analysis

Treatment models are also analytic models, which specify independent, dependent, and mediating variables and depict causal pathways. Judd & Kenny (47) show how modern multivariate statistical techniques can be used to test the relationships posited by a treatment theory. Lipsey (57) argues that the use of treatment theory to select appropriate, sensitive outcome measures may mitigate the common problem of insufficient statistical power in social evaluations by increasing the true effect size associated with effective treatments.

Treatment Theory and the Interpretation of Evaluation Results

Community-based prevention programs that address health-related behaviors may not always produce dramatic effects. Evaluation findings have often been mixed (28), controversial (70), or negative (94) and are likely to continue to be so. Treatment theory may clarify the meaning of findings by delineating the role of the treatment, or aspects of the treatment, as the cause of a positive or negative result. Concomitantly, treatment theory may play a crucial role in disentangling bad evaluation methods from bad treatment ideas from bad treatment implementations (57).

Treatment Theory and the Advancement of Treatment Effectiveness

Most community-based prevention programs resemble each other, at least in general ways. Evaluations based on treatment theory should advance the state of the art by identifying the details of good ideas for replication or enhancement and bad ideas for a return trip to the drawing board.

COMMUNITIES AS UNITS OF ALLOCATION

Under our definition, community-based interventions are aimed at entire communities. Hence, an evaluation that uses a concurrently studied control group must generally use entire communities as controls. The unit of allocation in this design is thus the community, even though many outcome measures (including all those discussed in this section), such as smoking status or dietary fat intake, may originate with observations on individuals in those communities. Sometimes, communities are actually randomized to intervention and control groups (34, 89), as we discuss later. However, nonrandomized designs must also deal with the consequences of community-level allocation, and they require added attention to the possibility of community-level confounding factors.

Probably, the most important consequences of allocation by community are reduced statistical power and added complexity in estimating sample size requirements or statistical power. When we have person-level outcome measures, but community-level allocation and analysis, two sources of random variation must be considered and estimated: individual-level variation within a community and community-level variation within a treatment group. We must also consider two kinds of sample sizes: the number of individuals per community and the number of communities per treatment group. For a fixed total number of individuals studied, statistical power is almost always lower when allocation is by community (or cluster) rather than by individual, as shown in a short and accessible paper by Cornfield (17). At least under classical methods of analysis, part of the loss of power occurs because the number of degrees of freedom for a statistical test of treatment effect depends on the number of communities studied, not on the number of individuals studied in those communities (17, 48). When the number of communities is small, this number of degrees of freedom is also small, and the critical value that a test statistic must achieve is higher than for studies that allocate individuals. This effect on power can grow large when the number of communities falls below about ten.

More specifically, the power to detect an effect of the intervention depends directly on the precision with which the mean level of the relevant outcome can be estimated for each treatment group. For a simple design involving randomization of c communities to an intervention group and c more to a control group, with n individuals studied per community, the expected sampling variance of the mean for each treatment group is:

$$\frac{\sigma_C^2 + \dfrac{\sigma^2}{n}}{c},$$

where σ_C^2 is the community-level variance component (i.e. variance in the true mean level of the outcome variable among communities) and σ^2 is the individual-level variance component (i.e. variance in the outcome variable among individuals within a community). As a rule, the evaluator has little control over the size of σ_C^2 or σ^2, but must estimate them both to estimate study power.

The above expression also shows that if σ_C^2 is at all large relative to σ^2, there are likely to be only modest gains from studying more individuals per community (i.e. increasing n), but potentially major gains in power from studying more communities per treatment group (i.e. increasing c). Of course, these two options for enhancing power may have quite different cost implications. In some situations, the marginal cost of each intervention site may be large, but the marginal cost of a control site may be more modest. If so, the evaluator may wish to form unequal-sized treatment groups, with more control sites than intervention sites.

An equivalent way of considering this issue (23) is to note that, under community allocation, observations on the individuals in each treatment group cannot be considered statistically independent of each other, as they can under individual allocation. Instead, observations on individuals who reside in the same community tend to be correlated. For continuous variables, the appropriate measure of correlation is the intraclass correlation, which can be expressed as

$$\frac{\sigma_C^2}{\sigma_C^2 + \sigma^2}.$$

The formulation based on correlated observations is thus closely linked to that based on variance components, as the intraclass correlation can be viewed as a measure of the relative sizes of the two variance components. Mickey et al

(61) discuss this issue in terms of the design effect and show how its magnitude can depend on study duration.

Specific Methods for Estimating Sample Size and Power

Statistical tools useful for study planning have been developed for a variety of study designs that involve allocation by community. Donner and colleagues (22, 23) and Hsieh (43) provide guidelines for studies of simple, two-group comparisons that involve continuous or dichotomous outcome measures. Shipley et al (81) describe and illustrate methods for designs involving randomization of matched pairs of communities. Hsieh (43) discusses an approach for power calculations when communities are to be randomized within two or more strata, and when treatment effects are to be measured in terms of a pretest/posttest comparison over time. Koepsell et al (48) suggest an approach that can be used when the time path of a program effect is of central interest, as may be true for an evaluation developed around a specific intervention model. They also discuss different approaches for longitudinal versus repeated cross-sectional samples of individuals studied over time. Earlier work by Gillum et al (35) also considers the problem of allowing for dropouts over time.

Obtaining Estimates of Community-Level Variance

One of the greatest challenges in estimating power and sample-size requirements in community-based studies is providing estimates of the community-level variance component, σ_C^2. [For a design involving comparison of changes over time, the evaluator would instead supply an estimate of σ_{CT}^2, the community-by-time interaction variance, against which treatment-by-time interactions would be tested. See Koepsell et al (48).] Depending on the outcome variable of interest, suitable estimates can sometimes be derived from public data sources, such as the Centers for Disease Control Behavioral Risk Factor Survey, or from previous studies.

Several statistical methods for estimation of variance components have been proposed (77). Particularly when the number of individuals studied varies across communities, these methods can yield different estimates. As a practical matter, both the BMDP and SAS computer packages have procedures for computing variance components. In BMDP, procedure P3V provides both maximum likelihood or restricted maximum likelihood (REML) estimation methods. In SAS, the corresponding procedure is PROC VARCOMP.

For illustration, Table 1 presents estimates of σ_C^2 and of σ^2 for current smoking status, as derived from three studies that involved data collection across several communities: the evaluation of the Kaiser Family Foundation Community Health Promotion Grant Program (89), the RAND Health Insurance Experiment (64), and a survey of cancer-related risk behaviors conducted in Washington State by the Cancer Prevention Research Program at the Fred Hutchinson Cancer Research Center (1990, unpublished data). In each of those studies, cities or counties were the communities of interest, and smoking status was coded as 0=nonsmoker, 100=smoker to yield estimates in a convenient numerical range. Within each study, estimates of σ_C^2 obtained by the three statistical methods are generally similar, e.g. they range from 8.8 to 10.7 for the Kaiser data. However, the point estimates are quite different across studies; REML estimates range from 5.4 for the RAND data to 30.3 for the Washington State data. Despite the relatively large number of individuals studied, estimates of σ_C^2 from these data sets are based on small numbers of communities and thus have rather wide confidence limits. When such data are used in study planning, it may be wise to use several estimates of σ_C^2, which vary through a plausible range and yield "optimistic" and "pessimistic" estimates of sample size or statistical power.

Particularly for large data sets, the task of computing variance component estimates can be time-consuming and costly, and an investigator may lack the resources to do so. Sometimes, only published, community-level means or prevalences may be available. In these situations, an investigator can obtain a crude point estimate of σ_C^2 by simply computing the variance of the set of community-level means or prevalences. On average, such an estimate tends to

Table 1   Examples of individual- and community-level variance components for current smoking status

	Kaiser Community Health Promotion Grants Program	RAND Health Insurance Experiment (at entry)	Washington State Cancer-Related Behavioral Risk Factor Survey
No. communities	15	6	35
Total no. individuals	8726	5094	1642
Prevalence of smoking	24%	37%	26%
Individual-level variance (σ^2)			
Point estimate	1800.7	2342.3	1990.7
95% conf. limits	(1746.2, 1855.1)	(2249.5, 2435.3)	(1850.9, 2130.7)
Community-level variance (σ_C^2)			
REML Method			
Point estimate	10.7	5.4	30.3
95% conf. limits	(0, 21.7)	(0, 16.5)	(0, 79.9)
ML Method			
Point estimate	8.8	3.8	25.1
95% conf. limits	(0, 17.6)	(0, 12.1)	(0, 67.2)
Method of Moments			
Point estimate	10.0	5.0	20.1

be conservative (i.e. too large) and probably still has wide confidence limits if based on a small number of communities. But, at least the estimate gives an investigator an idea of σ_C^2 for use in study planning.

Analysis Strategies

Oft-quoted advice by Cornfield (17) is: "Randomization by cluster accompanied by an analysis appropriate to randomization by individual is an exercise in self-deception . . . and should be discouraged." Whiting-O'Keefe & Simborg (91) have also commented on the all-too-common practice of ignoring the proper unit of analysis in studies that involve assignment of aggregates to treatment conditions.

Space limitations permit only brief mention of several suitable analysis techniques. Randomization tests (65) provide a valid method to test for program effects with minimal statistical assumptions. These tests are more feasible to implement with small numbers of study units, especially in the present era of cheap computing power. However, they have the decided disadvantage of never being able to reject the null hypothesis if the number of possible assortments of study communities into treatment groups is very small. Traditional analysis-of-variance methods for hierarchial (nested) study designs may be used and are readily implemented when the number of observations per community is relatively constant across communities (25). Analysis using community means as though they were elementary observations can also be a straightforward and valid approach for such "balanced" designs. The above-mentioned BMDP procedure P3V can accommodate designs with unequal sample sizes (20). The analysis of variance is most applicable for continuous outcome measures, but it may also be suitable for dichotomous outcomes if the number of observations per community is reasonably large and if community prevalences are not too close to 0 or 1.

Donald & Donner (21) have suggested a method that accounts for randomization by cluster when combining 2×2 contingency tables across communities. Donner & Donald (24) have proposed analytic methods when randomization by cluster has been carried out within strata. Zeger et al (95) have described powerful and flexible analysis methods for correlated dichotomous outcomes by using generalized estimating equations in the context of longitudinal studies. Software to implement their approach is not yet widely available, however.

ALLOCATION OF A SMALL NUMBER OF COMMUNITIES

Often, funding agencies or communities themselves decide whether a program is to be mounted in a particular community or set of communities, and an evaluator may have little say in the matter. On other occasions, a multi-community program may be set up as a planned social experiment, thus allowing evaluation considerations to affect the process by which communities are designated as intervention or nonintervention sites. But, even when an evaluator has the luxury of allocating communities to treatment groups, it may be far from clear how best to do so. Here, we consider two aspects of the decision.

Should Communities Be Randomized?

When only a few study communities are available to be allocated randomly to an intervention and a control group, there is an increased risk of a major imbalance between groups on important confounding factors, whether these factors are known or unknown. One can argue that some possible outcomes of simple randomization would be unacceptable, such as those that put intervention and control communities into the same media market and lead to cross-contamination. For that reason, for example, and to minimize investigator travel, communities close to study headquarters are sometimes chosen as intervention sites, thus leaving communities farther away as controls.

Nonetheless, even when only a few communities are available for study, a random allocation process has much to recommend it (51), especially when processes other than simple random allocation are considered. The difficulty of creating acceptably balanced treatment groups results chiefly from the limited number of communities available for assignment, and that difficulty remains whether randomization is used or not. Other methods for achieving balance, such as matching or stratification, can be used in conjunction with randomization. In the COMMIT project, for example, 11 pairs of communities were formed, and one member of each pair was chosen at random to be the intervention site (34); in the Kaiser Health Promotion Evaluation Project, a form of restricted randomization was used after study communities were arranged into strata (89). Restricted randomization can also be sued to deal with the problem of shared media markets by ruling out certain unacceptable study group configurations in advance and selected one of the remaining acceptable configurations at random, as long as each community ultimately has an equal chance of becoming an intervention or a control site. (This may be a particularly suitable context in which to use a randomization test for statistical inference.) In brief, although a carefully designed random allocation process may not prevent problems of treatment group comparability as neatly as it does with larger samples, it need not complicate them either. And, randomization offers other advantages: namely, a firm basis for formal hypothesis testing and a public perception of even-handedness in forming the comparison groups that is hard to achieve any other way.

Should Communities Be Matched?

As noted above, matching can be used with or without randomization to achieve some degree of comparability between intervention and control groups or to enhance power. Theoretically, the best factor on which to match is one that is highly correlated with change in the outcome variable; in practice, there may be limited knowledge about which community character-istics qualify as good matching factors on this basis. Freedman et al (34) showed that a matching scheme that incorporated geographic proximity and community size appeared to perform well in forming matched pairs that were similar with regard to the prevalence of the target behavior at baseline. However, Martin et al (59) suggest that when the number of study communi-ties is small, matching should be used only in the presence of a very good matching factor, chiefly because the loss of degrees of freedom that results from using the community pair (rather than the individual community) as the unit of analysis can seriously compromise power and, in fact, weaken the comparison.

LONGITUDINAL VERSUS REPEATED CROSS-SECTIONAL SAMPLES

A central goal of most community-based health promotion programs is to reduce risky health behaviors in study communities. Surveys of community residents at two or more points in time are often required to obtain direct evidence on whether this goal is met. These surveys may use either longitu-dinal samples, which consist of a panel of individuals in each community who are surveyed repeatedly, or repeated cross-sectional samples, which consist of a fresh sample of individuals from each community on each survey occasion (usually with only a small probability of repeated selection of the same individual). Although this discussion is in terms of samples of individuals, similar comments apply to other possible subunits within a community, such as restaurants or schools.

Several writers (1, 29, 36, 73) have commented on the relative merits of the longitudinal and repeated cross-sectional sampling approaches. The choice between the two depends on the correspondence between sample type and program objectives, on relative susceptibility to biases, on statistical power trade-offs, and on cost. Table 2 summarizes factors to be considered in this section.

Correspondence with Program Objectives

An important question is whether the intervention seeks primarily to change the health behavior of individuals, or to change the prevalence of risky behaviors in the community. These two kinds of changes are not the same, as

Table 2 Factors influencing a choice between longitudinal and repeated cross-sectional samples

Factor	Longitudinal	Cross-sectional
Program objective	Directly measures change in individual health characteristics	Directly measures change in community prevalence of health characteristics
Selection bias at recruitment	May be worse because participation is not anonymous	Participation may be anonymous
Attrition	Losses to follow-up may be related to behavior being evaluated	Not a problem
Testing	Repeated questioning may be a co-intervention	Not a problem
Maturation	Panel gets older, while community at large may not	Not a problem
History	Panel consists of more long-term community residents with exposure to "local history"	Less a problem
Cross-contamination	Not a problem	Movement between intervention and control communities may dilute intervention effect
Statistical power	Higher for fixed sample size and intervention effect	Lower

communities are dynamic populations whose membership can change over time because of births, deaths, and in- and out-migration. A decline in the community prevalence of a behavior over time may occur, even in the absence of any individual-level behavior change, if individuals who join or leave the community differ systematically from other community residents in terms of their health behavior. Community-based programs usually do seek individual-level behavior change. But, sometimes, they may also change the social environment, deliberately or otherwise, through recruitment of persons with healthy behavior and out-migration of those with risky behavior, e.g. a worksite health promotion program may succeed in institutionalizing a preference for nonsmokers in hiring decisions, and it may make workplace smoking policies uncomfortable for smokers so that they seek jobs elsewhere. Other factors being equal, longitudinal samples are theoretically better suited to isolating program effects on individual behavior change, whereas repeated cross-sectional samples are better suited to measuring program effects on community-wide prevalence.

If the survey involves a large fraction of the community, and if population turnover is low, one may, in fact, generate a longitudinal subsample within the cross-sectional samples by repeated selection of the same individuals. In other situations, there may be ways to circumvent limitations of a specific sampling approach by altering other aspects of the survey methodology. For example, respondents in a follow-up cross-sectional survey can be asked about their length of residence in the community and about any changes in their health behavior that occurred during the study period. It may also be possible to supplement a longitudinal sample or to replace those lost to follow-up with newcomers during the study to render its composition more representative of the community at each time point, even though this option complicates data analysis.

Susceptibility to Bias

Table 2 also highlights certain sources of bias that can affect longitudinal and repeated cross-sectional samples differently; thus, "bias" means any systematic difference between measured characteristics of the sample and the corresponding true characteristics of the population supposedly represented by the sample.

Self-selection at recruitment can occur under either sampling approach because of nonresponse. Active refusal to participate is an important component of nonresponse (31, 42, 88), and concerns about privacy account for many refusals in some surveys (19). Although respondents can participate anonymously as part of a single cross-sectional sample, members of a longitudinal sample must reveal their identities and consent to be recontacted. These additional demands may further jeopardize willingness to participate.

Attrition affects longitudinal, but not repeated cross-sectional, samples. Attrition can be large: In the Stanford Five-City Project, 39% of the baseline cohort completed three follow-up surveys over a five-year period (28). Several longitudinal studies have found that individuals who smoke at baseline are more likely to drop out than those who do not (41, 45, 46). Other studies have found that subjects who are harder to follow are more likely to have worse exercise habits (54) or higher levels of substance abuse at follow-up (41, 53, 69). These findings suggest that losses from a cohort often occur preferentially among those with worse health habits.

Testing effects occur when changes in reported behavior are caused (or inhibited) by the act of repeated questioning. They affect longitudinal samples only. Although the possibility of such effects has long been known by psychologists (8, 16) and shown for nonhealth behaviors, such as voting (49), little evidence is available concerning testing effects on reported health characteristics. In the MRFIT STUDY (63), a larger discrepancy between self-reported and thiocyanate-adjusted quit rates for smoking in the intervention group compared with the control group at follow-up suggested the possibility of testing-treatment interaction. A study by Bridge et al (7) suggests that repeated questioning resulted in shifting attitudes about cancer. Murray et al (62) found greater declines in smoking in a repeatedly questioned cohort of adolescents compared with a single, comparably aged cross-sectional sample. They inferred that the surveys themselves may have accounted for part of the difference.

Maturation occurs in a longitudinal sample, which ages over time, whereas the age distribution in the community and in repeated cross-sectional samples may change very little. Any age-related phenomenon may thus appear to change in a longitudinal sample over time, even if the change had no relation to a community intervention.

History may also preferentially affect longitudinal samples, which necessarily consist of longer-term community residents. Stable members of the community may have more exposure to local, nonprogram-related events that cause behavior change.

Cross-contamination of treatment groups is at least a theoretical possibility, if mobility among study communities is high. With repeated cross-sectional samples, a follow-up survey participant may have recently moved from a control community to a study community, or vice versa, thus rendering the subject's exposure status unclear. This kind of bias can be more of a concern if "community" is broadly defined to include such settings as workplaces or schools.

Although these sources of bias can interfere with the degree to which the sample reflects the community at a given time point, they do not necessarily result in a biased estimate of program effect. If attrition affects longitudinal samples similarly in intervention and control communities, for example, this source of error would "cancel out" in a comparison between study groups. Likewise, bias that remains stable over time could still allow accurate estimation of a change in the prevalence of a characteristic over time. The strongest evaluation designs used to date have assessed program effect by comparing changes over time between intervention and control groups. Under such a design, the estimate of program effect would be biased only if there is interaction among size of bias, treatment group, and time, e.g. if repeated surveying renders a person more susceptible to an intervention effect, or if attrition of persons with unhealthy behavior occurs differently in the intervention group versus the control group. Unfortunately, little empirical evidence is available to judge how serious such potential threats to validity are in practice.

Statistical Power

A major attraction of the longitudinal-sample approach is its greater statistical power to detect change. This gain in power results from, and is quantitatively dependent on, intertemporal correlation in health characteristics at the individual level: The more stable the characteristic, the greater the advantage of a longitudinal sample for detecting a hypothesized change of a given size. Schlesselman (76) and Cook & Ware (15) discuss the statistical principles that underlie this conclusion. Koepsell et al (48) discuss performance of sample-size calculations for both sampling approaches.

Given that the longitudinal-sample approach may be more susceptible to a variety of biases, as discussed above, Martin et al (58) derived a simple inequality that shows how large the added bias must be to outweigh the power advantages of a longitudinal sample, at least for a simple design situation. Specifically, consider a design in which r = the correlation between individual's baseline and follow-up health behavior status, n = the number of individuals surveyed per occasion, b_L = the amount of bias in the estimate of mean change from baseline to follow-up based on a longitudinal sample, b_X = the corresponding bias for a cross-sectional sample, and s^2 = the overall variance in behavior. Martin showed that when $r < n(b_L^2 - b_X^2)/2s^2$, then a cross-sectional sample approach yields a lower expected mean-squared error than a longitudinal-sample approach.

Unfortunately, a confident choice between sampling approaches depends on having good advance estimates of the likely extent of several kinds of bias and of the expected intertemporal correlation in the characteristics being measured. Moreover, all of these factors can be expected to vary from one behavior to another, so that the superior sampling approach for studying one behavior may be inferior for studying another. Perhaps for these reasons, several evaluations of large-scale community interventions have used both longitudinal and cross-sectional samples; these evaluations usually let the baseline survey sample serve both as the longitudinal sample and as the first cross-sectional sample (29, 44, 89). Building on this practical stratagem of safety through redundancy, Thornquist & Anderson (86) have recently proposed what they nickname a "belt and suspenders" method for combined analysis of data from longitudinal and cross-sectional samples, which uses generalized estimating equations.

VALIDITY OF SELF-REPORTED HEALTH CHARACTERISTICS

In community-based health promotion and disease prevention studies, information about health behavior is often gathered directly from individuals through interviews or self-administered questionnaires. There is a widespread belief that people are inclined to overreport desirable health behaviors and underreport undesirable health behaviors. As more attention is paid to health behaviors in the media, in public places, in worksites, and in clinical practice, individuals, families, and different social groups may become sensitized to socially desirable forms of behavior. Therefore, methodologies to investigate and improve the validity of self-reports are important to develop and apply.

One major approach is to search for "objective" measures of behavior, on the assumption that they are free of subjective bias. Biochemical validation tests, such as those used in smoking research, are prized for their criterion validity. These "gold standard" measures, however, may be too costly, as well as vulnerable to between-individual variation in absorption, metabolism, and excretion (37). One investigative team even concludes that ". . . questionnaire response appears to be the standard against which physiologic test of smoking must be judged, not vice versa" (68). Self-reports often become the only feasible method for collecting data on health behaviors. We summarize here published evidence for the validity of self-reports for two forms of health behavior that have been common targets of community-based interventions: cigarette smoking and dietary behavior. We also discuss the major methodologies for evaluating and improving these reports.

Cigarette Smoking

A recent review and meta-analysis of studies, which uses biochemical validation of smoking behavior, suggests that self-reports of cigarette smoking obtained by in-person interviews have fairly high sensitivity and specificity among adult respondents who participate in community studies, when examined in relation to a biochemical measure of smoking status (66). Similar validation studies, which have been carried out among students, suggest that self-reports among adolescents involved in smoking cessation interventions are less accurate. Biochemical validation remains desirable in evaluations of smoking cessation interventions.

Biochemical validation cannot determine, however, the accuracy of reports regarding smoking consumption, i.e. the number of cigarettes smoked (85). Nor can biochemical tests be used to validate smoking histories that yield estimates of risk in terms of pack-years. Lifetime smoking consumption is likely underreported, given the difficulties of long-term recall.

Several methodological techniques have been used to evaluate and improve self-reports of smoking behavior. Studies of surrogate reports of behavior, usually next-of-kin and particularly spouses, indicate that self-reports of cigarette smoking correlate highly with surrogate reports (60).

Other studies have suggested that informing subjects that a biochemical measure of cigarette smoking, such as salivary cotinine or expired carbon monoxide, is to be obtained improves the validity of self-reports (4, 26). In some instances, bogus measurement procedures are used, or biochemical samples are obtained but never analyzed. This approach has been called the "bogus pipeline." When genuine objective measures were used in research with adolescents, Bauman & Dent (4) found that adolescents who had recently smoked reported significantly greater amounts of smoking if they were informed about the biochemical measure before completing the questionnaire.

Unfortunately, published studies evaluating self-reports of cigarette smoking seldom contain the actual questions used to classify smokers and nonsmokers. Thus, the form and content of the questions themselves are difficult to evaluate. The actual wording of questions can influence the responses given and, hence, the categorization of respondents as smokers (87). Therefore, studies asking about smoking should report or reference the questions used, so that this potential source of invalidity can be examined and controlled. They should also report whether subjects were told before answering questions that they would later be asked to provide a specimen for biochemical validation.

Dietary Behavior

A problem with assessing dietary behavior through self-report is that eating is a mundane, frequent behavior that a person does with relatively little attention. At least three methods have been used in community-based studies to assess dietary change: nutrient intake (diet records, 24-hour recall, and food-frequency questionnaires); biochemical measures (primarily serum cholesterol); and approaches aimed at the specific targets of the intervention (measures of individual behavior, such as "Yesterday, did you eat a vegetable with dinner?", or environmental measures as discussed below, such as percent of supermarket milk shelf space devoted to lowfat milk) (50).

The lack of a criterion measure of dietary intake in free-living persons is the major problem in evaluating the validity of these measures. Assessing convergent validity (concurrence among different measures) is a common alternative. In general, correlations among various nutrient intake measures are rarely above 0.6 and, depending upon the nutrient, are frequently as low as 0.3 (55). Even for food frequency questionnaires, which are designed to minimize intra-individual variability, test-retest correlations are rarely above 0.65 and may be as low as 0.2 (84).

A special threat to validity arises from the nonblinded nature of most community dietary intervention studies. If the intervention program has an effective public education component, residents of intervention communities understand the relationship between food and health better and pay greater attention to food and food choices. These intervention effects could influence measurements in the absence of behavior change, thus confounding any interpretation of contrasts between intervention and control communities. The act of retesting a cohort may also produce biases in reported behaviors, as discussed earlier. Unfortunately, there are few data with which to substantiate or estimate the magnitude of these potential biases.

In practice, 24-hour recalls and food records have usually been deemed too expensive, time-consuming, and difficult to administer for use in large-scale

community studies. Food frequency questionnaires and abbreviated questionnaires of behavior specifically targeted by the intervention, methods that rely
upon retrospective reports of dietary habits, are most often the only practical
means for assessing dietary change. The cognitive processes that underlie
responding to these methods are complex. For example, food frequency
judgments require individuals to assign "typical frequency" and portion size
judgments for what is often a long list of food items. An inferential process,
by which a frequency judgment is derived at the time the question is asked,
must occur. Little research has been done to investigate these cognitive
processes and their potential for biasing reported dietary behaviors (82, 83).

Epidemiologic studies of dietary behavior (93) have found that respondents' reports of current dietary behaviors, or recall of previous behaviors,
depend on whether the foods are perceived as socially desirable or personally
relevant. Comparisons with daily food records have indicated overestimates
of up to 50% on food frequency judgments for "healthy" foods and underestimates of up to 30% for "unhealthy" foods (74).

Various approaches need to be investigated to both assess and minimize
these biases in dietary recall. For example, social desirability and food
salience scales may be included in evaluation schemes (18). Less direct
approaches include making the dietary intake assessment an adjunct to some
other task not so closely related to health habits (e.g. embedding it in a longer
series of questions about consumer buying behavior). Another approach
might be to include bogus foods (e.g. lowfat olive oil) in food frequency
questionnaires to estimate the overreporting of "healthy" foods.

Both laboratory-based and community-level studies are needed to advance
our understanding of how individuals evaluate and report health behaviors,
and whether any biases we find differ for persons in community intervention
and control communities. Over the last few decades, the accumulated research suggests that self-reports of smoking require biochemical validation in
intervention studies, particularly with adolescents in school-based cessation
programs. The lack of such biochemical measures for self-reported dietary
behavior adds considerable complexity to the assessment of an inherently
complicated and multifaceted behavior.

MEASURES OF COMMUNITY ENVIRONMENT

Several complicating factors that arise in assessing the outcome of community-level interventions enhance the attractiveness of a class of measures
that we call "environmental" indicators. This section briefly describes the
complicating factors, defines environmental indicators and places them in the
context of other community-level measures, and gives some examples. Cheadle et al (12) provide a more complete discussion of this class of measures.

As noted above, two difficulties arise in assessing community-level interventions: the impossibility of blinding individual subjects to the presence of the intervention, which threatens the validity of self-reported attitudes, behaviors, and outcomes; and the complexity of the mechanism of action by which community programs change individual behaviors, with many intermediate steps in the behavior change process. As illustrated by the causal model shown Figure 1, these intermediate steps often involve modifying that which can be labeled the "community environment," defined broadly to include the legal, social, and economic, as well as the physical, environment. Components of the health-related community environment include institutions (stores, worksites, political institutions), geography (air, water quality), media messages (TV, radio, print), laws, and regulations (smoking ordinances).

Environmental indicators thus serve two functions in an evaluation. First, they provide an indicator of shared attitudes and/or collective behavior that does not rely on self-reports. Second, they capture features of the environmental link in the chain that connects health-promotion programs to changes in health-related behavior.

Environmental indicators are derived from observations of the community context in which people live. To clarify this notion, it is useful to relate them to other "community-level measures," i.e. approaches to characterizing the community as a whole as opposed to individuals or subgroups within it. Community-level measures can be divided into three sub-categories: "individual-disaggregated"—information originally obtained on individuals for whom individual-level covariate data (e.g. demographic characteristics) are available that can be considered in analyzing and interpreting community-level summary statistics; "individual-aggregated"—measures derived from individual-level information, but available only in aggregated form; and "environmental indicators"—measures based on observations of the community environment.

Most community-level measures that have been used in evaluating health promotion programs fall into the first category, i.e. are based on individual-level measures (e.g. interview surveys, physiologic measures) through which additional information on each respondent is available. These data are most frequently gathered by investigators who are evaluating a particular health-promotion program, but could easily include other public-use data available at the individual level (birth and death tapes, hospital discharge abstracts). Community-level measures formed by aggregating individual-level data, devoid of identifiers, to the community level include data collected by agencies other than the program evaluators. Examples of aggregate measures include census data, mortality rates, traffic-accident statistics, and most economic data (e.g. sales information).

Environmental indicators, the third class of community-level measures, are derived from observations of aspects of the community environment that, like other community-level measures, are then aggregated to the level of the community. For example, the number, type, and visibility of nonsmoking signs in a workplace (which can be regarded as a small community) are an environmental indicator of the attitudes of the workers and management in that workplace toward smoking. Greater degrees of militancy toward smoking among employees and management will probably be associated with more and better-advertised no-smoking areas. In addition, the number and character of workplace no-smoking signs are indicators of the environmental influences acting on employees.

There are several strands in the existing literature relevant to environmental indicators. Since the mid-1960s, a substantial literature on social indicators and social indicator models has accumulated in sociology (9, 52, 72). For example, Carley (9) presents indicators derived from the Social and Economic Accounts System (SEAS) developed by Fitzsimmons & Lavey (32), which organizes 477 community indicators into 15 sectors. Health sector social indicators in the SEAS include individual-aggregated measures (e.g. number of deaths per 1000 live births), as well as measures that could be classified as environmental indicators: number of full-time equivalent physicians, hospitals, and hospital beds.

Another close relative to environmental indicators in the existing literature are the "unobtrusive" or "nonreactive" measures first collected and categorized by Webb et al (90). A measure is unobtrusive if the object of interest is unaware of being observed. Nonreactive measures do not suffer from the problem of reactivity bias, i.e. the "true" response is not altered by the process of measurement. All unobtrusive measures are nonreactive, but some nonreactive measures may be highly obtrusive (e.g. blood tests). In many cases, these unobtrusive measures would be classified as individual-level measures under our scheme, as the observations are made on individuals and then aggregated to get an estimated mean or proportion for the group of interest. However, several other measures reported in the literature are based on characteristics of the community environment [e.g. graffiti (78)] and can, therefore, be classified as environmental indicators.

Table 3 provides examples of community-level measures related to tobacco use. These measures are categorized along two dimensions: the measurement category (individual-disaggregated, individual-aggregated, and environmental) and the obstrusiveness and reactivity bias likely to be associated with the measure. The environmental measures are further subdivided according to the component of the environment being measured (e.g. workplace, restaurant).

The examples in Table 3 may help clarify the earlier discussion of terminology. The newspaper poll of attitudes could, in principle, be shifted to the

Table 3 Examples of community-level measures of smoking-related attitudes and behavior

Measurement Category[a]	Obtrusive		Unobtrusive
	Reactive	Nonreactive	
Individual-Disaggregated	Phone survey of smoking status, attitudes toward smoking in public places	Cotinine, other biochemical measures of smoking status	Sample of household garbage to count cigarette butts
Individual-Aggregated	Published results of newspaper poll of attitudes toward smoking in public places	Classroom-level cotinine measures	Cigarette sales; Election results from a vote over a nonsmoking ordinance
Environmental			
Worksite	Interview with company CEO; his/her views on smoking policy	Survey of company smoking policies	Prevalence of designated nonsmoking areas
Restaurants and other public spaces	Staff response to customers who smoke in nonsmoking areas	Proportion of restaurants with some nonsmoking seating	Ashtray prevalence; visibility of non-smoking signs
Community as a whole	Interviews with key informants: community attitudes	Interviews with key informants: legislative history of ordinances	Does community have a nonsmoking ordinance?

[a] See text for discussion of measurement categories.

individual-disaggregated category, if the newspaper collected demographic information on the respondents and made the individual-level information available to outside investigators. The worksite environmental indicators cover aspects of company smoking policy. The interview with the company president is likely to be colored by concern about public relations, and thus subject to a considerable amount of reactivity bias. The company will also be aware that a survey is being conducted of its smoking policy, but because the assessment could focus on written policy statements, there is less chance of an untruthful response. The observation of the prevalence of no-smoking areas could be made unobtrusively, if admittance were gained for some reason other than to conduct such a survey (e.g. the observations could be made by an employee).

The advantages of environmental indicators have already been noted: They are frequently unobtrusive and, therefore, not subject to response bias. And, they are measurements of important intermediate factors in health-promotion interventions. The drawbacks of environmental indicators are the same ones that have held back the development of unobtrusive measures in social psychology: lack of persistent and credible efforts to assess and improve the validity and reliability of candidate measures (78). An effort to overcome this lack of evidence for environmental indicators has begun, however. For example, the reliability of a grocery store instrument designed as an environmental indicator of dietary habits has been assessed as part of the evaluation of the Kaiser Family Foundation Community Health Promotion Grants Program (11, 89). The validity of the grocery store instrument has also been assessed, by comparing the results of the survey with a phone survey of individuals in the same communities (10). Only through such a process of accumulating information about validity, reliability, and responsiveness to change can a fair test of these measures be conducted.

CONCLUSIONS

At present, the community-based approach to health promotion appears to be in an expansion phase, spurred in part by the apparent success of several large-scale, community-wide programs aimed at prevention of cardiovascular disease. New programs are now being developed for a wider array of health conditions, the definition of "community" is being broadened to include both larger and smaller social units, and the range of target populations is being widened demographically and socioeconomically. Many newer community-based programs are being mounted with fewer resources and a different mix of intervention modalities than their predecessors. All of these factors emphasize the importance of rigorous evaluation to determine when, where, how, and for whom the community-based approach succeeds. We hope that the above discussion helps sensitize evaluators to the special challenges they face in attempting to answer those important questions and kindles the interest of methodologists to develop new and better evaluative tools.

ACKNOWLEDGMENT

This work was supported by Grant No. CA 34847 from the National Cancer Institute.

Literature Cited

1. Altman, D. C. 1986. A framework for evaluating community-based heart disease prevention programs. *Soc. Sci. Med.* 22:479–87
2. Bandura, A. 1971. *Social Learning Theory.* Morristown, NJ: Gen. Learning
3. Bang, A. T., Bang, R. A., Tale, O., Sontakke, P., Solanki, J., et al. 1990. Reduction in pneumonia mortality and total childhood mortality by means of community-based intervention trial in Gadchiroli, India. *Lancet* 336:201–6
4. Bauman, K. E., Dent, C. W. 1982. Influence of an objective measure on self-reports of behavior. *J. Appl. Psychol.* 67:623–28
5. Bickman, L. 1987. The functions of program theory. *New Directions for Program Evaluation* 33:5–18. San Francisco: Jossey-Bass
6. Bracht, N., ed. 1990. *Health Promotion at the Community Level.* Newbury Park, Calif: Sage
7. Bridge, G. R., Reeder, L. G., Kanouse, D., Kinder, D. R., Nagy, V. T., et al. 1977. Interviewing changes attitudes-sometimes. *Public Opin. Q.* 41:56–64
8. Campbell, D. T., Stanley, J. C. 1963. *Experimental and Quasi-experimental Designs for Research,* Boston: Houghton Mifflin
9. Carley, M. 1981. *Social Measurement and Social Indicators: Issues of Policy and Theory.* London: George, Allen & Unwin
10. Cheadle, A., Psaty, B., Curry, S., Wagner, E., Diehr, P., et al. 1991. Community-level comparisons between the grocery store environment and individual dietary practices. *Prev. Med.* 20:250–61
11. Cheadle, A., Psaty, B. M., Wagner, E. W., Diehr, P. H., Koepsell, T. D., et al. 1990. Evaluating community-based nutrition programs: assessing the reliability of a survey of grocery store product displays. *Am. J. Public Health* 80:709–11

12. Cheadle, A., Wagner, E. W., Koepsell, T. D., Kristal, A., Patrick, D. 1991. Environmental indicators: A tool for evaluating community-based health-promotion programs. *Am. J. Prev. Med.* In press
13. Chen, H. T., Rossi, P. H. 1983. Evaluating with sense: The theory-driven approach. *Eval. Rev.* 7:283–302
14. Chen, H. T., Rossi, P. H. 1980. The multi-goal, theory-driven approach to evaluation: a model linking basic and applied social science. *Soc. Forces* 59:106–22
15. Cook, N. R., Ware, J. H. 1983. Design and analysis methods for longitudinal research. *Annu. Rev. Public Health* 4:1–23
16. Cook, T. D., Campbell, D. T. 1979. *Quasi-experimentation: Design and Analysis Issues for Field Settings,* Boston: Houghton Mifflin
17. Cornfield, J. 1978. Randomization by group: a formal analysis. *Am. J. Epidemiol.* 108:100–2
18. Crowne, D. P., Marlowe, D. 1964. *The Approval Motive: Studies in Evaluative Dependence,* New York: Wiley
19. DeMaio, T. J. 1980. Refusals: who, where, why. *Public Opin. Q.* 44:223–33
20. Dixon, W. J., Brown, M. B., eds. 1990. *BMDP Statistical Software Manuals,* Vols. 1, 2. Berkeley: Univ. Calif. Press
21. Donald, A., Donner, A. 1987. Adjustments to the Mantel-Haenszel chi-square statistic and odds ratio variance estimator when the data are clustered. *Stat. Med.* 6:491–99
22. Donner, A. 1984. Approaches to sample size estimation in the design of clinical trials-a review. *Stat. Med.* 3:199–214
23. Donner, A., Birkett, N., Buck, C. 1981. Randomization by cluster. Sample size requirements and analysis. *Am. J. Epidemiol.* 114:906–14
24. Donner, A., Donald, A. 1987. Analysis of data arising from a stratified design

with the cluster as unit of randomization. *Stat. Med.* 6:43–52

25. Dunn, O. J., Clark, V. A. 1987. *Applied Statistics: Analysis of Variance and Regression,* New York: Wiley

26. Evans, R. I., Hansen, W. B., Mittelmark, M. B. 1977. Increasing the validity of self-reports of smoking behavior in children. *J. Appl. Psychol.* 62:521–23

27. Farquhar, J. W. 1978. The community-based model of life style intervention trials. *Am. J. Epidemiol.* 108:103–11

28. Farquhar, J. W., Fortmann, S. P., Flora, J. A., Taylor, C. B., Haskell, W. L., et al. 1990. Effects of community education on cardiovascular disease risk factors. The Stanford five-city project. *J. Am. Med. Assoc.* 264:359–65

29. Farquhar, J. W., Fortmann, S. P., Maccoby, N., Haskell, W. L., Williams, P. T., et al. 1985. The Stanford five-city project: design and methods. *Am. J. Epidemiol.* 122:323–34

30. Farquhar, J. W., Wood, P. D., Breitrose, H., Haskell, W. L., Meyer, A. J., et al. 1977. Community education for cardiovascular health. *Lancet* 1:1192–95

31. Fitzgerald, R., Fuller, L. 1982. I hear you knocking but you can't come in. The effects of reluctant respondents and refusers on sample survey estimates. *Soc. Method Res.* 11:3–32

32. Fitzsimmons, S. J., Lavey, W. G. 1975. Social economic accounts system (SEAS) toward comprehensive community-level assessment procedure. *Soc. Indic. Res.* 2:389–452

33. Fortmann, S. P., Haskell, W. L., Williams, P. T., Varady, A. N., Hulley, S. B., et al. 1986. Community surveillance of cardiovascular diseases in the Stanford five city project. *Am. J. Epidemiol.* 123:656–69

34. Freedman, L. S., Green, S. B., Byar, D. P. 1990. Assessing the gain in efficiency due to matching in a community intervention study. *Stat. Med.* 9:943–52

35. Gillum, R. F., Williams, P. T., Sondik, E. 1980. Some considerations for the planning of total-community prevention trials—when is sample size adequate? *J. Community Health* 5:270–78

36. Glass, G. V., Willson, V. L., Gottman, J. M. 1975. *Design and analysis of time-series experiments,* Boulder: Colorado Assoc. Univ. Press

37. Gordis, L. 1976. Methodologic issues in the measurement of patient compliance. In *Compliance with Therapeutic Regimens,* ed. D. Sackett, R. Haybnes, pp. 51–68. Baltimore: Johns Hopkins Univ. Press.

38. Green, L. W., Lewis, F. M. 1986. *Measurement and Evaluation in Health Education and Health Promotion,* Palo Alto, Calif: Mayfield

39. Green, L. W., McAlister, A. L. 1984. Macro-intervention to support health behavior: some theoretical perspectives and practical reflections. *Health Educ. Q.* 11:323–39

40. Green, L. W., Raeburn, J. M. 1988. Health promotion. What is it? What will it become? *Health Promot.* 3:151–59

41. Hansen, W. B., Collins, L. M., Malotte, C. K., Johnson, C. A., Fielding, J. E. 1985. Attrition in prevention research. *J. Behav. Med.* 8:261–75

42. Hawkins, D. F. 1975. Estimation of nonresponse bias. *Soc. Method Res.* 3:461–83

43. Hsieh, F. Y. 1988. Sample size formulae for intervention studies with the cluster as unit of randomization. *Stat. Med.* 8:1195–1201

44. Jacobs, D. R., Luepker, R. V., Mittelmark, M. B., Folsom, A. R., Pirie, P. L., et al. 1986. Community-wide prevention strategies: evaluation design of the Minnesota Heart Health Program. *J. Chronic Dis.* 39:775–88

45. Jooste, P. L., Yach, D., Steenkamp, H. J., Botha, J. L., Rossouw, J. E. 1990. Drop-out and newcomer bias in a community cardiovascular follow-up study. *Int. J. Epidemiol.* 19:284–89

46. Josephson, E., Rosen, M. A. 1978. Panel loss in a high school drug study. In *Longitudinal Research on Drug Use: Empirical Findings and Methodological Issues,* ed. D. Kandel. Washington, DC: Hemisphere

47. Judd, C. M., Kenny, D. A. 1981. Process analysis: Estimating mediation in treatment evaluation. *Eval. Rev.* 5:602–19

48. Koepsell, T. D., Martin, D. C., Diehr, P. H., Psaty, B. M., Wagner, E. W., et al. 1991. Data analysis and sample size issues in evaluations of community-based health promotion and disease prevention programs: a mixed-model approach. *J. Clin Epidemiol.* 44:701–14

49. Kraut, R. E., McConahay, J. B. 1973. How being interviewed affects voting: an experiment. *Public Opin. Q.* 37:398–407

50. Kristal, A. R., Abrams, B. F., Thornquist, M. D., Disogra, L., Croyle, R. T., et al. 1990. Development and validation of a food use checklist for evaluation of community nutrition interventions. *Am. J. Public Health* 80:1318–22

51. Lachin, J. M. 1988. Statistical proper-

ties of randomization in clinical trials. *Control. Clin. Trials* 9:289–311

52. Land, K. C. 1975. *Social Indicator Models*. New York: Sage

53. LaPorte, D. J., McLellan, A. T., Erdlen, F. R., Parente, R. J. 1981. Treatment outcome as a function of follow-up difficulty in substance abusers. *J. Consult. Clin. Psychol.* 49:112–19

54. Lee, C., Owen, N. 1986. Community exercise programs: follow-up, difficulty and outcome. *J. Behav. Med.* 9:111–17

55. Lee-Han, H., Mcguire, V., Boyd, N. F. 1989. A review of methods used by studies of dietary measurement. *J. Clin. Epidemiol.* 42:269–79

56. Lefebvre, R., Lasater, T., Carleton, R., Peterson, G. 1987. Theory and delivery of health programing in the community: The Pawtucket Heart Health Program. *Prev. Med.* 16:80–95

57. Lipsey, M. W. 1990. Theory as method: small theories of treatment. *AHCPR Conference Proceedings, Research Methodology: Strengthening Causal Interpretations of Nonexperimental Data*, ed. L. Sechrest, E. Perrin, J. Bunker, pp. 33–51. DHHS Publ. No. (PHS) 90–3454

58. Martin, D. C., Diehr, P. H., Koepsell, T. D., Wagner, E. W., Cheadle, A., et al. 1990. *A comparison of bias and precision in cohort and cross-sectional designs in community intervention studies*. Presented at Symp. Stat. Methods Eval. Interv. Prev. Strateg., Atlanta

59. Martin, D. C., Diehr, P. H., Perrin, E. B., Koepsell, T. D. 1990. *The effect of matching on the power of randomized community intervention studies*. Presented at Symp. Stat. Methods Eval. Interv. Prev. Strateg., Atlanta

60. McLaughlin, J. K., Mandel, J. S., Mehl, E. S., Blot, W. J. 1990. Comparison of next-of-kin with self-respondents regarding questions on cigarette, coffee, and alcohol consumption. *Epidemiology* 1:408–12

61. Mickey, R. M., Goodwin, G. D., Costanza, M. C. 1991. Estimation of the design effect in community intervention studies. *Stat. Med.* 10:53–64

62. Murray, M., Swan, A. V., Kiryluk, S., Clarke, G. C. 1988. The Hawthorne effect in the measurement of adolescent smoking. *J. Epidemiol. Community Health* 42:304–6

63. Neaton, J. D., Broste, S., Cohen, L., Fishman, E. L., Kjelsberg, M. O., et al. 1981. The Multiple Risk Factor Intervention Trial (MRFIT) VII. A comparison of risk factor changes between

the two study groups. *Prev. Med.* 10: 519–43

64. Newhouse, J. P., Manning, W. G., Morris, C. N., Orr, L. L., Duan, N., et al. 1981. Some interim results from a controlled trial of cost sharing in health insurance. *N. Engl. J. Med.* 305:1501–7

65. Noreen, E. 1989. *Computer-intensive Methods for Testing Hypotheses: An Introduction*, New York: Wiley

66. Patrick, D. L., Thompson, D., Cheadle, A., Koepsell, T. D., Kinne, S. 1990. *Validity of self-reported smoking: meta-analysis and review*. Presented at Int. Conf. Meas. Errors Surv., Tucson

67. Pentz, M. A., Dwyer, J. H., Mackinnon, D. P., Flay, B. R., Hansen, W. B., et al. 1989. A multi-community trial for primary prevention of adolescent drug abuse. Effect on drug use prevalence. *J. Am. Med. Assoc.* 261:3259–66

68. Pettiti, D. B., Friedman, G. D., Kahn, W. 1981. Accuracy of information on smoking habits provided on self-administered research questionnaires. *Am. J. Public Health* 71:308–11

69. Pirie, P. L., Murray, D. M., Luepker, R. V. 1988. Smoking prevalence in a cohort of adolescents, including absentees, dropouts, and transfers. *Am. J. Public Health* 78:176–78

70. Puska, P., Nissinen, A., Tuomilehto, J. 1986. The community-based strategy to prevent coronary heart disease: conclusions from the ten years of the North Karelia Project. *Prev. Med.* 15:176–91

71. Puska, P., Salonen, J. T., Nissinen, A., Tuomilehto, J., Vartiainen, E., et al. 1983. Change in risk factors for coronary heart disease during 10 years of community intervention programme (North Karelia project). *Br. Med. J.* 287:1840–44

72. Rossi, R. J., Gilmartin, K. J. 1980. *The Handbook of Social Indicators: Sources, Characteristics and Analysis*. New York: Garland STPM

73. Saloneon, J. T., Kottke, T. W., Jacobs, D. R., Hannan, P. J. 1986. Analysis of community-based cardiovascular disease prevention studies-evaluation issues in the North Karelia Project and the Minnesota Heart Health Program. *Int. J. Epidemiol.* 15:176–82

74. Salvini, S., Hunter, D. J., Sampson, L., Stampfer, M. J., Colditz, G. A., et al. 1989. Food-based validation of dietary questionnaires: the effects of week-to-week variation in food consumption. *Int. J. Epidemiol.* 18:858–67

75. Scheirer, M. A. 1987. Program theory and implementation theory: implications

for evaluators. *New Directions for Program Evaluation* 33:59–76. San Francisco: Jossey-Bass

76. Schlesselman, J. J. 1973. Planning a longitudinal study. I. Sample size determination. *J. Chronic Dis.* 26:553–60

77. Searle, S. R. 1987. *Linear Models for Unbalanced Data.* New York: Wiley

78. Sechrest, L., Belew, J. 1983. Nonreactive measures of social attitudes. In *Applied Social Psychology Annual,* ed. L. Bickman, 4:23–63. Beverly Hills, Calif: Sage

79. Shea, S., Basch, C. E. 1990. A review of five major community-based cardiovascular disease prevention programs. Part I: rationale, design, and theoretical framework. *Am. J. Health Promotion* 4:203–13

80. Shea, S., Basch, C. E. 1990. A review of five major community-based cardiovascular disease prevention programs. Part II: Intervention strategies, evaluation methods, and results. *Am. J. Health Promotion* 4:279–87

81. Shipley, M. J., Smith, P. G., Dramaix, M. 1989. Calculation of power for matched pair studies when randomization is by group. *Int. J. Epidemiol.* 18:457–61

82. Smith, A. F., Jobe, J. B., Mingay, D. J. 1991. Question-induced cognitive biases in reports of dietary intake. *Health Psychol.* In press

83. Smith, A. F., Jobe, J. B., Mingay, D. J. 1991. Retrieval from memory of dietary information. *Appl. Cogn. Psychol.* 5:1–27

84. Sorenson, A. W. 1982. Assessment of nutrition in epidemiologic studies. In *Cancer Epidemiology and Prevention,* ed. D. Schottenfeld, J. F. Fraumeni, pp. 434–74. Philadelphia: Saunders

85. Strecher, V. J., Becker, M. H., Clark, N. M., Prasada-Rao, P. 1989. Using patients' descriptions of alcohol consumption, diet, medication, compliance,

and cigarette smoking: the validity of self-reports in research and practice. *J. Gen. Int. Med.* 4:160–66

86. Thornquist, M., Anderson, G. L. 1990. *Analysis of the belt and suspenders design in community analysis.* Presented at Joint Meeting of Am. Stat. Assoc. and Biom. Soc., Anaheim

87. US Dep. Health Human Serv. 1990. *The health benefits of smoking cessation,* Public Health Serv: Cent. Dis Control, DHHS Publ. No. (CDC) 90–8416

88. Vernon, S. W., Roberts, R. E., Lee, E. S. 1984. Ethnic status and participation in longitudinal health surveys. *Am. J. Epidemiol.* 119:99–113

89. Wagner, E. H., Koepsell, T., Anderman, D., Cheadle, A., Curry, S., et al. 1991. The evaluation of the Kaiser Family Foundations Health Promotion Grants Program: overall design. *J. Clin. Epidemiol.* 44:685–700

90. Webb, E. J., Campbell, D. T., Schwartz, R. D., Sechrest, L. 1966. *Unobtrusive Measures: Non-reactive Research in the Social Sciences,* Chicago: Rand McNally

91. Whiting-O'Keefe, Q., Simborg, D. 1984. Choosing the correct unit of analysis in medical care experiments. *Med. Care* 22:1101–14

92. Worden, J. K., Flynn, B. S., Solomon, L. J., Costanza, M. C., Foster, R. S. Jr., et al. 1987. A community-wide breast self-exam education program. In *Advances in Cancer Control: The War on Cancer—15 Years of Progress,* pp. 27–37. New York: Liss

93. Worsley, A., Baghurst, K. I., Leitch, D. R. 1984. Social desirability and dietary inventory responses. *Human Nutr: Appl. Nutr.* 38A:29–35

94. Yeaton, W. H. 1990. See Ref. 57, pp. 85–99

95. Zeger, S. L., Liang, K. Y., Self, S. G. 1985. The analysis of binary longitudinal data with time-independent covariates. *Biometrika* 72:31–38

Annu. Rev. Publ. Health 13:59–78

PUBLIC HEALTH ASSESSMENT IN THE 1990s

Michael A. Stoto

Institute of Medicine, Washington, DC 20418

KEY WORDS: health objectives, *Healthy People 2000,* surveillance, health status indicators

INTRODUCTION

In 1990, the Secretary of Health and Human Services unveiled *Healthy People 2000: National Health Promotion and Disease Prevention Objectives* (46), which is a milestone in public health. *Healthy People 2000* identifies three national health goals: increase the span of healthy life, reduce health disparities among Americans, and achieve access to preventive services for all Americans. The report also details 300 specific objectives for health promotion and disease prevention programs with quantitative targets to be achieved by the year 2000. Meeting these objectives requires agreement by public health statisticians on measures of individual and community health status to guide public health policy development and priorities, especially for state and local areas, and improvement in the methods for tracking these measures.

Healthy People 2000 challenges public health practitioners to develop surveillance systems that are both meaningful in a public health sense and statistically sound. To clarify this challenge and outline some possible responses, I begin with some background on the public health assessment activities on which the year 2000 health objectives build and considerations that should guide public health assessment efforts. The next section presents general statistical issues in formulating measurable and meaningful objectives. Other sections are devoted to two specific issues: the development of a small set of health status indicators that is both meaningful and feasible to monitor and special issues associated with setting objectives and determining appropriate targets for state and local areas.

59

0163-7525/92/0501-0059$02.00

BACKGROUND

"Public health assessment," as used in the Institute of Medicine report *The Future of Public Health,* is the regular and systematic collection, assembly, analysis, and dissemination of information on the health of the community. This information includes statistics on health status, community health needs, and epidemiologic and other studies of health problems (15, p. 7).

The 300 objectives in *Healthy People 2000* indicate the information needed to guide public health policy at the state and local, as well as the national, levels. *Healthy People 2000* explicitly calls for strengthened public health assessment efforts by devoting one of its 22 priority areas to specific objectives for surveillance and data systems.

Healthy People 2000 also provides a means of communicating achievable health goals and the means for achieving them. Moreover, the report provides a means of measuring progress towards the national goals, of taking credit for battles won, and of assigning responsibility for further efforts (25).

The "Year 2000 Health Objectives Planning Act" (PL 101–582) requires the Secretary of Health and Human Services to implement the surveillance objectives and funds states to develop plans to monitor and improve the health status of their populations.

The information base for public health assessment is broad. The World Health Organization, for example, has published a report on the development of health indicators for its *Health For All* goal, which has guided national efforts in a number of countries (53). A decade ago, the US Public Health Service published national goals in the original *Healthy People* (44), as well as 226 specific health objectives for 1990 (48). In 1987, the National Committee on Vital and Health Statistics reviewed the status of health promotion and disease prevention data at the state and local levels and made recommendations to improve the use of existing data, to develop and promote strategies for sharing expertise in the use of this data, and to develop alternative methodologies to meet state and local data requirements (30). Many state and local health officers use the Model Standards for Community Preventive Health Services, a collaborative effort of the Centers for Disease Control, the American Public Health Association, and several other public health professional associations to guide local assessment efforts (1). The Public Health Foundation has developed core data sets for reporting on state public health activities related to the objectives (34), and the National Association of County Health Officials' APEX program has developed methods for assessing public health needs and resources at the local level (29).

Individual efforts to develop health status indicators must also be acknowledged (9, 19, 26). Among many such efforts, Murnaghan (28) has reviewed the status and priorities for health information systems needed for *Health for All by the Year 2000* with a special focus on developing countries.

CONSIDERATIONS FOR PUBLIC HEALTH ASSESSMENT

The twentieth century has seen a shift in the major causes of death from infectious to chronic diseases (6), which requires an increased emphasis on behavioral and environmental risk factors and on preventive medicine. Individual and community interventions can help prevent important health problems, such as injuries, teenage childbearing, and mental health problems. Efforts are still needed to sustain and improve on our historical successes in preventing infectious disease and to find ways to address such emerging problems as AIDS.

One aspect of this shift in focus is that changes in mortality rates can no longer be thought of as proxies for changes in morbidity or health status. When infectious diseases represented the major health problems, before modern medicine was able to control them effectively, mortality was a good proxy for the incidence of the disease that caused it. Modern medical care, however, has broken the link between incidence and mortality.

Furthermore, the chronic diseases and conditions that have replaced infectious diseases as the major causes of death and disability are more complex and require new outcome measures (21, 33). Individuals live longer with these conditions, often in poor health and with a low quality of life. The diseases typically have long asymptomatic stages. Thus there is a need for prevalence and incidence measures, as well as measures of severity and disease staging, functional limitations and disability, and quality of life.

These changes also bring a new focus on the antecedent risk factors for injuries and chronic diseases and conditions. By one estimate, two thirds of all deaths and years of life lost before age 65 are attributable to a preventable precursor, and are thus unnecessary or premature (2). Behavioral risk factors, such as smoking, can themselves be thought of as negative aspects of an individual's health status. Furthermore, the physical and social environments are increasingly viewed as important risk or protective factors, and thus they are also targets of intervention.

There is, however, danger in confusing ends and means. Risk factor objectives are useful because they show the impact of behavioral interventions long before there are any changes in chronic disease mortality rates. However, risk-related behaviors, the use of preventive services, and the availability of community health protection programs should be monitored as intermediate outcomes and indicators of program success or failure, but not as alternatives to direct health status measures.

STATISTICAL ISSUES IN SETTING OBJECTIVES

Responding to the change in mortality and morbidity patterns, the national objectives in *Healthy People 2000* suggest areas in which health status measures are possible and needed. The objectives spell out not only specific health status targets, but also changes in individual risk factors and in the physical and social environment that can help reach the goals. The range of topics covered by the objectives is extensive. It includes personal behavior and risk factors, including physical fitness and activity, nutrition, tobacco, and alcohol and other drugs; psychosocial factors, including mental health and violent and abusive behavior; the physical environment, including unintentional injuries, occupational safety and health, environmental health, and food and drug safety; infectious diseases, including HIV infection, and sexually transmitted diseases; reproductive and infant health, including family planning and maternal and infant health; chronic diseases, such as heart disease and stroke, cancer, diabetes, and oral health problems, and chronic disabling conditions; and services and protection, including educational and community-based programs, as well as clinical preventive services.

The comprehensive list of topics offers a catalog of health status measures from which states and local areas can choose. In setting forth its national objectives, *Healthy People 2000* also identifies almost 100 separate data sources and many measurement tools for public health assessment. The report contains 300 separately stated objectives, some of which have multiple parts, thus leading to almost 400 statistical series that must be monitored. Unfortunately, those testifying at hearings organized by the Public Health Service and the Institute of Medicine identified the large number of 1990 objectives as an impediment to effective assessment and implementation efforts (42). With the more than 200 additional special population targets for high risk groups, quantity alone makes monitoring the year 2000 objectives at the national, state, and local levels a formidable challenge.

Stating the objectives in quantitative terms is one of their great strengths, but the availability of data to measure progress has been a problem since the beginning of the Healthy People process. Green and colleagues (13), for instance, reviewed the data available in the early 1980s to track progress towards the 1990 objectives and found numerous gaps and statistical problems. Data were eventually acquired for several objectives that were published in 1980 with no baseline information. Indeed, this was one of the intended outcomes of setting the objectives (37). At mid-decade, however, there were no tracking data on more than one quarter of the 1990 national objectives (47). Despite explicit criteria in the development of the year 2000 objectives aimed at mitigating these problems (24), about one quarter of the year 2000 objectives in *Healthy People 2000* cite no currently available baseline data (40). The large number of objectives in this situation calls into question the availability of sufficient data to assess progress in the 1990s.

Andersen & Mullner (3) identify several other statistical problems with the 1990 health objectives, and many of these problems persist in *Healthy People*

2000. For instance, about one quarter of the year 2000 objectives list baseline data that do not correspond to the stated objective. One objective calls for 75% of primary care providers to "provide nutrition assessment and counseling and/or referral to qualified nutritionists or dietitians," but states as baseline data that "physicans provided diet counseling for an estimated 40–50% of patients" (46, p. 128). This baseline and objective disagree in terms of which type of provider is to provide the service, the service they provide, and the population to which the percentage is applied (40). The lack of precision in this objective might reflect underlying uncertainty among health professionals about who should provide which services.

Three specific statistical issues are discussed below: the specification of individual objectives, the interpretation of trends, and standardization.

Specification of Individual Objectives

In many respects, the individual objectives are similar to items on a survey questionnaire. If the results are to be interpreted with confidence, careful development and testing are needed to ensure that the objectives are operationalized in a clear and unambiguous way. Most of the objectives in *Healthy People 2000* are carefully written in this respect, but others exhibit several statistical problems that should be avoided.

Some of the objectives are not written in a statistically operational form; that is, even with all of the information in hand it will be difficult to tell if the objective has been met. For example, objective 7.17 calls for local jurisdictions to have "coordinated, comprehensive violence prevention programs: (46, p. 240). Although a long list of attributes of coordinated and comprehensive programs is given in the text, no operational definition is provided by which to judge whether a particular jurisdiction's program is coordinated and comprehensive.

Other objectives address very complex questions that are difficult to monitor through population surveys. For example, objective 5.8 is to "increase to at least 85% the proportion of people aged 10 through 18 who have discussed human sexuality, including values surrounding sexuality, with their parents and/or have received information through another parentally endorsed source, such as youth, school, or religious programs" (46, p. 198). Although survey data could provide information on aspects of this objective, it is difficult to imagine how questions could be designed to assess the proportion of adolescents that meet the specific implied criteria.

These problems arise because *Healthy People 2000* often does not distinguish between general health issues and operational measures of these issues. Rarely are data available in the precise form that policymakers prefer, so concessions must be made to data constraints. The presentation of the objectives should reflect this compromise by separately identifying the issues to be monitored and the best available data or proxy variables for these issues, and by stating targets in terms of the measurable quantities. Some objectives state two or more separate goals. For example, objective 20.1 calls for reductions in the number of cases of each of eight vaccine-preventable diseases (46, p. 513). Such multibarreled objectives are troublesome because they implicitly increase the number of objectives and contribute to the surveillance problems discussed above.

Some multibarreled objectives are especially vague because the target groups are not clearly identified. For example, objective 9.19 states: "Extend requirement of the use of effective head, face, eye, and mouth protection to all organizations, agencies, and institutions sponsoring sporting and recreation events that pose risk of injury: (46, p. 285). Such objectives are very difficult to monitor for two reasons. First, data must be obtained for all of the groups mentioned or implied in the list of target populations. In many cases, it is not clear where this list ends. Second, the data from the different populations must be combined into one overall percentage to compare against the objective target; often, the stated objective does not say how to do this.

Multibarreled objectives reflect a resistance to reducing the list of objectives to a manageable number. Public health issues are complex and admit to many solutions, so such resistance is understandable, but the cost in terms of resources needed to measure the additional measures and reduced comprehension of the overall message can be high. Priorities must be set among the measures, perhaps by using the approach discussed in the section on health status indicators.

Interpretation of Trends

Population-based health interview surveys provide many of the core health-status measures used in the year 2000 objectives. However, health interview data, especially trend data, can be difficult to interpret (50). The US National Health Interview Survey, an important source of data for the year 2000 objectives, measures the annual incidence of acute conditions and the prevalence of chronic conditions through a combination of open- and closed-ended questions about the presence of specific diseases and conditions. A common finding from these data has been that chronic illness and disability have been increasing at the same time that mortality (even for related diseases) has been falling. At least part of this increase does not reflect actual worsening in physical illness. Methodological explanations that may explain the trend include improved survey design that may have increased the proportion of the population reporting diseases and conditions that exist; improved access to medical care and better screening efforts that may have increased the proportion of the population diagnosed with, and therefore aware of, asymptomatic disease; and changing role expectations and improved disability benefits that may have increased the proportion of the population that reports work-related disability (50).

Several objectives rely on numbers of individuals who receive treatment for the disease in question, because of the lack of population-based data on the incidence or prevalence of specific diseases. For instance, objective 15.3 calls for a reversal in the increasing number of persons with "end-stage renal disease (requiring dialysis or transplantation)" (46, p. 397). The baseline figures cited, however, count the number of persons who receive dialysis or transplantation, not those who require it. Thus, these trends reflect changes in diagnostic and treatment patterns, as well as access through an expanding federal program. It is doubtful whether future changes in the data can be attributed to the success of the prevention activities intended by *Healthy People 2000*.

Standardization

Standardization methods are used to account for demographic changes in a single population over time (12). For instance, if there were no changes in the age-specific cancer rates between 1987 and 2000, aging of the population alone would cause the overall death rate to increase from 195.9 to 217.1 per 100,000, assuming the Census Bureau's median population projection for the US (38).

Standardization also serves a second, and very different, purpose. Because state and other geographic areas differ in the age, race, and sex composition of their population, they have different unadjusted rates. For example, Florida has a large population of elderly people and a high unadjusted death rate. Adjusted rates provide a fairer comparison among areas.

For some purposes, however, standardization could lead to difficulties. Standardized rates can present a different impression about the relative importance of the different causes of death, depending on the standard used. For example, accidents and adverse effects have a somewhat higher mortality rate than cerebrovascular diseases when adjusted to the 1940 population (35.0 versus 29.7 per 100,000), but the crude cerebrovascular mortality rate is more than 50% higher than the crude accident mortality rate (61.2 versus 39.5 per 100,000).

The difference is even greater for the overall cancer death rate. The 1987 rate is 50% higher (199.9 compared with 132.9 per 100,000) when the 1990 population, rather than the 1940 population, is chosen as the standard. The choice of standard also affects trends. If we use the 1990 standard, the cancer death rate increased by 6.2% between 1970 and 1987; with the 1940 standard, however, the increase is only 2.3% Neither one of these standards is "correct" in any absolute sense, but they give a very different impression.

Many statisticians favor using the 1940 US population as a standard, primarily because it would be consistent with the long-term practice of the National Center for Health Statistics and others in reporting mortality rates. Using this standard would facilitate the efforts of states that try to monitor their own progress on the objectives. Others argue against adjusting, especially to the 1940 population, because it masks the public health impact of the levels seen in crude death rates. One compromise would be to standardize the rates to a more recent population, such as the 1990 US population. This would give a better picture of the current public health impact of the various diseases (as measured by the relative numbers of deaths) and would provide the analytical benefits of age-adjustment. The difficulty with using a new standard is that special calculations are needed to adjust past data for trend analyses. The need for general changes in statistical reporting systems associated with *Healthy People 2000,* however, might provide an opportunity to switch all mortality reporting to a more current standard.

HEALTH STATUS INDICATORS

The 300 specific objectives in *Healthy People 2000* are useful for public health officials who try to design programs in particular areas, but they are too numerous for the public and political leaders to follow on a regular basis. A short list of health status indicators that can be understood and followed on a regular basis is necessary to maintain public and professional attention (15, 42). For instance, at a 1990 hearing on the year 2000 health objectives, Senator Jeff Bingaman called for the development of a short list of objectives that could be used for annual health "check-ups" at the national, state, and, perhaps, substate levels (31).

Healthy People 2000 recognizes this need. It calls for the development and implementation of "a set of health status indicators appropriate for Federal, State, and local health agencies," and an initial set of indicators was published by the Public Health Service in 1991 (7a). In light of the importance of the indicators and the likelihood that they will continue to be developed and refined throughout the 1990s, the following suggestions are offered about criteria for selecting the indicators. I also present a potential list of measures and discuss alternative approaches.

Criteria for Health Status Indicators

Health status indicators should sum up, almost at a glance, the health status of the community to which they apply: the nation, a state or local area, or some other defined population. Although policy makers and the media might prefer a single index of the health of the community that could be monitored on a regular basis (much like the nation follows the Gross National Product to assess the health of the economy), the multidimensional nature of health status means that no single, all-encompassing health index can paint a complete picture of the health status of the community. It should be possible, however, to construct a relatively short list of indices that, taken as a group, sum up most of the important aspects of the community's health.

Based on the work of the social indicators movement, Andrews (4, p. 27) has summarized some of the key characteristics of health indicators: "a *limited* yet *comprehensive* set of *coherent* and *significant* indicators which can be *monitored* over time, and which can be *disaggregated* to the level of the relevant social unit."

Organizing the health status indicators by age offers several advantages. First, this structure reflects life cycle patterns in health problems and priorities and the frequent use of age as an organizing principle in discussions of health promotion and disease prevention. This organization also provides continuity with the original *Healthy People* (44) and the 1990 health objectives (48). Furthermore, as Chapter 2 of *Healthy People 2000* (46) shows, organizing the objectives by age groups makes it easier to identify the issues to include; looking at one age group at a time obviates the need for imponderable comparisons between, say, reduction in teenage fertility and improvements in the quality of life for older persons.

Finally, the individual indicators must accurately reflect changes in the health of the community, rather than changes in health delivery systems or reporting systems. The indicators should be, to the extent possible, available and interpretable at the state and local levels, and the number of indices should be small enough so that both the public and public health policy makers can understand the message that the indicators carry.

The health status indicators are not a substitute for a comprehensive public health assessment system; they are intended to help a community compare the health of its population with other communities as a means of identifying problems and goals. Indeed, comprehensive information on particular health problems and risk factors are needed to follow up on the leads suggested by the indicators.

Proposed Health Status Indicators

To illustrate the tradeoffs necessary in developing a short list of health status indicators and to serve as a point of departure for further development of indicators, Table 1 contains a list of 23 particular measures. The list is organized in five age groups, and the table gives the major health issue to be addressed ("low birth weight," for example) as well as the specific measure(s) of it in the text that follows (percent of live births that weigh less than 2500 grams).

To reflect the national goal of reducing disparities between population groups, special target groups for some of the measures in which the dispari-

Table 1 Proposed health status indicators

Infants (Under 1 year)
  Deaths: Infant mortality rate (9.1 deaths of infants under 1 year per 1000 live births in 1990)
  Low birth weight: Births of babies weighing less than 2500 g (6.9% of live births)
  Prenatal care: Proportion of infants born to women who received prenatal care in the first trimester of pregnancy (76%)

Children (Ages 1–14)
  Deaths from injury: Death rate for accidents, homicide, and suicide combined (16.6 deaths per 100,000 children ages 1–14)
  Immunization: Proportion of children ages 1–4 reported immunized for measles, rubella, DPT, polio, and mumps (55.3–64.9% for each immunization separately in 1985)
  Toxic exposures: Prevalence of blood lead levels exceeding 15 μg/dL among children ages 6 months through 5 years (15.4 per 100,000 in 1984)

Adolescents/Young Adults (Ages 15–24)
  Deaths from injury: Death rate for accidents, homicide, and suicide combined (75.8 deaths per 100,000 persons ages 15–24)
  Teenage childbearing: Birth rate at ages 15–17 (33.8 live births per 1000 women ages 15–17 in 1988)
  Use of dangerous substances: Proportion of adolescents ages 12–17 who used the following substances in the month
    Tobacco: (12% in 1990)
    Alcohol: (25% in 1990)
    Cocaine: (0.6% in 1990)
  Sexually transmitted diseases: Incidence of gonorrhea (1123 cases reported per 100,000 adolescents ages 15–19 in 1989)

Adults (Ages 25–64)
  Premature chronic disease mortality: Death rate for cancer, heart disease, stroke, and diabetes combined (264.5 deaths per 100,000 persons ages 25–64)
  AIDS/HIV: Incidence of AIDS (16.6 new cases reported per 100,000 persons ages 13 and over in 1990)
  Smoking: Prevalence of cigarette smoking (28.8% of current smokers among persons ages 20 and older)
  Nutrition/physical activity: Prevalence of overweight (21% of persons ages 18 and over with body mass index greater than 27.8 kg/m(2) for men and 27.3 kg/m(2) for women)
  Workplace injury: Incidence of injuries resulting in medical treatment, lost time from work, or restricted work activity (8.1 cases per 100 full-time workers)
  Chronic disease screening:
    Breast cancer: Proportion of women ages 50 and over who received a clinical breast exam and a mammogram within the preceding year (19%)
    Serum cholesterol: Proportion of persons ages 18 and over who have ever had their blood cholesterol level checked (59% in 1988)

Older Adults (Ages 65 and over)
  Activity restrictions: Proportion of the noninstitutionalized population age 65 and over with partial or complete limitation of major activity from chronic conditions (22.8% in 1989)
  Disabling injury: Incidence of hip fractures (714 hospital discharges per 100,000 persons age 65 and over in 1988)
  Immunization: Proportion of persons ages 65 and over who receive an influenza vaccination in the preceding 12 months (34%)
  Dental health: Proportion of persons ages 65 and over who have lost all of their natural teeth (36% in 1986)

ties are especially great could be identified. To reflect the other two national goals, indicators were chosen to ensure that each age group includes measures that address mortality and morbidity, disability and quality of life, and access to preventive services. Some of the measures are intended to be comprehensive measures for a particular age group; the death rate for cancer, heart disease, stroke, and diabetes combined for ages 25–64, for instance, is a comprehensive measure of preventable chronic disease mortality. Other measures are sentinel in nature. For instance, breast cancer and serum cholesterol screening are indicators of the general availability and use of preventive services for adults.

The proposed health status indicators incorporate measures of health status, risk reduction, and use of preventive services. Year 2000 objectives from *Healthy People 2000* are used when possible. In some cases, other measures are proposed to match the age-based structure or the summary nature of the health status indicators. The indicators were also chosen to relate to as many priority areas as possible and to be available at the state and local levels.

For infants, mortality is a standard summary measure of both mortality and access to health care. Low birth weight is included because it is both an important health status outcome in itself and a proxy for disability and a broader set of problems than infant mortality. Use of prenatal care appears as the critical access issue for infants.

For children, the death rate from accidents, homicide, and suicide combined is a summary measure of mortality and a proxy for morbidity and disability from unintentional and intentional injuries. Together, these causes represent about half of the deaths in the age group.

Immunization of children below school age is used as a key clinical preventive service measure. Lead exposure is included as a sentinel measure for toxic exposures in general, even though data may not be available on a regular, national basis, because it is one of the most important environmental toxins.

The adolescents and young adults group covers a period of transition from parental to individual responsibility for health and safety and is one in which important high risk behaviors are, or are not, initiated. The death rate for accidents, homicide, and suicide combined is included because injuries are the leading cause of death and disability in this age group. As for children, the mortality rate is taken as a proxy for the disability caused by injuries. The teenage fertility rate is used as a key indicator of the future quality of life of both the mother and child. Unlike in *Healthy People 2000*, the fertility rate, rather than the pregnancy rate, is used because it is available from vital statistics for even small areas. We identify the use of tobacco, alcohol, and cocaine because of their direct health consequences and because they are risk factors for both immediate threats to health and chronic disease later in life.

We also include sexually transmitted diseases because the incidence rate peaks for this age group. Gonorrhea serves as a sentinel measure because it is a reportable disease (other potentially important ones, such as pelvic inflammatory disease, are not) and it is more common than syphilis.

Among adults, the death rate from the four leading chronic diseases (heart disease, cancer, stroke, and diabetes) combined provides a summary measure of premature mortality in this age group. This mortality rate is also a proxy for disability caused by the same chronic conditions. AIDS incidence is also included with this age category because its effect peaks among adults. Smoking prevalence and obesity are included as risk factors for chronic disease. Obesity is a proxy for both nutrition and physical activity and is more easily measured through population surveys. Workplace injuries are also included in this group as a key factor in disability and because such injuries peak in this age group. Breast cancer screening and cholesterol screening are chosen as measures of the use of preventive services. Both are important in their own right and have more room for improvement than the more universally accepted Pap smears or hypertension screening.

For older adults, both a general disability measure—limitations of major activities because of chronic conditions—and a major preventable cause of disability in this age range—hip fractures—are included. Loss of teeth is also an important cause of disability and has ramifications for such issues as nutrition and social isolation. Influenza vaccination is included as an indicator of access to and use of preventive services. No mortality measures are included for this age range, so we can focus on improving the quality of life, rather than simply prolonging it.

Alternative Approaches

Both the objectives in *Healthy People 2000* and the proposed indicators come out of the public health tradition. Recent work on "health status assessment" by health services researchers and others concerned with assessing the outcomes of health care for policy and medical purpose may eventually be useful for public health assessment.

According to Patrick & Bergner (32), "health-related" quality of life can be thought of in five concepts or domains: duration of life; impairments, such as subjective complaints, physical signs, self-reported disease, physiological measures, and medical diagnoses; functional status in physical, psychological, and social domains; health perceptions, including satisfaction with health and more general perceptions; and opportunity, including social or cultural handicaps and individual resilience. By using this framework, researchers have developed measurement tools to assess health status in general and for particular conditions. For instance, the RAND Medical Outcomes Study has developed a comprehensive measurement tool with only 20 questions suitable for use in self-administered population surveys (39). More specific indices have been developed for several particular populations, diseases, and conditions (22).

In health services research, the multidimensional nature of health status has been approached in at least two ways. First, weights for combining scores on multiple dimensions have been determined so that the aggregate score reflects the overall preferences of some reference population for tradeoffs between different disease and disability states. The Quality of Well Being (QWB) scale, for instance, is a preference weighted measure of symptoms and functioning that provides a score ranging from 0.0 for death to 1.0 for asymptomatic, optimum functioning (18). To weigh an individual's risk factors, perhaps some variant of the statistical methodology used in health risk appraisals (8) could be developed.

Another approach is to combine mortality and health status in a single index, often known as "Quality-Adjusted Life Years." This is a cohort measure in which the life table proportion that survives to each age is multiplied by a weight, such as the average QWB score, that expresses the average "health status" of individuals who reach that age. Erickson and colleagues (11) describe how such a statistic can be calculated for national populations based on data from health interview surveys, and a version has been incorporated into objective 17.1 of *Healthy People 2000*. Kaplan & Anderson (17) have proposed a model for integrating risk factors and health status information over time to form a comprehensive measure of health related quality of life. Although theoretically promising, these approaches have not been applied on a national scale, but their use on a population basis deserves further development and testing.

DATA FOR STATE AND LOCAL AREAS

If *Healthy People 2000* is to achieve its potential, communities of all sizes—states, counties, municipalities, and such groups as a company's employees and their families—must adopt their own objectives and measure their progress toward them through the 1990s (42, pp. 15–27). States and smaller communities, however, often find that data are unavailable or of poorer quality than national data. By assessing the ability of states to monitor the draft year 2000 objectives prepared in 1989, for instance, the Public Health Foundation found that on average states could only monitor 39% of the objectives. The proportion that could be monitored ranged from 27% to 58% across states (35). Data problems are more severe when information on racial, ethnic, and socioeconomic groups are needed.

The problems of state and local health departments cannot be solved simply by disaggregating national data. No national survey is likely to have a large enough sample to provide reliable direct estimates for all of the sub-populations required. Furthermore, current denominator data by race, ethnicity, and social-economic status are not generally available from the US Census Bureau. Rather than a single national survey, common survey methodology that can be replicated easily at the state and local levels, such as the Centers for Disease Control's Behavioral Risk Factor Surveillance System (36), needs to be developed.

Even when data are available for small geographical areas, as they are for vital statistics, the rates are unreliable because the events are infrequent. One approach to the sparse data problem is to use measures that are stable at the local level as proxies for the measures used in the national objectives. For instance, a local health department might choose to monitor infant health in terms of the proportion of low birth weight babies, rather than the infant mortality rate. Because the proportion of babies born with low birth weight is higher than the proportion that dies, this rate is more reliable for small areas. In choosing such proxy measures, however, it is important to verify that changes in the proposed measure truly reflect changes in the health characteristic to be monitored.

Another approach is to use formal statistical methods designed for small areas. These are not yet commonly used in public health assessment, but are discussed below because they warrant further development.

Statistical Models for Small Areas

For measures that are too variable at the state or local levels, three, five, or more years of numerator data can be aggregated into one or a running series of calculated rates. Such measures are slower to show the impact of interventions because they include data from past years, but they may be stable enough to show meaningful trends. When rates change over time, aggregated rates are not comparable unless all of the rates are based on the same number of years. Thus, standards are needed to judge whether the variability of rates and measures is sufficiently small for tracking purposes and to ensure that the results are comparable within states and the nation.

Kalton (16) has proposed four statistical models for small area estimation that have potential for public health assessment. "Synthetic estimation" uses information on the age, sex, and race distribution within a small area in combination with national race-, age-, and sex-specific rates of the outcome in question to estimate the prevalence in the small area. Elston and colleagues (10), for instance, have applied this approach to estimate the number of functionally dependent individuals for states and counties. "Regression estimation" uses information from a sample of small areas with complete data on a continuous outcome variable, e.g. the maternal mortality rate, and other generally available predictor variables to estimate a regression equation; these results then provide predicted values of the maternal mortality rate in other communities for which the predictor variables are available. "Structure preserving estimation" techniques use the methods of discrete data analysis, such as iterative proportional fitting (5), to combine survey-based information on the age and sex structure of an outcome, such as disability, with census information on the number of individuals in a community to estimate the prevalence of disability in a small community. "Composite estimation" combines information from the community in question (which might have a high degree of variability, depending on the size of the population) with a model-based estimate, such as those described above according to an empirical Bayes model (27). Manton and colleagues (23), for instance, describe the use of such a model to stabilize cancer mortality rates for counties in the US.

As Kalton points out, all of these approaches depend on a statistical model, so the choice of a good model and effective auxiliary variables is important. Unless the auxiliary variables are strongly related to the outcome variable in question, the small area estimates will vary little from one area to another (16). In practice, the choice of the model and auxiliary variables is limited by the data available. Thus, although these approaches may be useful for health planners in predicting health care needs, they will be helpful for public health assessment purposes only if auxiliary variables are available to reflect changes over time and local differences from national levels accurately.

Setting Targets and Priorities

Although *Healthy People 2000* presents numerical targets for most of the national objectives, it offers only limited information on how these targets were chosen. Progress reviews have no meaning if the targets are not reasonably chosen and the rationale is not clearly explained to the public. When other groups set their own targets, they need guidance in determining what is achievable.

The objective on coronary heart disease exemplifies the problem. The national objective calls for an annual coronary heart disease mortality rate of no more than 100 deaths per 100,000 population. This target implies a 2.3% annual decline, compared with the 3.0–3.1% annual decline (depending on the starting year) in the last two decades. The target is said to be "chosen on the basis of trend evaluation and expert judgment, and reflects the continuing downward trend in the overall coronary heart disease death rate" (46, p. 395), but *Healthy People 2000* offers no reason for the deceleration. The target for this particular objective is particularly important; the difference between this target and one slightly more optimistic than the historical trend—90 per 100,000—is equivalent to about seven months in life expectancy for the total population (43).

To set meaningful and feasible targets, state and local areas must consider differences from national values in baseline rates and trends in the measures in question, in addition to standardizing for population composition. Targets can also be set by comparison with other geographic areas or with epidemiological models that account for important risk factors in the population.

There are several statistical methods that can help the working groups set meaningful numerical targets. None of these can be used on a strictly mechanical basis, and all require significant subject matter judgment. However, these methods can give some idea of what will probably happen in the absence of further interventions or indicate the likely impact of interventions on outcomes. Thus, models can help set or fine-tune the targets.

The most straightforward statistical model is simple trend analysis. Such models can predict the level of various objective measures—assuming that current trends continue—as well as provide statistical confidence intervals. Objectives should usually be somewhat more favorable than what the trend analysis suggests will happen anyway. Projections should not be blindly accepted as the year 2000 target; rather, the target should be set higher or lower than the projected value, according to a subjective assessment of the progress that is possible (41).

Models that identify the lowest possible morbidity and mortality rates that have been observed in specific groups could also be useful in setting targets. The specific groups could be other countries or geographic, racial, ethnic, or socioeconomic subpopulations of the United States. Woolsey (51), for instance, has proposed a version of this. Hahn and colleagues (14) have estimated the possible reduction in mortality rates that can be expected with the elimination of the most important risk factors for chronic disease.

Mathematical models that relate health outcomes to specific interventions for many specific diseases and health behaviors can also be helpful in determining targets. These models provide insight into achievable health outcome levels and the relationship between the process and outcome objectives. For instance, the National Cancer Institute has developed a model to project cancer incidence and mortality under various cancer control programs, such as prevention programs, screening, and treatment (20). Such models require more data than simple trend analyses and take time to develop and verify. In addition, there can be substantial uncertainties in modeling the interventions and interactions among them. The modeling process itself, however, helps focus discussion and thinking and leads to a range of plausible targets. Similar models have been, or are being, developed for cardiovascular disease, AIDS, and other diseases (49). By using such models as appropriate, *Closing the Gap* synthesizes much of what is known about the potential health effects of health promotion and disease prevention (4).

Simple extrapolation models and process models, such as the one for cancer, form two extremes of a spectrum. Extrapolation models that consider age-period-cohort effects, projected demographic changes, and other factors (7) fall between the two and offer some promise.

IMPLEMENTATION

The national objectives in *Healthy People 2000* provide both the motivation and a good starting point for the development of public health assessment efforts at the national, state, and local levels. However, substantially more effort is needed in the 1990s if we are to achieve the promise of these objectives in the year 2000.

Because states and local areas are expected to develop objectives of their own that parallel the national objectives, *Healthy People 2000* itself is actually the first step in specifying a national public health data set. Recognizing this, the objectives and targets used in the national objectives must be documented to communicate to public health statisticians at all geographical levels the assumptions and methods used at the national level.

At the national level, documentation is needed on the technical characteristics of data sources used in *Healthy People 2000*; the detailed identifiers needed to adapt these data for the purposes of the objectives, such as ICD codes and hospital discharge codes; and the procedural definitions, such as the calculation of "body mass index" and the appropriate age- and sex-specific reference values.

For states, counties, and smaller localities, additional information is needed to implement comparable surveillance systems for the objectives. Model survey questions and survey methodologies for state and local use must be developed and disseminated. Careful consideration must also be given to identifying appropriate proxy measures and alternative methodologies for state and local level assessment, where events are infrequent and rates would be highly variable or where disaggregated geographical data are not available.

When data are available, methods are needed to translate the national numerical targets to the state and local levels. Such methods as age-adjustment and synthetic estimation should be explored. To determine feasible local targets, common methods for trend analysis, risk factor control analysis, and comparison with other geographic areas must be developed and made available. Modeled after the efforts of the European Regional Office of the World Health Organization (52), computer software could be developed to graph, analyze, and project state or local trends in conjunction with national data.

Because of its leadership role in health statistics, the federal government can help improve the surveillance tools needed to assess progress on the objectives and to set priorities for future actions. The Public Health Service acknowledges the need for strengthened public health assessment efforts and devotes Chapter 22 of *Healthy People 2000* to surveillance and data systems. Meeting these surveillance objectives will require vigorous national leadership and the collaboration of numerous federal agencies, state and local health agencies, and many private sector organizations. Because assessment is fundamental to the objectives process and public health in general, these activities surely deserve vigorous support.

ACKNOWLEDGEMENTS

This work was supported by funding from the Office of Disease Prevention and Health Promotion, Office of the Assistant Secretary for Health, Department of Health and Human Services under cooperative agreement no. HPV-87-002-03-0. It was conducted through the Division of Health Promotion and Disease Prevention of the Institute of Medicine, National Academy of Sciences. Much of the material in this paper is adapted from analyses prepared during the drafting of *Healthy People 2000*. I thank Michael Millman and others for comments on those analyses and the editors of this volume. Jane Durch deserves particular mention for her efforts in the preparation of the sample health status indicators in Table 1.

The analysis and opinions in this paper are mine; they do not necessarily reflect those of the Institute of Medicine, the National Academy of Sciences, or the US Public Health Service.

Literature Cited

1. Am. Public Health Assoc. 1991. *Healthy Communities 2000: Model Standards.* Washington: Am. Public Health Assoc. 3rd ed.
2. Amler, R. W., Dull, H. B., eds. 1987. *Closing the Gap: THe Burden of Unnecessary Illness.* New York: Oxford
3. Andersen, R., Mullner, R. 1990. Assessing the health objectives of the nation. *Health Aff.* 9:152–62
4. Andrews, F. M. 1989. Developing indicators of health promotion: Contributions from the social indicators movement. In *Health Promotion Indicators and Actions,* ed. S. B. Kar, pp. 23–49. New York: Springer
5. Bishop, Y. M. M., Fienberg, S. E., Holland, P. W. 1975. *Discrete Multivariate Analysis: Theory and Practice.* Cambridge, Mass: MIT
6. Breslow, L. 1990. A health promotion primer for the 1990s. *Health Aff.* 9:6–21
7. Brown, C. C., Kessler, L. G. 1988. Projections of lung cancer mortality in the United States: 1985–2025. *J. Natl. Cancer Inst.* 80:43–51

7a. Cent. Dis. Control. 1991. Concensus set of health status indicators for the general assessment of community health status—United States. *Morbid. Mortal. Wkly. Rep.* 40:449–51
8. DeFriese, G. H., Fielding, J. E. 1990. Health risk appraisal in the 1990s: Opportunities, challenges, and expectations. *Annu. Rev. Public Health* 11:401–18
9. Dever, G. E. A. 1991. *Community Health Analysis: Global Awareness at the Local Level.* Gaithersburg, Md.: Aspen
10. Elston, J. M., Koch, G. G., Weissert, W. G. 1991. Regression-adjusted small area estimates of functional dependency in the noninstitutionalized American population age 65 and over. *Am. J. Public Health* 81:335–43
11. Erickson, P., Kendall, E. A., Anderson, J. P., Kaplan, R. M. 1989. Using composite health status measures to assess the nation's health. *Med. Care* 27 (Suppl.):S66–76
12. Fleiss, J. L. 1981. *Statistical Methods*

for Rates and Proportions, pp. 237–55. New York: Wiley. 2nd ed.

13. Green, L. W., Wilson, R. W., Bauer, K. G. 1983. Data requirements to measure progress on the objectives for the nation in health promotion and disease prevention. *Am. J. Public Health* 73:18–24

14. Hahn, R. A., Teutsch, S. M., Rothenberg, R. B., Marks, J. S. 1990. Excess deaths from nine chronic diseases in the United States, 1986. *J. Am. Med. Assoc.* 264:2654–59

15. Inst. Med. 1988. *The Future of Public Health,* Washington, DC: Natl. Acad. Press

16. Kalton, G. 1991. Methods of small area estimation: A review. In *Proceedings of Consensus Conference on Small Area Analysis.* Washington, DC: Health Resour. Serv. Adm.

17. Kaplan, R. M., Anderson, J. P. 1990. The general health policy model: An integrated approach. in *Quality of Life Assessments in Clinical Trials,* ed. B. Spilker, pp. 131–49. New York: Raven

18. Kaplan, R. M., Bush, J. W., Berry, C. C. 1976. Health status: Types of validity and the index of well-being. *Health Serv. Res.* 11:478–507

19. Kar, S. B., ed. 1989. *Health Promotion Indicators and Actions,* pp. 23–49. New York: Springer

20. Levin, D. L., Gail, M. H., Kessler, L. G., Eddy, D. M. 1986. A model for projecting cancer incidence and mortality in the presence of prevention, screening, and treatment programs. In *Cancer Control Objectives for the Nation, 1985–2000* (NCI Monograph #2). Bethesda, Md: Natl. Cancer Inst.

21. Levine, D. B., Zitter, M., Ingram, L. eds. (Comm. Natl. Stat.) 1990. *Disability Statistics: An Assessment* (Report of a Workshop). Washington, DC: Natl. Acad. Press

22. Lohr, K. N. 1989. Advances in health status assessment: Overview of the conference. *Med. Care* 27 (Suppl.):S1–11

23. Manton, K. G., Woodbury, M. A., Stallard, E., Riggan, W. B., Creason, J. P., Pellom, A. C. 1989. Empirical Bayes procedures for stabilizing maps of US cancer mortality rates. *J. Am. Stat. Assoc.* 84:637–50

24. Mason, J. O. 1990. A prevention policy framework for the nation. *Health Aff.* 9:22–29

25. McGinnis, J. M. 1990. Setting objectives for public health in the 1990s: Experience and prospects. *Annu. Rev. Public Health* 11:231–49

26. Miller, C. A., Fine, A., Adams-Taylor, S. 1989. *Monitoring Children's Health.* Washington, DC: Am. Public Health Assoc. 2nd ed.

27. Morris, C. N. 1983. Parametric empirical Bayes inference: Theory and applications. *J. Am. Stat. Assoc.* 78:47–54

28. Murnaghan, J. H. 1981. Health indicators and information systems for the year 2000. *Annu. Rev. Public Health* 2:299–361

29. Natl. Assoc. County Health Officials. 1990. *National Profile of Local Health Departments.* Washington, DC: Natl. Assoc. County Health Officials

30. Natl. Comm. Vital Health Stat. 1987. Final report of the subcommittee on data gaps in disease prevention and health promotion. (Append. VI, NCVHS annu. rept.) Washington, DC: Natl. Comm. Vital Health Stat.

31. Natl. Inst. Health Div. Legis. Anal. 1990. The quality of US health promotion statistics to review year 2000 objectives. In *Highlights* 2:85–87. Bethesda, Md: Natl. Inst. Health

32. Patrick, D. L., Bergner, M. 1990. Measurement of health status in the 1990s. *Annu. Rev. Public Health* 11:165–83

33. Pope, A. M., Tarlov, A. R., eds. (Inst. Med.) 1991. *Disability in America: Toward a National Agenda for Prevention.* Washington DC: Natl. Acad. Press

34. Public Health Found. 1990. *Data for the Year 2000 National Health Objectives.* Washington, DC: Public Health Found.

35. Public Health Found. 1990. *A Report on the States' Ability to Measure Progress Toward Achievement of the Year 2000 Objectives.* Washington, DC: Public Health Found.

36. Remington, P. L., Smith, M. Y., Williamson, D. F., Anda, R. F., Gentry, E. M., Hogelin, G. C. 1988. Design, characteristics, and usefulness of state-based behavioral risk factor surveillance: 1981–87. *Public Health Rep.* 103:366–75

37. Sommers, K. B. 1990. The role of prevention objectives (letter). *Health Aff.* 9:204

38. Spencer, G. (US Bur. Census). 1989. *Projections of the Population of the United States, by Age, Sex, and Race: 1988 to 2080.* Current Population Reports, Ser. P-25, #1018. Washington, DC: GPO

39. Stewart, A. L., Hays, R. D., Ware, J. E. 1988. The MOS short-form general health survey: Reliability and validity in a patient population, *Med. Care* 26:724–35

40. Stoto, M. A. 1990. Measuring progress in health promotion (letter). *Health Aff.* 9:202–3
41. Stoto, M. A. 1989. Statistical issues in formulating the health objectives for the year 2000. In *Proc. of the 1989 Public Health Conf. on Records and Stat.* Washington: Natl. Cent. Health Stat.
42. Stoto, M. A., Behrens, R., Rosemont, C., eds. 1990. *Healthy People 2000: Citizens Chart the Course.* Washington, DC: Natl. Acad. Press
43. Stoto, M. A., Durch, J. S. 1991. National health objectives for the year 2000: The demographic impact of health promotion and disease prevention. *Am. J. Public Health* 81:1456–65
44. US Dep. Health Educ. Welf. 1979. *Healthy People: The Surgeon General's Report on Health Promotion and Disease Prevention.* Washington, DC: GPO
45. US Dep. Health Human Serv. 1991. *Health United States 1990.* Washington, DC: GPO
46. US Dep. Health Human Serv. 1991. *Healthy People 2000: National Health Promotion and Disease Prevention Objectives.* Washington, DC: GPO
47. US Dep. Health Human Serv. 1986. *The 1990 Health Objectives for the Nation: A Midcourse Review.* Washington, DC: GPO
48. US Dep Health Human Serv. 1980. *Promoting Health/Preventing Disease: Objectives for the Nation.* Washington, DC: GPO
49. Weinstein, M. C., Coxson, P. G., Williams, L. W., Pass, T. M., Stason, W. B., Goldman, L. 1987. Forecasting coronary heart disease incidence, mortality, and cost: The coronary heart disease policy model. *Am. J. Public Health* 77:1417–26
50. Wilson, R. W., Drury, T. F. 1984. Interpreting trends in illness and disability: Health statistics and health status. *Annu. Rev. Public Health* 5:83–106
51. Woolsey, T. D. 1981. *Toward an Index of Preventable Mortality,* Vital and Health Stat., Ser. 2, No. 85. Washington, DC: GPO
52. World Health Org. (Reg. Off. Eur.) 1989. HFA/PC (Computer program and data disk to monitor Health For All in the European Region). Copenhagen: World Health Org.
53. World Health Org. (Reg. Off. Eur.) 1985. *Targets for Health for All.* Copenhagen: World Health Org.

Annu. Rev. Publ. Health. 1992. 13:79–98

THE HANTAVIRUSES, ETIOLOGIC AGENTS OF HEMORRHAGIC FEVER WITH RENAL SYNDROME: A Possible Cause of Hypertension and Chronic Renal Disease in the United States[1]

J. W. LeDuc

Disease Assessment Division, United States Army Medical Research Institute of Infectious Diseases, Fort Detrick, Frederick, Maryland 21702

J. E. Childs and G. E. Glass

Department of Immunology and Infectious Diseases, School of Hygiene and Public Health, The Johns Hopkins University, Baltimore, Maryland 21205

KEY WORDS: rodent-borne zoonoses, nephropathia epidemica, Seoul virus, Puumala virus

---

INTRODUCTION

Although little is known in the United States about hemorrhagic fever with renal syndrome (HFRS), this disease is a significant cause of human morbidity and mortality across Eurasia. The severest form of HFRS is most prevalent

---

[1]In conducting the research described in this report, the investigator(s) adhered to the "Guide for the Care and Use of Laboratory Animals," as promulgated by the Committee on Care and Use of Laboratory Animals of the Institute of Laboratory Animal Resources, National Research Council. The facilities are fully accredited by the American Association for Accreditation of Laboratory Animal Care.

The views of the author(s) do not purport to reflect the positions of the Department of the Army or the Department of Defense.

The US Government has the right to retain a nonexclusive royalty-free license in and to any copyright covering this paper.

in Asia, where more than 150,000 cases occur annually (52), with consistent mortality rates of about 5%. The disease has been given a multitude of names (22), which has contributed to the confusion concerning its actual distribution and epidemiology. In China, the disease is known as epidemic hemorrhagic fever; in Korea, it is called Korean hemorrhagic fever. In Scandinavia, western USSR, and western Europe, a milder form of this disease occurs, with case-mortality rates of less than 1%. This form of HFRS is called nephropathia epidemica. The World Health Organization adopted the term "hemorrhagic fever with renal syndrome" to serve as a unifying name for these and related conditions (21).

This group of diseases is caused by a newly recognized group of viruses, the genus *Hantavirus,* of the family Bunyaviridae. These viruses are maintained in nature primarily in rodents of the superfamily Muroidea, which includes the common species of rats (*Rattus* spp.), house mice (*Mus musculus*), field or woodland mice (*Apodemus* spp.), and voles (*Microtus* and *Clethrionomys* spp.). Although other mammals are occasionally infected with these viruses, in each geographic region where distinctive forms of HFRS occur, each hantavirus is primarily associated with a single species of rodent (Table 1). Unlike other bunyaviruses that cause disease in humans (such as California encephalitis and Sandfly fever viruses), arthropod vectors are believed to play a negligible role in the transmission of hantaviruses. Human infection results from inhalation or contact with virus excreted or secreted in rodent urine, saliva, or feces. Rodent bite has rarely been implicated in human infection (17), although this route of transmission may play a role in rodent-

Table 1   Members of the genus *Hantavirus* (Bunyaviridae), their rodent reservoirs, geographical distribution, and associated human disease(s)

Virus	Primary rodent host	Distribution	Disease
Hantaan	*Apodemus agrarius* (Striped field mouse)	China, Korea, eastern USSR,	Epidemic hemorrhagic fever, Korean hemorrhagic fever
	Apodemus flavicollis (Yellow-necked mouse)	Balkans	Hemorrhagic fever with renal syndrome (severe)
Seoul	*Rattus norvegicus* (Common or brown rat)	Worldwide	Epidemic hemorrhagic fever[a] (mild type)
Puumala	*Clethrionomy glareolus* (Bank vole)	Scandinavia, western USSR, eastern Europe	Nephropathia epidemica
Prospect Hill	*Microtus pennsylvanicus* (Meadow vole)	United States (Maryland, Minnesota)	None known
Leakey[b]	*Mus musculus* (House mouse)	United States (Texas)	None known

[a] Disease associated with rat-borne hantaviruses is documented in Asia only.
[b] Proposed new virus.

to-rodent transmission (25). Humans do not excrete or secrete large amounts of virus during infection, and are thus unlikely to transmit the virus to other humans or rodents.

These viruses are of special interest because they occur in the United States, as well as foreign countries. At present, three differnt hantaviruses have been identified in the US; of these, the Seoul virus of Norway rats (*Rattus norvegicus*), is clearly associated with human disease in other countries. Residents of major cities in the US, especially those dwelling in the inner cities, are routinely exposed to rats infected with hantaviruses and may, in turn, become infected. There is increasing evidence that infection may cause an acute disease and predispose an individual to subsequent development of chronic renal disease or hypertension or increased risk of cerebrovascular accident (26). Thus, the hantaviruses represent an emerging viral disease that offers new challenges and, perhaps, explains some long-standing questions.

HFRS, HANTAVIRUSES, AND RODENT HOSTS

Hantaviruses and the diseases they cause can best be understood by examining the individual viruses and the ecological relationships to their rodent hosts.

Korean Hemorrhagic Fever and Hantaan Virus

Western physicians and scientists first became aware of human disease due to hantaviral infections during the Korean conflict, when more than 2400 United Nations forces were infected with a mysterious "new" disease, then called Korean hemorhagic fever (18, 73, 75). Although this disease was new to Western science, it was not new to the region: Japanese and Russian physicians had described an identical disease in Manchuria during the 1930s and 1940s, when the Japanese lost thousands of troops to the illness (75). The Allied Forces in Korea established the Hemorrhagic Fever Commission to investigate the disease; but, in spite of a massive effort, the causative agent, Hantaan virus, was not isolated until 1976.

Lee and colleagues (60, 62), working at Korea University in Seoul, were the first to detect and then isolate the etiological agent of Korean hemorrhagic fever. An antigen that reacted with convalescent sera from Korean hemorrhagic fever patients was found in the lungs of the striped field mouse, *Apodemus agrarius* (60). A virus was subsequently isolated from lung tissue from the same species and named "Hantaan virus" in recognition of the Hantaan River, which flows through the endemic region of Korea (62). Shortly thereafter, Hantaan virus was adapted to growth in cell culture (20), and an immunofluorescent antibody (IFA) test was developed. The availability of antigen and an assay allowed for rapid progress in defining the distribu-

Table 2   Chronology of selected events in the study of hemorrhagic fever with renal syndrome

Event	Approximate Dates
Clinical descriptions of HFRS in Asia and Europe	1930s–1950s
Isolation of Hantaan virus	1976
Cell culture adaptation	1981
Relatedness of agents causing KHF, EHF, and NE demonstrated	1980–1983
Global distribution of infected rodents	1982–1987
Grouping of agents in genus *Hantavirus* family Bunyaviridae	1983–1985
Widespread human infection and disease	1983–1988
Association with chronic disease	1990

tion and epidemiology of HFRS. Within five years, the diverse clinical entities, which occurred across Asia and Europe under several different names, were shown to be caused by viruses related to Hantaan virus (Table 2).

Extensive surveys of potential animal reservoirs in Korea, as well as investigations into the possible infection of ectoparasites associated with these species, failed to reveal additional hosts for Hantaan virus other than *A. agrarius* (61). Experimental infections of this natural rodent host revealed an unusual characteristic of Hantaan virus and, as it turned out, all hantaviruses. After *A. agrarius* were inoculated with Hantaan virus, a brief viremia developed in the animals at seven to ten days postinfection. Subsequently, viral antigen was detectable in many organs of the animals, including the kidney and lungs; virus was shed in their saliva, feces, and urine (57). Shedding of infectious virus persisted despite the presence of antibody capable of neutralizing Hantaan virus in in vitro assays (Figure 1). The persistent infection had no apparent detrimental effects on the host, and the rodent became a carrier of infectious virus, in a relationship similar to that previously described for arenavirus-rodent infections. Virus was persistently shed into the environment through contaminated urine and feces for periods of time that were probably equivalent to the natural lifespan of these rodents in the field. Investigators now suspect that excreted, infectious virus in urine and feces from infected rodents is the source of virtually all human infections. This also holds true for other hantaviruses discussed below (45, 93, 99).

The epidemiology of the hantaviruses and HFRS is intimately linked to the

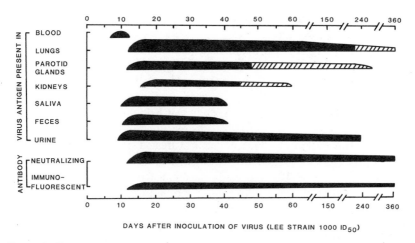

Figure 1   The course of infection and infectivity of Hantaan virus in *Apodemus agrarius*. Shaded area of bars for lung, parotid glands, and kidneys indicates presence of antigen, but not virus. Similar chronic infection and persistent shedding of virus is thought to occur in most primary hosts of hantaviruses. (From Ref. 57. Reproduced with permission.)

biology of the rodent host. Natural population cycles of rodents and certain human behaviors result in distinctive seasonal patterns of HFRS. In Asia, the disease is most common in late fall and early winter (51). These are the periods during which field mouse populations are maximal and the harvesting of crops places farmers in rodent-infested environments. The majority of HFRS cases are in the adult male population, as men are most likely to come into contact with rodents as part of their farming practices.

What is now called "classic" HFRS due to Hantaan virus in Asia is characterized by a mild to severe disease, which follows an incubation period of two to three weeks, with a range of 5 to 42 days (75, 92). The disease progresses in relatively well-defined successive stages (in chronological order): febrile, hypotensive, oliguric, diuretic, and convalescent (8, 74, 75). Convalescence can take two to three months. The major clinical signs and symptoms seen in each stage are fever, shock, renal impairment, relative hypovolemia, and fluid and electrolyte imbalance. A petechial rash may also be present, and a characteristic facial flushing develops in many patients. Among the more severely ill patients, hemorrhagic signs, including scleral injection, ecchymosis, and gastrointestinal bleeding, may be seen (75). In fatal cases, death is usually a consequence of shock or renal failure and occurs most frequently during the oliguric stage of disease. Recovery from infection was believed to be complete (54, 75); however, reports of chronic renal impairment exist (15, 42, 44, 78), and recent observations from our own studies show an association between past infection with a hantavirus and chronic renal disease (26).

Treatment of HFRS has traditionally been limited to careful supportive care, with special attention to fluid balance augmented by renal dialysis in the most critically ill patients (59). Recently, a double-blind, placebo-controlled efficacy trial of the antiviral drug, ribavirin, was conducted in Wuhan, China (31). This 1986–1988 collaborative study was held during the course of two transmission seasons. Of the 108 patients receiving placebo, ten deaths were recorded. However, only three of the 123 treated patients died (31). This significant difference in mortality indicated that ribavirin may be useful in the treatment of acute HFRS, especially if administered early in the course of disease. The drug also markedly reduced morbidity and frequently decreased the time patients spent in each stage of illness.

Severe HFRS of the Balkans

Recently, an extremely severe type of HFRS was recognized in the mountainous regions of Greece (3, 4, 46), Albania, parts of Yugoslavia (5, 28), and Bulgaria. This disease is far more severe than nephropathia epidemica seen elsewhere in Europe and more closely resembles the Asian form of HFRS. Although relatively few cases have been recorded, the mortality rate appears to be even greater than in Asia; preliminary reports suggest that 15–30% of patients hospitalized with this disease may succumb to their infection. The causative agent, originally named Porogia virus, is closely related to Hantaan virus (3). It is also maintained by a small rodent, the yellow-necked mouse, *Apodemus flavicollis* (27). Unlike HFRS in Asia and other parts of Europe, cases in the Balkans peak during the warmer months of the year, as most cases occur around August.

The origin of this severe form of HFRS is currently unknown, although the relatively wide geographic distribution of the virus throughout the Balkan Region, and its localization in sparsely populated rural habitats, suggests that human commerce was probably not involved in determining its present distribution. Nonetheless, serological analyses clearly indicate a very close relationship between isolates obtained from rodents and humans in the Balkans and Asian isolates of prototype Hantaan virus. Complete sequence information is not available for any Balkan isolate, but examination of small genomic sections of the M segment (365 base pairs), amplified by polymerase chain reaction (PCR) and digested by restriction endonucleases, suggests that at least the segment examined is highly conserved among both Balkan and Asian isolates (S.-Y. Xiao 1991, unpublished observations).

Nephropathia Epidemica and Puumala Virus

A less severe form of HFRS, with a case-mortality rate of less than 1%, is found in Scandinavia, western USSR, and other European countries (42, 43,

88). Although nephropathia epidemica was first described in Scandinavia in the 1930s, it is only now emerging as a relatively common cause of acute renal failure in France (35, 76), Italy (79), Belgium (96), and other European countries (36, 95, 97). As with Hantaan virus, the virus that causes nephropathia epidemica, Puumala virus, was only recently discovered and isolated.

Puumala virus is maintained in nature by the bank vole, *Clethrionomys glareolus* (7), which is widely distributed in western Europe and western USSR; its range overlaps that of this milder form of HFRS (Figure 2). The course of viral infection in the vole host is similar to that described for Hantaan, with long-term, somewhat sporadic, shedding of virus in feces and urine (102). The disease in humans is highly seasonal; most cases occur in the late fall and early winter. A correlation between high rodent numbers and increased annual incidence of disease has been shown in Sweden for the years 1961–1974 (70). In Sweden, for reasons which are unclear, nephropathia epidemica is largely limited to the northern half of the country: Infection in voles mirrors the distribution of human disease, although the same vole species occurs throughout the country (68). Again, adult men living in rural locations and engaged in outdoor employment, such as forestry workers, comprise the majority of cases (38). The vole host of viruses that cause nephropathia epidemica also moves into storage buildings and homes during cold weather; thus, indoor exposure can occur (70).

Although the disease spectrum of nephropathia epidemica is similar to that seen for Far Eastern forms of HFRS, some of the clinical signs or symptoms are less prominent or occur in fewer patients (43). Renal dysfunction is still the prominent clinical characteristic, but anuria is rare. Concentrating capacity of the kidney may be impaired from weeks to months, but serious hemorrhagic manifestations and mortality are generally absent (43).

Seoul Virus and Urban Rats

Certainly, the most significant event in the recent history of HFRS research, from the global public health perspective, was the recognition of HFRS among urban residents of Seoul, Korea, and the subsequent isolation of Seoul virus from city rats (56). Seoul virus was first discovered by Lee and colleagues during their investigations of Hantaan virus (56). They were intrigued by cases of HFRS that occurred in urban residents with no history of rural travel and no exposure to *A. agrarius*. These patients suffered from a disease indistinguishable from the milder forms of HFRS due to Hantaan virus, and they developed antibodies reactive with Hantaan virus in the IFA test. When rodents were captured in and around these patients' homes, no *A. agrarius* were trapped. However, both *R. norvegicus* and *R. rattus,* the black or roof rat, were present; when examined, they also possessed antibodies reactive by IFA tests with Hantaan virus. Later, through use of cross-neutralization tests, researchers discovered that the virus infecting rats and

Global Distribution of Rodent Reservoirs of HFRS

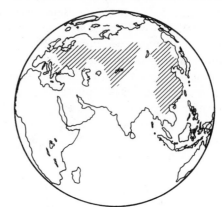

Distribution of *Apodemus agrarius*

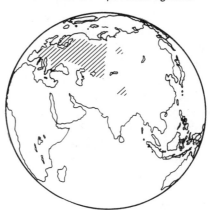

Distribution of *Clethrionomys glareolus*

Figure 2   Distribution of *Apodemus agrarius* and *Clethrionomys glareolus,* primary hosts of Hantaan and Puumala viruses, respectively.

urban residents was antigenically distinct from Hantaan; this virus was named Seoul virus.

After the discovery of Seoul virus in urban rats in Korea, the possibility of potential international dissemination of this zoonosis via the shipping industry was suggested. With the exception of Antarctica, Norway and black rats are now widely distributed on all continents, where they have been introduced from Europe and Asia. Within a few years, infected Norway rat were identi-fied in the United States within the port cities of Philadelphia and Houston (49), New Orleans (94), and Baltimore (13). Viruses similar or identical to Seoul virus were isolated from rats captured in each of these locations, and the search for infected rats was expanded to a global scale. Serological surveys documented the presence of infected rats in many parts of Asia, Europe, Africa, and South America (48). Detailed surveys for human infection and disease are not available from most of these locations.

Extensive investigations were initiated to study this Seoul-like virus in inner-city Baltimore rats. Infected rats were found widely distributed throughout the city (14), but were especially abundant in the lower-income neighborhoods, in which accumulated trash, litter, and garbage provided ideal conditions for rat infestations (13). Infections had been stably enzootic within the rats of Baltimore for at least ten years (J. E. Childs and G. E. Glass, unpublished data), based on long-term trapping in specific alleys. In addition, Norway rats do not move great distances in urban environments; therefore, widespread dissemination of a virus, without an arthropod vector, generally takes many years. Thus, Seoul-like viruses were not recent introductions to the US, but had been here for some time and had become widely disseminated. Rat populations of several areas were followed longitudinally over two years, and we were able to demonstrate that virus was transmitted among rats throughout the year. About 11% of the population became infected per month (11). As older cohorts of rats were examined, their antibody prevalence rates increased until virtually all of the oldest rats had become infected (Figure 3).

The infection of laboratory rat colonies and tissue lines derived from rats also pose a public health threat to certain occupational groups. Outbreaks of laboratory rat-associated HFRS have been documented in Korea (58), Japan (30), and the Soviet Union (41); sporadic cases have occurred in Belgium (16) and the United Kingdom (65). Generally, these infections are limited to animal handlers or laboratory personnel. In some countries, infection rates of laboratory rat colonies can be high and widespread among research facilities. In the US, there is no evidence that commercial or laboratory colonies of rats are infected with Seoul-like viruses (45), and the widely practiced methods of barrier breeding and cesarean derivation may reduce the risk of introducing and maintaining infection within colonies (45). Routine screening of laboratory animals for viral pathogens now usually includes serological tests for Hantaan (39).

Cell lines derived from tumors of rats can be infected with a hantavirus, and were the source implicated in a recent human infection (66). Again, there is no evidence that commercially available cell lines are contaminated in the US (50).

Prospect Hill Virus and Meadow Voles

Prospect Hill virus was isolated from meadow voles (*Microtus pennsylvanicus*) captured in Frederick, Maryland, in the early 1980s (63). This virus is antigenically distinct from other mouse, rat, or vole hantaviruses and co-

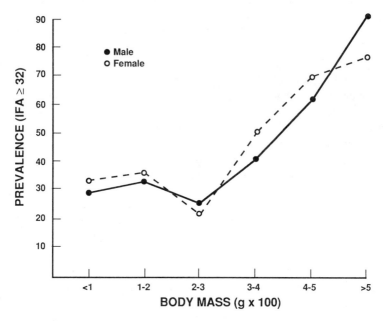

Figure 3   Relationship between antibody prevalence, as determined by IFA, and body mass for 525 Norway rats captured in Baltimore, 1980–1985. Rats were separated by sex, then grouped into 100 g mass classes. (From Ref. 13. Reproduced with permission.)

circulates in space and time with Seoul-like viruses in small mammal communities in the US (37). Typically, the prevalence of Prospect Hill viral infection in voles is around 20–25% and increases in older cohorts of voles (12, 103). This virus is not currently considered a public health problem. Specific neutralizing antibodies to this hantavirus have been detected in sera collected from professional mammalogists (104), who constitute a high-risk group for exposure to the reservoir. The infected individuals had no recollection of an illness compatible with HFRS.

Leakey Virus and House Mice

One of the most recently proposed additions to the *Hantavirus* genus is a virus isolated from the common house mouse *(Mus musculus)* in Texas (6). This virus can be differentiated from other hantaviruses by serological techniques. The public health relevance of this agent is unresolved; however, Baek et al (6) have reported human disease associated with serological evidence of Leakey virus infection. The geographic distribution, host specificity, and prevalence of this virus has not been adequately established for any region. We speculate that some of the hantaviral antibody found in house mice in recent surveys by IFA, and shown to be non-neutralizing for Hantaan and Seoul viruses, may be directed against Leakey virus.

MOLECULAR BIOLOGY, DIAGNOSTIC TESTS, AND VACCINE DEVELOPMENT

In conjunction with progress made in our understanding of the epidemiology of the hantaviruses, has come detailed molecular characterization of this new group of viruses. Some of the molecular techniques have provided powerful new tools to aid in the diagnosis (86, 98) and epidemiological study of HFRS and promise to provide novel vaccine candidates.

Hantaan and related viruses were placed in the family Bunyaviridae on the basis of physical characteristics and genetic determinations (32, 33, 82–84). These viruses show the characteristic tripartite RNA genome of other bunyaviruses, but were placed in a new genus by virtue of their unique 3' terminal sequences (83). The three segments, designated S, M, and L for small, medium, and large, code for nucleocapsid protein (85, 89), envelope glycoproteins (24, 72), and a presumed transcriptase (80), respectively. Various strains of hantaviruses have been cloned and sequenced (1, 2, 24, 34, 71, 72, 83–85, 87, 89), and both the surface glycoproteins and the core nucleocapsid protein have been expressed in different systems (81). These expressed proteins may be produced in large, relatively pure quantities and may eventually replace cell culture derived antigens for use in diagnostic tests for HFRS (77, 81).

Currently, definitive diagnosis of HFRS is relatively slow, as it depends on clinical presentation, coupled with appropriate serological tests and, in rare cases, virus isolation. Standard serological tests to confirm a diagnosis of HFRS are mostly based on immunofluorescent or enzyme-linked immunosorbent assays to detect immunoglobulin G (29, 64, 67, 69, 90). However, for epidemiological monitoring in regions where more than one hantavirus circulates, positive identification of the infecting agent may depend on cumbersome cross-plaque-reduction neutralization assays of serum performed on batteries of hantaviruses under laboratory containment conditions (91).

Serological tests for immunoglobulin M (IgM) antibody specific for hantaviruses are useful aids in diagnosing acute disease (47). Immunoglobulin M antibody is present very early during the course of the disease. In a study in Wuhan, China, the majority of patients had IgM on admission to the hospital (10). Based on limited study, other hantaviral infections show a similar pattern; thus, measuring specific anti-hantaviral IgM antibodies is the method of choice for diagnosis of acute HFRS.

Virus isolation is a difficult task with hantaviral infections. The advent of

PCR technology, and its adaptation to RNA viruses, may make it possible to diagnose and identify the type of hantavirus within a single day (98). Both M segment and S segment PCR tests are currently being investigated, and universal primers that bind to and amplify more than 20 strains of hantavirus have been identified. After amplification, restriction enzymes can be employed to differentiate isolates rapidly. Such analyses have shown tremendous power to group hantaviruses, and these methods hold great potential for future molecular epidemiological studies.

In addition to cloning sequences of hantaviral genomes for diagnostic purposes, researchers at the United States Army Medical Research Institute of Infectious Diseases have constructed an engineered vaccine for Hantaan virus by using vaccinia virus as a vector. Phase 1 testing of candidate vaccine constructs is planned for the near future. Currently, suckling mouse and suckling rat brain vaccines are available, or being tested, in North and South Korea (55); other inactivated vaccines are being developed (100).

HFRS IN THE UNITED STATES

Shortly after the recognition that hantaviral infections occurred in rats and other rodents in the US, seroepidemiological surveys were undertaken to determine the extent of human exposure and to search for evidence of human disease. Early studies showed that human infection occurred among shipyard workers (94), mammalogists (104), dialysis patients, and laboratory workers (23), as well as other populations. However, as no acute illness consistent with the then known presentation of HFRS was observed, investigators suggested that HFRS in the US may be a mild or atypical disease, or that the viruses present on this continent may be nonpathogenic (101). A recent survey of forestry workers and others with outdoor occupations suggests that infection from Prospect Hill-like viruses is rare (19).

However, the abundance of hantaviral infections among inner-city rats, their coexistence with the resident human population, and the recognition in Asia that this virus causes acute illness led us to search for human disease among the inner-city residents of Baltimore. Studies conducted in the intervening years since the initial identification of hantaviruses in the US had shown that HFRS due to rat-borne viruses in Asia caused an illness that was less severe in its hemorrhagic and renal manifestations than that caused by Hantaan virus. The disease associated with rat-borne viruses also showed a higher degree of hepatic involvement (9, 53).

We first conducted a serosurvey of more than 2000 persons who visited a venereal disease clinic, which was located in inner-city Baltimore. The population sampled was predominantly composed of black men in their mid-20s who were of lower socio-economic status. Several individuals in this group were found with antibody specific for the Baltimore strain of Seoul virus, which yielded an antibody prevalence rate of 2.4 per thousand. All of these individuals were born in Baltimore and resided in areas known to have infected rats; none had traveled outside of the US. These results indicated a low rate of indigenous exposure to hantaviruses within the city.

We next examined sera from more than 4500 patients seen at the Johns Hopkins Hospital. Patients with elevated proteinuria were selected for examination, as this has been a consistent laboratory finding in all forms of HFRS, regardless of the infecting virus (42). This population was also drawn primarily (> 75%) from inner-city Baltimore, where infected rats were common. This group was primarily composed of black women in their mid-40s who were also from lower socio-economic neighborhoods. The antibody prevalence rate at 12 per thousand was fivefold higher than that seen at the venereal disease clinic. As a control population, individuals using the Johns Hopkins Hospital emergency room were examined for exposure to hantaviruses. Age-corrected seroprevalence in the emergency room population did not differ significantly from the sexually transmitted disease clinic, but was 1.5–3.2 times lower than in the proteinuria group.

Most of the seropositive patients did not have IgM antibodies, and sequential samples failed to show rising titers, thus suggesting that these were previous infections. However, five patients showed either seroconversion, rising neutralizing titers, or elevated IgM titers and neutralizing titers, which indicated recent exposure. These patients consistently had nausea, vomiting, epigastric pain, and low-grade fever. Laboratory findings indicated renal and liver involvement, as measured by elevated BUN, serum creatinine, AST, ALT, total bilirubin, and LDH (G. E. Glass, A. J. Watson, and J. E. Childs 1991, unpublished information). Thrombocytopenia occurred in some patients, and pleural effusion was also observed. Hemorrhagic manifestations were rare and mild, although blood in the sputum and melena were reported. Thus, illness associated with changes in hantaviral antibody status was similar to reports of mild HFRS due to rat-borne hantaviruses from the Far East and Europe (9). This suggests that HFRS occurs in US populations exposed to infected rats, but the relative rarity of severe, acute illness may preclude its recognition. Among the Johns Hopkins group, the acute illness resolved spontaneously with supportive care. However, at least one patient continued to show evidence of chronic renal insufficiency 13 months after the illness, and the potential for sequelae from HFRS infection was of concern.

Many of the Johns Hopkins patients with antibodies to a hantavirus suffered some form of chronic disease. We matched each seropositive person (N=15) by age and sex to five seronegative controls from the same patient population, and found that the seropositive group was significantly more likely to suffer from a specific form of chronic renal disease, hypertension, or a history of stroke than were seronegative individuals with proteinuria (26). The association was specific for those conditions that could conceivably be linked to past kidney disease, whereas the rates of other chronic illnesses, such as diabetes, did not differ significantly. The differences could not be explained on the basis of race, residence, occupation, age, or sex.

Patients' charts were reviewed by a nephrologist, who lacked prior knowledge of the patients' serological status, for the primary diagnosis underlying their renal disease. Hypertensive nephrosclerosis was the most common diagnosis among the seropositive group (70%), and these findings differed significantly from those of the matched seronegative controls (9%), among whom diabetes mellitus was the most common cause of renal disease (50%). Other factors, such as drug abuse, polycystic disease, and glomerulonephritis, were secondary causes of renal dysfunction among the seronegative control group.

Finally, we examined more than 400 patients enrolled in a chronic renal dialysis program in Baltimore. The population age and sex distribution was similar to that of the Johns Hopkins Hospital sample. The rate of seropositivity for this group was 20 per 1000, the highest of any group sampled.

Encouraged by the discovery of an apparent association between seropositivity to hantaviruses and some forms of chronic disease, we encouraged our collaborators in Europe to consider the possibility of chronic renal damage among the patients they had diagnosed. Most initially felt that there was no significant sequelae after HFRS. When they specifically looked, however, they found that about 10% of their hospitalized patients left with some evidence of persistent renal dysfunction (A. Antoniadis and J. W. LeDuc 1990, unpublished observation). Few of these patients have been systematically followed over time, and those that have were only followed for a few years. Even so, several continue to have a demonstrable inability to concentrate urine, other indications of possible permanent kidney damage, or essential hypertension. We are actively investigating this facet of the disease to determine how frequently chronic disease follows HFRS.

These studies indicate that HFRS does occur within the US and produces an illness similar to that seen in other parts of the world where disease is due to rat-borne hantaviruses. They also suggest that infection may produce serious sequelae among populations that are exposed to rats in this country.

The possibility of long-term renal dysfunction after a hantaviral infection has not been well studied. One of the few studies examined Korean Conflict veterans who had suffered hantaviral infections and a group of matched controls in 1956, about three to five years after most cases would have been infected (78). This study found a significant increase in the rate of genitourinary hospital admissions among the HFRS cases, which increased with the severity of their original disease. Other findings included hyposthenuria, persistent mild albuminuria, and hypertension. Similarly, Lähdevirta (42, 44) examined patients with nephropathia epidemica 1–6.5 years after disease and found evidence of depressed renal tubular function and hypertension in some of these patients. Hypertension was especially common in his follow-up population; nearly 75% of the individuals were hypertensive. These indications of chronic renal dysfunction and hypertension are consistent with the hypothesis that their condition could evolve over time to condition similar to those seen among the Baltimore residents.

A planned experiment is to reexamine the Korean Conflict veterans now, nearly 40 years after their initial disease, to determine their present level of kidney function. The staff of the Medical Follow Up Agency, in collaboration with our laboratory, has initiated plans to conduct such a study, and those results may be available in the near future. Fortunately, the records from the original study by Rubini et al (78) are still intact at the Follow Up Agency, and we should be able to make some very interesting comparisons.

Providing the proof that infection with a hantavirus may predispose an individual to hypertension and chronic renal sequelae is of great relevance. In excess of $50 billion a year is spent in the US for medical care for kidney and urologic disease. About $3 billion of that total is for federal Medicare payments for dialysis and transplantation for persons with end-stage kidney disease (40). This total is growing, while the funds available for medical care, in general, are shrinking. If even a small portion of this burden is a consequence of past hantaviral infections, for example the 2% that we found in our Baltimore dialysis units, then we as a nation are spending about $100 million a year on a condition with opportunities for prevention, control, and clinical intervention. Clearly, this emerging disease requires our immediate attention and action.

CONCLUDING COMMENTS

The past decade has witnessed a tremendous growth in our knowledge regarding the epidemiology, molecular biology, and diseases caused by the hantaviruses. We now know that several different viruses are capable of causing clinically similar diseases. These viruses are maintained in nature primarily within rodent reservoirs, in which they cause chronic infections with persistent viral shedding in secretions or excretions. The hantaviruses are distributed far more widely than once suspected. The diagnosis of acute HFRS can now be made rapidly and accurately, and ribavirin, an antiviral drug, appears to be efficacious in its treatment, if given early in the course of disease. The molecular characterization of these viruses has progressed rapidly and holds the promise of novel vaccine design and manufacture in the near future. Finally, preliminary evidence suggests that past hantaviral infection may be associated with subsequent development of chronic renal disease, a phenomenon that may have considerable domestic and global public health and economic implications.

Literature Cited

1. Antic, D., Lim, B.-U., Kang, C. Y. 1991. Nucleotide sequence and coding capacity of the large (L) genomic RNA segment of Seoul 80-39 virus, a member of the Hantavirus genus. *Virus Res.* 19:59–65
2. Antic, D., Lim, B.-U., Kang, C. Y. 1991. Molecular characterization of the M genomic segment of the Seoul 80-39 virus; nucleotide and amino acid sequence comparisons with other hantaviruses reveal the evolutionary pathway. *Virus Res.* 19:47–58
3. Antoniadis, A., Grekas, D., Rossi, C. A., LeDuc, J. W. 1987. Isolation of a hantavirus from a severely ill patient with hemorrhagic fever with renal syndrome in Greece. *J. Infect. Dis.* 156:1010–13
4. Antoniadis, A., LeDuc, J. W., Daniel-Alexiou, S. 1987. Clinical and epidemiological aspects of hemorrhagic fever with renal syndrome (HFRS) in Greece. *Eur. J. Epidemiol.* 3:295–301
5. Avsic-Zupanc, T., Likar, M., Novakovic, S., Cizman, B., Kraigher, A., et al. 1990. Evidence of the presence of two hantaviruses in Slovenia, Yugoslavia. *Arch. Virol.* (Suppl. 1):87–94
6. Baek, L. J., Yanagihara, R., Gibbs, C. J. Jr., Miyazaki, M., Gajdusek, D. C. 1988. Leakey virus: a new hantavirus isolated from *Mus musculus* in the United States. *J. Gen. Virol.* 69:3129–32
7. Brummer-Korvenkontio, M., Vaheri, A., Hovi, T., von Bonsdorff, C.-H., Vuorimies, J., et al. 1980. Nephropathia epidemica: detection of antigen in bank voles and serologic diagnosis of human infection. *J. Infect. Dis.* 141:131–34
8. Bruno, P., Hassell, L. H., Brown, J., Tanner, W., Lau, A. 1990. The protean manifestations of hemorrhagic fever with renal syndrome. *Ann. Intern. Med.* 113:385–91
9. Chan, Y. C., Wong, T. W., Yap, E. H., Tan, H. C., Lee, H. W., et al. 1987. Haemorrhagic fever with renal syndrome involving the liver. *Med. J. Aust.* 147:248–49
10. Chen, L., Wang, H., Gu, X., Chen, S., Qin, G., et al. 1987. Early diagnosis of hemorrhagic fever with renal syndrome

by IgM ELISA technique. *Chin. Med. J.* 100:402–6
11. Childs, J. E., Glass, G. E., Korch, G. W., LeDuc, J. W. 1987. Prospective seroepidemiology of hantaviruses and population dynamics of small mammal communities of Baltimore, Maryland. *Am. J. Trop. Med. Hyg.* 37:648–62
12. Childs, J. E., Glass, G. E., Korch, G. W., LeDuc, J. W. 1988. The ecology and epizootiology of hantaviral infections in small mammal communities of Baltimore: a review and synthesis. *Bull. Soc. Vector Ecol.* 13:113–22
13. Childs, J. E., Korch, G. W., Glass, G. E., LeDuc, J. W., Shah, K. V. 1987. Epizootiology of hantavirus infections in Baltimore: isolation of a virus from Norway rats, and characteristics of infected rat populations. *Am. J. Epidemiol.* 126:55–68
14. Childs, J. E., Korch, G. W., Smith, G. A., Terry, A. D., LeDuc, J. W. 1985. Geographical distribution and age related prevalence of Hantaan-like virus in rat populations of Baltimore, Maryland, USA. *Am. J. Trop. Med. Hyg.* 34:385–87
15. Cizman, B., Ferluga, D., Kaplan-Pavlovcic, S., Koselj, M., Drinovec, J., et al. 1989. Renal involvement in hantavirus disease. *Adv. Exp. Med. Biol.* 252:173–80
16. Desmyter, J., LeDuc, J. W., Johnson, K. M., Brasseur, F., Deckers, C., et al. 1983. Laboratory rat associated outbreak of haemorrhagic fever with renal syndrome due to Hantaan-like virus in Belgium. *Lancet* ii:1445–48
17. Dournon, E., Moriniere, B., Matheron, S., Girard, P. M., Gonzalez, J. P., et al. 1984. HFRS after a wild rodent bite in the Haute-Savoie-and risk of exposure to Hantaan-like virus in a Paris laboratory. *Lancet* i:676–677
18. Earle, D. P. 1954. Symposium on epidemic hemorrhagic fever. *Am. J. Med.* 16:617–704
19. Forthal, D. N., Bauer, S. P., McCormick, J. B. 1987. Antibody to hemorrhagic fever with renal syndrome viruses (Hantaviruses) in the United States. *Am. J. Epidemiol.* 126:1210–13
20. French, G. R., Foulke, R. S., Brand, O.

A., Eddy, G. A., Lee, H. W., et al. 1981. Korean hemorrhagic fever: propagation of the etiologic agent in a cell line of human origin. *Science* 211:1046–48

21. Gajdusek, G. C. 1989. See Ref. 52, pp. 1–10

22. Gajdusek, D. C., Goldfarb, L. G., Goldgaber, D. 1987. *Bibliography of Hemorrhagic Fever with Renal Syndrome.* NIH Publ. No. 88-2603. Washington, DC: US Dep. Health and Human Serv. 290 pp. 2nd ed.

23. Gibbs, C. J. Jr., Takenaka, A., Franko, M., Gajdusek, D. C., Griffin, M. D., et al. 1982. Seroepidemiology of Hantaan virus. *Lancet* ii:1406–7

24. Giebel, L. B., Stohwasser, R., Zoller, L., Bautz, E. K. F., Darai, G. 1989. Determination of the coding capacity of the M genome segment of nephropathia epidemica Hallnas B1 by molecular cloning and nucleotide sequence analysis. *Virology* 172:498–505

25. Glass, G. E., Childs, J. E., Korch, G. W., LeDuc, J. W. 1988. Association of intraspecific wounding with hantaviral infection in wild rats *(Rattus norvegicus).* *Epidemiol. Infect.* 101:459–72

26. Glass, G. E., Childs, J. E., Watson, A. J., LeDuc, J. W. 1990. Association of chronic renal disease, hypertension, and infection with a rat-borne hantavirus. *Arch. Virol.* (Suppl. 1):69–80

27. Gligic, A., Frusic, M., Obradovic, M., Stojanovic, R., Hlaca, D., et al. 1989. Hemorrhagic fever with renal syndrome in Yugoslavia: Antigenic characterization of Hantaviruses isolated from *Apodemus flavicollis* and *Clethrionomys glareolus.* *Am. J. Trop. Med. Hyg.* 41:109–15

28. Gligic, A., Obradovic, M., Stojanovic, R., Vujosevic, N., Ovcaric, A., et al. 1989. Epidemic hemorrhagic fever with renal syndrome in Yugoslavia, 1986. *Am. J. Trop. Med. Hyg.* 41:102–8

29. Goldgaber, D., Lee, P.-W., Yanagihara, R., Gibbs, C. J. Jr., Gajdusek, D. C. 1985. Quantitation of Hantaan virus infectivity, antigen, and antibody by immunoenzyme methods. In *Proc. 1st Int. Symp. on Public Health in Asia and the Pacific Basin. Hemorrhagic Fever with Renal Syndrome,* ed. T. R. Bender, A. R. Diwan, J. S. Raymond, pp. 55–59. Honolulu: Univ. of Hawaii at Manoa

30. Hayashi, T., Kikuchi, K., Urasawa, S., Suzuki, A., Yachi, A., et al. 1981. Comprehensive reports of epidemic hemorrhagic fever (Korean hemorrhagic fever) observed in Sapporo Medical College in 1981. *Sapporo Med. J.* 51: (Suppl.):K1–K41

31. Huggins, J. W., Hsiang, C. M., Cosgriff, T. M., Guang, M. Y., Smith, J. I., et al. 1991. Prospective, doubleblind, concurrent, placebo-controlled, clinical trial of intravenous ribavirin therapy of hemorrhagic fever with renal syndrome (HFRS). *J. Infect. Dis.* In press

32. Hung, T., Xia, S.-M., Song, G., Liao, H.-X., Chao, T.-X., et al. 1983. Viruses of classical and mild forms of haemorrhagic fever with renal syndrome isolated in China have similar Bunyavirus-like morphology. *Lancet* i:589–91

33. Hung, T., Xia, S.-M., Zhao, T. X., Zhou, J. Y., Song, G., et al. 1983. Morphological evidence for identifying the viruses of hemorrhagic fever with renal syndrome as candidate members of the Bunyaviridae family. *Arch. Virol.* 78: 137–44

34. Isegawa, Y., Fujiwara, Y., Ohshima, A., Fukunaga, R., Murakami, H., et al. 1990. Nucleotide sequence of the M genome segment of hemorrhagic fever with renal syndrome virus strain B-1. *Nucleic Acids Res.* 18:4936

35. Kessler, M., Prieur, J. P., Hurault de Ligny, B., Schmit, J. L., Dureax, J. B. 1986. La fievre hemorragique avec syndrome renal a propos de treize cas observes en Lorraine. *Nephrologie* 4: 147–52

36. Koolen, M. I., Jansen, H. L. H., Assmann, K. J. M., Clement, J., Van Liebergen, F. J. H. M. 1989. A sporadic case of acute hantavirus nephropathy in The Netherlands. *Neth. J. Med.* 35:25–32

37. Korch, G. W., Childs, J. E., Glass, G. E., Rossi, C. A., LeDuc, J. W. 1989. Serological evidence of hantaviral infections within small mammal communities of Baltimore, Maryland: spatial and temporal patterns and host range. *Am. J. Trop. Med. Hyg.* 41:230–40

38. Korpela, H., Lähdevirta, J. 1978. The role of small rodents and patterns of living in the epidemiology of nephropathia epidemica. *Scand. J. Infect. Dis.* 10: 303–5

39. Kraft, V., Meyer, B. 1990. Seromonitoring in small laboratory animal colonies. A five year survey: 1984–1988. *Z. Versuchstierkd.* 33:29–35

40. Krakauer, H. 1986. Assessment of alternative technologies for the treatment of end-stage renal disease. *Isr. J. Med. Sci.* 22:245–59

41. Kulagin, C. M., Fedorova, H., Ketiladze, E. C. 1962. Laboratory outbreak

of hemorrhagic fever with renal syndrome (Clinico-epidemiological characteristics). *J. Microbiol. Epidemiol. Immunol.* 33:121–26 (in Russian)

42. Lähdevirta, J. 1971. Nephropathia epidemica in Finland. A clinical, histopathological, and epidemiological study. *Ann. Clin. Res.* 3 (Suppl. 8):1–154

43. Lähdevirta, J. 1982. Clinical features of HFRS in Scandinavia as compared with East Asia. *Scand. J. Infect. Dis.* (Suppl.) 36:93–95

44. Lähdevirta, J., Collan, Y., Jokinen, E. J., Hiltunen, R. 1978. Renal sequelae to nephropathia epidemica. *Acta Pathol. Microbiol. Scand. Sect. A* 86:265–71

45. LeDuc, J. W. 1987. Epidemiology of Hantaan and related viruses. *Lab. Anim. Sci.* 37:413–18

46. LeDuc, J. W., Antoniadis, A., Siamopoulos, K. 1986. Epidemiological investigations following an outbreak of hemorrhagic fever with renal syndrome in Greece. *Am. J. Trop. Med. Hyg.* 35:654–59

47. LeDuc, J. W., Ksiazek, T. G., Rossi, C. A., Dalrymple, J. M. 1990. A retrospective analysis of sera collected by the hemorrhagic fever commission during the Korean Conflict. *J. Infect. Dis.* 162:1182–84

48. LeDuc, J. W., Smith, G. A., Childs, J. E., Pinheiro, F. P., Maiztegui, J. I., et al. 1986. Global survey of antibody to Hantaan-related viruses among peridomestic rodents. *Bull. WHO* 64:139–44

49. LeDuc, J. W., Smith, G. A., Johnson, K. M. 1984. Hantaan-like viruses from domestic rats captured in the United States. *Am. J. Trop. Med. Hyg.* 33:992–98

50. LeDuc, J. W., Smith, G. A., Macy, M., Hay, R. J. 1985. Certified cell lines of rat origin appear free of infection with Hantavirus. *J. Infect. Dis.* 152:1082–83

51. Lee, H. W. 1982. Korean hemorrhagic fever. *Prog. Med. Virol.* 28:96–113

52. Lee, H. W. 1989. WHO collaborating center for virus reference and research. In *Manual of Hemorrhagic Fever with Renal Syndrome*, ed. H. W. Lee, J. M. Dalrymple, pp. 11–18. WHO Collaborating Center for Virus Reference and Research (Hemorrhagic fever with renal syndrome). Seoul: Korea Univ.

53. Lee, H. W. 1989. See Ref. 52, pp. 36–38

54. Lee, H. W. 1989. Hemorrhagic fever with renal syndrome in Korea. *Rev. Infect. Dis.* 11 (Suppl. 4):S864–76

55. Lee, H. W., Ahn, C. N., Song, J. W.,

Baek, L. J., Seo, T. J., Park, S. C. 1990. Field trial of an inactivated vaccine against hemorrhagic fever with renal syndrome. *Arch. Virol.* (Suppl. 1): 35–47

56. Lee, H. W., Baek, L. J., Johnson, K. M. 1982. Isolation of Hantaan virus, the etiologic agent of Korean hemorrhagic fever, from wild urban rats. *J. Infect. Dis.* 146:638–44

57. Lee, H. W., French, G. R., Lee, P. W., Baek, L. J., Tsuchiya, K., et al. 1981. Observations on natural and laboratory infection of rodents with the etiologic agent of Korean hemorrhagic fever. *Am. J. Trop. Med. Hyg.* 30:477–82

58. Lee, H. W., Johnson, K. M. 1982. Laboratory-acquired infections with Hantaan virus, the etiologic agent of Korean hemorrhagic fever. *J. Infect. Dis.* 146:645–51

59. Lee, H. W., Lee, M. C., Cho, K. S. 1980. Management of Korean haemorrhagic fever. *Med. Prog.* 2:15–21

60. Lee, H. W., Lee, P.-W. 1976. Korean hemorrhagic fever. I. Demonstration of causative antigen and antibodies. *Korean J. Intern. Med.* 19:371–83

61. Lee, H. W., Lee, P.-W., Baek, L. J., Song, C. K., Seong, I. W. 1981. Intraspecific transmission of Hantaan virus, etiologic agent of Korean hemorrhagic fever, in the rodent *Apodemus agrarius*. *Am. J. Trop. Med. Hyg.* 30:1106–12

62. Lee, H. W., Lee, P.-W., Johnson, K. M. 1978. Isolation of the etiologic agent of Korean hemorrhagic fever. *J. Infect. Dis.* 137:298–308

63. Lee, P.-W., Amyx, H. L., Yanagihara, R., Gajdusek, D. C., Goldgaber, D., et al. 1985. Partial characterization of Prospect Hill virus isolated from meadow voles in the United States. *J. Infect. Dis.* 152:826–29

64. Lee, P.-W., Meegan, J. M., LeDuc, J. W., Tkachenko, E. A., Tvanov, A. P., et al. 1989. See Ref. 52, pp. 75–106

65. Lloyd, G., Bowen, E. T. W., Jones, N., Pendry, A. 1984. HFRS outbreak associated with laboratory rats in UK. *Lancet* ii:1175–76

66. Lloyd, G., Jones, N. 1986. Infection of laboratory workers with hantavirus acquired from immunocytomas propagated in laboratory rats. *J. Infect.* 12:117–25

67. Niklasson, B., Kjelsson, T. 1988. Detection of nephropathia epidemica (Puumala virus)-specific immunoglobulin M by enzyme-linked immunosorbent assay. *J. Clin. Microbiol.* 26:1519–23

68. Niklasson, B., LeDuc, J. W. 1987. Epidemiology of nephropathia epidemica in Sweden. *J. Infect. Dis.* 155:269–76
69. Niklasson, B., Tkachenko, E., Ivanov, A. P., van der Groen, G., Wiger, D., et al. 1990. Haemorrhagic fever with renal syndrome: Evaluation of ELISA for detection of Puumala-virus-specific IgG and IgM. *Res. Virol.* 141:637–48
70. Nystrom, K. 1977. Incidence and prevalence of endemic benign (epidemic) nephropathy in AC County, Sweden, in relation to population density and prevalence of small rodents. *Umea Univ. Med. Diss. (New Ser.)* 30:1–92
71. Parrington, M. A., Kang, C. Y. 1990. Nucleotide sequence analysis of the S genomic segment of Prospect Hill virus: Comparison with the prototype Hantavirus. *Virology* 175:167–75
72. Parrington, M. A., Lee, P. W., Kang, C. Y. 1991. Molecular characterization of the Prospect Hill virus M RNA segment: a comparison with the M RNA segments of other hantaviruses. *J. Gen. Virol.* 72:1845–54
73. Paul, J. R., McClure, W. 1958. Epidemic hemorrhagic fever attack rates among United Nations troops during the Korean War. *Am. J. Hyg.* 68:126–28
74. Pon, E., McKee, K. T. Jr., Diniega, B. M., Merrell, B., Corwin, A., Ksiazek, T. G. 1990. Outbreak of hemorrhagic fever with renal syndrome among US Marines in Korea. *Am. J. Trop. Med. Hyg.* 42:612–19
75. Powell, G. M. 1954. Hemorrhagic fever: a study of 300 cases. *Medicine (Baltimore)* 33:97–153
76. Rollin, P. E., Laveran, H., Gonzalez, J. P., Coudrier, D., Sureau, P., et al. 1987. Fievre hemorrhagique avec syndrome renal dans le centre de la France. *Presse Med.* 16:175
77. Rossi, C. A., Schmaljohn, C. S., Meegan, J. M., LeDuc, J. W. 1991. Diagnostic potential of a baculovirus-expressed nucleocapsid protein for hantaviruses. *Arch. Virol.* (Suppl. 1):19–28
78. Rubini, M. E., Jablon, S., McDowell, M. E. 1960. Renal residuals of acute epidemic hemorrhagic fever. *Arch. Inst. Med.* 106:378–87
79. Salvadori, M., Lombardi, M., Bandini, S., Leoncini, F., Bartolozzi, D., et al. 1989. Acute renal involvement in Hantavirus infection: first report in Italy. *J. Nephrol.* 1:17–22
80. Schmaljohn, C. S. 1990. Nucleotide sequence of the L genome segment of Hantaan virus. *Nucleic Acids Res.* 18:6728
81. Schmaljohn, C. S., Chu, Y.-K., Schmaljohn, A. L., Dalrymple, J. M. 1990. Antigenic subunits of Hantaan virus expressed by baculovirus and vaccinia virus recombinants. *J. Virol.* 64:3162–70
82. Schmaljohn, C. S., Dalrymple, J. M. 1983. Analysis of Hantaan virus RNA: evidence for a new genus of Bunyaviridae. *Virology* 131:482–91
83. Schmaljohn, C. S., Hasty, S. E., Dalrymple, J. M., LeDuc, J. W., Lee, H. W., et al. 1985. Antigenic and genetic properties of viruses linked to hemorrhagic fever with renal syndrome. *Science* 227:1041–44
84. Schmaljohn, C. S., Hasty, S. E., Harrison, S. A., Dalrymple, J. M. 1983. Characterization of Hantaan virions, the prototype virus of hemorrhagic fever with renal syndrome. *J. Infect. Dis.* 148:1005–12
85. Schmaljohn, C. S., Jennings, G. B., Hay, J., Dalrymple, J. M. 1986. Coding strategy of the S genome segment of Hantaan virus. *Virology* 155:633–43
86. Schmaljohn, C. S., Lee, H. W., Dalrymple, J. M. 1987. Detection of hantaviruses with RNA probes generated from recombinant DNA. *Arch. Virol.* 95:291–301
87. Schmaljohn, C. S., Schmaljohn, A. L., Dalrymple, J. M. 1987. Hantaan virus M RNA: coding strategy, nucleotide sequence, and gene order. *Virology* 157:31–39
88. Sommer, A.-I., Traavik, T., Mehl, R., Berdal, B. P., Dalrymple, J. 1988. Hemorrhagic fever with renal syndrome (Nephropathia epidemica) in Norway: Seroepidemiology 1981–1985. *Scand. J. Infect. Dis.* 20:267–74
89. Stohwasser, R., Giebel, L. B., Zoller, L., Bautz, E. K. F., Darai, G. 1990. Molecular characterization of the RNA S segment of nephropathia epidemica virus strain Hallnas B1. *Virology* 174:79–86
90. Sugiyama, K., Matsuura, Y., Morita, C., Shiga, S., Akao, Y., et al. 1984. An immune adherence assay for discrimination between etiologic agents of hemorrhagic fever with renal syndrome. *J. Infect. Dis.* 149:67–73
91. Takenaka, A., Gibbs, C. J. Jr., Gajdusek, D. C. 1985. Antiviral neutralizing antibody to Hantaan virus as determined by plaque reduction technique. *Arch. Virol.* 84:197–206
92. Tsai, T. F. 1987. Hemorrhagic fever with renal syndrome: clinical aspects. *Lab. Anim. Sci.* 37:419–27
93. Tsai, T. F. 1987. Hemorrhagic fever

with renal syndrome: mode of transmission to humans. *Lab. Anim. Sci.* 37: 428–30

94. Tsai, T. F., Bauer, S. P., Sasso, D. R., Whitfield, S. G., McCormick, J. B., et al. 1985. Serological and virological evidence of a Hantaan virus-related enzootic in the United States. *J. Infect. Dis.* 152:126–36

95. van Ypersele de Strihou, C., Mery, J. P. 1989. Hantavirus-related acute interstitial nephritis in Western Europe. Expansion of a world-wide zoonosis. *Q. J. Med.*, New Ser. 73:941–50

96. van Ypersele de Strihou, C., Vandenbroucke, J. M., Levy, M., Doyen, C., Cosyns, J. P., et al. 1983. Diagnosis of epidemic and sporadic interstitial nephritis due to Hantaan-like virus in Belgium. *Lancet* ii:1493

97. Walker, E., Pinkerton, I. W., Lloyd, G. 1984. Scottish case of haemorrhagic fever with renal syndrome. *Lancet* ii:982

98. Xiao, S.-Y., Yanagihara, R., Godec, M. S., Eldadah, Z. A., Johnson, B. K., et al. 1991. Detection of hantavirus RNA in tissues of experimentally infected mice using reverse transcriptase-directed polymerase chain reaction. *J. Med. Virol.* 33:277–82

99. Xu, Z. Y., Gou, C. S., Wu, Y. L.,

Zhang, X. W., Liu, K. 1985. Epidemiological studies of hemorrhagic fever with renal syndrome: analysis of risk factors and of transmission. *J. Infect. Dis.* 152:137–44

100. Yamanishi, K., Tanishita, O., Tamura, M., Asada, H., Kondo, K., et al. 1988. Development of inactivated vaccine against virus causing haemorrhagic fever with renal syndrome. *Vaccine* 6:278–82

101. Yanagihara, R. 1990. Hantavirus infection in the United States: epizootiology and epidemiology. *Rev. Infect. Dis.* 12:449–57

102. Yanagihara, R., Amyx, H. L., Gajdusek, D. C. 1985. Experimental infection with Puumala virus, the etiologic agent of nephropathia epidemica, in bank voles *(Clethrionomys glareolus)*. *J. Virol.* 55:34–38

103. Yanagihara, R., Daum, C. A., Lee, P.-W., Baek, L. J., Amyx, H. L., et al. 1987. Serological survey of Prospect Hill virus infection in indigenous wild rodents in the USA. *Trans. R. Soc. Trop. Med. Hyg.* 81:42–45

104. Yanagihara, R., Gajdusek, D. C., Gibbs, C. J. Jr., Traub, R. 1984. Prospect Hill virus: serological evidence for infection in mammalogists. *N. Engl. J. Med.* 310:1325–26

Annu. Rev. Publ. Health. 1992. 13:99–126

HOW MUCH PHYSICAL ACTIVITY IS GOOD FOR HEALTH?

S. N. Blair, H. W. Kohl, and N. F. Gordon

Divisions of Epidemiology and Exercise Physiology, Institute for Aerobics Research, Dallas, Texas 75230

R. S. Paffenbarger, Jr.

Division of Epidemiology, Stanford University School of Medicine, Stanford, California 95305

KEY WORDS: physical fitness, cardiovascular disease, cancer, diabetes mellitus, musculoskeletal system

INTRODUCTION

Physical Activity from Prehistory to the Present

Remains of our early, human-like ancestors, *Australopithecus afarensis,* have been dated as 3.5–3.8 million years old. Nearly 4 million years of evolution of the human family, *Hominidae,* produced modern humans, *H. sapiens,* by approximately 35,000 years ago (71). The earliest hominids were scavengers; but, by about 1 million years ago, hunting and gathering was firmly established as a way of life for human beings. A hunting and gathering lifestyle involves high energy expenditure for several days a week, with peak bouts of strenuous physical activity (26, 93).

The next major change in human sociocultural development was the domestication of plants and animals and the rise of agriculture, which occurred only 10,000 years ago. Industrialization advances over the past 200 years led to further urbanization and the rise of the middle-class. But, even during this period, most individuals had relatively high energy expenditures compared with those of society at the end of the twentieth century.

Human energy expenditure requirements have declined over the twentieth century, a trend that has apparently accelerated during the technological era

99

0163-7525/92/0501-0000$02.00

following World War II (92). Increased automotive transportation, widespread adoption of sedentary activities, and labor-saving devices are major contributors to the decline in energy expenditure by individuals. The metabolic energy demands of previously strenuous jobs, such as working as a longshoreman or coal miner, are much lower today than in the past because of containerization, mechanization, and automation.

Humans evolved to be active animals and may not be able to adapt well to the modern sedentary lifestyle. This point is well stated by Eaton et al (27): "From a genetic standpoint, humans living today are Stone Age hunter-gatherers displaced through time to a world that differs from that for which our genetic constitution was selected." This teleological argument of human genetic selection and the need for physical activity does not prove that activity is necessary for health, but it may serve as a useful launching point for the review and discussion that follows.

Development of Exercise Science

The scientific study of exercise is a recent development (62). Physiologists in the latter part of the nineteenth century began to use exercise to perturb body systems to understand physiological functioning better. Indeed, three exercise physiologists, Meyerhof (muscle metabolism) and Krogh, and Hill (physiology of exercise), have been awarded the Nobel prize for their research (74).

Over the past 70 years, hundreds of studies have documented the type and extent of changes with physical training that occur in skeletal muscle, the circulatory system, pulmonary function, the heart and vascular system, and endocrine function. These studies have been done in the young and the elderly, in men and women, with different training protocols, and under varying environmental conditions. The earlier studies typically had small samples, frequently lacked control groups, were short-term, and had other design flaws. These shortcomings have been overcome in studies over the past 10–20 years.

Systematic studies on the health effects of physical activity are more recent, primarily confined to the past 30–40 years. Morris et al (75–77) are generally credited with a leading role in formulating the modern physical activity–coronary heart disease hypothesis with their studies on London transport workers and, later, on British civil servants.

Definitions

Several key terms, central to the purpose of this chapter, need to be defined. We adopt the definitions of Caspersen et al (17) for physical activity, exercise, and physical fitness:

1. Physical activity: Any bodily movement produced by skeletal muscles that results in energy expenditure.

2. Exercise: Planned, structured, and repetitive bodily movement done to improve or maintain one or more components of physical fitness.
3. Physical fitness: A set of attributes that people have or achieve that relates to the ability to perform physical activity.

The physical fitness component that has been most frequently studied for an association to health is aerobic power or, as it is measured in the physiology laboratory, maximal oxygen uptake. This attribute is also called cardiovascular, cardiorespiratory, or endurance fitness. Unless otherwise specified, we use the term physical fitness to refer to aerobic power.

The other major term that needs to be defined is health. In this chapter, we take a broad view of health, one that not only includes freedom from disease, but also the ability to achieve activities of daily living. Disease endpoints are frequently used in studies of physical activity. For our purposes, however, the definition of health goes beyond freedom from clinical disease to include a focus on functional capability or functional health status. This latter characteristic includes avoidance of functional disability, but also extends to higher levels of functional capability. One of the most well-documented effects of regular physical activity is a higher level of physical fitness. This permits a higher level of functional ability to participate in a wide array of life's activities with ease and enjoyment. The active and fit person is not likely to become fatigued by the routine activities of daily living and has a greater capacity to meet emergencies or participate in vigorous recreational activities.

Purpose of this Chapter

This chapter reviews existing clinical exercise studies and population-based investigations of physical activity and physical health. We concentrate on potential preventive etiologic associations, with little emphasis on therapeutic effects of physical activity on health and disease. We integrate the findings from these two research fronts, point out agreements and disagreements, and summarize the results to assess how much physical activity is required for health. The descriptive epidemiology of physical activity in the United States and the public health burden of a sedentary lifestyle is discussed, and public health recommendations for physical activity and physical fitness are presented.

CLINICAL EXERCISE STUDIES

Exercise and Physical Fitness

Exercise-trained individuals have higher levels of physical fitness, and the relation between activity and fitness was probably known in antiquity. Athletes and soldiers have long been trained to improve their capacity for performance. Carefully done studies to quantify the training required to produce an improvement in fitness are a recent phenomenon; in 1957, Karvonen et al (55) published one of the first of these studies. Dozens of studies over the past 35 years focused attention on three principles of exercise prescription: intensity, frequency, and duration (5).

INTENSITY   For the past several decades, the generally held view is that there is a minimum exercise intensity required to stimulate an improvement in physical fitness. The American College of Sports Medicine (ACSM) was the first scientific organization to publish official statements on exercise prescription. Their 1975 textbook set 70% of maximal oxygen uptake as the minimum recommended exercise intensity for improving physical fitness (4). Subsequent studies lowered recommendations for the intensity threshold, and the third edition of the ACSM book in 1986 (3) recommended a minimum exercise intensity of 50%. The 1991 fourth edition (2) recommends moderate exercise, defined as exercise between 40–60% of maximal capacity, as appropriate for many persons. A 1990 ACSM position stand states that "persons with a low fitness level can achieve a significant training effect with . . . 40–50%" of capacity (5). An alternate hypothesis to a threshold level of intensity is that the response to exercise training is primarily, if not exclusively, dependent upon the total energy expended in exercise and not intensity. This distinction is important and needs additional clarification. If a minimum intensity threshold exists, it probably varies depending upon the initial fitness level of the participant, the duration of the exercise session, the length of the training period, and perhaps other individual characteristics of the person undergoing training.

DURATION   The ACSM recommends 20–60 minutes of continuous aerobic activity for each exercise session (2, 5). There is an interrelationship between intensity and duration in their impact on fitness change. Low intensity activity must be sustained longer than high intensity activity to have the same effect on improvement in aerobic power. Again, the total energy expenditure of the exercise session is likely the critical determining factor for fitness change.

Investigators have challenged the belief that continuous aerobic activity is necessary to achieve a training effect. A recent study addresses the issue by comparing two different training regimens (21). One group trained five days per week with one 30-minute session per day. A second group trained five days per week with three 10-minute sessions per day. Improvements in physical fitness after eight weeks of training were similar, thus suggesting that the accumulation of activity over the course of the day can produce a training effect.

FREQUENCY   The ACSM recommends participation in exercise training three to five days per week (2, 5). Most studies show little change in physical fitness if exercise is done less than three days per week, unless the exercise is quite strenuous. And, exercising more than five days per week does not result in greater improvement in fitness than training five days per week (5).

Physiological Effects of Acute and Chronic Exercise

The potential beneficial effects of acute and chronic exercise on physical fitness and health have been intensely investigated in recent years. Existing laboratory and clinical studies have documented a broad array of physiologic benefits, including metabolic, hormonal, and cardiovascular adjustments that are evident at rest, as well as during and following both maximal and submaximal exertion (14). Acute and chronic exercise also reduce anxiety and depression and positively impact other psychological characteristics of both normal persons and those with clinical disorders (99). In this section, we focus only on those key physiological benefits that have been hypothesized to contribute toward a reduced risk for mortality, especially from cardiovascular disease and cancer.

IMPROVEMENT OF BALANCE BETWEEN MYOCARDIAL OXYGEN DEMAND AND SUPPLY   The myocardial oxygen requirement during exercise is determined by a variety of factors, the most important of which are reflected by the rate-pressure product (that is, the product of the heart rate and systolic blood pressure) (2). Because the rate-pressure product increases linearly during graded exercise, so too does the myocardial oxygen demand. Following exercise training, the rate-pressure product elicited by a given submaximal exercise intensity is usually substantially attenuated (117). This enables a specific physical activity to be performed with a lessened myocardial oxygen demand and, therefore, a reduced risk for myocardial ischemia.

Currently, there is no direct evidence that exercise conditioning induces the formation of coronary collaterals in humans, and this issue will probably not be resolved until more sophisticated techniques for assessing coronary collateralization are developed and utilized in clinical exercise training studies (56). However, there is now preliminary evidence that exercise training may indeed enhance myocardial oxygen delivery and/or utilization (29, 56).

ECCENTRIC VENTRICULAR HYPERTROPHY   Myocardial hypertrophy is an adaptive mechanism that develops in response to increased hemodynamic loading of the heart. Depending on the specific nature of the hemodynamic loading, the resultant increase in cardiac mass is associated with characteristic alterations in the volume of the cardiac cavities and in the thickness of their walls. As an adaptive response to volume overloading of the left ventricle, dynamic exercise training often produces an increase in left ventricular wall thickness and, to a greater degree, chamber size. This so-called eccentric hypertrophy is believed to be associated with an increase in myocyte vascularity that is commensurate with the degree of hypertrophy of the myocytes themselves and thereby improves myocardial function and assures myocyte health (123).

Left ventricular function is a principal determinant of the risk of mortality following an acute myocardial infarction. Because persons with eccentric hypertrophy could suffer relatively less impairment in left ventricular function for a given amount of myocardial damage, Ekelund et al (31) have hypothesized that they may be better able to survive an acute myocardial infarction.

REDUCED RISK FOR LETHAL VENTRICULAR ARRHYTHMIAS   Noakes et al (81) have shown that the exercise-trained rat heart has a reduced propensity for ventricular fibrillation during normoxia, hypoxia, and acute regional myocardial ischemia. They have further demonstrated that exercise training increases the ventricular fibrillation threshold of the previously infarcted isolated rat heart before and after the onset of reinfarction (96). These findings imply that regular exercise, before or after an acute myocardial infarction, may act directly on the myocardium to enhance its resistance to lethal ventricular arrhythmias. Although human studies are needed to substantiate this hypothesis, it is compatible with the finding of metaanalyses, which demonstrate that cardiac rehabilitation protects against mortality (which is mostly related to lethal ventricular arrhythmias) rather than reinfarction (82, 83), and epidemiologic studies, which link a physically active lifestyle with a reduced risk for sudden cardiac death (76, 84).

FAVORABLE EFFECT ON BLOOD COAGULABILITY   Total occlusion of a coronary artery as a result of thrombus formation at the site of an atherosclerotic stenosis is believed to be the final precipitating event in more than 90% of acute myocardial infarctions. Although conflicting findings have been reported and additional research is still needed, exercise training is thought to reduce the adhesiveness and aggregability of blood platelets (30, 101). Moreover, whereas physical inactivity appears to decrease fibrinolysis, exercise training tends to moderately augment it (30), which would improve the body's ability to dissolve thrombi if they form.

IMPROVED PLASMA LIPIDS AND LIPOPROTEINS   Table 1 presents a summary of the effect of acute and chronic exercise on plasma lipids and lipoproteins. Of these benefits, perhaps the most relevant is the increase in high density lipoprotein (HDL)-cholesterol. Generally, a single bout of moderate-to-long duration aerobic exercise evokes a 4–6 mg/dl increase in the HDL-cholesterol levels of men and women (41). Recent studies by Hughes et al (51, 52) further suggest that although exercise intensity does not appear to be a significant modifier of the acute impact of aerobic exercise on HDL-cholesterol levels in men, exercise duration does. In their study, the increase

Table 1 Results of studies investigating the relationship between aerobic exercise training and lipoprotein levels[a,b]

	Studies of acute exercise	Cross-sectional studies	Longitudinal studies
Total Cholesterol	↓	→ ↓	→ ↓
VLDL	↓	↓	↓
LDL	↓	→ ↓	→ ↓
HDL	↑	↑	↑
Total cholesterol/HDL	↓	↓	↓

[a] ↓ = generally, a decrease has been found; ↑ = generally, an increase has been found; → ↓ = generally, no change or a decrease has been found.
[b] Reproduced with permission from Ref. 41.

in serum HDL-cholesterol levels at 24 hours after a bout of exercise performed at an oxygen uptake of 20% below the anaerobic threshold was greater when the exercise duration was 45 minutes, as compared with 30 minutes (52).

Likewise, although not all studies are in agreement, results generally show a 5–15% increase in plasma HDL-cholesterol levels following chronic exercise training (41). In men, such increases appear to be directly related to both the intensity of exercise and total quantity of weekly energy expenditure (126). In women, recent research conducted at the Institute for Aerobics Research suggests that moderate intensity exercise training performed at approximately 55% of the maximal heart rate may be as effective in increasing HDL-cholesterol levels as higher intensity exercise training (25).

REDUCED RISK FOR HYPERTENSION AND LOWERING OF HIGH BLOOD PRESSURE   Epidemiologic studies have documented a reduced risk for the development of hypertension in physically active persons (42). Several studies have also demonstrated that the blood pressures of hypertensive patients are reduced for one to three hours following a single 30–45 minute bout of aerobic exercise (42). Moreover, a recent metaanalysis of 25 longitudinal studies has confirmed the efficacy of aerobic exercise training in lowering elevated systolic and diastolic blood pressures (43). The average sample-size-weighted reductions in resting systolic and diastolic blood pressures in this metaanalysis were 10.8 and 8.2 mmHg, respectively. Interestingly, in the studies included in the metaanalysis, moderate-intensity exercise appeared to be just as effective—if not more so—than higher-intensity exercise.

ENHANCED INSULIN SENSITIVITY   Findings from the Framingham study indicate that the incidence of cardiovascular disease among individuals with diabetes mellitus is approximately two to three times higher than that in normoglycemic individuals (53). Recent research has further shown that insulin enhances the proliferation of arterial smooth-muscle cells and stimulates lipogenesis in arterial tissue (34). Not surprisingly, hyperinsulinemia has also been linked to an accentuated risk for acute myocardial infarction, even in nondiabetic men (24).

Acutely, a single bout of submaximal aerobic exercise enhances insulin sensitivity in skeletal muscle and other tissues. Therefore, such exercise often results in a decline in the blood glucose levels of patients with insulin-dependent or noninsulin dependent diabetes mellitus (122). This exercise-induced improvement in glucose metabolism may persist from hours to days and is thought to be modulated by an increase in the cell membrane glucose transporter number, as well as an increase in the intrinsic activity of these transporters (59).

With chronic exercise training, glycemic control also improves in persons with noninsulin-dependent and, to a lesser degree, insulin-dependent diabetes (122). However, as is partly the case with plasma lipoproteins and blood pressure, it is unclear whether such improvements are largely due to the cumulative effects of the individual acute bouts of exercise, rather than a training-mediated change in fitness per se (122).

REDUCTION OF OBESITY AND IMPROVEMENT IN BODY FAT DISTRIBU-TION   Caloric restriction through dieting, in combination with caloric expenditure through regular exercise, appears to be the most effective means of preventing obesity and maintaining an ideal body weight. This approach, as compared with dieting alone, better preserves lean body mass and may possibly be linked to favorable chronic changes in resting metabolic rate (35, 94, 120). Regular exercise may also be associated with benefits in terms of both maintenance and stability of weight loss (57).

Recent studies have shown that many of the adverse consequences of obesity may be more closely coupled to the distribution of body fat than to the amount of body fat (8). Indeed, individuals with more fat on the trunk, especially intraabdominal fat, are at increased risk of death when compared with individuals who are equally fat, but whose fat is predominantly on the extremities (8). Although additional studies are needed, regular exercise appears capable of evoking favorable changes in body fat distribution (23). Indeed, preliminary exercise-training studies suggest a preferential mobilization of trunk subcutaneous fat as compared with peripheral subcutaneous fat (23).

ENHANCEMENT OF IMMUNOLOGIC FUNCTION   In view of existing evidence that physical activity decreases the risks of colon cancer (especially in men) and breast and reproductive cancer in women, together with the recognized importance of the immune system in the body's defense against neoplasia, it is understandable why the immunology of exercise is currently an active area of research (15, 108). Although both acute and chronic exercise have been associated with potentially beneficial immunologic consequences, the hypothesis that an exercise-induced enhancement of immunosurveillance contributes to a decreased cancer risk is currently controversial and in need of considerable future research. Indeed, many experts now believe that the mechanism by which regular physical activity may protect against certain types of cancer is nonimmunologic in nature (15, 108). Such nonimmunologic mechanisms are thought to include a reduction in intestinal transit time, in the case of colon cancer (61), and hormonal alterations (for example, decreased estrogen levels and consequently less end-organ stimulation), in the case of breast and reproductive cancers (15, 108).

Summary of Clinical Exercise Studies

Clinical studies confirm that exercise influences many bodily systems and functions. Several possibly healthful effects of exercise have been identified. Some of these effects are acute responses to a single bout of exercise; others result from chronic training adaptations.

EPIDEMIOLOGICAL STUDIES OF ACTIVITY OR FITNESS AND HEALTH

Cardiovascular Diseases

Increased risk of cardiovascular diseases caused by sedentary lifestyle has been evaluated in more epidemiological studies than for all other disease endpoints combined, and coronary heart disease (CHD) is by far the most frequently studied of the cardiovascular diseases. Numerous review papers are available on the risk of CHD associated with sedentary habits; in 1987, Powell et al (97) published one of the most comprehensive of these papers. As it has been established that sedentary habits are causally related to increased risk of CHD, we will not review this topic in detail.

HYPERTENSION   Cross-sectional studies show lower blood pressures in active and fit persons, compared with their unfit and sedentary peers (19, 40). The magnitude of differences in blood pressure across activity or fitness groups is modest, typically less than 10 mm Hg for systolic pressure and 5 mm Hg for diastolic pressure. This association appears to be independent of potential confounding variables, such as body fat, alcohol intake, family history of hypertension, and age. However, activity does not seem to normalize the blood pressure in all hypertensive persons (43).

One prospective epidemiological study evaluated change in physical fitness in relation to change in blood pressure (10). A total of 753 middle-aged men were followed for an average of 1.6 years, with physical fitness assessed at baseline and follow-up examinations by maximal exercise treadmill testing. Increases in fitness and decreases in body weight were associated with decreases in systolic and diastolic blood pressures. The association between fitness change and blood pressure change disappeared in multiple regression models when change in body weight was added. Thus, the effect of fitness change on blood pressure was largely mediated by changes in weight.

There are two prospective studies on sedentary habits or low levels of physical fitness on risk of developing physician-diagnosed hypertension. Both studies followed large groups [14,998 Harvard alumni (90) and 4820 men and 1219 women from the Cooper Clinic (11)] for up to 12 years. All study participants were free of diagnosed hypertension at baseline. The risk of developing physician-diagnosed hypertension during follow-up was increased by 35% in sedentary as compared with active alumni, and by 52% in unfit as compared with fit Cooper Clinic patients. These results were not due to confounding by such factors as age, smoking habit, family history of hypertension, or body composition.

STROKE   There are only a few epidemiological reports on physical activity or fitness and incidence of stroke, and the findings are equivocal. Results of these studies are displayed in Table 2. A problem in interpreting these data is that most studies do not distinguish between hemorrhagic and nonhemorrhagic (thromboembolic) stroke. We may reasonably expect that physical activity or fitness could have an impact on nonhemorrhagic stroke, as this disease seems to have a similar pathogenetic mechanism as that ascribed to CHD, and activity and fitness are inversely related to CHD. Activity and fitness might affect risk of hemorrhagic stroke indirectly via an association with blood pressure, but the association, if present, would likely be weak. Stroke incidence in the Harvard alumni study shows a strong inverse gradient across leisure time physical activity in kilocalories per week (86). Job-related activity shows a U-shaped relationship with stroke among Italian railroad workers. Workers in both sedentary and heavy activity categories have an elevated relative risk of 2.2 compared with workers in the moderate activity group (73). We consider the possible relationship between activity or fitness and stroke to be likely, but not established. As evidenced by Table 2, problems in further interpretation stem from varying definitions of physical activity (occupational/leisure time, lifetime versus point estimate), outcome, and differences in populations under study.

PERIPHERAL VASCULAR DISEASE   If an active and fit way of life reduces the risk of atherosclerotic coronary disease, it might also affect peripheral atherosclerotic disease. Investigators from the Framingham Heart Study examined the 14-year incidence of peripheral artery disease by physical activity index at baseline in men aged 35–64 years (54). Bivariate and multivariate analyses showed no relationship between activity and peripheral artery disease.

Cancer

Nearly 70 years ago, investigators noted that death rates from cancer among men classified by occupational assignment were inversely related to energy expenditure from muscular activity (18, 109). More recently, evidence has accumulated that physical activity may protect against colon, but not rectal, cancer (1, 38, 39, 61, 95, 107, 110, 121, 125, 127).

Physical activity assessment at a single time may not reflect activity over the long term, and long-term activity may be important for diseases such as cancer, which has a long development stage. Two points of activity assessment (1962 or 1966 and 1977) were obtained in 17,148 Harvard alumni who were followed prospectively for colon and rectum cancer occurrence by 1988 (67). Higher levels of physical activity, which were evaluated by using either assessment taken alone, were not associated with colon cancer risk. However, alumni who were highly active (energy expenditure of 2500 or more kcal per week) at both assessments had half the risk of developing colon cancer as those who were inactive (less than 1000 kcal per week) at both assessments. Thus, either consistently higher levels of activity are necessary to protect against colon cancer, or combining two assessments increases the precision of the physical activity measurement. No evidence was found that higher levels of activity protected against rectum cancer.

Clinical and laboratory studies have suggested a role of testosterone in the development of prostate cancer. Exercise may have physiologic affects on sex hormone production and utilization. Accordingly, these same Harvard alumni were followed for the incidence of this cancer in the same 26-year period (68). Although men who were highly active (expending 4000 or more kcal per week at both assessments) were at reduced risk of prostate cancer, there was no gradient response of protection at lower levels of energy expenditure, and these findings need to be repeated.

In like fashion, observations suggesting a lower risk of breast cancer among women athletes as compared with nonathletes (36) are based on small numbers and must be interpreted cautiously. Further, this particular study is based on interviews with women who have survived breast cancer, and selection or survival biases cannot be ruled out in interpreting the findings.

Physical fitness, as assessed by maximal exercise tolerance on a treadmill test, is inversely associated with cancer mortality in the Aerobics Center Longitudinal Study (12). There were 64 cancer deaths in 10,224 men and 18 cancer deaths in 3120 women who were followed for an average of eight years (total of 110,482 person-years of observation). Age-adjusted cancer death rates per 10,000 person-years of observation across low, moderate, and high

Table 2 Summary of studies assessing the relationship between physical activity and stroke

Study (ref.)	Population	Definition of Exposure	Definition of Stroke	Result	Comments
Paffenbarger & Williams (88)	>50,000 male college alumni survivors' age range 30–70 years	Participation in varsity college athletics (yes/no)	Death due to stroke (hemorrhagic and occlusive) (n = 171)	Inverse association	Twofold higher rate of stroke among non-varsity athletes; no confounding assessment
Kannel & Sorlie (54)	1909 men aged 35–64 at fourth biennial examination, Framingham; 14-year follow-up	Physical activity index based on hours/day at specific activity intensity	Cerebrovascular accident (n = 87)	Inverse association	No statistically significant association after controlling for age, systolic BP, serum cholesterol, glucose intolerance, cigarette habit, and left ventricular hypertrophy
Salonen et al (105)	3829 women and 4110 Eastern Finnish men aged 30–59 years; approximately 7-year follow-up	Physical activity at work and during leisure time low/high	Cerebral stroke ICD-8 430-437 morbidity and mortality (n = 71 men and 56 women)	Inverse association Women: leisure time work Men: work Null association Men: leisure time	Statistically significant RR (1.6, 95% CI = 1.1–2.5) for men and women (1.7, 95% CI = 1.1–2.7) who were inactive at work. No significant association for leisure time physical activity, multivariate adjustment for age, serum cholesterol, diastolic BP, body mass index, and tobacco habit
Herman et al (49)	132 hospital-based stroke cases and 239 age/sex matched controls; Dutch men and women aged 40–74 years	Physical activity during leisure time (greatest portion of one's lifetime) ranging from little to regular-heavy	Rapidly developed clinical signs of focal or global disturbance of cerebral function lasting more than 24 hours or leading to death, with no apparent cause other than vascular origin	Inverse association	Statistically significant association (compared with the least active category) with an apparent dose-response across increasing levels of physical activity. Adjusted for a variety of possible confounders. Relative odds (relative to lowest activity category): light, 0.72 (95% CI = 0.37–1.42); heavy, 0.41 (95% CI = 0.21–0.84)

Study	Population	Exposure measure	Outcome	Association	Comments
Paffenbarger et al (86)	16,936 male college alumni entering college between 1916 and 1950 followed from 1962–1978	Physical activity index (kcal/wk) estimated from reports of stairs climbed, city blocks walked, and sports-play each week	Fatal stroke (n = 103)	Inverse association	Statistically significant association after adjustment for age, cigarette habit, and physician-diagnosed hypertension, dose-response gradient across physical activity index
Lapidus & Bengtsson (66)	1462 Swedish women aged 38–60, follow-up between 1968 and 1981	Physical activity at work and during leisure hours, lifetime and during previous years	Fatal and nonfatal stroke (n = 13)	Inverse association	Statistically significant association for work and leisure physical activity in past year. No statistical association for measures of lifetime exposure during work and leisure
Menotti & Seccareccia (73)	99,029 male Italian railroad employees aged 40–59 years, followed for five years	Job classification of physical activity at work (heavy, moderate, and sedentary)	Fatal stroke (n = 187)	"U" association	Lowest stroke death rate in "moderate" physical activity category. No control for confounding influences
Menotti et al (72)	8287 men aged 40–59 in six of seven countries from seven-country study; 20-year follow-up	Job classification of physical activity at work (heavy, moderate, and sedentary)	Fatal stroke	Null association	No association after statistical adjustment for risk factors
Harmsen et al (45)	7495 Swedish men aged 47–55 years at baseline and followed an average of 11.8 years	Physical activity at work and leisure hours	Fatal stroke (n = 230)	Null association	No association after adjustment for a variety of risk factors. Relative odds = (inactive versus all others) 1.2, 95% CI = 0.8–1.8

Note: CI = confidence interval

physical fitness categories were 20, 7, and 5 in men and 16, 10, and 1 in women, and these trends are statistically significant. The number of deaths in this study is relatively small at this time and precludes an evaluation of the association of fitness with site-specific cancer deaths. All patients in the analysis were apparently healthy at baseline; persons with a history or evidence of several chronic diseases were excluded. However, some individuals probably had subclinical cancer already present at baseline. Undetected disease could cause lassitude and inactive habits and result in lower fitness levels. Thus, some of the association between fitness and cancer mortality may have been due to cancer, thus causing low fitness. However, the inverse gradient of cancer mortality across fitness groups is striking and indicates a need for additional research.

Diabetes (NIDDM)

Noninsulin-dependent diabetes mellitus (NIDDM), which affects 10–12 million persons age 20 years or older, is a complex disorder characterized by increased insulin resistance and impaired insulin secretion. This disorder leads to increased risk of mortality from CHD and to other vascular complications, such as peripheral vascular disease, kidney disease, and blindness (22, 28, 80). Along with proper control of body weight and a prudent diet, physical activity is commonly advocated in the management of NIDDM (50, 80, 106, 128), but it has been little studied in the prevention or deferment of this disease. Certain indirect lines of evidence support the contention that physical activity lowers risk of NIDDM. For example, physically active societies have less NIDDM than more sedentary societies (7, 26, 124); as populations have become less active, the incidence of this disease has increased steadily. Physical activity increases insulin sensitivity (103, 112), and regular endurance exercise induces weight loss and positive changes in glucose metabolism (59, 100). Physical activity has also been inversely associated with the prevalence of diabetes in several cross-sectional studies (37, 58, 78, 116).

Direct evidence of a protective role of physical activity against NIDDM has been demonstrated in a prospective study of University of Pennsylvania alumni (47, 89). By using mail questionnaires, contemporary physical activity patterns and other life-style habits were examined in relation to the incidence of NIDDM in 5990 men; the disease developed in 202 of these men in 15 years of follow-up.

Leisure-time physical activity, expressed as kilocalories (kcal) in walking, stair climbing, and recreational activities, was inversely related to the development of NIDDM. Incidence rates declined as energy expenditure increased from less than 500 to 3500 or more per week. For each 500 kcal increment in energy expenditure, diabetes was reduced by about 6%, and this inverse relationship persisted when body composition, weight gain since college, history of hypertension, and parental history of diabetes were considered. The protective effect of physical activity was strongest with moderate to vigorous sports play. The effect was also strong in individuals considered at higher risk of NIDDM because they were overweight-for-height or hypertensive, or had parental history of diabetes.

This study among college alumni supports the concept that prevention or delay of NIDDM may be achieved by increasing overall activity and that vigorous activities (swimming, brisk cycling, running, etc.) may induce a stronger effect than more moderate activities.

Osteoarthritis

Osteoarthritis is a major public health problem in the United States (79), and some investigators are concerned that vigorous exercise may increase risk of the disease developing. The title of a recent editorial in the *Journal of Internal Medicine,* "Jogging—for a healthy heart and worn-out hips?," expresses a common concern that exercise may increase the risk of osteoarthritis (32). Cross-sectional studies show no differences in the prevalence of osteoarthritis between runners and control subjects (64, 91). A two-year follow-up study by Lane et al (63) also shows similar progression rates for osteoarthritis in runners and controls.

A preliminary analysis of data from the Aerobics Center Longitudinal Study shows no increase in osteoarthritis of the hip or knee across levels of exposure to running (13). The six-year incidence of osteoarthritis in a group of 1039 women and 4429 men was higher in older and more obese subjects. But, the incidence was not higher in subjects who had run more miles in their lifetimes, had been running for more years, and had run more miles in the year before the beginning of the study. Although selection/protection competition cannot be unraveled in these early data, available indications are that running and jogging are not associated with an increased risk of osteoarthritis of the hip or knee.

Osteoporosis

Osteoporosis, and the associated fracture risk, are major public health problems, especially for older individuals. Peak bone mass is attained early in life, probably by the second or third decade (111). A gradual decline in bone mineral density occurs throughout middle-age and is markedly accelerated in women after menopause, especially during the first five postmenopausal years (111). Numerous studies on the relation of physical activity to bone mineral density have been conducted over the past several years. Two reviews (111, 119) provide an excellent summary of these reports.

The current research supports a few general conclusions. Clearly, bone responds to the physical stress of exercise. Regular physical activity is likely to boost peak bone mass in young women, probably slows the decline in bone mineral density in middle-aged and older women, and may increase bone mineral density in patients with established osteoporosis (111). Much additional research is needed to clarify the specific type and amount of exercise that most efficaciously promotes bone health at various stages of life. There is a paucity of studies of men, and this void also needs to be addressed. It is not clear how physical activity and other proven or suspected effective interventions, such as calcium supplementation and estrogen replacement therapy, might interact to promote or maintain bone health.

Regular physical activity may provide benefits beyond a direct impact on bone mineral density. Active individuals have greater muscle mass and are stronger, which might reduce the risk of falling and protect against fractures when falls occur. Sorock et al (113) report a reduced risk of fracture (relative risk = 0.41 in men and 0.76 in women) in active individuals when compared with sedentary ones.

Musculoskeletal Disability

Musculoskeletal disorders are common, especially in older individuals. These disorders may contribute to inability to perform routine activities or to risk of falling. The high prevalence of relative disability in older persons is manifested by problems with walking, doing household chores, and accomplishing personal activities (20). Falls are a major health problem for the elderly. The etiology of falling is complex, and multiple factors are identified as possible causes; but, limitations in musculoskeletal function, such as low levels of muscle strength, balance, and flexibility, may be contributors (118).

Runners report fewer limitations in routine activities and lower levels of disability than control subjects (65). Muscle dysfunction and problems with mobility are strongly associated with low levels of muscular strength (33). Furthermore, even elderly individuals (86–96 years) improve muscle strength with an eight-week, weight training program (33); in fact, average gains in strength of 175% were noted. Increases in strength were also associated with objective improvements in mobility tests.

At present, data are limited, and more studies, including intervention trials, are needed to evaluate the possible impact of increased physical activity on the incidence of musculoskeletal disorders. However, older persons in particular are clearly likely to suffer relative disability, decreased function, falls, and specific musculoskeletal disorders; some of these problems may be due to a progressive loss of musculoskeletal function caused by decades of sedentary living habits. Future work should focus on quantifying levels of activity and fitness required to prevent dysfunction and on appropriate and acceptable intervention programs to restore function.

Summary of Epidemiological Studies

DOSE-RESPONSE RELATIONSHIP   Most of the general public and many health professionals believe that regular exercise is an important health habit. For the past two decades, exercise scientists have promoted a scientific approach to exercise prescription that specifies exercise intensity, duration, and frequency (2–5). These recommendations are based on numerous controlled trials of exercise training that have characterized the shape of the dose-response relationship of exercise to short-term improvements in physical fitness. The exercise prescription emphasizes relatively vigorous, large muscle activity for at least 20 minutes at a minimum of three times per week. This dose of exercise was adopted by the Surgeon General of the United States for the 1990 health objectives (98). Many public education campaigns, books, and articles have presented the exercise prescription approach as advice to the public. We believe that these activities have led both the public and health professionals to adopt a dichotomous view of exercise. That is, unless a person achieves the specified exercise prescription, there are no benefits or responses to the training program. In our opinion, this is an incorrect view, especially in terms of the health effects of physical activity.

The relation between various levels of physical activity or physical fitness to mortality from five recent prospective studies is presented in Figure 1. These studies indicate that there is a gradient of risk across activity or fitness levels and that moderate levels of activity or fitness are associated with important and clinically significant reductions in risk. This observation opposes the widely believed threshold concept, which asserts that there is no benefit from physical activity until the exercise prescription level is reached and that there are further improvements across higher levels of exercise. Figure 2 illustrates an idealized benefit curve *(solid line)* across activity or fitness levels based on current studies, and a second hypothetical curve *(dotted line)* that probably represents the prevailing opinion of the public and health professionals.

The dose-response relationship indicated by the five studies is good news for sedentary individuals. They can have hope that a moderate physical activity program is likely to yield some important health benefits. The public health message should be "Doing some physical activity is better than doing none at all." That is, a little is better than none, and, to a degree, more is better than less. The moderate level of physical fitness that is associated with much lower death rates than the low fitness level in the Aerobics Center Longitudinal Study (12) can be achieved with relatively little activity. A brisk, two-mile walk in 30–40 minutes (3–4/mph) taken on most days would be sufficient to produce the moderate fitness level defined in the study. A recent randomized clinical trial suggests that three ten-minute walks over the course of the day have about the same impact on physical fitness as one 30-minute walk (21). Thus, exercise recommendations can emphasize the accumulation of 30 minutes of walking (or the energy expenditure equivalent in some other activity) over the day as sufficient to have important health and functional benefits. This approach may be less intimidating and easier to follow than the prescription of a continuous exercise session and should be

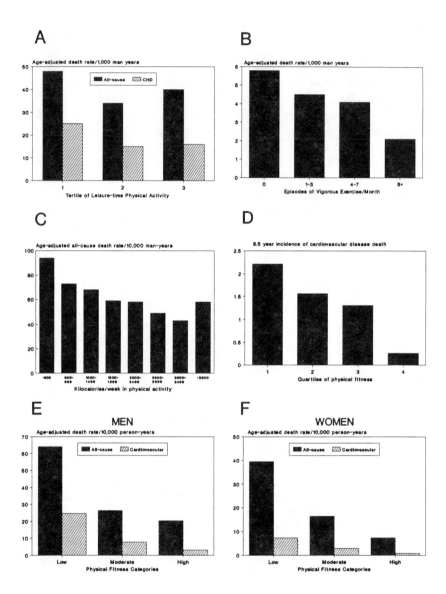

Figure 1   Rates for coronary heart disease, cardiovascular disease, or all-cause mortality are plotted on the vertical axis. The horizontal axis indicates exposure to various levels of physical activity or physical fitness. The figure is constructed from data taken from five prospective epidemiological studies: A (69); B (75); C (87); D (31); E and F (12). The rates in the different panels cannot be compared directly because of different methodology, endpoints, and study populations.

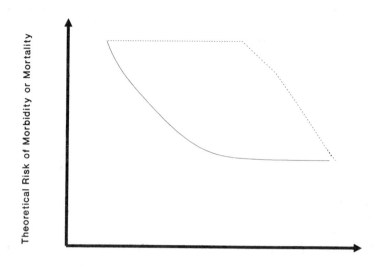

Level of Physical Activity or Physical Fitness

Figure 2   The solid line indicates change in risk across levels of activity of fitness; this line is idealized from published prospective studies. The dashed *(upper)* line indicates the relation of disease endpoints to level of activity or fitness on the assumption that the traditional exercise prescription is required to obtain health benefits and that higher levels of activity or fitness produce additional benefits, as indicated by the decline in risk beyond the threshold point.

considered for intervention programs (9, 46). A five-minute walk after breakfast and before dinner, a ten-minute walk at lunchtime, and a few minutes of stair climbing spread across the day would result in the accumulation of a dose of activity that should improve health and function in previously sedentary and unfit individuals.

METHODOLOGIC ISSUES IN POPULATION STUDIES OF PHYSICAL ACTIVITY
Design and methodological concerns are sometimes raised regarding the interpretation of data from epidemiological studies. In this section, we discuss the issues of bias and physical activity assessment.

Bias   Much has been written about bias in population studies, and most standard texts treat the topic thoroughly (48, 102). Epidemiological studies of physical activity, physical fitness, and health have been typically conducted in opportunistic cohorts, such as college alumni (86, 87, 90), preventive medicine clinic patients (11, 12), or high risk men (69). Frequently, results from such studies are questioned because of possible selection bias. Selection bias is not a major problem in these studies, however, because persons enrolled in such studies come under observation before knowledge of any outcome. As in most epidemiological investigations, care must be taken when generalizing the results, and replications in other groups are needed. One possible bias in existing studies is that the sedentary or unfit subjects may be in those categories because they may already have some disease, which in turn causes inactivity and concomitantly increases risk of death. Investigators have dealt with these problems by evaluating the relationship between activity or fitness to mortality in early and later follow-up intervals (12, 75, 87), or by considering changes in classifications of work activity (84).

Assessment Issues   Efforts have been made to validate physical activity assessment instruments used in population studies (60, 104, 115), but there are several important issues that need further attention. First is the temporality of the physical activity exposure, as it may be positioned in the etiologic pathway or constellation of diseases and disorders. All studies to date have typically relied on a single, point estimate of physical activity (or inactivity) as a measure of exposure. Earlier studies (77, 84, 85) assessed relative and absolute energy expenditure needs on the job, whereas the more recent studies focused on leisure-time physical activity (69, 86, 87, 90). As in the study of dietary intake and disease, investigators have assumed that these point estimates of activity are correlated with the habitual, or lifetime, exposure to physical activity that is more plausibly in an etiologic pathway; this assumption has not yet been confirmed. The problem of misclassification of exposure to physical activity (either by a change in behavior during a follow-up period or by real assessment error) based on a single baseline measure is one that should serve to underestimate the true point estimate of risk. Thus, we may argue that any increased risk demonstrated with a single, point estimate of physical activity should only be strengthened with a more complete and accurate, and less variable, measure of physical activity exposure. This has not often been demonstrated; a notable exception is the above-mentioned study of physical activity and colon cancer incidence (67).

   The second issue is that even if the assumption of a single, point-estimate of physical activity is etiologically valid, it is unknown how many days (or views) of assessment are necessary to build a picture of true habitual energy expenditure. As with dietary intake (70), we can reasonably assume a certain degree of intraindividual variation in energy expenditure. Thus, how many assessment days are needed to minimize this intraindividual variation and provide unbiased estimates of physical activity habits? Such work has been done in the area of dietary intake (6, 70), but nothing is yet available for energy expenditure. This problem relates to measurement error and subsequent misclassification of exposure in much the same way as was discussed above, and must be solved to provide more precise estimates of physical activity exposure. New approaches to physical activity assessment need to be developed to address these problems to approximate appropriate physiologic parameters of interest in different populations better.

DESCRIPTIVE EPIDEMIOLOGY OF PHYSICAL ACTIVITY IN THE UNITED STATES

Physical Activity Within Demographic Groups

The contributions of physical activity to a healthful lifestyle have received an increasing amount of emphasis over the past two or three decades. Casual observation that adults are becoming more physically active can be supported by data from national surveys that show small increases in the percentage of individuals who are active and decreases in the percentage who are sedentary (114). We are, however, not an active society; seven out of eleven of the Surgeon General's objectives for activity and fitness for 1990 were probably not achieved (98). Data from the 1985 National Health Interview Survey show that 25% of adult men and 30% of adult women were sedentary (no reported physical activity in the past month) (16). Another 30% of men and women were classified as irregularly active, and only 8% of the men and 7% of the women were exercising at the level recommended in the 1990 objectives. Physical activity levels generally were inversely related to age and directly related to educational level and income. Whites appeared to be somewhat more active than blacks and persons with race not specified.

Population Attributable Risks of Low Activity and Fitness

The epidemiological studies reviewed above support the inference that low levels of physical activity and physical fitness are strong and independent risk factors for cardiovascular, cancer, and all-cause mortality. The high prevalence of sedentary habits in the US thus leads to a high population attributable risk for sedentary lifestyle. Paffenbarger et al (87) calculate the population attributable risk for all-cause mortality for sedentary habits ($<$ 2000 kilocalories per week in physical activity; approximately 60% of the Harvard alumni were at risk by this definition) to be 16%, compared with 6% for hypertension, 22% for cigarette smoking, and 5% for a positive family history of early parental death. Low physical fitness (least fit quintile) in the Aerobics Center Longitudinal Study was associated with population attributable risks of 9% in men and 15% in women (12). These risk estimates were comparable to, or higher than, the estimates for other well established risk factors, such as cigarette smoking, elevated blood cholesterol or blood pressure, high fasting blood glucose, high body mass index, and a history of premature coronary heart disease death in a parent.

Hahn et al (44) recently estimated the number of deaths attributed to several risk factors for nine chronic diseases. The estimates were based on published studies and death rates in the US in 1986. The number of deaths attributed to sedentary habits [sedentary or irregularly active as described by Caspersen et al (16)] was 256,686. This number was exceeded by the estimates for smoking (361,911) and obesity (261,988), but was greater than the numbers estimated for elevated cholesterol (253,194) or hypertension (225,962).

Population-attributable risk estimates for sedentary habits and low physical fitness are high. Inactivity in the US appears to be a public health problem that is of comparable magnitude to cigarette smoking, obesity, high blood pressure, and high blood cholesterol levels.

SUMMARY

Research studies over the past several decades confirm the health benefits of regular physical activity, a concept with foundations in antiquity. The effects of activity on certain individual health conditions, the precise dose of activity that is required for specific benefits, the role (if any) of intensity of effort, and the elucidation of biological pathways whereby activity contributes to health are topics for further research. Although details remain to be clarified, it is now clear that regular physical activity reduces the risk of morbidity and mortality from several chronic diseases and increases physical fitness, which leads to improved function. Table 3 outlines the relationship of activity to several diseases, a judgment on the strength of the evidence, and a rough determination of the amount of research extant. Results from clinical exercise studies and epidemiological investigations can be integrated into a consistent and coherent theory of healthful physical activity. However, some differences between these two research streams need to be reconciled. Exercise physiologists have generally recommedned relatively intensive activity and a formal approach to exercise prescription. The epidemiological studies suggest a linear dose-response relationship, at least up to a point, between physical activity and health and functional effects. These data support public health recommendations directed toward the most sedentary and unfit stratum of the population and emphasize doing at least moderate physical activity. If this group of adults would accumulate 30 minutes of walking per day (or the equivalent energy expenditure in other activities), they would receive clinically significant health benefits. An important point is that it does not matter what type of physical activity is performed: Sports, planned exercise, household or yard work, or occupational tasks are all beneficial. The key factor is total energy expenditure; if that is constant, improvements in fitness and health will be comparable. There are probably 40 million adults in the US whose sedentary habits place them at considerably increased risk of morbidity and mortality from several diseases. These same individuals also are more likely to have functional limitations, especially as they move into the later years of life.

The sizable independent relative risk for impaired health in sedentary persons, and the large number at risk, leads to a substantial public health

Table 3 Summary results of studies investigating the relationship of physical activity or physical fitness to selected incidences of chronic diseases[a,b]

Disease	Number of studies	Trends across activity or fitness categories and strength of evidence
Obesity	***	↓ ↓ ↓
Coronary artery disease	***	↓ ↓ ↓
Hypertension	**	↓ ↓
Stroke	**	↓
Peripheral vascular disease	*	→
Cancer (all sites)	*	↓
colon	***	↓ ↓
rectum	***	→
breast	*	↓
prostate	*	↓
lung	*	↓
Non-insulin dependent diabetes	*	↓ ↓
Osteoarthritis	*	→
Osteoporosis	**	↓ ↓
Musculoskeletal disability	**	↓ ↓

[a] *Few studies, probably less than 5; **several studies, approximately 5–10; ***many studies, more than 10.

[b] → No apparent difference in disease rates across activity or fitness categories; ↓ some evidence of reduced disease rates across activity or fitness categories; ↓ ↓ good evidence of reduced disease rates across activity or fitness categories, control of potential confounders, good methods, some evidence of biological mechanisms; ↓ ↓ ↓ excellent evidence of reduced disease rates across activity or fitness categories, good control of potential confounders, excellent methods, extensive evidence of biological mechanisms, relationship is considered causal.

burden. This problem deserves continued and increased attention by physicians and other health professionals, scientists, and the public health establishment.

ACKNOWLEDGMENTS

We thank Laura Becker for providing secretarial support and Chris Ensmann and Shannon Jackson for assistance with the literature review. This work was supported in part by grants from the National Institutes of Health (AG06945, AR39715, HL34174, CA44854).

Literature Cited

1. Albanes, D., Blair, A., Taylor, P. R. 1989. Physical activity and risk of cancer in the NHANES I population. *Am. J. Public Health* 79:744–50

2. Am. Coll. Sports Med. 1991. *Guidelines for Exercise Testing and Prescription*. Philadelphia: Lea & Febiger. 314 pp. 4th ed.

3. Am. Coll. Sports Med. 1986. *Guidelines for Exercise Testing and Prescription*. Philadelphia: Lea & Febiger. 179 pp. 3rd ed.

4. Am. Coll. Sports Med. 1975. *Guidelines for Graded Exercise Testing and Exercise Prescription*. Philadelphia: Lea & Febiger. 116 pp.

5. Am. Coll. Sports Med. Position Stand. 1990. The recommended quantity and quality of exercise for developing and maintaining cardiorespiratory and muscular fitness in healthy adults. *Med. Sci. Sports Exerc.* 22:265–74

6. Beaton, G. H., Milner, J., Corey, P., McGuire, V., Cousins, M., et al. 1979. Sources of variance in 24-hour dietary recall data: implications for nutrition study design and interpretation. *Am. J. Clin. Nutr.* 32:2546–59

7. Bjorntorp, P., De Jounge, K., Sjostrom, L., Sullivan, L. 1970. The effect of physical training on insulin production in obesity. *Metabolism* 19:631–37

8. Bjorntorp, P., Smith, U., Lönnroth, P., eds. 1988. Health implications of regional obesity. *Acta Med. Scand.* 723 (Suppl.). 237 pp.

9. Blair, S. N. 1991. *Living with Exercise.* Dallas: American Health Publishing Company. 119 pp.

10. Blair, S. N., Cooper, K. H., Gibbons, L. W., Gettman, L. R., Lewis, S., et al. 1983. Changes in coronary heart disease risk factors associated with increased treadmill time in 753 men. *Am. J. Epidemiol.* 118:352–59

11. Blair, S. N., Goodyear, N. N., Gibbons, L. W., Cooper, K. H. 1984. Physical fitness and incidence of hypertension in healthy normotensive men and women. *J. Am. Med. Assoc.* 252:487–90

12. Blair, S. N., Kohl, H. W. III, Paffenbarger, R. S. Jr., Clark, D. G., Cooper, K. H., et al. 1989. Physical fitness and all-cause mortality: a prospective study of healthy men and women. *J. Am. Med. Assoc.* 262:2395–2401

13. Blair, S. N., Kohl, H. W. III, Powell, K. E., Caspersen, C. J., Barlow, C. E. 1990. Running and incidence of osteoarthritis (abstract). *Med. Sci. Sports Exerc.* 22(Suppl.):S116

14. Bouchard, C., Shephard, R. J., Stephens, T., Sutton, J., McPherson, B., eds. 1990. *Exercise, Fitness and Health. A Consensus of Current Knowledge.* Champaign: Human Kinetics. 720 pp.

15. Calabrese, L. H. 1990. Exercise, immunity, cancer and infection. See Ref. 14, pp. 567–79

16. Caspersen, C. J., Christenson, G. M., Pollard, R. A. 1986. Status of the 1990 Physical Fitness and Exercise Objectives—evidence from NHIS 1985. *Public Health Rep.* 101:587–92

17. Caspersen, C. J., Powell, K. E., Christenson, G. M. 1985. Physical activity, exercise, and physical fitness: definitions and distinctions for health-related

research. *Public Health Rep.* 100:126–31

18. Cherry, T. 1922. A theory of cancer. *Med. J. Aust.* 1:425–38

19. Cooper, K. H., Pollock, M. L., Martin, R. P., White, S. R. 1976. Physical fitness levels vs. selected coronary risk factors. *J. Am. Med. Assoc.* 236:166–69

20. Cornoni-Huntley, J., Brock, D. B., Ostfeld, A. M., Taylor, J. O., Wallace, R. B., eds. 1986. *Established Populations for Epidemiologic Studies of the Elderly.* Bethseda: Natl. Inst. Health. 428 pp.

21. DeBusk, R. F., Stenestrand, U., Sheehan, M., Haskell, W. L. 1990. Training effects of long versus short bouts of exercise in healthy subjects. *Am. J. Cardiol.* 65:1010–13

22. Defronso, R. A., Ferrannin, E., Koivisto, V. 1983. New concepts in the pathogenesis and treatment of non-insulin-dependent diabetes mellitus. *Am. J. Med.* 74(Suppl. 1A):52–81

23. Després, J.-P., Tremblay, A., Nadeau, A., Bouchard, C. 1988. Physical training and changes in regional adipose tissue distribution. *Acta Med. Scand.* 723(Suppl.):205–12

24. Ducimetiere, P., Eschwege, E., Papoz, L., Richard, J. L., Claude, J. R., et al. 1980. Relationship of plasma insulin levels to the incidence of myocardial infarction and coronary heart disease mortality in a middle-aged population. *Diabetologia* 19:205–10

25. Duncan, J. J., Gordon, N. F., Scott, C. B., Vaandrager, K., Rudling, K., et al. 1991. Walking for cardiovascular fitness—walking for health: how much is enough? (abstr.) *Natl. Conf. Cholesterol and High Blood Pressure Control—program book*, pp. 97–98

26. Eaton, S. B., Konner, M., Shostak, M. 1988. Stone agers in the fast lane: chronic degenerative disease in evolutionary perspective. *Am. J. Med.* 84: 739–49

27. Eaton, S. B., Shostak, M., Konner, M. 1988. *The Paleolithic Prescription: A Program of Diet and Exercise and a Design for Living.* New York: Harper & Row

28. Editorial: Type 2 Diabetes or NIDDM. Looking for a better name. 1989. *Lancet* i:588–91

29. Ehsani, A., Heath, G., Hagberg, J., Burton, E., Holloszy, J. 1981. Effects of 12 months of intense exercise training on ischemic ST-segment depression in patients with coronary artery disease. *Circulation* 64:1116–24

30. Eichner, E. 1986. Coagulability and rheology: hematologic benefits from exercise, fish, and aspirin: implications for athletes and nonathletes. *Physician Sportsmed.* 14:102–10

31. Ekelund, L., Haskell, W. L., Johnson, J. L., Whaley, F. S., Criqui, M. H., et al. 1988. Physical fitness as a predictor of cardiovascular mortality in asymptomatic North American men: the Lipid Research Clinics Mortality Follow-up Study. *N. Engl. J. Med.* 319: 1379–84

32. Ernst, E. 1990. Jogging—for a healthy heart and worn-out hips? *J. Int. Med.* 228:295–97

33. Fiatarone, M. A., Marks, E. C., Ryan, N. D., Meredith, C. N., Lipsitz, L. A., et al. 1990. High-intensity strength training in nonagenarians: effects on skeletal muscle. *J. Am. Med. Assoc.* 263:3029–34

34. Flodin, N. 1986. Atherosclerosis: an insulin-dependent disease? *J. Am. Coll. Nutr.* 5:417–27

35. Frey-Hewitt, B., Vranizan, K. M., Dreon, D. M., Wood, P. D. 1990. The effect of weight loss by dieting and exercise on resting metabolic rate in overweight men. *Int. J. Obes.* 14:327–34

36. Frisch, R. E., Wyshak, G., Albright, N. L., Albright, T. E., Schiff, I., et al. 1985. Lower prevalence of breast cancer and cancers of the reproductive system among former college athletes compared to non-athletes. *Br. J. Cancer* 52:885–91

37. Frisch, R. E., Wyshak, G., Albright, T. E., Albright, N. L., Schiff, I. 1986. Lower prevalence of diabetes in female former college athletes compared to non-athletes. *Diabetes* 35:1101–5

38. Garabrant, D. H., Peter, J. M., Mack, T. M., Bernstein, L. 1984. Job activity and colon cancer risk. *Am. J. Epidemiol.* 119:1005–14

39. Gerhardsson, M., Norell, S. E., Kiviranta, H., Pedersen, N. L., Ahlbom, A. 1986. Sedentary jobs and colon cancer. *Am. J. Epidemiol.* 123:775–80

40. Gibbons, L. W., Blair, S. N., Cooper, K. H., Smith, M. 1983. Association between coronary heart disease risk factors and physical fitness in healthy adult women. *Circulation* 67:977–83

41. Gordon, N. F., Cooper, K. H. 1988. Controlling cholesterol levels through exercise. *Compr. Ther.* 14:52–57

42. Gordon, N. F., Scott, C. B., Wilkinson, W. J., Duncan, J. J., Blair, S. N. 1990. Exercise and mild essential hypertension. Recommendations for adults. *Sports Med.* 10:390–404

43. Hagberg, J. M. 1990. Exercise, fitness, and hypertension. See Ref. 14, pp. 455–66

44. Hahn, R. A., Teutsch, S. M., Rothenberg, R. B., Marks, J. S. 1990. Excess deaths from nine chronic disease in the United States, 1986. *J. Am. Med. Assoc.* 264:2654–59

45. Harmsen, P., Rosengren, A., Tsipogianni, A., Wilhelmsen, L. 1990. Risk factors for stroke in middle-aged men in Göteburg, Sweden. *Stroke* 21:223–29

46. Harris, S. S., Caspersen, C. J., DeFriese, G. H., Estes, H. Jr. 1989. Physical activity counseling for healthy adults as a primary preventive intervention in the clinical setting: report for the US Preventive Services Task Force. *J. Am. Med. Assoc.* 261:3590–98

47. Helmrick, S. P., Ragland, D. R., Leung, R. W., Paffenbarger, R. S. Jr. 1991. Physical activity and reduced occurrence of non-insulin-dependent diabetes mellitus. *N. Engl. J. Med.* 325: 147–52

48. Hennekens, C. H., Buring, J. E. 1987. *Epidemiology in Medicine.* Boston: Little Brown. 383 pp.

49. Herman, B., Schmitz, P. I. M., Leyten, A. C. M., Van Luijk, J. H., Frenken, C. W. G. M., et al. 1983. Multivariate logistic analysis of risk factors for stroke in Tilburg, The Netherlands. *Am. J. Epidemiol.* 118:514–25

50. Horton, E. S. 1988. Role and management of exercise in diabetes mellitus. *Diabetes Care* 11:201–11

51. Hughes, R. A., Thorland, W. G., Eyford, T., Hood, T. 1990. The acute effects of exercise duration on serum lipoprotein metabolism. *J. Sports Med. Phys. Fitness* 30:37–44

52. Hughes, R. A., Thorland, W. G., Housh, T. J., Johnson, G. O. 1990. The effect of exercise intensity on serum lipoprotein responses. *J. Sports Med. Phys. Fitness* 30:254–60

53. Kannel, W. B., McGee, D. 1979. Diabetes and cardiovascular disease: The Framingham Study. *J. Am. Med. Assoc.* 241:2035–38

54. Kannel, W. B., Sorlie, P. 1979. Some health benefits of physical activity: the Framingham Study. *Arch. Intern. Med.* 139:857–61

55. Karvonen, M., Kentala, K., Mustala, O. 1957. The effects of training heart rate: a longitudinal study. *Ann. Med. Exp. Biol. Fenn.* 35:307–15

56. Kavanagh, T. 1989. Does exercise improve coronary collateralization? A new

look at an old belief. *Physician Sports-med.* 17:96–114

57. King, A. C., Frey-Hewitt, B., Dreon, D. M., Wood, P. D. 1989. Diet vs. exercise in weight maintenance: the effects of minimal intervention strategies on long-term outcomes in men. *Arch. Intern. Med.* 149:2741–46

58. King, H., Zimmet, P., Raper, L. R., Balkau, B. 1984. Risk factors for diabetes in three Pacific populations. *Am. J. Epidemiol.* 119:396–409

59. King, P., Hirshman, M., Horton, E. D., Horton, E. S. 1989. Glucose transport in skeletal muscle membrane vesicles from control and exercised rats. *Am. J. Physiol.* 257:C1128–34

60. Kohl, H. W., Blair, S. N., Paffenbarger, R. S. Jr., Macera, C. A., Kronenfeld, J. J. 1988. A mail survey of physical activity habits as related to measured physical fitness. *Am. J. Epidemiol.* 127:1228–39

61. Kohl, H. W., LaPorte, R. E., Blair, S. N. 1988. Physical activity and cancer: an epidemiological perspective. *Sports Med.* 6:222–37

62. Koplan, J. P., Powell, K. E. 1984. Physicians and the Olympics. *J. Am. Med. Assoc.* 252:529–30

63. Lane, N. E., Bloch, D. A., Hubert, H. B., Jones, H., Simpson, U., et al. 1990. Running, osteoarthritis, and bone density: initial 2-year longitudinal study. *Am. J. Med.* 88:452–59

64. Lane, N. E., Bloch, D. A., Jones, H. H., Marshall, W. H. Jr., Wood, P. D., et al. 1986. Long-distance running, bone density, and osteoarthritis. *J. Am. Med. Assoc.* 255:1147–51

65. Lane, N. E., Bloch, D. A., Wood, P. D., Fries, J. F. 1987. Aging, long-distance running, and the development of musculoskeletal disability: a controlled study. *Am. J. Med.* 82:772–80

66. Lapidus, L., Bengtsson, C. 1986. Socioeconomic factors and physical activity in relation to cardiovascular disease and death. A 12-year follow-up of participants in a population study of women in Gothenburg, Sweden. *Br. Heart J.* 55:295–301

67. Lee, I.-M., Paffenbarger, R. S. Jr., Hsieh, C-c. 1991. Physical activity and risk of colorectal cancer among college alumni. *J. Natl. Cancer Inst.* In press

68. Lee, I.-M., Paffenbarger, R. S. Jr., Hsieh, C-c. 1991. Physical activity and risk of prostatic cancer among college alumni. *Am. J. Epidemiol.* In press

69. Leon, A. S., Connett, J., Jacobs, D. R. Jr., Rauramaa, R. 1987. Leisure-time physical activity levels and risk of

coronary heart disease and death: the Multiple Risk Factor Intervention Trial. *J. Am. Med. Assoc.* 258:2388–95

70. Liu, K., Stamler, J., Dyer, A., McKeever, J., McKeever, P. 1978. Statistical methods to assess and minimize the role of intra-individual variability in obscuring the relationship between dietary lipids and serum cholesterol. *J. Chron. Dis.* 31:399–418

71. Malina, R. M. 1988. Physical activity in early and modern populations: an evolutionary view. In *Physical Activity in Early and Modern Populations*, ed. R. Malina, H. Eckert, 21:1–12. Champaign: Human Kinetics. 114 pp.

72. Menotti, A., Keys, A., Blackburn, H., Aravanis, C., Dontas, A., et al. 1990. Twenty-year stroke mortality and prediction in twelve cohorts of the Seven Countries Study. *Int. J. Epidemiol.* 19:309–15

73. Menotti, A., Seccareccia, F. 1985. Physical activity at work and job responsibility as risk factors for fatal coronary heart disease and other causes of death. *J. Epidemiol. Community Health* 39:325–29

74. Montoye, H. J. 1991. Health, exercise and athletics: a millennium of observations—a century of research. *Am. J. Human Biol.* In press

75. Morris, J. N., Clayton, D. G., Everitt, M. G., Semmence, A. M., Burgess, E. H. 1990. Exercise in leisure time: coronary attack and death rates. *Br. Heart J.* 63:325–34

76. Morris, J. N., Everitt, M., Pollard, R., Chave, S., Semmence, A. 1980. Vigorous exercise in leisure-time: protection against coronary heart disease. *Lancet* ii:1207–10

77. Morris, J. N., Heady, J. A., Raffle, P. A. B., Roberts, C. G., Parks, J. W. 1953. Coronary heart disease and physical activity of work. *Lancet* ii: 1053–1120

78. Morsiani, M. 1989. *Epidemiology and Screening of Diabetes*. Boca Raton, Fla: CRC

79. Natl. Cent. Health Stat., Collins, J. G. 1986. Prevalence of selected chronic conditions, United States, 1979–81. *Vital and Health Statistics*. Ser. 10, No. 155. DHHS Publ. No. (PHS) 86-1583. Public Health Serv. Washington, DC: GPO

80. Natl. Inst. Health. 1987. Consensus Development Conference statement on diet and exercise in non-insulin-dependent Diabetes Mellitus. *Diabetes Care* 10: 639–44

81. Noakes, T., Higginson, L., Opie, L.

1983. Physical training increases ventricular fibrillation thresholds of isolated rat hearts during normoxia, hypoxia and regional ischemia. *Circulation* 67:25–30

82. O'Connor, G., Buring, J., Yusaf, S., Goldhaber, S. Z., Olmstead, E. M., et al. 1989. An overview of randomized trials of rehabilitation with exercise after myocardial infarction. *Circulation* 80: 234–44

83. Oldridge, N. B., Guyatt, G. H., Fischer, M. S., Rimm, A. A. 1988. Cardiac rehabilitation after myocardial infarction: combined experience randomized clinical trials. *J. Am. Med. Assoc.* 260:945–50

84. Paffenbarger, R. S. Jr., Hale, W. E. 1975. Work activity and coronary heart disease mortality. *N. Engl. J. Med.* 292:545–50

85. Paffenbarger, R. S. Jr., Hale, W. E., Brand, R. J., Hyde, R. T. 1977. Work-energy level, personal characteristics, and fatal heart attack: a birth-cohort effect. *Am. J. Epidemiol.* 105:200–13

86. Paffenbarger, R. S. Jr., Hyde, R. T., Wing, A. L., Steinmetz, C. H. 1984. A natural history of athleticism and cardiovascular health. *J. Am. Med. Assoc.* 252:491–95

87. Paffenbarger, R. S. Jr., Hyde, R. T., Wing, A. L., Hsieh, C-c. 1986. Physical activity, all-cause mortality, and longevity of college alumni. *N. Engl. J. Med.* 314:605–13

88. Paffenbarger, R. S. Jr., Williams, J. L. 1967. Chronic disease in former college students V. Early precursors of fatal stroke. *Am. J. Public Health* 57:1290–99

89. Paffenbarger, R. S. Jr., Wing, A. L. 1973. Chronic disease in former college students XII. Early precursors of adult-onset diabetes mellitus. *Am. J. Epidemiol.* 97:314–23

90. Paffenbarger, R. S. Jr., Wing, A. L., Hyde, R. T., Jung, D. L. 1983. Physical activity and incidence of hypertension in college alumni. *Am. J. Epidemiol.* 117: 245–57

91. Panush, R. S., Schmidt, C., Caldwell, J. R., Edwards, N. L., Longley, S., et al. 1986. Is running associated with degenerative joint disease? *J. Am. Med. Assoc.* 255:1152–54

92. Park, R. J. 1989. Healthy, moral, and strong; educational views of exercise and athletics in 19th century America. In *Fitness in American Culture; Images of Health, Sport, and the Body 1830–1940,* ed. K. Grover, pp. 123–68. Amherst, Mass: Amherst Univ.

93. Park, R. J. 1988. How active were early

populations? In *Physical Activity in Early and Modern Populations,* ed. R. Malina, H. Eckert, 1:13–21. Champaign: Human Kinetics. 114 pp.

94. Pavlou, K., Steffee, W., Lerman, R., Burrows, B. 1985. Effects of dieting and exercise on lean body mass, oxygen uptake, and strength. *Med. Sci. Sports Exerc.* 17:466–71

95. Peters, R. K., Garabrant, D. H., Yu, M. C., Mack, T. M. 1989. A case-control study of occupational and dietary factors in colorectal cancer in young men by subsite. *Cancer Res.* 49:5459–68

96. Posel, D., Noakes, T., Kantor, P., Lambert, M., Opie, L. H. 1989. Exercise training after experimental myocardial infarction increases the ventricular fibrillation threshold before and after the onset of reinfarction in the isolated rat heart. *Circulation* 80:138–45

97. Powell, K. E., Thompson, P. D., Caspersen, C. J., Kendrick, J. S. 1987. Physical activity and the incidence of coronary heart disease. *Annu. Rev. Public Health* 8:253–87

98. Progress toward achieving the 1990 National Objectives for Physical Fitness and Exercise. 1989. *Morbid. Mortal. Wkly. Rept.* 38:449–53

99. Raglin, J. S. 1990. Exercise and mental health. Beneficial and detrimental effects. *Sports Med.* 9:323–29

100. Rauramaa, R. 1984. Relationship of physical activity glucose tolerance and weight management. *Prev. Med.* 13:37–46

101. Rauramaa, R., Salonen, J. T., Seppanen, K., Salonen, R., Veralainen, J. M., et al. 1986. Inhibition of platelet aggregability by moderate-intensity physical exercise: a randomized clinical trial in overweight men. *Circulation* 74:939–44

102. Rothman, K. J. 1987. *Modern Epidemiology.* Boston: Little Brown. 358 pp.

103. Ruderman, N. B., Ganda, O. P., Johansen, K. 1978. The effect of physical training on glucose tolerance and plasma lipids in maturity-onset diabetes. *Diabetes* 28 (Suppl.):89–92

104. Sallis, J. F., Haskell, W. L., Wood, P. D., Fortmann, S. P., Rogers, T., et al. 1985. Physical activity assessment methodology in the Five-City Project. *Am. J. Epidemiol.* 121:91–106

105. Salonen, J. T., Puska, P., Tuomilehto, J. 1982. Physical activity and risk of myocardial infarction, cerebral stroke, and death: a longitudinal study in Eastern Finland. *Am. J. Epidemiol.* 115: 526–37

106. Schneider, S. H., Ruderman, N. B. 1986. Exercise and physical training and the treatment of diabetes mellitus. *Compr. Ther.* 12:49–56
107. Severson, R. K., Nomura, A. M. Y., Grove, J. S., Stemmermann, G. N. 1989. A prospective analysis of physical activity and cancer. *Am. J. Epidemiol.* 130:522–29
108. Simon, H. B. 1990. Discussion: exercise, immunity, cancer and infection. See Ref. 14, pp. 581–88
109. Sivertsen, I., Dahlstrom, A. N. 1922. The relation of muscular activity to carcinoma. A preliminary report. *J. Cancer Res.* 6:365–78
110. Slattery, M. L., Schumacher, M. C., Smith, K. R., West, D. W., Abd-Elghany, N. 1988. Physical activity, diet, and risk of colon cancer in Utah. *Am. J. Epidemiol.* 128:989–99
111. Snow-Harter, C., Marcus, R. 1991. Exercise, bone mineral density, and osteoporosis. In *Exercise and Sport Sciences Reviews*, ed. J. O. Holloszy, 19:351–88. Baltimore: Williams & Wilkins. 606 pp.
112. Soman, V. R., Veikko, K. A., Deibert, D., Feliz, P., De Fronzo, R. 1979. Increased insulin sensitivity and insulin binding to monocytes after physical training. *N. Engl. J. Med.* 301:1200–4
113. Sorock, G. S., Bush, T. L., Golden, A. L., Fried, L. P., Breuer, B. et al. 1988. Physical activity and fracture risk in a free-living elderly cohort. *J. Gerontol.: Med. Sci.* 43:M134–39
114. Stephens, T. 1987. Secular trends in adult physical activity: exercise boom or bust? *Res. Q. Exerc. Sport* 58:94–105
115. Taylor, H. L., Jacobs, D. R. Jr., Schucker, B., Knudsen, J., Leon, A. S., et al. 1978. A questionnaire for the assessment of leisure time physical activities. *J. Chron. Dis.* 31:741–55
116. Taylor, R., Ram, P., Zimmet, P., Raper, L. R., Ringrose, H. 1984. Physical activity and prevalence of diabetes in Melanesian and Indian men in Fiji. *Diabetologia* 27:578–82
117. Thompson, P. 1988. The benefits and risks of exercise training in patients with chronic coronary artery disease. *J. Am. Med. Assoc.* 259:1537–40
118. Tinetti, M. E., Speechley, M., Ginter, S. F. 1988. Risk factors for falls among elderly persons living in the community. *N. Engl. J. Med.* 319:1701–7
119. Tipton, C. M., Vailas, A. C. 1990. See Ref. 14, pp. 331–34
120. Van Dale, D., Saris, W., Ten Hoor, F. 1990. Weight maintenance and resting metabolic rate 18–40 months after a diet-exercise treatment. *Int. J. Obes.* 14: 347–59
121. Vena, J. E., Graham, S., Zielezny, M., Swanson, M. K., Barnes, R. E., Nolan, J. 1985. Lifetime occupational exercise and colon cancer. *Am. J. Epidemiol.* 122:357–65
122. Vranic, M., Wasserman, D. 1990. Exercise, fitness, and diabetes. See Ref. 14, pp. 467–90
123. Weber, J. R. 1988. Left ventricular hypertrophy: its prime importance as a controllable risk factor. *Am. Heart J.* 116:272–79
124. West, K. M. 1978. *Epidemiology of Diabetes and Its Vascular Lesions.* New York: Elsevier. 579 pp.
125. Whittemore, A. S., Wu-Williams, A. H., Lee, M., Zheng, S., Gallagher, R. P. 1990. Diet, physical activity, and colorectal cancer among Chinese in North American and China. *J. Natl. Cancer Inst.* 82:915–26
126. Wood, P., Haskell, W., Blair, S., Williams, P. T., Krauss, R. M. 1983. Increased exercise level and plasma lipoprotein concentrations: a one-year, randomized controlled study in sedentary, middle-aged men. *Metabolism* 32: 31–39
127. Wu, A. H., Paganini-Hill, A., Ross, R. K., Henderson, B. E. 1987. Alcohol, physical activity and other risk factors for colorectal cancer: a prospective study. *Br. J. Cancer* 55:687–94
128. Zinman, B., Vranic, M. 1985. Diabetes and exercise. *Med. Clin. North Am.* 69:145–57

Annu. Rev. Publ. Health 1992. 13:127–50

THE HEALTH EFFECTS OF LOW-LEVEL IONIZING RADIATION

Arthur C. Upton, Roy E. Shore, and Naomi H. Harley

New York University Medical Center, Institute of Environmental Medicine, New York, NY 10016

KEY WORDS: carcinogenesis, mutation, radionuclide, radon, x-ray

INTRODUCTION

Within months after Roentgen's discovery of the x-ray in 1895, burns of the skin and other acute injuries were encountered in pioneer radiation workers (12, 27), thus prompting efforts to reduce the levels of occupational exposure. In subsequent years, as the thresholds for different types of reactions gradually became better known, the exposure limits for radiation workers underwent a series of further reductions (82, 83). As a result, protection standards ultimately evolved that now suffice to prevent gross damage of tissue, barring radiation accidents (37). Although today's protection standards are adequate to prevent gross injury, they are not presumed to protect completely against the mutagenic and carcinogenic effects of radiation, which may have no thresholds (57, 87).

The concept that the mutagenic effects of radiation might have no threshold dates from the 1940s, when classical experiments on the fruitfly suggested that the frequency of mutations increases in proportion to the dose of x-rays, without a threshold (54). In the 1950s, apprehension that future generations might suffer genetic harm from the global increases in environmental radiation caused by atmospheric testing of nuclear weapons prompted national (55) and international (94) assessments of the risks, which have been periodically updated (87, 89–93).

Concern about the hazards associated with low-level irradiation was further

127

0163/7525/92/0501-0127$02.00

heightened in the 1950s by the suggestion that the risk of leukemia may also increase in proportion with the radiation dose, and that a significant percentage of such cancers in the general population may, therefore, result from natural background irradiation (44). This suggestion was reinforced at about the same time by the observation of an association between childhood leukemia and prenatal diagnostic x-irradiation (47, 79, 80). Since then, the non-threshold dose-incidence hypothesis has also been extended to other malignancies; the risks of radiation-induced cancer are now thought to exceed the risks of heritable effects in the low dose domain (57, 87).

Because assessments of the risks of low-level irradiation are highly uncertain, they have been a subject of ongoing scientific controversy. As a result of such controversy, the fact that the risk estimates have continued to change with the evolution of new information, and confusion over terminology (e.g. the introduction of new units of measure), the assessments have failed to gain public understanding and credibility. To put the pertinent public health issues into perspective, we review the status of our knowledge of the effects of low-level ionizing radiation, with particular reference to the implications of recent revisions in the relevant risk assessments by national and international committees.

SOURCES AND LEVELS OF RADIATION IN THE ENVIRONMENT

Radiation Quantities and Units

Radiation quantities and doses are expressed in various units (35). The unit now used internationally for expressing the dose of radiation that is absorbed in tissue is the gray (Gy). The unit formerly used for the same purpose is the rad (1 Gy = 1 joule per kg of tissue = 100 rad).

Because particulate radiations generally cause greater injury than x-rays or gamma rays for a given dose in Gy, another unit, the sievert (Sv), is used in radiological protection to enable doses of different types of radiation to be normalized in terms of biological effectiveness. Thus, the dose equivalent of any radiation in sieverts is the dose in Gy multiplied by an appropriate weighting factor, so that one seivert of any radiation represents, in principal, the dose that is equivalent in biological effectiveness to one gray of gamma rays. The unit formerly used for the same purpose is the rem (1 Sv = 100 rem).

Because the probability of injury from a given dose equivalent varies with the organ or tissue irradiated, a further unit—the effective dose equivalent—is also used. This unit, expressed in Sv, denotes the dose equivelent to the tissue of interest, weighted by the ratio between the resulting risk of injury and the risk of injury that would be attributable to the same dose equivalent if it were delivered to the body as a whole.

For expressing the collective dose equivalent to a population, the person-Sv (or person-rem) is used; this unit represents the product of the average dose equivalent per person times the number of persons exposed, e.g. 1 sievert to each of 100 persons = 100 person-sievert (= 10,000 person-rem). A collective dose equivalent that is expected to be received over a period of time extending into the future, as from an internally deposited radionuclide, is called the committed collective dose equivalent, or collective dose equivalent commitment.

The amount of radioactivity that is present at any one time in a given sample of matter is expressed in bequerels; one becquerel (Bq) corresponds to that quantity of radioactivity in which there is one atomic disintegration per second. Another unit that has been used for the same purpose is the curie (Ci); one Ci represents that quantity of radioactivity in which there are 3×10^{10} atomic disintegrations per second ($1 \text{ Bq} = 2.7 \times 10^{-11} \text{ Ci}$).

Sources and Levels of Exposure

Natural background radiation, which exists at varying intensities throughout the environment, comes from three main sources: cosmic rays; radium, thorium, uranium, and other radioactive elements in the earth's crust; and potassium-40, carbon-14, and other radionuclides contained in living cells themselves. The three components of natural background radiation—cosmic rays, external gamma radiation, and internal radiation—each account for about one third of the total annual dose of slightly less than 1.0 mSv (100 mrem) received on average by a person who resides at sea level in the US (Table 1). In certain locations, one of the components may be increased by a factor of two. For example, living at a mile-high elevation may increase the cosmic ray dose to 0.50 mSv (50 mrem) per year; living in an area where the earth is rich in radium may increase the external gamma-ray dose to 0.60 mSv (60 mrem) per year. However, both components are rarely doubled at the same time, and the dose from internal emitters (other than radon) is quite constant, so that the total annual dose is unlikely to increase by more than 30%, depending on location (62).

Moreover, the average dose to the bronchial epithelium from inhaled radon and its daughters greatly exceeds the dose to any other soft tissue of the body (Table 1), and regions of the bronchial epithelium in smokers receive additionally even larger doses from polonium-210, which is present naturally in tobacco smoke (65). Also, at the high altitudes of modern jet aircraft travel, the hourly dose-equivalent may exceed 0.005 mSv (0.5 mrem) on northerly routes, thus reaching levels many times higher during solar flares (62).

Table 1 Average amounts of ionizing radiation received annually from different sources by members of the US population[a]

Source	Dose Equivalent[b]		Effective Dose	
	(mSv)	(mrem)	(mSv)	(%)
Natural				
Radon[c]	24	2,400	2.0	55
Cosmic	0.27	27	0.27	8
Terrestrial	0.28	28	0.28	8
Internal	0.39	39	0.39	11
Total natural	—	—	3.0	82
Artificial				
Medical				
x-ray diagnosis	0.39	39	0.39	11
Nuclear medicine	0.14	14	0.14	4
Consumer products	0.10	10	0.10	3
Other				
Occupational	0.009	0.9	<0.01	<0.3
Nuclear fuel cycle	<0.01	<1.0	<0.01	<0.03
Fallout	<0.01	<1.0	<0.01	<0.03
Miscellaneous[d]	<0.01	<1.0	<0.01	<0.03
Total artificial	0.63	0.63	0.63	18
Total natural and artificial	—	—	3.6	100

[a] From 57, 63, 64.
[b] Average dose equivalent to soft tissues.
[c] Dose equivalent to bronchial epithelium from radon daughter products. The assumed weighting factor for the effective dose equivalent, relative to whole-body exposure, is 0.08.
[d] Department of Energy facilities, smelters, transportation, etc.

In addition to the dose received from natural background radiation, the population is exposed to radiation from various anthropogenic sources, the most important of which is the use of x-rays in medical diagnosis (Table 1). Lesser amounts of man-made radiation are received from various other sources, including radioactive minerals in building materials, phosphate fertilizers, and crushed rock; radiation-emitting components of TV sets, smoke detectors, and other consumer products; radioactive fallout from atomic weapons; and nuclear power (Table 1).

NATURE AND MECHANISMS OF INJURY BY LOW-LEVEL IRRADIATION

Through random collisions with atoms and molecules in cells, radiation gives rise to ions and reactive radicals, which, in turn, break chemical bonds and cause other molecular alterations that lead to injury. The distribution of the ionization events along the path of an impinging radiation depends on the energy, mass, and charge of the radiation; x-rays and gamma rays produce ions sparsely along their tracks—that is, they are characterized by a low rate of linear energy transfer (LET)—in contrast to charged particles, which are densely ionizing.

Any molecular constituent of the cell can be altered by radiation, but DNA is the most critical biological target because of the limited redundancy of the genetic information it contains, i.e. damage to a single gene, if unrepaired, may kill or profoundly alter the affected cell. A dose of radiation large enough to kill the average dividing cell (~ 2 Sv, or 200 rem) causes hundreds of lesions in its DNA molecules; however, because most such lesions are reparable, the ultimate fate of a given lesion depends on the outcome of the cell's DNA repair processes, as well as on the initial lesion itself (103). For a given dose, the probability of an irreparable lesion is far higher with a densely ionizing radiation (e.g. a proton or an alpha particle) than with a sparsely ionizing radiation (e.g. an x-ray or a gamma ray) (28).

Unrepaired or misrepaired damage to DNA, in the form of mutations, has been well documented in many types of cells, including human lymphocytes (29) and erythrocyte precursors (42). At a given genetic locus, the frequency of mutations tends to increase linearly in the low-to-intermediate dose range, approximating 10^{-5} to 10^{-6} per Sv (57, 87). The linear nonthreshold nature of the dose-response relationship implies that a mutation can, in principle, occasionally result from the traversal of the genetic target by a single ionizing particle.

Radiation-induced damage may also break chromosomes, thus leading to changes in chromosome structure and number. The combined frequency of translocations, dicentrics, rings, and other chromosome rearrangements increases as a linear, nonthreshold function of the radiation dose in the low-to-intermediate dose range, approximating 0.1 per cell per Sv (100 rem) in human lymphocytes scored soon after irradiation in vitro (45). It is not astonishing, therefore, that the aberration frequency increases in the lymphocytes of atomic bomb survivors, radiation workers, and persons residing in areas of elevated natural background radiation. Because the dose-response relationship has been well characterized, the aberration frequency can serve as a crude biological dosimeter in radiation accident victims (45).

Radiation-induced damage to genes, chromosomes, and other vital organelles may be lethal to the affected cells, especially dividing cells, which are highly radiosensitive as a class. Measured in terms of proliferative capacity, the survival of dividing cells tends to decrease exponentially with increasing dose; 1–2 Sv (100–200 rem) generally suffices to reduce the surviving fraction by about 50% (89). The killing of individual cells is a stochastic process, but because too few cells are killed by a dose below 0.5 Sv (50 rem) to cause detectable tissue damage in most human organs, except those of the embryo (37), such effects are not considered further in this report.

HERITABLE (GENETIC) EFFECTS

Heritable mutations and chromosomal abnormalities increase in frequency with the dose of radiation to the germ cells in Drosophila, laboratory mice, and various other organisms (57, 87). However, such effects of radiation have not yet been detected in humans. Most strikingly, an intensive study of more than 76,000 children of atomic bomb survivors of Hiroshima and Nagasaki, carried out over four decades, has failed to detect heritable effects of radiation, as measured by untoward pregnancy outcomes, neonatal deaths, malignancies, balanced chromosomal rearrangements, sex-chromosome aneuploids, alterations of serum or erythrocyte protein phenotypes, changes in sex ratio, or disturbances of normal growth and development (70). Although negative, these findings are not incompatible with the data from the mouse, given the limited size of the study population and the comparatively small average gonadal radiation dose in question. Therefore, the findings are not interpreted to indicate that human germ cells are resistant to radiation mutagenesis, but rather that a dose of at least 1.0 Sv (100 rem) is required to double their mutation rate (57, 70).

The limited data that are now available permit only tentative estimates of the risks of radiation-induced heritable abnormalities in humans. These data imply that the percentage of all genetic diseases attributable to natural background irradiation is small (Table 2); however, the estimates are fraught with

Table 2 Estimates of the extent to which the frequencies of different heritable disorders are attributable to natural background irradiation[a]

Type of Disorder	Prevalence	Contribution From Natural Background Radiation[b]	
		First Generation	Equilibrium
		(per million live births)[c]	
Autosomal dominant	180,000	20–100	300
X-linked	400	<1	<15
Recessive	2,500	<1	very slow increase
Chromosomal	4,400	<20	very little increase
Congenital abnormalities	20,000–30,000	30	30–300
Other disorders of complex etiology			
Heart disease	600,000	not estimated	not estimated
Cancer	300,000	not estimated	not estimated
Selected others	300,000	not estimated	not estimated

[a] From 57.
[b] Equivalent to 1 mSv per year, or 30 mSv per generation (30 yrs).
[c] Values rounded.

uncertainty, owing to the lack of dose-response data for radiation-induced mutations in human germ cells and inadequate knowledge of the mutational component of many common disorders. No estimates are available for diseases of complex inheritance, which comprise the largest category of genetically related diseases (Table 2).

CARCINOGENIC EFFECTS

Ionizing irradiation causes neoplasms of many types in humans and laboratory animals (57, 87, 97). Such neoplasms characteristically take years or decades to develop and possess no features by which they can be distinguished individually from those induced by other causes. Moreover, with few exceptions, their induction has mainly been detectable after relatively large doses (>0.5 Sv) (50 rem) and has varied with the type of neoplasm, as well as with the age and sex of the exposed population (57, 87).

The available data indicate that radiation carcinogenesis is a multistage process and that the dose-incidence curves for different neoplasms can differ in shape, as well as in slope. For certain human neoplasms, the dose-incidence data are compatible with linear, nonthreshold relationships, but other relationships cannot be excluded (57). Assessment of the extent to which the risk of cancer may be increased by low-level irradiation is therefore dependent on the use of extrapolation models, based on assumptions about the relevant dose-incidence relationships.

Of various mathematical models that have been used to assess the risks of low-level radiation, the one judged to provide the best fit to the available data is of the form:

$$R(d) = R_0 [1 + f(d)g(b)] \qquad\qquad 1.$$

where R_0 denotes the age-specific background risk of death from a specific type of cancer; d denotes the radiation dose; $f(d)$ denotes a function of dose that is linear for cancers other than leukemia and linear-quadratic for leukemia [i.e. $f(d) = a_1d$ or $f(d) = a_2d + a_3d^2$]; and $g(b)$ denotes a risk function dependent on other parameters, such as sex, age at exposure, and time after exposure (57). Somewhat different risk models were used by the United Nations Scientific Committee on the Effects of Atomic Radiation (UNSCEAR) in its latest assessment (87); namely, a simple additive risk model of the form:

$$R(d) = R_0 + f(d) \qquad\qquad 2.$$

and a simple multiplicative risk model of the form:

$$R(d) = R_0 [1 + f(d)] \qquad\qquad 3.$$

both of which assumed the risk to vary as a linear nonthreshold function of the dose.

The estimates of lifetime radiation-induced cancer risks derived with the above three models provide a range of projections (Table 3). As emphasized by the Biological Effects of Ionizing Radiation (BEIR) V Committee, the upper limit of the estimates is about twice the values shown, and the data do not "rigorously exclude the existence of a threshold," or zero risk, in the low (mSv) dose domain (57).

The tabulated risk estimates are appreciably higher than the "preferred" estimates that were published by the BEIR III Committee (60) in 1980, owing primarily to revised estimates of the doses of A-bomb radiation received by the survivors of Hiroshima and Nagasaki; the use of a multiplicative risk projection model in preference to an additive projection model; and the use of a linear dose-incidence model for all cancers other than leukemia, rather than a linear-quadratic model for all cancers (57). On the other hand, the tabulated estimates are not appreciably higher than those derived by the BEIR I Committee in 1972 (61), which were based on the use of analogous risk models. Thus, the tabulated values may provide a reasonably stable range of estimates, given the existing uncertainties in the data. The source of uncertainty that accounts for most of the difference between the upper and lower estimates concerns the extent to which the risks of radiation-induced cancers can be expected to remain elevated long after irradiation. Although the risks of leukemia reach a peak and then decrease within 25 years after irradiation, it

Table 3 Estimated lifetime risks of cancer attributable to 0.1 Sv rapid whole-body irradiation

Type or Site of Cancer	Cancer Deaths Per 100,000[a]
Lung	60^b–170^c
Stomach	90^b–130^d
Leukemia	90^b–100^d
Colon	30^b– 80^d
Breast (female)	20^b– 40^c
Urinary tract	20^b– 40^d
Esophagus	20^b– 30^d
Ovary	20^b– 20^d
Multiple myeloma	10^b– 20^d
Thyroid	10^b– 15^d
Remainder	90^b–135^d
Total	460^b–780^c

[a] Values (rounded) for a population of both sexes and all ages at time of irradiation.
[b] Estimate based on simple additive risk model (87).
[c] Estimate based on modified multiplicative risk model (57).
[d] Estimate based on simple multiplicative risk model (88).

is not known how long the risks of other types of cancer may remain elevated. The extent to which the risks of cancer in persons irradiated during childhood may remain elevated after they have reached the age at which cancer becomes prevalent in the general population can be determined only by further long-continued follow-up of the atomic bomb survivors and other suitable populations.

Apart from the uncertainty about the length of time that the risk of cancer may remain elevated after irradiation, other issues that complicate assessment of the risks of low-level irradiation include uncertainty about the shape of the relevant dose-incidence curve; uncertainty about the extent to which the carcinogenic effects of a given dose may be influenced by variations in its distribution within time and space; uncertainty about the degree to which the risks may vary with age at irradiation, sex, smoking habits, diet, and other factors that affect susceptibility to carcinogenesis; and uncertainty about the accuracy of the dose measurements, diagnoses, and other data on which the estimates are based. Because of these issues, the tabulated risk estimates must be interpreted with caution.

Particular caution must be exercised in extrapolating from the estimates (Table 3) to predict the risk of cancer following the gradual accumulation of a given dose over a period of weeks, months, or years. Experiments on laboratory animals have demonstrated that the carcinogenic effects of low-LET radiation may be reduced by a factor of two-to-ten if the period of exposure is sufficiently prolonged (68, 88). The fact that no comparable reduction occurs with high-LET irradiation implies that the decrease does not result merely from age-dependent changes in susceptibility (88). In the absence of adequate human data on the comparative carcinogenicity of protracted low-LET irradiation, the UNSCEAR Committee (87) and the BEIR V Committee (57) were unable to specify the extent to which their projections may overestimate the risks of a dose of radiation that is accumulated over long periods of time. Insofar as the animal data are predictive for humans, the tabulated risk estimates (Table 3) may exaggerate by a factor of two or more the risks of cancer attributable to irradiation at low dose rates.

As noted above, radiation-induced cancers do not possess any characteristics by which they can be distinguished individually from those arising through other causes. However, the probability that a given cancer may have resulted from previous irradiation can, in principle, be estimated on the basis of the aforementioned risk models, if the radiation dose, age at exposure, and time since exposure are known and if the susceptibility of the affected individual is assumed to be no different from average. This approach, known as the probability of causation method, was the basis of a report mandated by the US Congress to provide a scientifically defensible method for evaluating compensation claims filed by citizens exposed to radioactive fallout downwind from the Nevada test site (59, 69).

TERATOGENIC EFFECTS

Since the pioneer observations of Bergonie and Tribondeau early in this century, we have known that the embryo is highly radiosensitive. During critical stages in organogenesis, which characteristically occupy a few days or weeks for each organ, irradiation of the embryo causes various malformations and other developmental disturbances. Such teratogenic effects are generally thought to result from radiation-induced injury or death of substantial numbers of cells, and not to result unless an appreciable threshold dose is exceeded. Nevertheless, malformations of many types have been produced in laboratory animals by doses as low as 50 mGy (5 rem) delivered during critical stages of organogenesis (88). A limited number of malformations in human infants has also been clinically associated with prenatal irradiation in the past, following the use of older radiological techniques and equipment that delivered higher doses to the embryo than are received in current practice (10).

Among the teratogenic effects observed in humans, especially noteworthy is a dose-dependent increase in the frequency and severity of impairment in brain development in A-bomb survivors who were irradiated between the eighth and the fifteenth weeks after conception. The pertinent data do not define the shape of the dose-effect curve, but are compatible with a nonthreshold function for impairment of intelligence and for severe mental retardation (88). In this cohort (and, to a lesser extent, in the cohort irradiated between the sixteenth and the twenty-fifth week after conception) there is also a dose-dependent downward shift of IQ test scores, which amounts to as much as 25 points per Sv (100 rem) (57, 88). The data are not robust enough to define whether there is a theshold for this effect.

PUBLIC HEALTH IMPLICATIONS

Radon

Environmental radon (^{222}Rn) exposure was first recognized as a significant carcinogen in 1984. However, follow-up studies of underground miners had previously indicated that radon at the high concentrations encountered in mines of many types (i.e., iron, zinc, lead, fluorspar, and uranium) was the primary cause of the elevated incidence of lung cancer in such workers (66, 67). The basic data for estimation of the lung cancer risks come from follow-up studies of four groups of underground miners: uranium miners in Colorado, Ontario, and Czechoslovakia, and iron miners in Malmberget, Sweden (58, 66). From the excess lung cancer risk (above that expected from smoking) in miners, we can estimate the resulting residential lung cancer risks by modeling lifetime radon exposures in the home, as the dose per unit radon exposure is essentially the same in homes as in mines (31, 56). In the three main published estimates of the risk of lung cancer arising from environmental radon exposure (36, 58, 66), the risk models have differed significantly in basic assumptions, but the quantitative estimates of lung cancer risk have agreed within a factor of three (Table 4) and are consistent with the preliminary results of case-control studies on the risks arising from environmental exposure (5).

In view of the risks associated with exposure to radon, and the fact that surveys in Sweden, the UK, the Federal Republic of Germany, Canada, and the US imply that radon contributes more than 50% of the annual effective dose equivalent to the population from natural sources (Table 1), many countries have issued guidelines for limiting exposure to radon. These countries have also recommended methods for reducing long-term exposure to radon in future housing stock (22).

Environmental Background Radiation Other than Radon

Exclusive of the dose to the bronchial epithelium from radon, the average dose of radiation received by members of the US population from other natural sources approximates 1 mSv (100 mrem) per year (Table 1). The risks, if any, that may be associated with this level of irradiation can be estimated only by extrapolation, based on the dose-response models discussed above. The risk estimates for heritable disorders, presented in Table 2, imply that only a small percentage of all such diseases is attributable to natural background irradiation; however, the estimates are fraught with uncertainty, for reasons already mentioned. The corresponding risk estimates for carcinogenic effects imply that no more than 1–3% of all cancers in the general population are caused by natural background irradiation (57).

Epidemiological studies of the extent to which the rates of disease vary

Table 4 Estimated lifetime risk of lung cancer attributable to continuous life-long exposure to indoor ^{222}Rn at a concentration of 150 Bq per m^3 (4 pCi per liter)[a]

Source (Reference)	Lifetime Risk (%)[b]
National Council on Radiation Protection and Measurements (66)	0.9
International Commission on Radiological Protection (36)	1.6
National Academy of Sciences (58)	3.4 (Men)
	1.4 (Women)

[a] 150 Bq per m^3 (4 pCi per liter) corresponds to the EPA guideline for maximum acceptable ^{222}Rn concentration in indoor air.

[b] Risk values shown apply to the general population, including both smokers and nonsmokers, unless otherwise specified.

correspondingly in relation to natural background radiation have yielded results that are generally consistent with the above estimates. The largest such study, which involves a sizable population residing in an area of elevated natural background radiation in Yanjiang County, China, has failed to detect a significant variation in disease frequencies attributable to differences in natural background radiation levels. However, this study did find the frequency of cytogenic abnormalities in the circulating lymphocytes of persons in the high-background area to be increased (102). Studies of disease rates in other high-background areas in the US, England, and other countries have produced varying results, which must be considered inconclusive because of the possible influence of confounding factors (57). Although several studies have found that the rates of cancer and other diseases vary inversely with natural background radiation levels, which some investigators have interpreted as evidence of beneficial (or "hormetic") effects of low-level irradiation, the relationship does not persist after the effects of altitude and other confounding variables have been adequately controlled (57, 105).

The occurance of clusters of childhood leukemia in the vicinity of Sellafield, Dounreay, and other nuclear installations in the UK has aroused concern over the possibility that the leukemias may have been caused by radiation released from the plants (6, 14). The releases are estimated to have increased the total radiation dose to surrounding populations by less than 2% (19), however, thus prompting the search for other possible causes. The possibility of an infective etiology has been suggested by the finding of a comparable excess of childhood leukemia in the New Town of Glenrothes, which contains no radiation facility but otherwise resembles Sellafield, Dounreay, and other nuclear plant sites that have recently experienced a large influx of population (41). Also supporting the hypothesis that some factor other than radiation may be responsible for the leukemia excesses is the finding that villages near potential sites of nuclear plants in the UK have shown similar excesses of leukemia (15).

An additional putative explanation has emerged from a case-control study by Gardner et al (24), which suggested that the excess leukemias near the Sellafield plant may have resulted from occupational irradiation of the fathers of the affected children. This inference, although based on a statistically significant odds ratio, rests on only four cases with significantly exposed fathers. Arguing against this interpretation is the fact that children of A-bomb survivors who were conceived postirradiation have shown no excess of childhood leukemia (111); mutations are not induced by radiation at a high enough frequency to account for the leukemias in question (1); and epidemiological studies of other populations in the UK have failed to confirm the association between paternal irradiation and the occurrence of childhood leukemia (50, 98). It is noteworthy that the rates of mortality from childhood leukemia in US counties that contain nuclear installations have shown no excess (38).

Although the rates of leukemia in southwestern Utah have increased in association with the deposition of radioactive fallout from nuclear weapons tests during 1952–1958, no consistent trend for all forms of leukemia or other types of cancer has been evident (57). Nevertheless, a significant excess of acute leukemia has been reported in those who have received as much as 6–30 mGy (600–3000 mrad) before age 20 and who died before 1964 (78). The excess appears somewhat larger than that which would be predicted on the basis of the risk models in Table 3, but the discrepancy is not statistically significant (75).

Occupational Irradiation

Early radiation workers were among the first to demonstrate carcinogenic effects of irradiation (95). Historic examples include carcinomas of the skin in pioneer radiologists and x-ray workers (23); leukemias in early radiologists (86); osteogenic sarcomas and carcinomas of cranial sinuses in early radium dial painters (48); and lung cancers in pitchblende and other underground hard-rock miners (99, 106). With the evolution of modern radiation protection standards, the occupational risks of such cancers have been drastically reduced, but the extent to which they may still be elevated remains a subject of ongoing study. Radiation has thus continued to be one of the most thoroughly investigated of occupational carcinogens.

Of the various forms of human cancer induced by irradiation, leukemia (excluding chronic lymphocyte leukemia) has the highest relative risk per unit dose (57). However, only one of 17 recent studies of radiation workers has found a significant overall excess of leukemia (Table 5). Furthermore, although an excess in an isolated subgroup has been reported in one study, a significantly positive dose-response relationship for the disease has not been observed in any of the nine studies in which individual radiation exposure data were analyzed (Table 5). These findings suggest that the average risk of leukemia in today's radiation workers is no larger than would be predicted on the basis of the extrapolation models discussed above.

Multiple myeloma is another form of cancer for which the relative risk following low-level irradiation is comparatively high (18). Indeed, the rate is elevated in several occupationally exposed cohorts, including workers of the Hanford nuclear facility (26), but in the majority of cohorts investigated the disease has shown no increased frequency (Table 6). Again, there is little reason to conclude that the risk of multiple myeloma in radiation workers is any higher than would be predicted on the basis of the extrapolation models discussed above.

Other forms of cancer have also been occasionally reported to be increased

Table 5 Relative risks of leukemia in radiation workers, as estimated from recent epidemiological studies

Study Group (Reference)	No. of Subjects (Rad; Controls)	Average Dose (mSv)	Observed/ Expected Leukemias[a]	Relative Risk (95%CI)	Average Follow-up (Yr)	Comments
Medical Technologists						
X-ray technologists	105,000	50–200	61/51	1.2 (0.9–1.5)	5–60 range	— (9)
US Army Rad technologists (39)	Rad, 6500; controls, 6800	Unknown; probably	12/6.7	1.8 (0.7–4.4)	29 >100	—
Nuclear Workers						
Nuclear shipyard workers (72, 77)	Rad, 7/610; controls, 15,580	28	7/8.3	0.8 (0.3–1.7)	≈15	Dose-response nonsignificant.
Hanford workers (25, 26)	36,235	23	42/57.3	0.7 (0.5–1.0)	21	Few internal depositions. Dose-response slope <negative.
Oak Ridge Natl Lab workers (109)	Rad, 6189; no recorded dose, 2/129	17	28/17.2	1.4 (0.6–3.2)	≈26	Leukemia excess for entire workforce. Dose-response slope not significant.
Oak Ridge fabrication (Y12) workers (13)	6780	10	4/8.5	0.5 (0.1–1.2)	20	51% with internal monitoring. Dose-response nonsignificant.

Oak Ridge fabrication (Y-12/TEC) workers (71)	18,869		40/43.57	0.9 (0.7–1.2)	26	—
Savannah River workers (17)	9860	(Low); Uranium dust exposures ≈40	18/13.3	1.4 (0.8–2.1)	24	≈15% of dose from internal deposition.
Mound workers (107)	Rad, 3299; unbadged, 953	30	Myeloid, 1/0.4	2.4 (0.1–63)	19	Some exposures to ^{210}Po, ^{238}Pu and ^{3}H.
UK Atomic Weapons Estab. workers (7)	Rad, 9390; unbadged, 13,160	7.8	4/9.2 (9.16)	0.4 (0.2–2.4)	18	40% with internal nuclides. Dose-response slope < negative.
UK Atomic Energy Auth. workers (8)	Rad, 20, 380; 19,160	32	18/15.4	1.2 (0.7–1.8)	16	Dose-response slope ~0.
Sellafield/BNF workers (75)	Rad, 10,150; unbadged, 3840	124	10/12.2	0.8 (0.4–1.5)	22	Dose-response slope nonsignificant.
Rocky Flats workers (25,108)	5410	41	4/5.4	0.7 (0.2–1.8)	14	Dose-response nonsignificant.
Miscellaneous Groups						
US uranium mill workers (104)	2002	(?)	0/4.5	0 (0,0.7)	21	—
Linde (84)	8146	(?)	11/11.0	1.0 (0.5–1.7)	>20	—
Small occupational studies (2, 3, 30, 34)	—	—	13/12.6	1.0 (0.6–1.7)	—	—

[a] All types of leukemia unless specified otherwise.

Table 6   Estimated relative risks of multiple myeloma in radiation workers, as indicated by recent epidemiological studies[a]

Study (References)	Observed/Expected	Ratio	Mean Tissue Dose (mSv)
Early US radiologists (49)	11/7.9	1.4	2400–6000
Early UK radiologists (74)	0/1.0	0	50–100/yr
Japanese radiation technologists (4)	2/0.7	2.9	≈600[b]
Chinese x-ray workers (101)	0/1.3	0	≈1000[b]
US Hanford workers (25, 26)	4/2.1	2.0	23
US Oak Ridge National Lab (109)	1/≈3.4[b]	≈0.3	17
US Oak Ridge fabrication workers (13)	4/2.8	1.4	≈10[b]
US Linde fabrication workers (84)	3/3.2	0.9	(?)
US uranium millers (104)	1/≈1.5[b]	0.7	(?)
US Rocky Flats (25, 108)	1/0	∞	41
UK Atomic Energy Authority (8)	3/5.3	0.6	32
UK Atomic Weapons Establishment (7)	2/3.6	0.6	8
UK Sellafield (75)	7/4.2	1.7	124
Atomic Energy of Canada, Ltd. (34)	1/2.1	0.5	47
US radium-dial painters (76)	6/2.2	2.8	26

[a] Portions of this table are adapted from Miller & Beebe (51) or Cuzick (18).
[b] ≈ denotes approximate values estimated for this tabulation.

in frequency in some cohorts of radiation workers. Mortality from lung cancer and leukemia, for example, increased with increasing dose in workers of the Oak Ridge National Laboratory (109). However, data on the smoking habits of the workers were not available, the increase in lung cancer was not significant in nonmonthly workers, there were no deaths from lung cancer in male monthly workers whose accumulated doses exceeded 40 mSv, lung cancer mortality in the group as a whole was less than two thirds of that which would have been expected from national rates, and the analysis of mortality from leukemia did not exclude deaths from chronic lymphocytic leukemia, which bear no known relation to previous irradiation. Hence, as has been emphasized elsewhere (81), the findings must be interpreted with caution. Excesses of other forms of cancer have also been reported occasionally in various occupationally exposed cohorts; however, because of methodological problems and other sources of uncertainty, the findings are of equivocal public health significance (57).

Radiation Accidents

In view of the many powerful sources of radiation in the modern world, the low frequency with which persons are accidentally irradiated attests to the effectiveness of existing safeguards. In spite of elaborate precautions, however, some 285 nuclear reactor accidents were reported in various countries between 1945 and 1987 (excluding the Chernobyl accident), thus resulting in the exposure of more than 1350 persons, with 33 fatalities (46). In most such accidents, the public has not been directly affected, but in each of the two most serious recent reactor accidents—the one at Three Mile Island (TMI) in 1978 and the one at Chernobyl in 1986—enough radiation material was released into the environment to pose a potential threat to the health of off-site populations.

Fortunately, in the TMI accident the largest dose to anyone residing near the reactor was no larger than the annual dose normally received from natural background irradiation (96). Not unexpectedly, therefore, the accident resulted in no detectable increase in birth defects or infant mortality in the surrounding population (85). Nevertheless, those living in the vicinity of TMI have shown evidence of persistent psychological stress (11), which has been implicated as a possible explanation for the temporary rise in the annual incidence of cancer during 1982–1984 in those residing closest to the plant (33). Because there was no associated increase in cancer mortality in this population, the possibility that the rise in incidence may have resulted from early ascertainment, as a consequence of heightened surveillance prompted by postaccident concern, has also been suggested (33).

In the Chernobyl accident, a far larger release of radioactivity occurred, thus necessitating the evacuation of tens of thousands of people and farm animals from the surrounding area. The accident caused a collective dose commitment to the population living within 30 km of the plant that is estimated to approximate 16,000 person-Sv (1,600,000 person-rem) (20). A dose commitment of this magnitude can be projected, on the basis of the aforementioned risk models (Table 3), to increase the lifetime risk of cancer in the population by as much as 4–8%, i.e. to multiply the natural risk by a factor of 1.04–1.08. Beyond 30 km, the accident resulted in a collective dose equivalent commitment to the Northern Hemisphere of approximately 600,000 person-Sv (60,000,000 person-rem) (87), which can be projected to cause as many as 30,000 excess cancers within the next 70 years, more than one third of which would occur in Byelorussia alone. Although such a large number of excess cancers would be a public health disaster, the projected excess in Byelorussia corresponds to less than the 1% of the cancers expected to occur there "spontaneously" during the next 70 years. Except in the most heavily exposed subpopulation, therefore, the excess is unlikely to be detectable.

Medical Irradiation

Diagnostic medical irradiation accounts for the largest part by far—over 80%—of population exposure to radiation from man-made sources (Table 1).

Although the use of radiography for diagnostic purposes has now been widely accepted, mammographic screening for breast cancer in asymptomatic women was challenged initially because its benefits were not well documented and the doses it delivered to the breast were appreciable. In the past 20 years, improved film-screen and xeromammographic methods have reduced breast doses significantly. Meanwhile, the evidence from several randomized trials has clearly shown reductions in breast cancer mortality of roughly 30% from mammographic screening for women over age 50, and the benefits in terms of mortality prevented are five to 100 times as great (depending upon age and dose) as the corresponding radiation risks (65). For women under age 50, the evidence for benefits from mammographic screening remains equivocal (16), an issue that needs to be resolved in view of the recommendations by some organizations to conduct routine mammographic screening at ages 40–49, although the ongoing randomized mammographic trials may contain too few women under age 50 to resolve this issue. In women with a familial or personal history of breast cancer, however, it is still recommended that mammographic screening begin at age 35 (16).

The thyroid gland appears to be unusually susceptible to radiation carcinogenesis, especially in childhood, judging from the effects of acute irradiation in A-bomb survivors and in patients treated with x-rays to the head and neck (57). Medical exposure to iodine-131 (^{131}I), which concentrates in the thyroid gland and has a seven-day effective biological half life, is therefore a matter of concern, as is the potential for exposure to ^{131}I released from nuclear plant accidents or in nuclear bomb fallout. Also of concern is the potential for exposure to ^{125}I, which is widely used for laboratory purposes in science, medicine, and industry. Although one animal study has suggested that ^{131}I is no less effective than x-rays in inducing thyroid cancer (43), the human data suggest that it may be three to ten times less effective (73). Unfortunately, because the available follow-up data on children who have received ^{131}I are sparse, there is considerable uncertainty in the estimate. The experience of the USSR population exposed to moderate or large doses of ^{131}I in the Chernobyl accident can advance our understanding of the effects of ^{131}I if investigated by carefully controlled, long-term studies.

Early reports by Stewart (79) and others, which suggested that the induction of childhood leukemia by in utero exposure to only a few mSv from maternal abdominal diagnostic x-ray examinations, were controversial because no excess leukemia had been seen in Japanese A-bomb survivors who were irradiated in utero (60). The earlier case-control studies have since been essentially confirmed by a large cohort study and several studies of twins (32, 52, 53). The fact that adult cancers are now also occurring with increased frequency among prenatally exposed A-bomb survivors (110) attests further to the radiosensitivity of the fetus.

IMPLICATIONS FOR EXPOSURE LIMITS

With the abandonment of the threshold hypothesis for mutagenic and carcinogenic effects of radiation, the setting of permissable exposure limits has become inextricably linked to assessment of the risks of such effects at low levels of exposure. In recognition of the possible existence of such risks, contemporary radiation protection practices are guided by the following principles (35):

1. Justification: Any activity that causes radiation exposure should produce a sufficient benefit to offset the harm it may cause.
2. Optimization: For any source of radiation, the likelihood of exposure and the dose it may deliver should be as low as reasonably achievable, and economic and social factors should be considered.
3. Dose limits: The dose to each individual, as well as the likelihood of exposure from all sources, should be subject to control.

In keeping with these principles, the system of radiation protection that has evolved includes exposure limits for every organ of the body. Furthermore, because the latest risk estimates (Table 3) imply that annual exposure of radiation workers to 50 mSv (5 rem) per year (the present maximum permissible dose limit) would ultimately increase the lifetime risk of cancer in such workers by more than 30%, the International Commission on Radiological Protection has recommended that the dose limit for workers be reduced to 20 mSv (2 rem) per year averaged over a period of five years, with no more than 50 mSv (5 rem) in any one year (35).

Although these new recommendations will probably not affect the majority of radiation workers greatly, as their exposures are already well below the present maximum permissible dose limit, implementation of the recommendations could reduce the level of exposure for the small subpopulation (<1%) of workers who now approach the dose limit repeatedly. In reducing the exposure of this subpopulation, it is important that its collective exposure not merely be redistributed over a larger fraction of the total workforce, as the same numbers of radiation-induced cancers would ultimately be expected to result.

Reduction of the dose to the patient is an important goal in the medical uses of radiation, because a 15% reduction in exposures from diagnostic radiology would reduce the total exposure of the population as much as the elimination of all other man-made sources of ionizing radiation (100). Perhaps the greatest room for improvement lies in the disparity between the state of the art in administering diagnostic radiation and the prevailing practices of the radiological medical community as a whole (21). A national survey of diagnostic exposures has shown that a small but significant fraction of radiologic practices delivers doses in common radiologic diagnostic procedures that are more than five times larger than the norm (40). Also, a recent report has noted that, in spite of technological advances, there has been relatively little change in patient diagnostic exposure levels since the 1970s (62). Finally, as noted above, measures to limit residential exposure to radon also are indicated.

ACKNOWLEDGEMENT

The authors are grateful to Ms. Lynda Witte and Ms. Eileen Santan for assistance in the preparation of the manuscript. Preparation of this report was supported in part by Grants ES 00260 and CA 13343 from the US Public Health Service and Grant SIG 09 from the American Cancer Society.

Literature Cited

1. Abrahamson, S. 1990. Commentary. Childhood leukemia at Sellafield. *Radiat. Res.* 123:237–38
2. Acquavella, J. F., Wiggs, L., Waxweiler, R., McDonell, D., Tietjen, G., Wilkinson, G. 1985. Mortality among workers at the Pantex weapons facility. *Health Phys.* 48:735–46
3. Acquavella, J. F., Wilkinson, G., Wiggs, L., Tietjen, G., Key, C. 1983. An evaluation of cancer incidence among employees at the Los Alamos National Laboratory. In *Epidemiology Applied to Health Physics*, Proc. of the 16th Midyear Topical Meeting, pp. 338–45. Albuquerque: Health Phys. Soc.
4. Aoyama, T. 1989. Radiation risk of Japanese and Chinese low dose-repeatedly irradiated population. *J. Univ. Occup. Environ. Health Jpn.* 11:432–42
5. Axelson, O. 1991. Occupational and environmental exposure to radon: Cancer risks. *Annu. Rev. Public Health* 12:235–55
6. Beral, V. 1990. Leukaemia and nuclear installations. *Br. Med. J.* 300:411–12
7. Beral, V., Fraser, P., Carpenter, L., Booth, M., Brown, A., Rose, G. 1988. Mortality of employees of the atomic weapons establishment. *Br. Med. J.* 297:757–70
8. Beral, V., Inskip, H., Fraser, P., Booth, M., Coleman, D., Rose, G. 1985. Mortality of employees of the United Kingdom atomic energy authority. *Br. Med. J.* 291:440–47
9. Boice, J., Morin, M., Mandel, J. 1990. Cancer risk in x-ray technologists. In

Proc. of the Board of Scientific Counselors, March 1–2, pp. 110–13, Washington, DC: Div. of Cancer Etiology, US Nat. Cancer Inst.
10. Brill, A. B., Forgotson, E. H. 1964. Radiation and congenital malformations. *Am. J. Obstet. Gynecol.* 90:1149–68
11. Bromet, E. J., Parkinson, D. K., Dunn, L. D. 1990. Long-term mental health consequences of the accident at Three Mile Island. *Int. J. Mental Health* 19:48–60
12. Brown, P. 1936. *American Martyrs to Sciences Through the Roentgen Rays*. Springfield, Ill: Thomas
13. Checkoway, H., Peare, N., Crawford-Brown, D., Cragle, D. 1988. Radiation doses and cause-specifric mortality among workers at a nuclear materials fabrication plant. *Am. J. Epidemiol.* 127:255–66
14. Committee on Medical Aspects of Radiation in the Environment (COMARE). 1989. *Third Report: Report on the Incidence of Childhood Cancer in the West Berkshire and North Hampshire Area, in Which are Situated the Atomic Weapons Research Establishment, Aldermaston and the Royal Ordinance Factory, Burghfield*. London: HM Stationery Office
15. Cook-Mozaffari, P., Darby, S., Doll, R. 1989. Cancer near potential sites of nuclear installations. *Lancet* 2:1145–47
16. Council On Scientific Affairs. 1989. Mammographic screening in asymptomatic women aged 40 years and older. *J. Am. Med. Assoc.* 261:2535–42
17. Cragle, D. L., McLain, R., Qualters, J.,

Hickey, J., Wilkinson, G., et al. 1988. Mortality among workers at a nuclear fuels production facility. *Am. J. Ind. Med.* 14:370–401

18. Cuzick, J. 1981. Radiation-induced myelomatosis. *N. Engl. J. Med.* 304: 204–20

19. Darby, S. C., Doll, R. 1987. Fallout, radiation doses near Dounreay, and childhood leukaemia. *Br. Med. J.* 294: 603–7

20. Dep. of Energy (DOE). 1987. *Health and Environmental Consequences of the Chernobyl Nuclear Power Plant Accident.* DOE/ER-0332. Washington, DC: Nat. Tech. Information Serv. US Dep. of Commerce.

21. Editorial. 1988. Radiation protection in the UK: An opportunity missed. *Lancet* 2:315–316

22. Environmental Protection Agency (EPA). 1986. *A Citizens Guide to Radon.* Washington, DC: EPA

23. Frieben, A. 1902. Demonstration lines cancroids des rechten handruckens, das sich nach langdauernde einwirkung von rontgenstrahlen entwickelt hatte. *Fortschr. Geb Roentgenstr* 6:106

24. Gardner, M. J., Snee, M., Hall, A., Powell, C., Downes, S., Terrell, J. 1990. Results of case-control study of leukemia and lymphoma among young people near Sellafield nuclear plant in West Cumbria. *Br. Med. J.* 300:423–29

25. Gilbert, E. S., Fry, S., Wiggs, L., Voelz, G., Cragle, D., Petersen, G. 1989. Analysis of combined mortality data on workers at the Hanford site, Oak Ridge National Laboratory, and Rocky Flats nuclear weapons plant. *Radiat. Res.* 120:19–35

26. Gilbert, E. Peterson, G., Buchanan, J. 1989. Mortality of workers at the Hanford site: 1945–1981. *Health Phys.* 56: 11–25

27. Glasser, O. 1933. *The Science of Radiology.* Springfield, Ill: Thomas

28. Goodhead, D. T. 1988. Spatial and temporal distribution of energy. *Health Phys.* 55:231–40

29. Grosovsky, A. J., Little, J. B. 1985. Evidence for linear response for the induction of mutations in human cells by x-ray exposure below 10 rads. *Proc. Natl. Acad. Sci. USA* 82:2092–95

30. Hadjimichael, O., Ostefeld, A., D'Atri, D., Brubaker, R. 1983. Mortality and cancer incidence experience of employees in a nuclear fuels fabrication plant. *J. Occup. Med.* 25:48–61

31. Harley, N. H. 1984. Comparing radon daughter dose: Environmental versus underground exposure. *Radiat. Prot. Dosim.* 7:371

32. Harvey, E., Boice, J., Honeyman, M., Flannery, J. 1985. Prenatal x-ray exposure and childhood cancer in twins. *N. Engl. J. Med.* 312:541–45

33. Hatch, M. C., Wallenstein, S., Beyla, J., Nieves, J., Susser, M. 1991. Cancer rates after the Three Mile Island nuclear accident and proximity to the plant. *Am. J. Public Health* 81:719–24

34. Howe, G. R., Weeks, J., Miller, A., Chiarelli, A., Etezadi-Amoli, J. 1987. *A Study of the Health of Employees of Atomic Energy of Canada Limited. IV. Analysis of Mortality During the Period 1950–1981.* Pinawa, Manitoba: Atomic Energy of Canada Ltd

35. Int. Comm. Radiol. Prot. (ICRP). 1991. Recommendations of the International Commission on Radiological Protection. ICRP Publ. No. 60. *Ann. ICRP* 21: 1–3

36. Int. Comm. Radiol. Prot. (ICRP). 1986. *Lung Cancer Risk from Indoor Exposure to Radon Daughters.* ICRP Publ. No. 50. Oxford: Pergamon

37. Int. Comm. Radiol. Prot. (ICRP). 1984. *Nonstochastic Effects of Radiation.* ICRP Publ. No. 41. Oxford: Pergamon

38. Jablon, S., Hrubec, Z., Boice, J. 1991. Cancer in populations living near nuclear facilities. A survey of mortality nationwide and incidence in two states. *J. Am. Med. Assoc.* 265:1403–8

39. Jablon, S., Miller, R. 1978. Army technologists: 29-year follow up for cause of death. *Radiology* 126:677–79

40. Johnson, D., Goetz, W. 1986. Patient exposure trends in medical and dental radiography. *Health Phys.* 50:107–16

41. Kinlen, L. 1988. Evidence for an infective cause of childhood leukemia: Comparison of a Scottish new town with nuclear reprocessing sites in Britain. *Lancet* 2:1323–27

42. Langlois, R. G., Bigbee, W. L., Kyoizumi, S., Nakamura, N., Bean, M. A., et al. 1987. Evidence for increased somatic cell mutations at the glycophorin A locus in atomic bomb survivors. *Science* 236:445–48

43. Lee, W., Chiacchierini, R., Shleien, B., Telles, N. 1982. Thyroid tumors following I-131 or localized X irradiation to the thyroid and pituitary glands in rats. *Radiat. Res.* 92:307–19

44. Lewis, E. B. 1957. Leukemia and ionizing radiation. *Science* 125:965–75

45. Lloyd, D. C., Purrott, R. J. 1981. Chromosome aberration analysis in radiological protection dosimetry. *Radiat. Prot. Dosim.* 1:19–28

46. Lushbaugh, C. C., Fry, S. A., Ricks, R. C. 1987. Nuclear reactor accidents: preparedness and consequences. *Br. J. Radiol.* 60:1159–83

47. MacMahon, B., Hutchison, G. B. 1964. Prenatal X-ray and childhood cancer: A review. *Acta Unio Int. Contra Cancrum* 20:1172–74

48. Martland, H. S. 1931. The occurrence of malignancy in radioactive persons. A general review of data gathered in the study of the radium dial painters, with special reference to the occurrence of ostogenic sarcoma and the interrelationship of certain blood diseases. *Am. J. Cancer* 15:2435–2516

49. Matanoski, G., Seltser, P., Sartwell, P., Diamond, E., Elliott, E. 1975. The current mortality rates of radiologists and other physician specialists: Specific causes of death. *Am. J. Epidemiol.* 101:199–210

50. McKinney, P. A., Alexander, F. E., Cartwright, R. A., Parker, L. 1991. Parental occupations of children with leukemia in west Cumbria, north Humberside, and Gateshead. *Br. Med. J.* 302: 681–87

51. Miller, R. W., Beebe, G. 1986. Leukemia, lymphoma, and multiple myeloma. In *Radiation Carcinogenesis*, ed. A. C. Upton, R. Albert, F. Burns, R. Shore, pp. 245–60. New York: Elsevier

52. Mole, R. H. 1974. Antenatal irradiation and childhood cancer. Causation or coincidence. *Br. J. Cancer* 30: 199–208

53. Monson, R., MacMahon, B. 1984. Prenatal x-ray exposure and cancer in children. In *Radiation Carcinogenesis: Epidemiology and Biological Significance,* ed. J. Boice, J. Fraumeni, pp. 97–105. New York: Raven

54. Muller, H. J. 1954. The manner of production of mutations by radiation. In *Radiation Biology, Vol. 1: High Energy Radiation,* ed. A. Hollaender, pp. 475–626. New York: McGraw-Hill

55. Nat. Acad. Sci. 1956. Advisory Committee of the Biological Effects of Ionizing Radiation. *The Biological Effects of Atomic Radiation.* Washington, DC: Nat. Acad. Sci.

56. Nat. Acad. Sci.-Nat. Res. Council. 1991. Panel on Dosimetric Assumption Affecting the Application of Radon Risk Estimates. *Comparative Dosimetry of Radon in Mines and Houses.* Washington, DC: Nat. Acad. Press

57. Nat. Acad. Sci.-Nat. Res. Council. 1990. Committee on the Biological Effects of Ionizing Radiation. (BEIR V).

Health Effects of Exposure to Low Levels of Ionizing Radiation. Washington, DC: Nat. Acad. Press

58. Nat. Acad. Sci.-Nat. Res. Council. 1988. Committee on Biological Effects of Ionizing Radiation (BEIR IV). *Health Risks of Radon and Other Internally Deposited Alpha-Emitters.* Washington, DC: Nat. Acad. Press

59. National Academy of Sciences-National Research Council. 1984. *Assigned Share for Radiation as a Cause of Cancer.* Washington, DC: Nat. Acad. Press

60. Nat. Acad. Sci.-Nat. Res. Council. 1980. Committee on Biological Effects of Ionizing Radiation (BEIR III). *The Effects on Populations of Exposure to Low Levels of Ionizing Radiation.* Washington, DC: Nat. Acad. Press

61. Nat. Acad. Sci.-Nat. Res. Council. 1972. Committed on Biological Effects of Ionizing Radiation (BEIR I). *Effects on Populations of Exposure to Low Levels of Ionizing Radiation.* Washington, DC: Nat. Acad. Sci.

62. Nat. Counc. Radiat. Prot. Meas. (NCRP). 1989. *Exposure of the U.S. Population from Diagnostic Medical Radiation.* Rep. No. 100. Bethesda: Nat. Counc. Radiot. Prot. Meas.

63. Nat. Counc. Radiat. Prot. Meas. (NCRP). 1987. *Exposure to the Population in the United States and Canada from Natural Background Radiation.* Rep. No. 94. Bethesda: Nat. Counc. Radiat. Prot. Meas.

64. Nat. Council on Radiation Protection and Measurement (NCRP). 1987. *Ionizing Radiation Exposure of the Population of the United States.* Rep. No. 93. Bethesda: Nat. Counc. Radiat. Prot. Meas.

65. Nat. Counc. Radiat. Prot. Meas. (NCRP). 1986. *Mammography—A User's Guide.* Rep. No. 85. Bethesda: Nat. Counc. Radiat. Prot. Meas.

66. Nat. Counc. Radiat. Protect. Meas. (NCRP). 1984. *Evaluation of Occupational and Environmental Exposures to Radon and Radon Daughters in the United States.* Rep. No. 78. Bethesda: Nat. Counc. Radiat. Prot. Meas.

67. Nat. Counc. Radiat. Prot. Meas. (NCRP). 1984. *Exposures From the Uranium Series with Emphasis on Radon and Its Daughters.* Rep. No. 77. Bethesda: Nat. Counc. Radiat. Prot. Meas.

68. Nat. Counc. Radiat. Prot. Meas. (NCRP). 1980. *Influence of Dose and Its Distribution in Time on Dose-Response Relationships for Low LET Radiations.*

Rep. No. 64. Washington, DC: Nat. Counc. Radiat. Prot. Meas.
69. Nat. Inst. Health (NIH). 1985. *Rep. of Nat. Inst. Health Ad Hoc Working Group to Develop Radioepidemiological Tables.* NIH Publ. No. 85–2748. Washington DC: GPO
70. Neel, J. V., Schull, W., Awa, A., Staoh, C., Otake, M., et al. 1990. The children of parents exposed to atomic bombs: Estimates of the genetic doubling dose of radiation for humans. *Am. J. Hum. Genet.* 46:1053–72
71. Polednak, A. P., Frome, E. 1981. Mortality among men employed between 1943 and 1947 at a uranium-processing plant. *J. Occup. Med.* 23:169–78
72. Rinsky, R. A., Zumwalde, R., Waxweiler, R., Murray, W. Jr., Bierbaum, P., et al. 1981. Cancer mortality at a naval nuclear shipyard. *Lancet* 1:231–35
73. Shore, R. E. 1991. The epidemiology of radiation-induced thyroid cancer: Research issues and needs. *Br. Inst. Radiol. Rep.* In press
74. Smith, P., Doll, R. 1981. Mortality from cancer and all causes among British radiologists. *Br. J. Radiol.* 54:187–94
75. Smith, P., Douglas, A. 1986. Mortality of workers at the Sellafield plant of British Nuclear Fuels. *Br. Med. J.* 293:845–54
76. Stebbings, J. H., Lucas, H., Stehney, A. 1983. Multiple myeloma, leukemia, and breast cancer among the US radium dial workers. In *Epidemiology Applied to Health Physics.* Albuquerque: Health Phys. Soc.
77. Stern, F., Waxweiler, R., Beaumont, J., Lees, J., Rinsky, R., et al. 1986. A case-control study of leukemia at a naval nuclear shipyard. *Am. J. Epidemiol.* 123:980–92
78. Stevens, W., Thomas, D. C., Lyon, J. L., Till, J. E., Kerber, R. A., et al. 1990. Leukemia in Utah and radioactive fallout from the Nevada test site. *J. Am. Med. Assoc.* 264:585–91
79. Stewart, A. M., Webb, J., Giles, D., Hewitt, D. 1956. Preliminary communication: Malignant disease in childhood and diagnostic irradiation in utero. *Lancet* 2:447–48
80. Stewart, A., Webb, J., Hewitt, D. 1958. A survey of childhood malignancies. *Br. Med. J.* 1:1495
81. Strom, D. J. 1991. A critique of "mortality among workers at Oak Ridge National Laboratory." *Nucl. News* 34:67–70

82. Taylor, L. S. 1958. History of the International Commission on Radiological Units and Measurements (ICRU). *Health Phys.* 1:306–14
83. Taylor, L. S. 1931. X-ray protection. *J. Am. Med. Soc.* 116:136–40
84. Teta, M. J., Ott, M. 1988. A mortality study of a research, engineering, and metal fabrication facility in western New York State. *Am. J. Epidemiol.* 127:540–51
85. Tokuhata, G. K. 1985. Three Mile Island nuclear accident and its effect on the surrounding population. In *Management of Radioactive Materials and Wastes: Issues and Progress,* ed. S. K. Majumdar, E. W. Miller, pp. 326–41. Harrisburg: Penn. Acad. Sci.
86. Ulrich, H. 1946, The incidence of leukemia in radiologists. *N. Engl. J. Med.* 234:45–46
87. Sci. Comm. Effects At. Radiat. (UNSCEAR). 1988. *Sources, Effects and Risks of Ionizing Radiation.* New York: UN
88. UN Sci. Comm. Effects At. Radiat. (UNSCEAR). 1986. *Genetic and Somatic Effects of Ionizing Radiation.* Report to the General Assembly, with annexes. (Forty-first Session, Suppl. No. 16). New York: UN
89. UN Sci. Comm. Effects At. Radiat. (UNSCEAR). 1982. *Ionizing Radiation: Sources and Biological Effects.* Report to the General Assembly, with annexes. New York: UN
90. UN Sci. Comm. Effects At. Radiat. (UNSCEAR). 1977. *Sources and Effects of Ionizing Radiation,* Report to the General Assembly, with annexes. (Thirty-second Session, Suppl. No. 40). New York: UN.
91. UN Sci. Comm. Effects At. Radiat. (UNSCEAR). 1972. *Ionizing Radiation: Levels and Effects.* (Official Records: Twenty-seventh Session, Suppl. No. 25). New York: UN
92. UN Sci. Comm. Effects At. Radiat. (UNSCEAR). 1966. *Report of the United Nations Scientific Committee on the Effects of Atomic Radiation.* (Official Records: Twenty-first Session, Suppl. No. 14). New York: UN
93. UN Sci. Comm. Effects At. Radiat. (UNSCEAR). 1962. *Report to the General Assembly,* (Official Records: Seventeenth Session, Suppl. No. 16). New York: UN
94. UN Sci. Comm. Effects At. Radiat. (UNSCEAR). 1958. *Report to the General Assembly,* (Official Records:

Thirteenth Session, Suppl. No. 17). New York: UN
95. Upton, A. C. 1986. Historical perspectives on radiation carcinogenesis. In *Radiation Carcinogenesis,* ed. A. C. Upton, R. E. Albert, F. J. Burns, R. E. Shore, pp. 1–10. New York: Elsevier
96. Upton, A. C. 1981. Health impact of the Three Mile Island accident. *Ann. NY Acad. Sci.* 365:63–70
97. Upton, A. C., Albert, R. E., Burns, F. J., Shore, R. E., eds. 1986. *Radiation Carcinogenesis.* New York: Elsevier
98. Urquhart, J. D., Black, R. J., Muirhead, M. J., Sharp, L., Maxwell, M., et al. 1991. Case-control study of leukaemia and non-Hodgkin's lymphoma in children in Caithness near the Dounreay nuclear installation. *Br. Med. J.* 302:687–92
99. Wagoner, J. K., Archer, V. E., Lundin, F. E. Jr., Holaday, D. A., Lloyd, J. W. 1965. Radiation as the cause of lung cancer among uranium miners. *N. Engl. J. Med.* 273:181–88
100. Wall, B., Rae, S., Darby, S., Kendall, G. 1981. A reappraisal of the genetic consequences of diagnostic radiology in Great Britain. *Br. J. Radiol.* 54:719–30
101. Wang, J. X., Inskip, P., Boice, J. Jr., Li, B. 1990. Cancer incidence among medical diagnostic X-ray workers in China, 1950–1985. *Int. J. Cancer* 45:889–95
102. Wang, Z., Boice, J. D., Wei, L., Gilbert, G. W., Zha, Y., et al. 1990. Thyroid nodularity and chromosome aberrations among women in areas of high background radiation in China. *J. Natl. Cancer Inst.* 82:478–85
103. Ward, J. F. 1988. DNA damage produced by ionizing radiation in mammalian cells: identities, mechanisms of

formation and repairability. *Prog. Nucleic Acid Res. Mol. Biol.* 35:96–128
104. Waxweiler, R., Archer, V., Roscoe, R., Watanabe, A., Thun, M. 1983. Mortality patterns among a retrospective cohort of uranium mill workers. In *Epidemiology Applied to Health Physics (Proc. Health Phys. Soc.),* pp. 428–35. Albuquerque: Health Phys. Soc.
105. Weinberg, C. R., Brown, K. G., Hoel, D. G. 1987. Altitude, radiation, and mortality from cancer and heart disease. *Radiat. Res.* 112:381–90
106. Weller, C. V. 1956. *Causal Factors in Cancer of the Lung,* pp. 43–47. Springfield, Ill: Thomas
107. Wiggs, L. D., Cox-Devore, C., Wilkinson, G., Reyes, M. 1991. Mortality among workers exposed to external ionizing radiation at a nuclear facility in Ohio. *J. Occup. Med.* 33:632–37
108. Wilkinson, G., Tietjen, G., Wiggs, L., Galke, W., Acquavella, J., et al. 1987. Mortality among plutonium and other radiation workers at a plutonium weapons facility. *Am. J. Epidemiol.* 125:231–50
109. Wing, S., Shy, C., Wood, J., Wolf, S., Cragle, D., Frome, E. 1991. Mortality among workers at Oak Ridge National Laboratory. Evidence of radiation effects in follow-up through 1984. *J. Am. Med. Assoc.* 265:1397–1402
110. Yoshimoto, Y., Kato, H., Schull, W. 1988. Risk of cancer among children exposed in utero to A-bomb radiations, 1950–84. *Lancet* 2:665–69
111. Yoshimoto, Y., Neel, J. V., Schull, W. J., Kato, H., Sado, M., et al. 1990. Malignant tumors during the first 2 decades of life in the offspring of atomic bomb survivors. *Am. J. Hum. Genet.* 46:1041–52

Annu. Rev. Publ. Health. 1992. 13:151–71

OCCUPATIONAL HEALTH CONCERNS OF FIREFIGHTING

Tee L. Guidotti and Veronica M. Clough

Occupational Health Program, University of Alberta Faculty of Medicine, Edmonton, Alberta T6G 2G3

KEY WORDS: firefighters, combustion gases, ergonomics, stress

INTRODUCTION

The health effects of exposures related to fighting fires has long been a major interest of occupational health investigators. Municipal firefighters are an unusually accessible and well-documented group of workers, as there are extensive records on their health and work history. The occupation has been studied intensively for evidence of chronic health effects. Interest in the health problems of firefighting increased considerably during the 1980s. A substantial body of work is now available that may lead to a reevaluation of many unresolved issues.

Firefighters are exposed to serious chemical and physical hazards, to a degree that is unusual in the modern work force. The acute hazards of firefighting, primarily trauma, thermal injury, and smoke inhalation, are obvious. A large literature has been developed on acute pulmomary injury associated with inhalation of hot air and toxic constituents of smoke, particularly the combustion products of commonly used plastics (18, 30, 63). The hazards of carbon monoxide and cyanide are particularly well recognized (4, 18). Although the acute health effects of these life-threatening hazards and the risk of physical injury in structures affected by fire are indisputable, the chronic health effects that follow recurrent exposure are not clear (3). Studies that directly address the health experience of firefighters have not yielded consistent results until relatively recently. This uncertainty has led to a patchwork of employment and workers' compensation board policies.

151

Firefighting is an unusual occupation, as it is perceived as dirty and dangerous, but indispensable and admirable. Firefighters, almost universally, enjoy public admiration and gratitude to a degree unmatched by other occupations, particularly in the public sector (90). Their occupation is rich in stories of personal courage, spirit in the face of adversity, and teamwork. However, firefighters also experience a constant awareness of imminent danger and the feeling that the next alarm may challenge them to the limit (100). The health of firefighters, and their willingness to face the hazards, cannot be fully understood without appreciating this psychological dimension (105).

HAZARDS

Occupational hazards experienced by firefighters may be categorized for convenience as physical, thermal and ergonomic, chemical, and psychological. The level of exposure experienced by a firefighter in a given fire depends on what is burning, the combustion characteristics of the fire, the structure on fire, the presence of nonfuel chemicals, the measures taken to control the fire, the presence of victims requiring rescue, and the position or line of duty held by the firefighter while fighting the fire. The hazards and levels of exposure experienced by the first firefighter to enter a burning building are different from those of the firefighters who enter later or who clean up after the flames are extinguished. However, the career exposure profiles of firefighters tend to average out the longer they spend in a particular rank. There is rotation among the active firefighting jobs in each platoon and a regular transfer of personnel between fire halls. Firefighters therefore have a similar probability of exposure in typical fire situations as long as they stay classified as a "firefighter"; "captains" accompany and direct the crews, but are still actively involved in fighting the fire on site. Thus, firefighting exposures tend to become similar over a longer period of time, although individual firefighters may still experience unusual exposures in particular incidents.

Within the last 20 years, the introduction of the self-contained breathing apparatus (SCBA) and other protective equipment has created a much safer working environment for the firefighter. However, the added weight of the equipment increases the physical exertion required. The protective clothing also becomes much heavier when it gets wet.

Thermal Hazards

Heat stress is compounded in firefighting by the combination of insulating properties of the protective clothing and physical exertion, which results in endogenous heat production (6).

Hot air alone is not usually a great hazard to the firefighter. Air heated above body temperature cools as it passes through the larynx (38). Dry air also does not have much capacity to retain heat and delivers little to the lower respiratory tract, so that heat-induced inhalation injury is not usually a risk when the air is dry. However, inhaled steam or hot wet air can cause serious burns to the lower airway simply because of the high latent heat capacity. Much more heat energy can be stored in water vapor than in dry air. Fortunately, steam inhalation is not common (91).

Radiant heat is typical of a fire situation and may be associated with skin changes, particularly erythema and telangiectasia, in the absence of obvious burns (107).

Chemical Hazards

Firefighters on the scene of a fire are frequently exposed to carbon monoxide, hydrogen cyanide, nitrogen dioxide, sulphur dioxide, hydrogen chloride, aldehydes, and such organic compounds as benzene (41, 59, 113). Before arriving and on return, firefighters are exposed to diesel exhausts at the fire station (37).

In the 1970s, about 80% of injuries of firefighters in service resulted from smoke inhalation or oxygen deficiency. More than 50% of fire-related fatalities are the result of smoke exposure, rather than burns (4, 18, 30, 77). One of the major contributing factors to mortality and morbidity in fires is hypoxia because of oxygen depletion in the affected atmosphere, which leads to loss of physical performance, confusion, and inability to escape (91). Another factor is the toxicity of the constituents of smoke, singly and in combination.

The study of the toxicology of smoke as a complex mixture and its individual constituents has advanced in recent years and has led to better designs for personal protective and fire management strategies. Smoke is a variable mixture of compounds, each possessing specific toxicological properties and contributing to interactive toxic effects. Therefore, the toxicity of smoke varies greatly, depending primarily on the fuel, the heat of the fire, and whether or how much oxygen is available for combustion. However, all smoke, including that from simple wood fires, is hazardous and potentially lethal with concentrated inhalation (26). The complexity of the chemical composition of smoke is also due, in part, to the presence of secondary products; after the products of combustion are formed, they remain chemically active and continue to react long after the fire has ceased to burn. The list of chemicals of toxicological concern is long (21, 26). Smoke from burning oil has been characterized and found to have mutagenic activity in in vitro assays (5); this is undoubtedly also true for other common types of fires.

Smoke is made up of two components, particulates and gases, which are suspended or dissolved in a third component, hot air. (Table 1) The degree of exposure experienced by a firefighter is determined by the chemistry and quantity of gases produced at the fire, the concentrations reached, the size

Table 1   Products of combusion of commonly burnt materials

Combusted material	Fuel component of original material	Toxic decomposition products[a]
wood, paper, cotton, jute	cellulose	aldehydes, acrolein
clothing, fabric, blankets, furniture	wool, silk	hydrogen cyanide, ammonia, hydrogen sulfide
tires	rubber	sulphur dioxide, hydrogen sulfide, methyl mercaptan, benzene-related compounds
upholstery material, wire, pipe coating, wall, floor, furniture coverings	polyvinyl chloride	hydrogen chloride, phosgene
insulation, upholstery material	polyurethane	hydrogen cyanide, isocyanates, oxides of nitrogen
clothing, fabric	polyester	hydrogen chloride
upholstery material, carpeting	polypropylene	acrolein
appliances, engineering plastics	polyacrylonitrile	hydrogen cyanide, nitriles, oxides of nitrogen
carpeting, clothing	polyamide (nylon)	hydrogen cyanide, ammonia, oxides of nitrogen
household and kitchen goods	melamine resins	hydrogen cyanide, ammonia, formaldehyde, oxides of nitrogen
aircraft windows, textiles	acrylics	acrolein
kitchen goods, electrical insulation, gaskets	polytetrafluorethylene (Teflon®)	octafluoroisobutylene
photographic film	nitrocellulose	oxides of nitrogen

[a] Carbon monoxide and carbon dioxide are produced in all cases. Other gases, such as the aldehydes, methane, and low-molecular-weight organic acids, are common in most fires.

distribution of the particulate phase, solubility properties of the gaseous constituents as a predictor of the degree of penetration to the lower respiratory tract, and the duration of exposure (24).

Particulates generated from burning wood or other organic matter are composed of chemically inert carbon particles that become adsorbed (coated) with other chemical substances. These agents produce an irritating effect and cause cough and an acute bronchitis. The particles may also become carriers of less volatile substances, such as chlorinated hydrocarbons, depending on the composition of the combustion products (16, 91).

The chemical components of the gaseous phase of smoke, many of which are adsorbed onto the particulates and thereby penetrate more deeply into the lower respiratory tract than they otherwise would, are responsible for most of the toxicological effects that result from smoke inhalation (38). Laboratory simulations of different fire conditions have permitted the characterization of many of the combustion products given off by burning natural and synthetic materials commonly found in building structures and furnishings. The exact composition of the combustion products vary, depending upon the composition of the burning material and the temperature at which each material undergoes thermal decomposition (54).

Carbon monoxide is considered the most common, characteristic, and serious acute hazard of firefighting. Carboxyhemoglobin accumulates rapidly with duration of exposure as a result of the affinity of carbon monoxide for hemoglobin, and high levels may result, particularly when heavy exertion increases minute ventilation and increases delivery of carbon monoxide to the lung during unprotected firefighting (42, 62, 98). Not surprisingly, levels of carbon monoxide measured on the scene at fires often exceed the Occupational Safety and Health Administration's short-term exposure levels (8). Carbon monoxide and carbon dioxide, which are natural products of combustion, are necessarily present at every fire. Hydrogen cyanide is also formed from the lower temperature combustion of nitrogen-rich materials, including such natural fibers as wool and silk and such common synthetics as polyurethane and polyacrylonitrile (92, 109, 115). Although elevated levels of thiocyanate as a marker for cyanide exposure are less common among firefighters than elevated carboxyhemoglobin levels (61), there is a close relationship between the two in firefighters who have sustained clinically significant smoke inhalation (20).

Light-molecular-weight hydrocarbons, aldehydes (such as formaldehyde), and organic acids may be formed by hydrocarbon fuels that burn at lower temperatures (78). The oxides of nitrogen are also formed in large quantity when temperatures are high, as a consequence of the oxidation of atmospheric nitrogen, and in lower temperature fires in which the fuel contains significant nitrogen. When the fuel contains chlorine, particularly in the form of polyvinyl chloride (PVC), hydrogen chloride is formed (24, 30).

Most toxic components of smoke, with the exception of carbon monoxide and hydrogen cyanide, are only rarely produced in lethal concentrations. Different gas combinations are likely to present different degrees of hazard (91).

The toxic products of polymeric, plastic materials have come under increasing scrutiny. Since the 1950s, these materials have been used in building construction and furnishings in Europe and North America in large amounts (83, 114). They were soon found to combust into particularly hazardous products. Acrolein, formaldehyde, and volatile fatty acids are common in smoldering fires of several polymers, including polyethylene and natural cellulose (78). These products were characterized in a series of elegant studies by Wooley, who found a close relationship between the temperature of combustion and the mix of nitrogen-containing products released from polyurethane. Generally, cyanide levels increase with temperature; acrylonitrile, acetonitrile pyridine, and benzonitrile occur in large quantity above 800°C but below 1000°C (114, 116, 124, 125). Combusted polyacrylonitrile is even richer in cyanide and nitriles (116). Polyvinyl chloride has been proposed as desirable polymer for furnishings because of its self-extinguishing characteristics, caused by the high chlorine content. Unfortunately, the material produces large quantities of hydrochloric acid when fires are sustained, as they are when PVC is only part of the fire (33).

Since the 1970s, there has been much interest in the relative toxicity of the mixed products of combusted materials, along with the recognition that no two fires are exactly alike (49, 54). Alarie and Anderson (1, 2), have conducted extensive research on the decomposition products of polymeric materials, by comparing the toxic effects to those of the wood of Douglas fir as a standard. Some materials, such as PVC, decompose rapidly and are rapidly lethal, but others, like polytetrafluoroethylene (PTFE), which also decomposes rapidly, kill more slowly even though they are ultimately more lethal over the duration of exposure than PVC. When rating the toxicity hazard of materials, one must consider the period of evaluation. Table 2 rates the toxicity of a variety of materials compared with a standard of 100 representing Douglas fir, and considers both the time and exposure level required to produce a lethal effect (2).

Within the last 20 years, the toxicity of smoke and its hazard to the firefighting profession have been fully recognized. In the early 1970s, the

Table 2 Index for burning components of original products summarizing several characteristics that contribute to or suppress toxicity (lower the index, the higher the toxicity)

Burning material	Index
Douglas fir	100.00
compressed spruce, pine, fir slab	65.92
fiberglass insulation	63.59
polyester resin	41.58
cellulose fiber	17.80
polyurethane foam	12.95
phenol formaldehyde-phenol resin	8.98
isocyanate foam	7.57
modacrylic	6.28
PVC	5.85
wool	5.77
polystyrene	5.47
acrylonitrile/butadiene/styrene	4.04
urea formaldehyde foam	3.91
PTFE	0.36

National Fire Prevention Association published a report, "Breathing Apparatus for the Fire Service," which, through increased recognition of the problem, led to the introduction of SCBA (127). Fire departments, such as Boston's, adopted mandatory use regulations that markedly reduced the number of smoke inhalations in subsequent years by as much as 80% (113). In 1976, an evaluation of the effectiveness of SCBA showed that blood levels of carboxyhemoglobin in firefighters, as a measure of carbon monoxide exposure, were lowest in firefighters who used SCBAs, but roughly the same for intermittent uses or nonusers. This study and others showed that firefighters who do not wear SCBAs during the "knock-down" and "overhaul" phases are at risk; unfortunately, this is the phase in which the flames are out, and the hazard only seems to be reduced (30, 93).

Firefighters judge the level of hazard they face by the intensity of smoke and decide whether to use an SCBA solely on the basis of what they see. This may be very misleading, especially in the clean-up phase after the flames are extinguished (112). On superficial inspection, the fire setting may appear safe at this stage; however, it can be dangerous (112). There is no apparent correlation between the intensity of smoke and the amount of carbon monoxide in the air (23, 60). Synthetic materials are most dangerous during smoldering conditions, as opposed to conditions of high heat (30, 53, 123). Concrete retains heat very efficiently and may act as a "sponge" for trapped gases that then out-gas from the porous material, thus releasing hydrogen chloride or other toxic fumes long after a fire has been extinguished (30, 108). Firefighters should also be cautioned against cigarette smoking during the clean-up phase, as this adds to the already elevated levels of carbon monoxide in the blood (65, 110). The hazards presented by unusual constituents in smoke are too variable and complex for detailed discussion here. The combustion products of many industrial chemicals and mixtures are unknown or only poorly characterized. A major problem with fires that involve chemical sources or storage facilities is knowing how to fight them with the least potential danger to the firefighter and local residents. Recent studies have suggested novel approaches to such situations. In the case of fires in an insecticide storage facility, Jeffries & Schiefer (52) have suggested that optimal management might be to enhance combustion intentionally to produce a fast, hot fire that combusts the material more completely and carries the airborne toxic products away from the vicinity vertically by convection currents.

Psychological Hazards

There are many sources of psychological stress in the life of a firefighter, in addition to the viscissitudes of daily life and career advancement (29, 70, 72). A firefighter regularly steps into a situation that others flee, thus accepting a level of personal risk that would be unacceptable in most other occupations. Although this risk is controlled to the extent possible with fire equipment and personal protection, the reality of firefighting is that much can go wrong in any fire, and the course of a serious fire is often unpredictable (51, 70).

Besides personal security, the firefighter must be concerned with the safety of others threatened by the fire and is sometimes a witness to pain, injury, and strong emotion. Rescuing victims is an especially stressful activity. The loss of a victim, especially a child, is reported in numerous anecdotes to be the most stressful experience a firefighter can endure.

The professional life of a firefighter is not an endless round of anxious waiting punctuated by stressful crises, however. Firefighters enjoy the many positive aspects of their work. The work is intrinsically interesting and, during alarms, presents a great deal of stimulation and variety. Few occupations are so unequivocally favored by public opinion or so respected by the community. Job security is largely assured in urban fire departments once a firefighter is hired, the pay usually compares well with other jobs, and the schedule allows ample opportunities for "moonlighting" between shifts. When a firefighter answers an alarm, there is a degree of apprehension and stress, but there is also exhilaration and a sense of purpose. These positive aspects of the job mitigate the stressful aspects and tend to protect the firefighter against the emotional consequences of repeated stress (51).

At the sound of an alarm, firefighters experience a degree of immediate anxiety because of the inherent unpredictability of the situation that they are about to encounter. Some investigators believe that the psychological stress experienced at this moment is as great and, perhaps, greater than any of the stresses that follow during the course of responding to an alarm. En route, hazardous traffic maneuvers and high noise levels from the sirens contribute to stress (94). Physiological and biochemical indicators of stress have also been assessed among firefighters (29).

HEALTH EFFECTS

Some jurisdictions attempt to justify cases of health disorders on an individual basis, and others prescribe selected chronic diseases as compensable occupational disorders among firefighters. The problem is compounded by changes in technology over several decades; the risks and their outcomes vary with the era during which the firefighters entered the workforce. Generally speaking, firefighters who entered service before the 1960s were exposed to smoke of less acute toxicity, but lacked personal protection equipment of acceptable effectiveness. Those entering within the last two decades have primarily been exposed to smoke of greater toxicity, but have had more effective respiratory protection available. Firefighters who joined the force in the last few years may have the benefit of both fire-retardant materials produced under more stringent safety codes and also respiratory protection meeting contemporary standards of effectiveness.

Acute Effects

INJURIES   Injuries associated with firefighting are predictable: burns, falls, and injury from falling objects. Jobs with a high risk of burns include those involving early entry and close-in firefighting, such as holding the nozzle. Burns are more commonly associated with basement fires, recent prior injury, and training outside the fire department of present employment. Falls tend to be associated with SCBA use, assignment to truck companies with climbing equipment, and, suggestively, childlessness. (Without dependent children, an individual may be more likely to take risks.) However, age and experience do not seem to be associated with risk of injuries in service (47).

RESPIRATORY DISORDERS   The respiratory effects of exposure to smoke and fumes from fires have been a major concern. Acute smoke inhalation carries a high mortality for unprotected victims (19) and is often combined with burns and other trauma. Fatal and overwhelming smoke inhalation has been reviewed extensively in the clinical literature (18, 22), and its manifestations are not unique to firefighting.

Transient changes have been associated with unremarkable fires (59, 82, 100), as well as fires involving certain chemicals (14), such as burning polyvinyl chloride (30), silicone plastic (39), butyl rubber insulation (82), and isocyanates (6, 73). In those cases in which the fires did not present an unusual hazard, the decrement in airflow (measured as the reduction in FEV_1, the forced expiratory volume in one second, between the beginning of a shift and return after an alarm) correlated with the concentration of particulate matter in the smoke cloud and the presence of eye irritation, but not the duration of exposure, work shift, or smoking history. Persistent effects, including neurological impairment, have been noted following exposures that involve isocyanate fumes (6), but in only a subset of firefighters exposed to burning polyvinyl chloride (30, 69, 111). In at least one case, these changes mimicked asthma, with wheezing and refractory bronchoconstriction (14).

Airway responsiveness increases after firefighting exposures (56, 82, 100, 101). Increased airways reactivity following minor smoke inhalation during routine firefighting is a complex response, more complicated than bronchoconstriction, which results from irritation. The response is persistent, does not correlate with baseline methacholine sensitivity, and is associated with acute but transient increases in airways responsiveness (82, 100, 101). In at least one case, exposure resulted in airflow obstruction—initially responsive to bronchodilators—that became progressively more severe despite treatment, until the patient died of respiratory failure two years later (14). In this case, the pathology may have resembled mucoid impaction syndrome.

There are very few studies of the pulmonary response to smoke in controlled situations in firefighting. Minty et al (74) studied nonsmoking firefighting instructors in the Royal Navy, by obtaining data on smoke composition, pulmonary function, and alveolar-capillary permeability following brief exposure to wood and diesel fires in training exercises. They found no change in pulmonary function; but, they did find an elevated permeability measure, which suggests that exposure to the smoke either damaged the integrity of the alveolar-capillary barrier or initiated a low-grade inflammatory response that in turn had the same effect because of release of proteolytic enzymes.

Chronic Health Effects

Several early studies examined firefighting, along with numerous other occupations, by using vital records for large populations (43, 45, 77, 88, 117, 118, 120, 121). These have sometimes been difficult to interpret because of methodological issues and misclassification (43). Two early cohort studies have been recognized for their usefulness in evaluating the health risks of firefighters: Mastromatteo's 1959 study on a cohort of firefighters in Toronto (71) and Musk et al's 1978 study on a large cohort from Boston (79). The Mastromatteo study was a pioneer effort in the field, which illustrated the use of basic techniques that have been adopted in many studies since. Because of its date, however, the findings have uncertain application to the current situation. Since these early landmarks, other major cohort studies have recently been contributed by Eliopulos et al (31) on a cohort from Western Australia, Feuer & Rosenman (36) on a cohort from New Jersey, Vena & Fiedler (122) on a cohort from Buffalo, New York, Heyer et al (48) and Rosenstock et al (96) on a cohort from Seattle, Beaumont et al (13) on a cohort from San Francisco, and Guidotti (44) on a cohort from the Canadian province of Alberta.

The chronic effects of greatest concern in studies of firefighters have been lung cancer, heart disease, and chronic obstructive pulmonary diseases. Recently, however, other forms of cancer, particularly genitourinary and colon and rectal, have emerged as likely associations.

A chronic effect that has only recently been documented is that of an increased risk of congenital cardiac defects in the offspring of male firefighters. The responsible exposure is not known (85).

CANCER   Lung cancer has been the most difficult cancer site to evaluate in epidemiologic studies of firefighters. Despite the obvious exposure to carcinogens inhaled in smoke (15), it has been difficult to document an excess in mortality from lung cancer of a magnitude and consistency compatible with occupational exposure. Without question, cigarette smoking is a confounding exposure that complicates the analysis, but the prevalence of smoking among firefighters does not appear to be excessive compared with other blue collar occupations (40). Respiratory protection has probably reduced individual exposure levels since the 1970s, although it was not optimally used for many years in most fire departments. An effective form of respiratory protection was probably introduced too late to have substantially modified lung cancer rates that are currently observed. A major issue is whether the above-mentioned introduction of synthetic polymers into building materials and furnishings has increased the risk of cancer among firefighters because of exposure to the combustion products.

The empirical findings on lung cancer from recent, well-designed epidemiological studies have been inconsistent. One study from Denmark (46), in which the comparison population is unusual, reported a standardized mortality ratio of 317 for older firefighters, whereas studies on cohorts from San Francisco and Buffalo showed no excess (13, 122). The possibility that an association is obscured, in comparison to the general population by the healthy worker effect, is probably less likely for this cause of death than for other chronic diseases; over the long periods of observation typical for these studies, the mortality experience of initially selected workers can be expected to approach that of the general population more closely, especially for noncardiovascular causes of death. Most studies have shown an excess of lung cancer on the order of 20–80% (48, 97), a magnitude not uncommon in studies of other blue collar occupations with less plausible exposure levels (43). In the most detailed analyses to date, a nonsignificant excess showed no clear distribution that would be consistent with duration of employment, exposure opportunity, or era of entry into the occupation (44, 122).

Documentation of an association between lung cancer and occupational exposure as a firefighter remains elusive; many investigators continue to believe that an association exists. Markers of genotoxic effect suggest that carcinogenicity is likely to occur (64). An effect probably does exist, but it is likely to be heavily obscured by confounding factors and may not be as strong as anticipated.

Other cancer sites have recently emerged as more consistent associations with firefighting. Evidence for an association with genitourinary cancers seems strong (97, 122). There is a less strong suggestion in the literature for colon and rectal cancers and for leukemia, lymphoma, and multiple myeloma (97, 122).

PULMONARY DISEASE   Most epidemiological studies of firefighters that report on mortality from chronic obstructive airways disease do not show an excess. There has been some concern that comparison to the general population may obscure a relative excess offset by the healthy worker effect. In one study, comparison with police showed a nonsignificant excess, but the police in this study showed an unusually low mortality (87).

Although excess mortality and morbidity are difficult to demonstrate, there is evidence from serial studies of pulmonary function that firefighters are at risk for airways obstruction. Reports of progressive abnormalities in lung function among firefighters have suggested as much as a doubling of the expected rate of decline in lung function that normally affects aging adults, and this difference is associated with an increased frequency of respiratory symptoms (87, 103, 106). These reports sparked a wave of concern in the mid-1970s because they suggested an eventual appearance of chronic lung disease among firefighters (3). This effect is most apparent following unusually severe exposures (119) and is associated with the number of fires fought over the first year or so. Declines of this magnitude have been associated with an increased risk for chronic obstructive airways disease (emphysema or chronic bronchitis) in other populations. Intense exposures have produced chronic changes in at least one case (63). If these findings are significant, one would expect an increase in mortality from chronic airways disorders compared with the general population. The above-mentioned studies show no such effect. The cohort study by Musk et al (79), for example, showed a standardized mortality ratio of 93, 83 for active firefighters and 101 for retired firefighters, which is well within the expected range. Significant abnormalities in pulmonary function have been reported in current firefighters among smokers only (28), and even that seems to represent minimal small airways disease in asymptomatic firefighters employed for at least 25 years (63). Thus, the weight of evidence suggests that firefighters are not at greatly increased risk of chronic respiratory disease unless they experience an unusual exposure (82, 126).

In the past, there had been some concern that firefighters with early lung disease leave the occupation and that the remaining firefighters are, therefore, selected for respiratory health (89). This effect may be less pronounced than initially assumed (104, 106). Fire departments, in effect, protect their own most vulnerable members by transferring them into positions with less opportunity for exposure, so that career firefighters with mild respiratory impairment may easily remain employed (102). Transfer patterns within the fire department result in a steady exit of those individuals most at risk for decline in airflow velocity from active firefighting positions and movement into positions in which their duties involved fighting few or no fires. A powerful selection bias at work apparently protects firefighters with abnormalities of pulmonary function from further exposure (80, 81).

The contribution of cigarette smoking to the overall picture remains difficult to sort out. Horsfield et al (50) studied 96 British firefighters and 69 nonsmoking, nonfirefighter control subjects over four years to evaluate the progression of their pulmonary function and any respiratory symptoms. The firefighters were regularly interviewed with respect to their smoking habits and the degree to which they felt affected by exposure to smoke on the job. This index was admittedly subjective, but took into account the situations in which personal protection may have failed. The authors found no evidence for functional abnormality on spirometry; indeed, pulmonary function in these firefighters deteriorated at a rate slower than in the controls. They did observe a consistent and suggestive pattern of reported symptoms: Symptoms, predominantly productive cough, were reported least often among the controls; more often among the nonsmoking, smoke-unaffected firefighters; at an intermediate frequency among smokers who were smoke-unaffected, as well as nonsmoking smoke-affected firefighters; and most often among smoking smoke-affected firefighters. Indeed, despite the crudely subjective index of occupational smoke exposure, the pattern strongly suggested a multiplicative interaction. The authors concluded that occupational exposure to smoke in firefighting is a determinant of respiratory symptoms almost as strong as cigarette smoking, with which it interacts, but that it does not appear to affect pulmonary function given current use of personal protection.

   These investigations were extraordinary in detail, perspicacity, and tenacity. The picture now seems to be fairly clear: Within the firefighting profession, there is an effective, but largely tacit, mechanism that works by administrative means to protect the most vulnerable members. It now seems safe to conclude that occupational exposure can indeed cause respiratory disorders alone in extreme situations or in combination with cigarette smoking. That this was not reflected in greater mortality from respiratory diseases in past years may reflect the effectiveness of the administrative measures described above. The risk of death from respiratory causes in future will be further reduced by increasing compliance with and technical effectiveness of the use of personal protection devices.

CARDIOVASCULAR DISEASE   Despite a presumption of occupational association in many jurisdictions when a firefighter dies of a myocardial infarction, firefighters have not been consistently shown to be at elevated risk for death from heart disease. Recent studies suggest that mortality is about that expected (13, 27, 44, 46, 96, 122), although some studies have suggested elevations of 50% (99). There is ergonomic evidence that some firefighters may be stressed to the limit during the exertions of their work. That this stress does not result in increased mortality probably reflects a strong healthy worker effect and the decreasing levels of exertion required with seniority and advancement beyond captain.

Two lines of reasoning suggest that cardiovascular disorders may be a problem among firefighters. The first is the documented presence of high degrees of cardiovascular stress during the response to alarms and the process of fighting the fire (10). The second is the known presence of carbon monoxide at high concentrations in smoke inhaled by firefighters (4, 18, 63). Several experiments have indicated that carbon monoxide exposure reduces the threshold for angina.

The cardiovascular response to an alarm is pronounced. Firefighters show a marked increase in heart rate during the response to a fire alarm. This increase averages about 50 beats within 30 seconds of the alarm sounding, which persists until arrival at the fire. The elevation in heart rate is much greater than that which would be expected in response to the exertion alone. During firefighting, heart rates of 150–160 beats/min were the norm, but occasional peaks of 175–195 occur, especially during the first 3–5 minutes of a fire and during stressful and dangerous crises. These are very high levels, associated with maximal exertion or anxiety. The response in heart rate does not show any consistent association with age or fitness of the firefighter, and there is great variation from person to person and in the same person from time to time (10, 55).

Electrocardiogram (EKG) changes suggesting coronary artery disease were found by Barnard et al (11) in nine of 90 randomly selected firefighters aged 40–59 in the city of Los Angeles. This level of prevalence of EKG-demonstrable coronary artery disease was comparable to that expected for a large group of middle-aged men but this in itself is surprising because firefighters, who are selected by stringent criteria for fitness, demonstrated a reduced prevalence of cardiovascular risk factors (12). Four of six firefighters with EKG abnormalities suggestive of ischemic changes had no evidence of advanced coronary artery disease, but three had abnormal left ventricular wall function (11). This raised the possibility that firefighters may be at risk for nonischemic myocardial injury on the basis of exposure to carbon monoxide or elevated circulating catecholamines (8–11). Indeed, of the original group tested, two had myocardial infarcts within two days of testing, an alarming experience (12).

Barnard and coworkers (9, 12) also described an ischemic response in healthy young men, including firefighters, who engaged in sudden, vigorous exercise without warm-up. They suggested a transient mismatch in oxygen supply and demand at the subendocardial level caused by temporarily inadequate perfusion for the suddenly increased demand for myocardial oxygen. Arterial pressure measurement confirmed that the relaxation time available for restoring coronary blood supply during diastole was markedly reduced during cold start-up exercise. Although this mechanism is probably not a cause of persistent or cumulative myocardial injury, it may play a role in unusual and emergent situations that require sudden maximal exertion.

The experience of firefighters who were studied in large groups has been quite different. Dibbs et al (27) examined a similarly "healthy" group of 171 firefighters in Boston enrolled in a cohort study on aging effects. They found a distribution of risk factors similar to that seen by Barnard and coworkers, but the incidence of detectable coronary heart disease and its complications over ten years of observation was no different than that for nonfirefighters of the same age in the study. The discrepancy suggests that Barnard's group of subjects, and the group studied before him by Felton (35) from the county of Los Angeles (distinct from the city, but recruited from the same population) differed in some important ways from the Boston firefighters.

ERGONOMIC ISSUES

Firefighting is a very strenuous occupation, which is often performed under extreme environmental conditions (67). The demands of firefighting are sporadic and unpredictable, characterized by long periods of waiting between bouts of intense activity. This irregular pattern of activity is an important feature of firefighting, as it adds to the component of stress that is probably caused by anxiety and responses to psychogenic stress.

There are several components to the physiological demands of firefighting, including energy cost of performing firefighting activities, heat stress associated with heat from the fire, and encumbrance by personal protection equipment. A detailed understanding of the physiological demands of firefighting must consider the contribution of each component and changes in each over time. For example, the use of personal protection equipment has imposed new physiological demands on firefighters, but has removed other demands by reducing exposure levels; personal protection equipment is also improving over time with advances in technology (66).

Energy Costs and Performance

Among common firefighting activities, climbing the aerial ladder is one of the most strenuous. Other strenuous activities include climbing stairs, dragging hose, rescuing a victim, and raising the ladder (58, 84, 95).

Firefighters adjust their levels of exertion in a characteristic pattern during simulated fire conditions, as reflected by heart rate. Initially, their heart rate increases rapidly to 70–80% of maximal within the first minute (68). As firefighting progresses, they maintain their heart rates at 85–100% maximal until the fire is out. With the addition of equipment and SCBA apparatus, they adjust their levels of exertion to remain at this intense level of activity. In other words, firefighters maintain their level of exertion at a relatively constant, intense level once active firefighting begins. Any additional burden, such encumbrance by the necessary protective equipment or victim rescue, reduces performance because firefighters are already exerting themselves to the maximum.

The energy requirements for firefighting are complicated by the adverse conditions in many inside fires. The metabolic demands of coping with heat transfer and fluid balance add to the existing demands of physical exertion. A major issue is the combined effect of the accumulation of internally generated heat during strenuous exercise and the external heat during fire conditions (38, 109).

Fitness and Performance Capacity

Numerous studies have evaluated the physiological characteristics of firefighters, usually in the context of other studies to determine the response to firefighting-related demands. Studies of the fitness of firefighters have shown fairly consistently that most firefighters are as or somewhat more fit than the general adult male population. However, they are not fit to an athletically trained level (17, 25, 57, 86). Fitness and health maintenance programs have been developed for firefighters, but have not been convincingly evaluated for their effectiveness.

The entrance of women applicants into firefighting caused a reevaluation of performance tests and studies comparing the sexes. Misner et al examined the performance of 37 men and 25 women on nine job-related tasks used as a screening battery in Chicago. The subjects were recruited from among athletes in training and individuals known to be highly physically fit. The intent was to compare the performance of suitably trained individuals who could achieve their potential maximum performance, rather than the assessment of typical applicants. They found that women demonstrated lower scores on average than men in all performance items, but that a subgroup of women performed nearly as well in some tasks. The overall difference in performance was primarily attributed to lower absolute lean body weight, which correlated most strongly and consistently with performance difference (76). The most difficult items for women were the stair-climbing exercises. Leg strength appears to be predicted by lean body weight, but not by other anthropometric measurements (75).

Given the potential for heat stress, toxic exposure, and hypoxia, Evanoff & Rosenstock (32) have suggested that women firefighters who are pregnant should cease firefighting activity sometime during the second trimester, and that contract policies facilitate pregnancy leave and temporary reassignment.

CONCLUDING REMARKS

The demands and harzards of firefighting have changed over the past decades (1, 4, 26, 34, 49, 90, 124), but the high quality and standard of service have remained the same (105). The use of highly sophisticated firefighting equipment and the introduction of innovative firefighting techniques, safer personal protective equipment (60), and better communications and information systems, as well as healthier life-styles (25, 40, 67), have helped meet public demands for service and, at the same time, have provided a safer and healthier working environment for the firefighter. In spite of these advances, firefighting continues to be a very hazardous occupation (47, 83, 90, 119).

Literature Cited

1. Alarie, Y. C. 1985. The toxicity of smoke from polymeric materials during thermal decomposition. *Annu. Rev. Pharmacol. Toxicol.* 25:325–47
2. Anderson, R. C., Alarie, Y. C. 1978. Screening procedures to recognize "supertoxic" decomposition products from polymeric materials under thermal stress. *J. Combust. Technol.* 5:54–63
3. Anon. 1975. Firemen's lungs. *Lancet.* 1:439
4. Anon. 1974. Fire-fighting: An insidious hazard. *Lancet.* 2:91
5. Atlas, E. L., Donnelly, K. C., Giam, C. S., McFarland, A. R. 1985. Chemical and biological characterization of emissions from a fireperson training facility. *Am. Ind. Hyg. Assoc. J.* 46:532–40
6. Axford, A. T., McKerrow, C. B., Parry-Jones, A., Le Quesne, P. M. 1976. Accidental exposure to isocyanates fumes in a group of firemen. *Br. J. Ind. Med.* 33:65–71
7. Deleted in proof
8. Barnard, R. J. 1979. Carbon monoxide: A hazard to firefighters. *Arch. Environ. Health.* 34:255–57
9. Barnard, R. J. 1975. Fire fighters—A fit population with ischemic heart disease. *Sports Med. Bull.* 10:7–9
10. Barnard, R. J., Duncan, H. W. 1975. Heart rate and ECG responses of firefighters. *J. Occup. Med.* 17:247–50
11. Barnard, R. J., Gardner, G. W., Diaco, N. V. 1976. "Ischemic" heart disease in firefighters with normal coronary arteries. *J. Occup. Med.* 18:818–20
12. Barnard, R. J., Gardner, G. W., Diaco, N. V., Kattus, A. A. 1978. Near-maximal ECG stress testing and coronary artery disease risk factor analysis in Los Angeles City fire fighters. *J. Occup. Med.* 17:693–95
13. Beaumont, J., Chu, G., Jones, J., Schenker, M., Singleton, J., et al. 1991. An epidemiologic study of mortality from cancer and other causes of death in San Francisco firefighters *Am. J. Ind. Med.* 19:357–72
14. Bergstrom, C. E., Tornling, G., Unge, G. 1988. Acquired progressive asthma in a fire fighter. *Eur. Respir. J.* 1:469–70
15. Brandt-Rauf, P. W., Cosman, B., Fallon, L. F. Jr., Tarantini, T., Idema, C. 1988. Health hazards of firefighters: Acute pulmonary effects after toxic exposures. *Br. J. Ind. Med.* 45:606–12
16. Bumb, R. R., Crummett, W. B., Cutie, S. S., Gledhill, J. R., Hummell, R. H., et al. 1980. Trace chemistries of fire: A source of chlorinated dioxins. *Science* 210(24):385–90
17. Byrd, R., Collins, M. 1980. Physiologic characteristics of fire fighters. *Am. Correct. Ther. J.* 34:106–9
18. Cahalane, M., Demling, R. H. 1984. Early respiratory abnormalities from smoke inhalation. *J. Am. Med. Assoc.* 251:771–73
19. Clark, W. R., Nieman, G. F. 1988. Smoke inhalation. *Burns* 14:473–94
20. Clark, C. J., Campbell, D., Reid, W. H. 1981. Blood carboxyhaemoglobin and cyanide levels in fire survivors. *Lancet* 1:1332–35
21. Cohen, M. A., Guzzardi, L. J. 1983. Inhalation of products of combustion. *Ann. Emerg. Med.* 12:628–32
22. Coleman, D. L. 1981. Smoke inhalation. *West J. Med.* 135:300–9
23. Corlett, R. C., Cruz, G. A. 1975. Smoke and toxic gas production in enclosed fires. *JFF/Combust. Toxicol.* 2:8–33
24. Crapo, R. O. 1981. Smoke-inhalation injuries. *J. Am. Med. Assoc.* 246 (15):1694–96
25. Davis, P. O., Biersner, R. J., Barnard, R. J., Schamadan, J. 1982. Medical evaluation of fire fighters: How fit are they for duty? *Postgrad. Med.* 72:241–45
26. Decker, W. J., Garcia-Cantu, A. 1986. Toxicology of fires: An emerging clinical concern. *Vet. Hum. Toxicol.* 28 (5):431–33
27. Dibbs, E., Thomas, H. E. Jr., Weiss, S. T., Sparrow, D. 1982. Fire fighting and coronary heart disease. *Circulation* 65:943–46

28. Douglas, D. B., Douglas, R. B., Oakes, E., Scott, G. 1985. Pulmonary functions of London firemen. *Br. J. Ind. Med.* 4:55–58

29. Dutton, L. M., Smolensky, M. H., Leach, C. S., Lorimer, R., Hsi, B. P. 1978. Stress levels of ambulance paramedics and firefighters. *J. Occup. Med.* 20:111–15

30. Dyer, R. F., Esch, V. H. 1976. Polyvinyl chloride toxicity in fires: Hydrogen chloride toxicity in firefighters. *J. Am. Med. Assoc.* 235:393–97

31. Eliopulos, E., Armstrong, B. K., Spickett, J. T., Heyworth, F. 1984. Mortality of firefighters in Western Australia. *Br. J. Ind. Med.* 41:183–87

32. Evanoff, B. A., Rosenstock, L. 1986. Reproductive hazards in the workplace: A case study of women firefighters. *Am. J. Ind. Med.* 9:503–15

33. Ezriel, N. 1973. PVC: Its known and expected behaviour in fire. *Fire Int.* 39:40–47

34. Faff, J., Tutak, T. 1989. Physiological responses to working with fire fighting equipment in the heat in relation to subjective fatigue. *Ergonomics* 32:629–38

35. Felton, J. S. 1973. Conducting cardiopulmonary evaluations of County of Los Angeles Safety Personnel. *Health Serv. Rep.* 88:515

36. Feuer, E., Rosenman, K. 1986. Mortality in police and firefighters in New Jersey. *Am. J. Ind. Med.* 9:517–27

37. Froines, J. R., Hinds, W. C., Duffy, R. M., LaFuente, E. J., Liu, W.-C. V. 1987. Exposure of firefighters to diesel emissions in fire stations. *Br. J. Ind. Med.* 48:200–7

38. Genovesi, M. G. 1980. Effects of smoke inhalation. *Chest* 77:335–36

39. Genovesi, M. G., Tashkin, D. P., Chopra, S., Morgan, M., McElroy, C. 1977. Transient hypoxemia in firemen following inhalation of smoke. *Chest* 71:441–44

40. Gerace, T. A. 1990. Road to a smoke-free service for Florida: Policies and progress. *J. Public Health Policy* 11:206–17

41. Gold, A., Burgess, W. A., Clougherty, E. V. 1978. Exposure of firefighters to toxic air contaminants. *Am. Ind. Hyg. Assoc. J.* 39:534–39

42. Griggs, T. R. 1977. The role of exertion as a determinant of carboxyhemoglobin accumulation in firefighters. *J. Occup. Med.* 19:759–61

43. Guidotti, T. L., Baser, M., Goldsmith, J. R. 1987. Comparing risk estimates from occupational disease monitoring data. *Public Health Rev.* 15:1–27

44. Guidotti, T. L. 1992. Mortality of urban firefighters in Alberta, 1927–1987. *Am. J. Ind. Med.* In press

45. Guralnick, L. 1963. Mortality by occupation and cause of death. *Vital Stat. Special Rep.* (US Public Health Serv.). 53(5):139

46. Hansen, E. S. 1990. A cohort study on the mortality of firefighters. *Br. J. Ind. Med.* 47:805–9

47. Heineman, E. F., Shy, C. M., Checkoway, H. 1989. Injuries in the fireground: Risk factors for traumatic injuries among professional fire fighters. *Am. J. Ind. Med.* 15:267–82

48. Heyer, N., Weiss, N. S., Demers, P., Rosenstock, L. 1990. Cohort study of Seattle fire fighters: 1945–1983. *Am. J. Ind. Med.* 17:493–504

49. Hilado, C. J., Cumming, H. J., Casey, C. J. 1978. Relative toxicity of materials in fire situations. *Mod. Plast.* 55:92–96

50. Horsfield, K., Cooper, F. M., Buckman, M. P., Guyuatt, A. R., Comming, G. 1988. Respiratory symptoms in West Sussex firemen. *Br. J. Ind. Med.* 45: 251–55

51. Hytten, K., Hasle, A. 1989. Fire fighters: A study of stress and coping. *Acta Psychiatr. Scand.* 80(Suppl.):355:50–55

52. Jeffries, C., Schiefer, H. B. 1985. Potential consequences of a fire in an insecticide storage facility. *Reg. Toxicol. Pharmacol.* 5:197–203

53. Kalman, D. A. 1986. Survey analysis of volatile organics released from plastics under thermal stress. *Am. J. Ind. Hyg. J.* 47:270–75

54. Kimmerle, G. 1974. Aspects and methodology for the evaluation of toxicological parameters during fire exposure. *JFF/Combust. Toxicol.* 1:4–50

55. Kuorinka, I., Korhonen, O. 1981. Firefighters' reaction to alarm, an ECG and heart rate study. *J. Occup. Med.* 23:762–66

56. Large, A. A., Owens, G. R., Hoffman, L. A. 1990. The short-term effects of smoke exposure on the pulmonary function of firefighters. *Chest* 97:806–9

57. Lemon, P. W. R., Hermiston, R. T. 1977. Physiological profile of professional fire fighters. *J. Occup. Med.* 19:337–40

58. Lemon, P. W. R., Hermiston, R. T. 1977. The human energy cost of firefighting. *J. Occup. Med.* 19:558–62

59. Le Quesne, P. M., Axford, A. T., McKerrow, C. B., Parry Jones, A. 1976. Neurological complications offer a single severe exposure to toluene diisocyanate. *Br. J. Ind. Med.* 33:72–78

60. Levine, M. S. 1979. Respirator use and protection from exposure to carbon monoxide. *Am. Ind. Hyg. Assoc. J.* 40:832

61. Levine, M. S., Radford, E. P. 1978. Occupational exposures to cyanide in Baltimore fire fighters. *J. Occup. Med.* 20:53–56

62. Levy, A. L., Lum, G., Abeles, F. J. 1976. Carbon monoxide in firemen before and after exposure to smoke. *Ann. Clin. Lab. Sci.* 6:455–58

63. Loke, J., Farmer, W., Matthay, R. A., Putnam, C. E., Smith, G. J. W. 1980. Acute and chronic effects of firefighting on pulmonary function. *Chest* 77:369–73

64. Liou, S.-H., Jacobson-Kram, D., Poirier, M. C., Nguyen, D., Strickland, P. T., Tockman, M. S. 1989. Biological monitoring of firefighters: Sister chromatid exchange and polycyclic aromatic hydrocarbon-DNA adducts in peripheral blood cells. *Cancer Res.* 49:4929–35

65. Loke, J., Farmer, W. C., Matthay, R. A., Virgulto, J. A., Bouhuys, A. 1976. Carboxyhemoglobin levels in firefighters. *Lung* 154:35–39

66. Louhevaara, V., Smolander, J., Korhonen, O., Tuomi, T. 1986. Effects of industrial respirators on breathing pattern at different work levels. *Eur. J. Appl. Physiol.* 55:142–46

67. Maki, J., Gibeau, C., Mills. June 1981. A review of firefighters' occupational health and safety information and information needs. *Edmonton, Alberta Workers' Health Safety and Compensation.* Occup. Health Safe. Div. Publ. No. 81–067/R

68. Manning, J. E., Griggs, T. R. 1983. Heart rates in fire fighters using light and heavy breathing equipment: Similar near-maximal exertion in response to multiple work load conditions. *J. Occup. Med.* 25:215–18

69. Markowitz, J. S. 1989. Self-reported short- and long-term respiratory effects among PVC-exposed firefighters. *Arch. Environ. Health* 44:30–33

70. Markowitz, J. S., Gutterman, A. M., Link, B., Rivera, M. 1987. Psychological response of firefighters to a chemical fire. *J. Hum. Stress* 13:84–93

71. Mastromatteo, E. 1959. Mortality in city firemen: II. A study of mortality in firemen of a city fire department. *Am. Med. Assoc. Arch. Ind. Health* 20:277–83

72. McFarlane, A. C. 1988. The phenomenology of post-traumatic stress disorders following a natural disaster. *J. Nerv. Ment. Dis.* 176:22–29

73. McKerrow, C. B., Davies, H. J., Parry

Jones A. 1970. Symptoms and lung function following acute and chronic exposure to toulene di-isocyanate. *Proc. R. Soc. Med.* 63:376–82

74. Minty, B. D., Royston, D., Jones, J. B., Smith, D. J., Searing, C. S. M., Beeley, M. 1985. Changes in permeability of the alveolar-capillary barrier in firefighters. *Br. J. Ind. Med.* 42:631–34

75. Misner, J. E., Boileau, R. A., Plowman, S. A., Elmore, B. G., Gates, M. A., et al. 1988. Leg power characteristics of female fire fighter applicants. *J. Occup. Med.* 30:433–37

76. Misner, J. E., Plowman, S. A., Boileau, R. A. 1987. Performance differences between males and females on simulated firefighting tasks. *J. Occup. Med.* 29:801–5

77. Milham, S. Jr. Occupational mortality in Washington State, 1950–1979. Cincinnati: US Public Health Serv., *DHHS (NIOSH).* Publ. No. 83-116

78. Morikawa, T. 1976. Acrolein, formaldehyde, and volatile fatty acids from smoldering combustion. *J. Combust. Toxicol.* 3:135–50

79. Musk, A. W., Monson, R. R., Peters, J. M., Peters, R. D. 1978. Mortality among Boston firefighters, 1915–1975. *Br. J. Ind. Med.* 35:104–8

80. Musk, A. W., Peters, J. M., Bernstein, L., Rubin, C., Monroe, C. B. 1982. Pulmonary function in firefighters: A six-year follow-up in the Boston Fire Department. *Am. J. Ind. Med.* 3:3–9

81. Musk, A. W., Peters, J. M., Wegman, D. H. 1977. Lung function in firefighters In: A three year follow-up of active subjects. *Am. J. Public Health* 67:626–29

82. Musk, A. W., Smith, T. J., Peters, J. M., McLaughlin, E. 1979. Pulmonary function in firefighters: Acute changes in ventilatory capacity and their correlates. *Br. J. Ind. Med.* 36:29–34

83. Narita, H., Kikuchi, I., Ogata, K., Inoue, S., Uehara, K., Takehara, Y. 1987. Smoke inhalation injury from newer synthetic building materials—a patient who survived 205 days. *Burns* 13:147–52

84. O'Connell, E. R., Thomas, P. C., Cady, L. D., Karwasky, R. J. 1986. Energy costs of simulated stair climbing as a job-related task in fire fighting. *J. Occup. Med.* 28:282–84

85. Olshan, A. R., Teschke, K., Baird, P. A. 1990. Birth defects among offspring of firemen. *Am. J. Epidemiol.* 131(2):312–21

86. Peabody, H. D. 1973. San Diego Fire Department Health Survey. In *Survival*

in the Fire Fighting Profession: 2nd Symp. on Occup. Health and Hazards of the Fire Serv., April 1973, Univ. of Notre Dame, Indiana. Redmond Mem. Fund, Int. Assoc. Fire Fighters

87. Peters, J. M., Theriault, G. P., Fine, L. J., Wegman, D. H. 1974. Chronic effect of firefighting on pulmonary function. *N. Engl. J. Med.* 291:1320–22

88. Petersen, G. R., Milham, S. Jr., et al. 1983. Occupational mortality in the State of California, 1959–1961. Cincinnati, US Public Health Serv. *DHHS (NIOSH)* Publ. No. 83–116

89. Phoon, W. O., Ong, C. N., Foo, S. C., Plueksawan, W. 1983. A cross-sectional study on the health of firefighters in Singapore. *Jpn. J. Ind. Health* 25:463–70

90. Polakoff, P. L. 1976. Attention should be given to limiting firefighting hazards. *Occup. Health Safe.* 53:55–56

91. Prien, T., Traber, T. L. 1988. Toxic smoke components and inhalation injury—a review. *Burns* 14(6):451

92. Purser, D. A., Grimshaw, P., Berrill, K. R. 1984. Intoxication by cyanide in fires: A study in monkeys using polyacrylonitrile. *Arch. Environ. Health* 39:394–400

93. Radford, E. P., Levin, M. S. 1976. Occupational exposures to carbon monoxide in Baltimore fire fighters. *J. Occup. Med.* 18(9):628–32

94. Reischl, U. W. E., Bair, H. S., Reischl, P. 1979. Firefighter noise exposure. *Am. Ind. Hyg. Assoc. J.* 40:482–89

95. Romet, T. T., Frim, J. 1987. Physiological responses to fire fighting activities. *Eur. J. Appl. Physiol.* 56:633–38

96. Rosenstock, L., Demers, P., Heyer, N. J., Barnhart, S. 1990. Respiratory mortality among firefighters. *Br. J. Ind. Med.* 47:462–65

97. Sama, S. R., Martin, T. R., Davis, L. K., Kriebel, D. 1990. Cancer incidence among Massachusetts firefighters, 1982–1986. *Am. J. Ind. Med.* 18:47–54

98. Sammons, J. H., Coleman, R. L. 1974. Firefighters' occupational exposure to carbon monoxide. *J. Occup. Med.* 16:543–46

99. Sardinas, A., Miller, J. W., Hansen, H. 1986. Ischemic heart disease mortality of firemen and policemen. *Am. J. Public Health* 76:1140–41

100. Sheppard, D., Distefano, S., Morse, L., Becker, C. 1986. Acute effects of routine firefighting on lung function. *Am. J. Ind. Med.* 9:333–40

101. Sherman, C. B., Barnhart, S., Miller,

M. F., Segal, M. R., Aitken, M., et al. 1989. Firefighting increases airway responsiveness. *Am. Rev. Respir. Dis.* 140:185–90

102. Sidor, R., Peters, J. M. 1974. Fire fighting and pulmonary function: An epidemiology study. *Am. Rev. Respir. Dis.* 109:249–54

103. Sidor, R., Peters, J. M. 1974. Prevalence of chronic non-specific respiratory disease in fire fighters. *Am. Rev. Respir. Dis.* 109:255–61

104. Sidor, R., Peters, J. M. 1973. Differences in ventilatory capacity of Irish and Italian firefighters. *Am. Rev. Respir. Dis.* 109:669–71

105. Smith, D. 1988. *Firefighters: Their Lives in Their Own Words.* New York: Doubleday

106. Sparrow, D., Bosse, R., Rosner, B., Weiss, S. T. 1982. The effect of occupational exposure on pulmonary function: A longitudinal evaluation of fire fighters and nonfirefighters. *Am. Rev. Respir. Dis.* 125:319–22

107. Stevenson, C. J. 1985. Effects of radiant heat in fire fighting instructors. *Br. J. Ind. Med.* 42:67–68

108. Sumi, K., Tsuchiya, Y. 1971. Toxic gases and vapours produced at fires. *Can. Build. Dig., Div. Build. Res.,* Natl. Res. Counc. Can. Dec.

109. Symington, I. S., Anderson, R. A., Oliver, J. S., Thomson, I., Harland, W. A., Kerr, J. W. 1978. Cyanimide exposure in fires. *Lancet* 2:91–92

110. Takano, T., Sasaki, J., Maeda, H. 1980. Occupational exposure of firefighters to carbon monoxide. *Jpn. J. Hyg.* 35(2):461–66

111. Tashkin, D. P., Genovesi, M. G., Chopra, S., Coulson, A., Simmons, M. 1977. Respiratory status of Los Angeles firemen: One-month follow-up after inhalation of dense smoke. *Chest* 71:445–49

112. Thomas, D. M. 1971. *The Smoke Inhalation Problem.* Proc. Symp. Occup. Health and Hazards of Fire Serv. Int. Assoc. Firefighters Symp. 1971

113. Treitman, R. D., Burgess, W. A., Gold, A. 1980. Air contaminants encountered by firefighters. *Am. Ind. Hyg. Assoc. J.* 41:796–802

114. Treitman, R. D., Gold, A., Burgess, W. A. 1979. *Air Contaminants Encountered By Firefighters.* 5th Symp. on the Health and Hazards of the Fire Service, Redmond Mem. Fund, San Diego

115. Tsuchiya, Y. 1977. Significance of HCN generation in fire gas toxicity. *J. Combust. Toxicol.* 4:271–82

116. Tsuchiya, Y., Sumi, K. 1977. Thermal decomposition products of polyacrylonitrile. *J. Appl. Biopolym. Sci.* 21:975–80
117. UK Regist. Gen. 1970. UK Registrar General's decennial report for England and Wales, 1970, London, HM Stationery Off.
118. UK Regist. Gen. 1960. UK Registrar General's decennial report for England and Wales, 1960, London, HM Stationery Off.
119. Unger, K. M., Snow, R. M., Mestas, J. M., Miller, W. C. 1980. Smoke inhalation in firemen. *Thorax* 35:838–42
120. US Natl. Inst. Occup. Safe. Health and US Soc. Secur. Adm. 1980. *Occupational Characteristics of Disabled Workers.* Cincinnati: US Public Health Serv. DHHS (NIOSH). Publ. No. 80–145
121. US Soc. Secur. Adm. and US Public Health Serv. 1967. *Occupational Characteristics of Disabled Workers, by Dis-abling Condition.* Washington, DC: GPO
122. Vena, J. E., Fiedler, R. C. 1987. Mortality of a municipal-worker cohort: IV. Firefighters. *Am. J. Ind. Med.* 11:671–84
123. Wojtczak-Jaroszowa, J., Jaroszz, D. 1986. Health complaints, sicknesses and accidents of workers employed in high environmental temperatures. *Can. J. Public Health* 77(Suppl. 1):132–35
124. Wooley, W. D. 1973. Toxic products from plastics materials in fires. *Plast. Polym.* 41:280–86
125. Wooley, W. D. 1972. Nitrogen-containing products from the thermal decomposition of flexible polyurethene forms. *Br. Polym. J.* 4:27–43
126. Young, I., Jackson, J., West, S. 1980. Chronic respiratory disease and respiratory function in a group of firefighters. *Med. J. Aust.* 1:654–58
127. Yuill, C. H. 1972. Smoke: What's in it? *Fire J.* 66:3, 47–55

Annu. Rev. Publ. Health 1992. 13:173–96

BIOLOGICAL INTERACTIONS AND POTENTIAL HEALTH EFFECTS OF EXTREMELY-LOW-FREQUENCY MAGNETIC FIELDS FROM POWER LINES AND OTHER COMMON SOURCES

T. S. Tenforde

Life Sciences Center, Pacific Northwest Laboratory, Richland, Washington 99352

KEY WORDS: mechanisms of interaction, cell and tissue effects, cancer, fetal development, exposure guidelines

INTRODUCTION

The possible relationship between human exposure to time-varying magnetic fields in the extremely-low-frequency (ELF) range and adverse health effects has become a subject of considerable public interest and concern. By definition, the ELF band is composed of electromagnetic fields with frequencies below 300 Hz and, therefore, encompasses the 50-Hz and 60-Hz frequencies used throughout the world for electric power transmission and distribution. Numerous reports have appeared in the literature during the past decade that claim to link exposure to ELF fields in the home and workplace to an apparent elevation in cancer risk. This chapter explores the biological interactions and potential human health effects of ELF magnetic fields and summarizes and critically evaluates the literature that has given rise to the public and scientific debate on this subject.

173

PHYSICAL QUANTITIES, UNITS, AND MEASUREMENT TECHNIQUES FOR ELF MAGNETIC FIELDS

Quantities and Units

The flux density, **B**, of a magnetic field is defined in terms of the force **F** exerted on a charge moving with velocity **v** (the Lorentz force law), $\mathbf{F} = Q(\mathbf{v} \times \mathbf{B})$. The term in parentheses is a vector cross-product equal in magnitude to $|\mathbf{v}| \, |\mathbf{B}| \sin \Theta$, where Θ is the angle between **v** and **B**. With **F** in newtons, Q in coulombs, and **v** in m/s, the metric unit for the magnetic flux density **B** is the tesla (T). The units of electric and magnetic field quantities are summarized in Table 1. It is important to note from the Lorentz force law that a maximum force is exerted on the moving charge Q when **v** and **B** are orthogonal, and no force is exerted when they are parallel. In addition, a magnetic field exerts no force (and, hence, does no work) on a charge that is not moving.

ELF Magnetic Field Measurements

A time-varying magnetic field induces a voltage in any electrically conductive circuit exposed to it. This fact is commonly used in magnetic field meters, which measure the voltage induced by an alternating magnetic field in a "search" coil (23, 54). Meters of this type that are sensitive to low-intensity fields are commercially available. Miniature magnetic field monitors can be worn by individuals for personal exposure measurements. One example is the EMDEX personal monitor, which contains an on-board microprocessor for logging a time history of field exposures (90). The Institute of Electrical and Electronics Engineers, Inc. has established standard methods for the measurement of time-varying magnetic fields from power line sources (39).

Table 1 Quantities and units of electric and magnetic fields

Quantity	MKS/SI Unit[a]	CGS Unit[b]	Equivalence[c]
Electric field intensity	volt/meter (V/m)	statvolt/centimeter (statv/cm)	1 V/m = 3.33×10^{-5} statv/cm
Magnetic field flux density	tesla (T)	gauss (G)	1 T = 10^4 G

[a] MKS/SI is the International System of metric units (m/kg/s).
[b] CGS is the Gaussian system of units (cm/g/s).
[c] Units most commonly used to describe magnetic fields in laboratory research and in typical human exposure conditions are mT and μT, which are equal to 10 G and 10 mG, respectively.

SOURCES OF ELF MAGNETIC FIELDS

Magnetic fields in the ELF range are present throughout the environment and originate from both natural and man-made sources (36, 72). The naturally occurring, time-varying fields in the atmosphere have several origins, including diurnally varying fields on the order of 0.03 μT associated with solar and lunar influences on ion currents in the upper atmosphere. The largest time-varying, atmospheric magnetic fields arise intermittently from intense solar activity and thunderstorms and reach intensities on the order of 0.5 μT during a large magnetic storm. Superimposed on the magnetic fields associated with irregular atmospheric events is a weak ELF field, which results from the Schumann resonance phenomenon (36). These fields are generated by lightning discharges and propagate in the resonant atmospheric cavity formed by the surface of the earth and the lower boundary of the ionosphere.

Extremely-low-frequency magnetic fields originating from man-made sources generally have much higher intensities than the naturally occurring atmospheric fields and, in some occupational settings, reach levels that approach 0.1 T. Two sources of ELF fields that have been the topics of considerable public interest are high-voltage transmission lines and land-based naval communication systems. The field at ground level beneath a 765-kV, 60-Hz power line carrying 1 kA per phase is 15 μT (87). The maximum field at ground level associated with the ELF antennae used in submarine communications is 14 μT (4). Household appliances operated from a 60-Hz line voltage source produce local magnetic fields in their immediate vicinity with flux densities as high as 2.5 mT (36). However, the magnetic field strength decreases rapidly as a function of distance from the surfaces of household devices (28), and the ambient field levels at most locations within a household environment are generally less than 0.3 μT (17, 57, 90). The video display terminals present in most offices generate local ELF magnetic fields with flux densities up to 5 μT, although the typical exposure level at the operator's location is less than 1 μT (93, 107). Several industrial heating processes produce ELF magnetic fields of high intensity within the occupational environment. For example, based on a survey of electrosteel and welding industries in Sweden, Lövsund et al (55) reported that the local fields near 50-Hz ladle furnaces reached a level of 8 mT. The authors also measured flux densities as high as 0.07 T near induction heating devices that operate in the 50-Hz to 10-kHz range.

Time-varying magnetic fields in the ELF frequency range are also employed in medical treatments, including the stimulation of bone fracture reunion (8, 113) and the measurement of blood flow rates (62). Magnetic resonance imaging also produces time-varying magnetic fields up to several T/s as a result of the switching of magnetic field gradients used for the localization of nuclei with magnetic moments, such as protons (15, 94).

INTERACTIONS OF ELF FIELDS WITH TISSUE

Extremely-low-frequency magnetic fields induce electrical currents in tissue that circulate in loops within planes that are orthogonal to the direction of incidence of the field. This relationship between a time-varying magnetic field and the circulating electric field that it induces is expressed formally by Faraday's law:

$$\frac{\partial \mathbf{B}}{\partial t} = - \nabla \times \mathbf{E} \qquad\qquad 1.$$

where $\nabla \times \mathbf{E}$ is the curl of the electric field vector. A magnetically induced electric field gives rise to currents that are predicted from Ohm's law, $\mathbf{J} = \sigma\mathbf{E}$, where $\mathbf{J}$ is the induced current density, expressed in the MKS/SI system in A/m^2, and σ is the tissue conductivity in S/m [Siemen (S) $=$ ohm^{-1}].

The magnitude of the induced current density can be calculated easily from Equation 1 and Ohm's law for simple geometries. Consider, for example, a model of the human body as a uniformly conductive ellipsoid of revolution with the major axis, z, parallel to the long axis of the body. If a sinusoidal magnetic field with an amplitude, B_o, is incident along the z axis, then the peak amplitude of the induced current density in a plane defined by the orthogonal x and y coordinate axes is given by:

$$J = \frac{2\pi f B_o \sigma}{a^2 + b^2} (b^4 x^2 + a^4 y^2)^{1/2} \qquad\qquad 2.$$

where a and b are the semi-axes of the ellipsoid. The induced currents circulate in closed loops within a plane defined by the x and y coordinates (orthogonal to the z axis).

Magnetically induced current densities in erect humans can be modeled to a good approximation by using Equation 2. A typical adult man has a height of 1.7 m, a mass of 70 kg, and a ratio of body width to thickness of about 2. An ellipsoid with semi-major axes of 0.85 m, 0.20 m, and 0.10 m has the same height, the same width-to-thickness ratio, and a body volume of 7.1×10^{-2} m^3. The maximum electric field and current density induced in this ellipsoidal model occur when the magnetic field lines are horizontal and perpendicular to the front of the body. By using Equation 2 with $a = 0.20$ m and $b = 0.85$ m, the calculated value of J is $1.2\, f B_o \sigma$. As an example, for a human with an average tissue conductivity of 0.2 S/m in a 60-Hz, 50-μT field (the highest value under a high-voltage transmission line), $J = 0.7$ mA/m^2.

Although the initial physical interaction of time-varying magnetic fields with living systems is the induction of electric currents in tissue, several secondary events may occur that involve biochemical and structural alterations at the cellular and subcellular levels. At present, there is convincing evidence that ELF magnetic fields do not produce DNA strand breaks or influence the repair of DNA damage caused by other agents (26, 75). There is also evidence that ELF fields do not produce cytogenetic alterations and are not directly mutagenic (18, 53). However, a growing body of evidence indicates that the pericellular currents established by ELF fields can alter ion binding to membrane macromolecules and influence ligand-receptor interactions at the cell surface (e.g. the binding of hormones or other mitogens) (2, 97, 102). These changes in membrane properties are envisioned as setting up transmembrane signaling events, possibly mediated by Ca^{++} or cyclic nucleotides, that trigger abnormal biochemical and cell growth states. Recent experiments have demonstrated that a magnetically induced electric field of 0.1 V/m can significantly increase Ca^{++} uptake in mitogen-activated thymocytes (112). In other experiments, investigators have observed that exposure to pulsed and sinusoidal ELF magnetic fields leads to altered RNA transcription patterns in dipteran salivary gland cells and in cultured human cells (30, 31, 33, 34, 115). This effect is accompanied by a significant change in the spectrum of cellular proteins synthesized by the exposed cells relative to control cells (33). The changes observed in RNA transcripts exhibit a strong dependence on the amplitude and frequency of the applied ELF magnetic field (34, 115). A possible explanation of these observations is that the field alters the rate constant for one (or more) of the intermediate sequential reactions that are involved in RNA synthesis and degradation (52). The threshold field level for producing such effects appears to be on the order of 1 mV/m or less (32, 34).

The findings of several cellular and membrane responses to relatively weak ELF fields have raised the question of how these signals compare with the thermally generated electrical noise (Nyquist noise) present in cell membranes (114). For fields in the ELF range, the minimum signal strength required to exceed the Nyquist noise in a cell membrane was estimated to be approximately 0.1 V/m. This calculation was based on the effective bandwidth, Δf, of a cell membrane represented as a parallel combination of a resistance, R, and a capacitance, C: $\Delta f = (4RC)^{-1}$. However, a considerably lower field threshold of approximately 0.1 mV/m was predicted if the membrane response to an applied field occurs only in a narrow band of frequencies (e.g. a 10-Hz bandwidth), and if the effects of signal-averaging are considered. These simple physical concepts add to the plausibility that relatively weak ELF fields can produce measurable responses in cellular functions mediated by the plasma membrane. However, the above analysis is confined to individual cells and does not address the confounding effects of endogenous

ELF background fields that are always present in the environment of cells and tissues in vivo (10).

In a recent theoretical paper, Adair (1) has questioned whether biological effects could occur in response to the weak ambient fields to which humans are routinely exposed in the home or workplace. He argues that the fields induced in tissue at the level of individual cells would be too weak to overcome the effects of Boltzmann thermal noise or electrical noise in cell membranes. This theoretical treatment, however, neglects the considerable signal amplification that can occur in large arrays of electrically coupled cells in tissue. It also fails to consider nonequilibrium phenomena, such as cooperative transitions (2, 95, 103), through which extremely weak signals could exert significant effects on cell membrane properties.

EFFECTS OF COMBINED STATIC AND ELF MAGNETIC FIELDS

Several experimental studies have provided evidence that the combination of a weak static magnetic field, comparable in strength to the geomagnetic field, and a time-varying magnetic field in the ELF frequency range can produce resonance interactions that influence ion movements through membrane channels and other biological phenomena. Five types of experiments have indicated that certain combinations of static magnetic field flux density and time-varying magnetic field frequency can produce alterations in the rate of calcium ion release from the surfaces of cells in brain tissue (12); the operant behavior of rats in a timing discrimination task (50, 105); calcium-dependent diatom mobility (74, 91); calcium ion uptake by human lymphocytes (49); and changes in fibroblast proliferation (77). Investigators have suggested that the physical mechanism underlying these effects is ion cyclotron resonance (22, 46, 47, 60). In this process, a resonant transfer of energy from a time-varying magnetic field occurs when its frequency matches the cyclotron resonance frequency of an ion moving within a static magnetic field. The resonance condition is formally expressed by the equation,

$$f_c = \frac{QB}{2\pi m} \qquad 3.$$

where f_c is the ion cyclotron resonance frequency, Q is the ion charge, and m is the ion mass. For the typical range of the geomagnetic field over the surface of the earth (30–70 μT), the resonant frequencies of many biologically important ions, such as Na^+, K^+, and Ca^{++}, fall within the ELF range.

Although several experimental results suggest a resonance mechanism through which weak static and ELF fields could produce measurable biological effects, the interpretation of this work presents theoretical difficulties. There are five major problems with the ion cyclotron resonance theory: the collision frequency of ions undergoing cyclotron resonance motion in membrane channels is required to be orders of magnitude less than the typical collision frequency in an aqueous solution at physiological temperatures; the interaction energy of the weak static magnetic field with biological ions is several orders of magnitude less than the Boltzmann thermal energy, kT (= 4.28 × 10^{-21} J at 310 K); the thermally generated electrical noise (Nyquist noise) present in ion transport channels that traverse biological membranes (114) is several orders of magnitude greater than the electric field induced in these channels by the resonant time-varying magnetic field; the radius calculated for a stable ion cyclotron orbit under the conditions used in the experiments cited above is approximately 50 m, which is more than 10 orders of magnitude greater than the typical dimensions of an ion channel in a cell membrane (79); and for ion motion that is constrained to lie along a prescribed path, such as the helical path envisioned by Liboff (46) for ion transport through membrane channels, it follows directly from the equation of motion for the particle that a static magnetic field cannot influence the ion movement and establish a resonance condition (38). The ion cyclotron resonance interaction is thus limited to unconstrained ion movements through membrane channels. All these factors would interfere with the establishment of ion cyclotron resonance conditions in combined static and time-varying magnetic fields. Obviously, there is a need to refine the theoretical description of this phenomenon before it can form a plausible basis for weak field interactions with biological membranes. Also, two recent studies have failed to observe an effect of combined fields on Na^+ and Ca^{++} transport under ion cyclotron resonance conditions (48, 69).

A recent theoretical model has been proposed in which the resonant effects of combined static and ELF fields are visualized as resulting from an effect on the vibrational energy levels of an ion, with a resulting effect on its interaction with ligand binding sites (45). This theory is physically more plausible than the ion cyclotron resonance model, but remains to be tested experimentally.

BIOLOGICAL EFFECTS OF ELF MAGNETIC FIELDS

An effect of ELF magnetic fields on humans, which was first described by d'Arsonval (20), is the induction of a flickering illumination within the visual field known as magnetophosphenes. This phenomenon occurs as an immediate response to stimulation by either pulsed or sinusoidal magnetic fields with frequencies less than 100 Hz, and the effect is completely reversible with no apparent influence on visual acuity. The maximum visual sensitivity to sinusoidal magnetic fields has been found at a frequency of 20 Hz in human subjects with normal vision. At this frequency, the threshold magnetic field flux density found by Lövsund et al (56) to elicit phosphenes is approximately 10 mT. The threshold field level increases rapidly as a function of frequency below and above 20 Hz. The corresponding time rate of change of the sinusoidal field is 1.26 T/s. In other studies, Silny (89) has observed thresholds for magnetophosphene perception in human volunteers as low as 5 mT with 18-Hz sinusoidal fields. In studies with pulsed fields that had a rise time of 2 ms and a repetition rate of 15 Hz, the threshold values of dB/dt for eliciting phosphenes ranged from 1.3 to 1.9 T/s in five adult subjects (14). A trend in the data suggested that the threshold was lower among younger subjects. In related studies, investigators also observed that the stimulus duration is an important parameter, because pulses of 0.9-ms duration with $dB/dt = 12$ T/s did not evoke phosphenes.

Several types of experimental evidence indicate that the magnetic field interaction that leads to magnetophosphenes occurs in the retina: magnetophosphenes are produced by time-varying magnetic fields applied in the region of the eye, and not by fields directed toward the visual cortex in the occipital region of the brain (5); pressure on the eyeball abolishes sensitivity to magnetophosphenes (5); the threshold magnetic field flux density required to elicit magnetophosphenes in human subjects with defects in color vision has a different dependence on the field frequency than that observed for subjects with normal color vision (56); and in a patient who had both eyes removed as the result of severe glaucoma, phosphenes could not be induced by time-varying magnetic fields, thereby precluding the possibility that magnetophosphenes can be initiated directly in the visual pathways of the brain (56).

Silny (89) also studied other phenomena related to the sensitivity of the visuosensory system to time-varying magnetic fields. In experiments with human subjects, distinct flickering could be elicited in the visual field by sinusoidal magnetic fields in the frequency range of 5–60 Hz. The threshold field intensity varied with the field frequency and background light level, but was as low as 5 mT under optimal conditions. Alterations in visually evoked potentials (VEP) were also reported to occur in sinusoidal magnetic fields at intensity levels that are five to ten times greater than those that produce magnetophosphenes (89). The change in VEP was characterized by a reversal of polarity and a decreased amplitude of the three major evoked potentials. These effects were observed within three minutes after onset of the magnetic field exposure, and the VEP returned to normal only after a recovery period of approximately 30–70 minutes following termination of the exposure. The relationship of these changes in the VEP to the mechanism of magnetophosphene induction is not clear from currently available evidence.

Time-varying magnetic fields that induce current densities above 1 A/m^2 in tissue lead to neural excitation and can produce irreversible biological effects, such as cardiac fibrillation (76, 102). Several investigators have achieved direct neural stimulation by using pulsed or sinusoidal magnetic fields that induced tissue current densities in the range of 1–10 A/m^2. In one study involving electromyographic recordings from the human arm, Polson et al (73) found that a pulsed field with dB/dt greater than 10^4 T/s was required to stimulate the median nerve trunk. The duration of the magnetic stimulus is also an important parameter in the excitation of nerve and nerve-muscle specimens. By using a 20-kHz sinusoidal field applied in bursts of 0.5- to 50-ms duration, Öberg (68) found that a progressive increase in the magnetic flux density was required to stimulate the frog gastrocnemius neuromuscular preparation when the burst duration was reduced to less than 2–5 ms. A similar rise in threshold stimulus strength has been observed for frog neuromuscular stimulation by using pulsed magnetic fields with pulse durations less than approximately 1 ms (109, 110).

Time-varying magnetic fields that induce tissue current densities less than approximately 1–10 mA/m^2 produce few, if any, irreversible biological effects. This general observation is not surprising, as the endogenous current densities present in many organs and tissues lie in the range of 0.1 to 10 mA/m^2, as discussed by Bernhardt (10). In contrast, time-varying magnetic fields that induce peak current densities greater than approximately 10 mA/m^2 reportedly produce various alterations in the biochemistry and physiology of cells and organized tissues. One example is the effect of the bidirectional pulsed fields used to facilitate bone fracture reunion in humans (8). Numerous laboratory investigations have also led to reports of a broad spectrum of alterations in cellular, tissue, and animal systems in which current densities exceeding 1–10 mA/m^2 were induced by ELF magnetic fields (96–100). These effects include altered cell growth rate; decreased rate of cellular respiration; altered metabolism of carbohydrates, proteins, and nucleic acids; effects on gene expression and genetic regulation of cell functions; teratological and developmental effects; morphological and other nonspecific tissue changes in animals, frequently reversible with time following exposure; endocrine alterations, including suppression of the nocturnal level of pineal melatonin; altered hormonal responses of cells and tissues, including effects on cell-surface receptors; and altered immune response to antigenic stimulation.

In assessing these reported effects of time-varying magnetic fields, it is important to recognize that very few of the observations have been independently replicated in a second laboratory. In many cases, in which attempts at replication were carried out, the results were contradictory. One notable example of this variability is the attempt by several groups of investigators to determine whether teratological effects result from the exposure of chicken embryos to pulsed magnetic fields of low intensity, as originally reported by Delgado et al (21). Widely divergent results, ranging from no effects to significant effects on embryo development, were obtained in these experiments (97). To resolve the question of whether Delgado et al's (21) original experimental results are replicable under controlled laboratory conditions, the Office of Naval Research and the US Environmental Protection Agency (EPA) recently sponsored an international cooperative effort, which involved six independent laboratories (9). Laboratories located in Spain, Sweden, Canada, and the US were equipped with identical pulsed magnetic-field exposure systems that had been constructed and tested by the same engineering team. The pulse parameters chosen for this study were 100-Hz repetition frequency, 500-μs pulse duration, 2-μs pulse rise and fall times, and peak magnetic flux density of 1.0 μT. Each of the six laboratories conducted ten separate experiments with 20 chick eggs, ten of which were exposed to the pulsed field for the first 48 hours of incubation; the remaining ten eggs were sham-exposed for the same time interval. Two of the six laboratories observed a statistically significant increase in the proportion of abnormal embryos (p < 0.001 and p = 0.03), whereas the other four laboratories did not observe a significant difference between the exposed and sham-exposed embryos. The overall data from the six different laboratories, however, did show a statistically significant increase in the proportion of abnormal embryos in the exposed groups of eggs. The interlaboratory variations observed in this series of experiments are indicative of the difficulty encountered in replicating the results of biological studies on ELF field effects, even when exceptional efforts are made to control the relevant experimental variables.

HUMAN HEALTH STUDIES

Many studies on human responses to ELF magnetic fields have been reported, primarily epidemiological studies on adverse reproductive outcomes and elevated cancer risk in more highly exposed groups of individuals (104, 111). The conclusions of many of these studies have been difficult to interpret. This problem has largely arisen because of a lack of information on the biologically effective exposure parameters for ELF fields, and because of the failure of many investigators to account for confounding variables. Only some highlights of the human studies are summarized here, as extensive reviews are available (64, 97, 104, 111).

Laboratory Investigations

Several studies have been made of the general health profiles of individuals who work in electrical occupations or who were exposed to ELF magnetic fields under controlled laboratory conditions. Medical examinations of 379 workers in electrical substations in Italy revealed no adverse clinical symptoms relative to a control group of 133 workers (7). Laboratory studies on humans exposed to ELF magnetic fields have also failed to reveal any adverse physiological or psychological symptoms in the exposed subjects. The strongest field used in these experiments was a 5-mT, 50-Hz field to which subjects were exposed for four hours by Sander et al (78). No field-associated changes were observed in serum chemistry, blood cell counts, blood gases and lactate concentration, electrocardiogram, pulse rate, skin temperature, circulating hormones (cortisol, insulin, gastrin, thyroxin), and various neuronal measurements, including visually evoked potentials recorded in the electroencephalogram. Graham et al (35) observed small changes in heart rate and motor responses in extensive studies on human subjects exposed to 60-Hz electric and magnetic fields with intensities comparable to those of fields in the vicinity of high-voltage transmission lines. These effects were reversible following termination of the exposure. Several other physiological and biochemical indices that were examined in this controlled human study did not exhibit significant changes during exposure to 60-Hz fields with intensities up to 12 kV/m and 30 μT.

Electric Blankets and Electrically Heated Beds

A study by Wertheimer & Leeper (116) led to evidence of seasonal changes in fetal growth and in abortion rate among women who used electrically heated beds during the winter months. The authors contended that these adverse effects on fetal development could result from exposure to the 60-Hz electromagnetic fields present at the surfaces of electrically heated beds. They pointed out, however, that the potentially harmful effect of excessive heat on fetal growth cannot be excluded on the basis of their data. In a more recent study on magnetic field exposures in the home and cancer incidence in children, Savitz et al (84) concluded that the use of electric blankets was weakly associated with childhood cancer. However, the elevated odds ratio of 1.3 was not statistically significant. Another study found no elevation in the risk of acute myelogenous leukemia as a result of electric blanket use (71). A recent report indicated that the nighttime urinary excretion of a melatonin metabolite, 6-hydroxymelatonin sulfate, is altered in human subjects who use electric blankets (120). The possible influence of this endocrine effect on human health remains to be determined. Many US manufacturers have recently introduced design changes in the wiring of electric blankets that lead to nearly complete cancellation of the surface 60-Hz magnetic fields. Blankets that are operated with a direct current supply (i.e. not varying with time) have also been produced.

Video Display Terminals

Goldhaber et al (29) have reported that the rate of miscarriages increased by approximately 80% among women who worked on video display terminals for more than 20 hours per week, as compared with women who did similar work without the use of these devices. No statistically significant risk of miscarriage was found among women who worked at video display terminals for less than 20 hours per week. Overall, the increase in rate of birth defects was about 40% for women who worked at video display terminals for more than five hours per week, but this increase was not statistically significant. Although the results of this study suggest that the fields from video display terminals may enhance the risk of miscarriage, the possible role of job stress or other unidentified factors cannot be excluded on the basis of the available information. In distinct contrast to the results of the Goldhaber et al (29) study, nine other epidemiological surveys have not obtained evidence for a significant elevation in spontaneous abortion rate or birth defects as the result of prolonged exposure during pregnancy to the electromagnetic fields from video display terminals (13, 16, 24, 25, 44, 58, 66, 67, 86). The latest of the studies with negative outcomes was a comprehensive analysis involving more than 2000 directory-assistance telephone operators who use video display terminals throughout the workday (86).

Residential Fields and Cancer Risk

One of the most controversial issues related to the interaction of electromagnetic fields with humans is the reported link between residential and occupational exposure to ELF fields and cancer risk. The first report on this subject was published by Wertheimer & Leeper (119), who found that cancer deaths (primarily leukemia and nervous system tumors) in children less than 19 years of age in the Denver, Colorado, area were correlated with the presence of high-current primary and secondary wiring configurations near their residences. This retrospective epidemiological study was based on 344 fatal childhood cancer cases from 1950 to 1973 and an equal number of age-matched controls chosen from birth records. The electrical power lines near the birth and death residences of the cancer cases and the residences of the controls were inspected and classified as being either high-current con-figurations (HCC) or low-current configurations (LCC), which are assumed to reflect the local intensity of the 60-Hz magnetic fields within the homes of the subjects. The percentage of the cancer cases whose birth and death residences were near HCC was significantly greater than for the control subjects, from which the authors concluded that an association may exist between the strength of magnetic fields from the residential power-distribution lines and the frequency of childhood cancer. In a subsequent publication, these authors reported that a similar association exists for the incidence of adult cancer

(117). This later study was based on 1179 cancer cases (78% fatal) in Denver, Boulder, and Longmont, Colorado, from 1967 to 1977.

Based on direct measurements of 60-Hz electric and magnetic fields in 434 homes in the Denver metropolitan area, Barnes et al (6) concluded that the magnetic field component was weakly correlated with the power line wiring code used by Wertheimer & Leeper (117, 119). Kaune et al (43) obtained a similar result in studies of homes in three counties in Washington state. The 60-Hz electric field component of electromagnetic fields measured within the homes was not correlated with the power line wiring code. This finding was not unexpected, as the electric fields emanating from power line sources are attenuated by trees, the walls of homes, and other objects. In contrast, the magnetic fields emanating from power lines are not influenced by materials that lack a significant amount of iron or other magnetic materials (e.g. trees or the walls of homes). Emphasis has therefore been placed on determining whether an association exists between cancer risk and exposure to the magnetic field component of ELF fields.

Following Wertheimer & Leeper's initial report on childhood cancer, five other epidemiological studies have been conducted to determine whether a relationship exists between residential magnetic fields from power line sources and the incidence of cancer in children. In the first of these studies, Fulton et al (27) used methodology that was matched as closely as possible to that of Wertheimer & Leeper, including the designation of HCC and LCC power lines. This study involved 119 leukemia patients with ages of onset from 0 to 20 years, whose address histories were obtained from medical records at Rhode Island Hospital, and 240 control subjects chosen from Rhode Island birth certificates. Fulton et al (27) concluded that no statistically significant correlation existed between the incidence of leukemia and the residential power line configurations. Wertheimer & Leeper (118) were critical of this study because the case and control groups had not been matched for interstate migration, for years of occupancy at residences, or for the ages of the children at the time their residential addresses were determined from birth records and hospital medical records. Reevaluating the data, Wertheimer & Leeper (118) excluded cases and controls aged 8 and older, which allowed them to define a complete residential history for the remaining subjects (53 cases and 71 controls). In this subset of the total population studied by Fulton et al (27), Wertheimer & Leeper found a weakly significant correlation (p = 0.05) between the incidence of leukemia and residential HCC power lines.

Another study of childhood cancer incidence was conducted in the county of Stockholm by Tomenius (108), who analyzed the residential 50-Hz magnetic fields for 716 cases that had a stable address from the time of birth to the time of cancer diagnosis, and for 716 controls who were matched for age, sex, and birth location. An evaluation was made of the electrical wiring configurations near the residences of the study population, and measurements were made of the magnetic-field flux density in the frequency range above 30 Hz at the entrance door to each residence. Among the residences within 150 m of 200 kV power lines, a statistically significant elevation was found in the incidence of cancer. The most frequently observed types of cancer were nervous system tumors and leukemia. There was, however, an inconsistency in the results of this study insofar as the cancer risk was greater in homes with magnetic field levels at the entrance less than 0.3 μT relative to homes in which the field level was more than 0.3 μT.

In contrast to the findings of Wertheimer & Leeper (119) and Tomenius (108), Myers et al (63) found no relationship between the risk of childhood cancer and residential proximity to overhead power lines. This study was conducted in the Yorkshire Health Region in England, and included 376 cancer cases diagnosed in children less than 15 years of age from 1970 to 1979. There were 590 age-matched controls in the study. Magnetic fields at the birth addresses were calculated on the basis of data from the electrical load records for the overhead lines. The results showed no significant elevation in the cancer risk ratio with increasing field strength, and no dependence of the risk ratio on distance from the overhead lines.

A case-control epidemiological study by Savitz et al (85) attempted to verify the initial findings of Wertheimer & Leeper (119) on childhood cancer in the Denver area. This study involved 357 cancer cases diagnosed between 1976 and 1983. The cancer incidence data were analyzed on the basis of both the Wertheimer/Leeper wiring code and spot measurements of 60-Hz magnetic fields in the homes. A correlation between cancer risk in children less than 14 years of age and the proximity of their residences to high-current wiring configurations was found. However, the authors observed no statistically significant association between the measured household fields and childhood cancer incidence. The results of this study are, therefore, ambiguous and suggest that the wire code developed by Wertheimer & Leeper may be an indicator of some unidentified carcinogenic factor, or factors, in the urban environment. This possibility is suggested by a recently completed study in Los Angeles (S. J. London et al 1991, unpublished) that led to results similar to those obtained in the Savitz et al (85) study.

Two other epidemiological surveys have failed to detect an association between residential exposure to power-frequency fields and cancer risk. In England, McDowall (59) found no correlation between cancer mortality and residential exposure to the fields from electrical utility installations (substations and overhead power lines). This study involved a retrospective analysis of mortality from 1971 to 1983 among a population of 7631 persons in East Anglia who were identified as living near electrical installations. The standardized mortality ratios for this large study population were lower than expected for three major causes of death: cancer, cardiovascular disease, and respiratory disease. The results of this study, therefore, did not support other claims of an elevated cancer risk associated with residential exposure to power-frequency fields.

A case-control study of the incidence of acute nonlymphocytic leukemia (ANL) in three counties in Washington state also failed to find a correlation between residential exposure to 60-Hz fields and cancer risk (88). For 164 cases of ANL and 204 controls from the same geographic area, residential wiring codes were analyzed by the Wertheimer/Leeper technique and direct measurements were made of the residential electric and magnetic fields (43). Several confounding variables, such as smoking habits and socioeconomic status of the case and control subjects, were analyzed. The overall results provided no evidence for a possible association between residential exposure to 60-Hz fields and the risk of ANL.

Occupational Exposure and Cancer Risk

The controversy surrounding the issue of exposure to ELF fields and cancer risk has been increased by numerous epidemiological reports published since 1982, in which an apparent association was found between employment in various electrical occupations and cancer risk (primarily leukemia and tumors of the nervous system). Many of these studies have been reviewed previously (19, 80, 97). Savitz & Calle (82) have attempted to collate the data from 11 of these published studies to estimate the average relative risk of all leukemias, acute leukemias, and acute myelogenous leukemias among workers in 12 different classes of electrical occupations. The overall relative risk and 95% confidence intervals for leukemia mortality were the following: total leukemias, 1.2 (1.1–1.3); acute leukemias, 1.4 (1.2–1.6); and acute myelogenous leukemias, 1.5 (1.2–1.8). Savitz & Calle (82) concluded that a correlation exists between employment in electrical occupations and leukemia risk. However, they pointed out that none of the epidemiological surveys conducted thus far has established that exposure to 60-Hz electromagnetic fields is the causal factor that leads to an elevated cancer risk among electrical workers. Similar results and conclusions were obtained by Coleman & Beral (19) in a meta-analysis of data on leukemia risk among workers in electrical occupations.

Four separate studies have reported an increased risk of brain tumors among workers in electrical occupations (51, 61, 92, 106). These epidemiological studies were based on data obtained from death certificates of workers in electrical occupations in different geographic areas within the US. Although the findings were reasonably consistent, none of these studies established a true causal relationship between exposure to 60-Hz fields and the risk of brain malignancies. In addition, the potential contribution to cancer risk of exposure to other agents, such as organic solvents, was not assessed in any of the epidemiological studies on brain tumor incidence among electrical workers.

Critique of Epidemiological Studies

Overall, the epidemiological studies on the possible correlation between cancer risk and residential exposure to electromagnetic fields do not support the conclusion of a strong association. In the earlier studies on this subject, especially those conducted by Wertheimer & Leeper (117, 119) in the Denver area, the control groups were chosen in a nonblind manner. In addition, quantitative measurements of the 60-Hz fields within the residences of the case and control subjects have been made only in the studies by Savitz et al (85) and Severson et al (88), and in the above-mentioned study by London et al. As discussed above, magnetic field levels measured in homes have shown a much weaker association with cancer risk than have the Wertheimer/Leeper wire codes. Finally, with the exception of these two studies, no attempt was made to analyze the role of confounding variables in the overall cancer risk of the case and control populations. Savitz & Feingold (83) have found that residential traffic density is strongly associated with childhood cancer, especially leukemia, among the same study population that was previously reported to have an association between cancer risk and power line configurations (85). They speculated that benzene, a known leukemogen, in automobile exhaust fumes may have been a contributing factor in the elevated incidence of childhood cancer. Savitz & Baron (81) have emphasized the importance of estimating and correcting for confounding variables in epidemiological studies. In the case of ELF fields, several large studies are currently underway in the US and other nations that are attempting to identify possible confounding variables (40, 111).

In view of limitations in the epidemiological studies conducted to date, it is not possible to conclude that a definite association exists between the exposure of individuals to ELF fields and their relative risk of contracting leukemia or other forms of cancer. The available evidence suggests that workers in electrical occupations have an increased risk of cancer, primarily leukemia and nervous tissue tumors. Similarly, individuals living in homes near high-current configurations of power distribution lines may have an elevated cancer risk, although the available data are not convincing. In a recent literature review (111), staff members at the EPA indicated that "with our current understanding, we can identify 60-Hz magnetic fields from power lines and perhaps other sources in the home as a possible, but not proven, cause of cancer in humans." The EPA report stated further that, in spite of methodological weaknesses, "the occupational studies tend to support the results of the childhood cancer studies, and excesses occur at the same sites." There exists a clear need for additional epidemiological surveys on large populations

of subjects, in which efforts are made to analyze the possible role of confounding variables and to conduct proper dosimetry measurements for exposure assessment. Approximately 20 epidemiological studies on cancer risk in
relation to power-frequency electromagnetic field exposure are currently
under way in Europe, Australia, and North America (40, 111).

EFFECTS OF ELF MAGNETIC FIELDS ON CARDIAC PACEMAKERS

Extremely-low-frequency magnetic and electric fields can produce
electromagnetic interference (EMI) in implanted medical electronic devices,
such as cardiac pacemakers (37, 101). The unipolar design of demand cardiac
pacemakers, in which the cathode lead is implanted in the heart and the
pacemaker case serves as the anode, is particularly susceptible to low-
frequency EMI. In experimental studies with a magnetic resonance imaging
system, Pavlicek et al (70) found that a rapidly-switched gradient field with a
time variation of 3 T/s can induce potentials up to 20 mV in the loop formed
by the electrode lead and the case of a unipolar pacemaker. Jenkins & Woody
(42) examined 26 pacemaker models for sensitivity to 60-Hz magnetic fields.
Twenty of these units reverted to an asynchronous mode or exhibited abnormal pacing characteristics in 60-Hz fields with amplitudes ranging from 0.1 to
0.4 mT. The average threshold flux density for producing pacemaker
malfunction was 0.2 mT. This level is high relative to common human
exposures, but is less than the magnetic flux densities near the surfaces of
many appliances and tools (28).

EXPOSURE GUIDELINES FOR ELF MAGNETIC FIELDS

Although many states in the US have established limits on human exposure to
60-Hz fields in the vicinity of high-voltage transmission lines, there are
currently no federal regulations on public or occupational exposures to fields
in the ELF range. However, guidelines for exposure to fields in this frequency
range have been established in West Germany and the United Kingdom. In
the West German guidelines (11), the exposure limit for magnetic fields was
set at the level of 20 mT for frequencies below 2 Hz. At frequencies from 2 to
10,000 Hz, the exposure limit was set in accord with the formula B (rms) =
$27.135/f^{0.4325}$ mT, which gives a limit of 5.0 mT at 50 Hz. In the United
Kingdom (65), the time-varying magnetic field limit recommended by the
National Radiological Protection Board (NRPB) for occupational exposures
was set at 10 mT for frequencies below 10 Hz. At frequencies in the range of
10 to 750 Hz, the occupational exposure limit was set in accord with the
formula B (rms) = $94/f$ mT, which gives a limit of 1.88 mT at 50 Hz. At

frequencies from 750 to 50,000 Hz, the exposure limit was set at 0.125 mT. The guideline also states that occupational personnel should not be exposed to the maximum permissible field levels for more than two hours per day. Significantly lower exposure limits were established in the NRPB guidelines for the general public.

In 1990, the International Non-Ionizing Radiation Committee (INIRC) of the International Radiation Protection Association (IRPA) recommended a set of exposure limits on 50/60 Hz electric and magnetic fields (41). The limit on magnetic flux density for occupational exposures was set at 0.5 mT for the entire workday, 5 mT for exposures of less than two hours duration, and 25 mT for exposure of the limbs throughout the workday. The IRPA/INIRC exposure limits for the general public were set at 0.1 mT for continuous exposures and 1.0 mT for exposures during periods of a "few hours per day."

In 1991, the American Conference of Governmental Industrial Hygienists (ACGIH) proposed guidelines for occupational exposure to time-varying magnetic fields with frequencies in the range of 1 Hz to 30 kHz (3). The maximum exposure level at 60 Hz was set at 1 mT, which limits the maximum induced current density within the body to a root-mean-square value of 10 mA/m^2. The rationale for the ACGIH guidelines was that, apart from the controversial issue of cancer risk in relation to occupational or residential exposure to 60-Hz fields, there is no strong evidence for harmful effects of ELF magnetic fields that induce current densities in the body of 10 mA/m^2 or less. The ACGIH also recommends that personnel wearing cardiac pacemakers should not be exposed to 60-Hz magnetic fields above 0.1 mT to avoid possible problems with electromagnetic interference.

SUMMARY AND CONCLUSIONS

Various different effects of ELF magnetic fields have been reported to occur at the cellular, tissue, and animal levels. Certain effects, such as the induction of magnetophosphenes in the visual system, have been established through replication in several laboratories. Many other effects, however, have not been independently verified or, in some cases, replication efforts have led to conflicting results. A substantial amount of experimental evidence indicates that the effects of ELF magnetic fields on cellular biochemistry, structure, and function can be related to the induced current density, with a majority of the reported effects occurring at current density levels in excess of 10 mA/m^2. These effects, therefore, occur at induced current-density levels that exceed the endogenous currents normally present in living tissues. From this perspective, it is extremely difficult to interpret the results of recent epidemiological studies that have reported a correlation between cancer incidence and exposure to 50-Hz or 60-Hz magnetic fields with very low flux densities. The levels of current density induced in tissue by occupational or residential exposure to these fields are, in nearly all circumstances, significantly lower than the levels found in laboratory studies to produce measurable perturbations in biological functions. There is a clear need for additional epidemiological research to clarify whether exposure to ELF magnetic fields is, in fact, causally linked to cancer risk. Laboratory animal studies conducted under controlled conditions are also needed to determine whether ELF magnetic fields can initiate or promote tumors. In addition, more studies of both a theoretical and experimental nature are needed to elucidate the molecular and cellular mechanisms through which low-intensity magnetic fields can influence living systems. A growing body of evidence indicates that cell membranes play a key role in the transduction and amplification of ELF field signals. Elucidation of the physical and biochemical pathways that mediate these transmembrane signaling events will represent a major advance in our understanding of the molecular basis of magnetic field effects on biological systems.

ACKNOWLEDGMENTS

The skillful assistance of Marianna Cross and Shirley Nolen in the preparation of this manuscript is gratefully acknowledged. Research support is received from the US Department of Energy under Contract DE-AC06-76RLO 1830 with the Pacific Northwest Laboratory. The Pacific Northwest Laboratory is operated for the US Department of Energy by the Battelle Memorial Institute.

Literature Cited

1. Adair, R. K. 1991. Constraints on biological effects of weak extremely-low-frequency electromagnetic fields. *Phys. Rev. A* 43:1039–48
2. Adey, W. R. 1981. Tissue interactions with nonionizing electromagnetic fields. *Physiol. Rev.* 61:435–514
3. Am. Conf. Gov. Ind. Hyg. 1990–1991. *Threshold Limit Values and Biological Exposure Indices.* Cincinnati: Am. Conf. Gov. Ind. Hyg.
4. Am. Inst. Biol. Sci. 1985. *Biological and Human Health Effects of Extremely Low Frequency Electromagnetic Fields.* Arlington, Va: Am. Inst. Biol. Sci.
5. Barlow, H. B., Kohn, H. I., Walsh, E. G. 1947. Visual sensations aroused by magnetic fields. *Am. J. Physiol.* 148:372–75
6. Barnes, F., Wachtel, H., Savitz, D., Fuller, J. 1989. Use of wiring configuration and wiring codes for estimating externally generated electric and magnetic fields. *Bioelectromagnetics* 10:13–21

7. Baroncelli, P., Battisti, S., Checcucci, A., Comba, P., Grandolfo, M., et al. 1986. A health examination of railway high-voltage substation workers exposed to ELF electromagnetic fields. *Am. J. Ind. Med.* 10:45–55
8. Bassett, C. A. L., Mitchell, S. N., Gaston, S. R. 1982. Pulsing electromagnetic field treatment in ununited fractures and failed arthrodeses. *J. Am. Med. Assoc.* 247:623–28
9. Berman, E., Chacon, L., House, D., Koch, B. A., Koch, W. E., et al. 1990. Development of chicken embryos in a pulsed magnetic field. *Bioelectromagnetics* 11:169–87
10. Bernhardt, J. 1979. The direct influence of electromagnetic fields on nerve and muscle cells of man within the frequency range of 1 Hz to 30 MHz. *Radiat. Environ. Biophys.* 16:309–23
11. Bernhardt, J. H., Haubrich, H. J., Newi, G., Krause, N., Schneider, K. H. 1986. Limits for electric and magnetic

192   TENFORDE

fields in DIN VDE standards: Considerations for the range 0 to 10 kHz. In *Proc. Int. Conf. Large High Voltage Electr. Syst.*, No. 36–10, 1–9 Sept. 1982, Paris

12. Blackman, C. F., Benane, S. G., Rabinowitz, J. R., House, D. E., Joines, W. T. 1985. A role for the magnetic field in the radiation-induced efflux of calcium ions from brain tissue in vitro. *Bioelectromagnetics* 6:327–37

13. Bryant, H., Love, E. 1989. Video display terminal use and spontaneous abortion risk. *Int. J. Epidemiol.* 15:132–38

14. Budinger, T. F., Cullander, C., Bordow, R. 1984. Switched magnetic field thresholds for the induction of magnetophosphenes. In *Abstr. Soc. Magn. Reson. in Med. 3rd Annu. Meet.*, pp. 118–19, 13–17 Aug., New York

15. Budinger, T. F., Lauterbur, P. C. 1984. Nuclear magnetic resonance technology for medical studies. *Science* 226:288–98

16. Butler, W. J., Brix, K. A. 1986. Video display terminal work and pregnancy outcome in Michigan clerical workers. Presented at Public Health Assoc. Annu. Meet., Las Vegas, Aug. 1986. Also published in *Humane Technology*, pp. 67–91. Nottingham, England

17. Caola, R. J., Deno, D. W., Dymek, V. S. W. 1983. Measurements of electric and magnetic fields in and around homes near a 500 kV transmission line. *IEEE Trans. Power Appl. Sys.* PAS-102:3338–47

18. Cohen, M. M., Kunska, A., Astemborski, J. A., McCulloch, D., Paskewitz, D. A. 1986. Effects of low-level, 60-Hz electromagnetic fields on human lymphoid cells: I. Mitotic rate and chromosome breakage in human peripheral lymphocytes. *Bioelectromagnetics* 7:415–23

19. Coleman, M., Beral, V. 1988. A review of epidemiological studies of the health effects of living near or working with electricity generation and transmission equipment. *Int. J. Epidemiol.* 17:1–13

20. d'Arsonval, M. A. 1896. Dispositifs pour la mesure des courants alternatifs à toutes frequences. *C.R. Soc. Biol. (Paris)* 3(100 Ser.):450–51

21. Delgado, J. M. R., Leal, J., Monteagudo, J. L., Garcia, M. G. 1982. Embryological changes induced by weak, extremely low frequency electromagnetic fields. *J. Anat.* 134:533–51

22. Durney, C. H., Rushforth, C. K., Anderson, A. A. 1988. Resonant AC-DC magnetic fields: Calculated response. *Bioelectromagnetics* 9:315–36

23. *Environ. Health Criteria 69: Magn. Fields.* 1987. Geneva: WHO

24. Ericson, A., Kallen, B. 1986. An epidemiological study of work with video display screens and pregnancy outcome: I. A registry study. *Am. J. Ind. Med.* 9:447–57

25. Ericson, A., Kallen, B. 1986. An epidemiological study of work with video display screens and pregnancy outcome: II. A case-control study. *Am. J. Ind. Med.* 9:459–75

26. Frazier, M. E., Reese, J. A., Morris, J. E., Jostes, R. F., Miller, D. L. 1990. Exposure of mammalian cells to 60-Hz magnetic or electric fields: Analysis of DNA repair of induced, single-strand breaks. *Bioelectromagnetics* 11:229–34

27. Fulton, J. P., Cobb, S., Preble, L., Leone, L., Forman, E. 1980. Electrical wiring configurations and childhood leukemia in Rhode Island. *Am. J. Epidemiol.* 111:292–96

28. Gauger, J. R. 1984. *Household Appliance Magnetic Field Survey.* IIT Res. Inst. Rep. No. E06549-3. Washington, DC: US Naval Electron. Sys. Command

29. Goldhaber, M. K., Polen, M. R., Hiatt, R. A. 1988. The risk of miscarriage and birth defects among women who use video display terminals during pregnancy. *Am. J. Ind. Med.* 13:695–706

30. Goodman, R., Abbott, J., Henderson, A. S. 1987. Transcriptional patterns in the X chromosome of *Sciara coprophila* following exposure to magnetic fields. *Bioelectromagnetics* 8:1–7

31. Goodman, R., Bassett, C. A. L., Henderson, A. S. 1983. Pulsing electromagnetic fields induce cellular transcription. *Science* 220:1283–85

32. Goodman, R., Henderson, A. S. 1988. Exposure of salivary gland cells to low frequency fields alters polypeptide synthesis. *Proc. Natl. Acad. Sci. USA* 85:3928–32

33. Goodman, R., Henderson, A. S. 1986. Sine waves enhance cellular transcription. *Bioelectromagnetics* 7:23–29

34. Goodman, R., Wei, L.-X., Xu, J.-C., Henderson, A. 1989. Exposure of human cells to low frequency electromagnetic fields results in quantitative changes in transcripts. *Biochim. Biophys. Acta* 1009:216–20

35. Graham, C., Cook, M. R., Cohen, H. D. 1990. *Immunological and Biochemical Effects of 60-Hz Electric and Magnetic Fields in Humans.* Midwest Res. Inst. Final Rep. Contract No. DE-FC01-84-CE-76246 (Order No. DE90006671).

Oak Ridge, Tenn: US Dep. Energy Off. Sci. Tech. Inf.

36. Grandolfo, M., Vecchia, P. 1985. Natural and man-made environmental exposures to static and ELF electromagnetic fields. In *Biological Effects and Dosimetry of Static and ELF Electromagnetic Fields*, ed. M. Grandolfo, S. M. Michaelson, A. Rindi, pp. 49–70. New York: Plenum

37. Griffin, J. C. 1985. The effects of ELF electric and magnetic fields on artificial cardiac pacemakers. In *Assessments and Viewpoints on the Biological and Human Health Effects of Extremely Low Frequency (ELF) Electromagnetic Fields*, pp. 173–83. Washington, DC: Am. Inst. Biol. Sci.

38. Halle, B. 1988. On the cyclotron resonance mechanism for magnetic field effects on transmembrane ion conductivity. *Bioelectromagnetics* 9:381–85

39. *IEEE Recommended Practices for Measurement of Electric and Magnetic Fields from AC Power Lines*. 1979. IEEE Standard 644-1979. New York: Inst. Electr. and Electron. Eng.

40. Int. Agency for Res. on Cancer *ad hoc* Working Group. 1990. Extremely low-frequency electric and magnetic fields and risk of human cancer. *Bioelectromagnetics* 11:91–99

41. Int. Non-ionizing Radiat. Comm. of the Int. Radiat. Prot. Assoc. 1990. Interim guidelines on limits of exposure to 50/60 Hz electric and magnetic fields. *Health Phys.* 58:113–22

42. Jenkins, B. M., Woody, J. A. 1978. Cardiac pacemaker responses to power frequency signals. *Proc. IEEE Int. Symp. Electromagn. Compat.* EMC-S 78:273–77

43. Kaune, W. T., Stevens, R. G., Callahan, N. J., Severson, R. K., Thomas, D. B. 1987. Residential magnetic and electric fields. *Bioelectromagnetics* 8: 315–35

44. Kurppa, K., Holmberg, P. C., Rantala, K., Nurminen, T., Saxen, L. 1985. Birth defects and exposure to video display terminals during pregnancy. *Scand. J. Work Environ. Health* 11: 353–56

45. Lednev, V. V. 1991. Possible mechanism for the influence of weak magnetic fields on biological systems. *Bioelectromagnetics* 12:71–75

46. Liboff, A. R. 1985. Geomagnetic cyclotron resonance in living cells. *J. Biol. Phys.* 13:99–102

47. Liboff, A. R., McLeod, B. R. 1988. Kinetics of channelized membrane ions in magnetic fields. *Bioelectromagnetics* 9:39–51

48. Liboff, A. R., Parkinson, W. C. 1991. Search for ion-cyclotron resonance in a Na^+-transport system. *Bioelectromagnetics* 12:77–83

49. Liboff, A. R., Rozek, R. J., Sherman, M. L., McLeod, B. R., Smith, S. D. 1987. $^{45}Ca^{++}$ cyclotron resonance in human lymphocytes. *J. Bioelectr.* 6:13–22

50. Liboff, A. R., Thomas, J. R., Schrot, J. 1989. Intensity threshold for 60-Hz magnetically induced behavioral changes in rats. *Bioelectromagnetics* 10:111–13

51. Lin, R. S., Dischinger, P. C., Conde, J., Farrell, K. P. 1985. Occupational exposure to electromagnetic fields and the occurrence of brain tumors: an analysis of possible associations. *J. Occup. Med.* 27:413–19

52. Litovitz, T. A., Montrose, C. J., Goodman, R., Elson, E. C. 1990. Amplitude windows and transiently augmented transcription from exposure to electromagnetic fields. *Bioelectromagnetics* 11:297–312

53. Livingston, G. K., Gandhi, O. P., Chatterjee, I., Witt, K., Roti Roti, J. L. 1986. *Reproductive Integrity of Mammalian Cells Exposed to 60 Hz Electromagnetic Fields*. Final Rep. NY State Power Lines Proj. #218209. Albany, NY: NYSPLP, Wadsworth Cent. for Lab. and Res.

54. Lo, C. C., Fujita, T. Y., Geyer, A. B., Tenforde, T. S. 1986. A wide dynamic range portable 60-Hz magnetic dosimeter with data acquisition capabilities. *IEEE Trans. Nucl. Sci.* 33:643–46

55. Lövsund, P., Öberg, P. Å., Nilsson, S. E. G. 1982. ELF magnetic fields in electrosteel and welding industries. *Radio Sci.* 17(5S):35S–38S

56. Lövsund, P., Öberg, P. Å., Nilsson, S. E. G., Reuter, T. 1980. Magnetophosphenes: a quantitative analysis of thresholds. *Med. Biol. Eng. Comput.* 18:326–34

57. Male, J. D., Norris, W. T., Watts, M. W. 1987. Exposure of people to power frequency electric and magnetic fields. In *Interaction of Biological Systems with Static and ELF Electric and Magnetic Fields*, ed. L. E. Anderson, B. J. Kelman, R. J. Weigel, pp. 407–18. Proc. 23rd Annu. Hanford Life Sci. Symp., Richland, Wash. CONF-841041. Springfield, Va: Natl. Tech. Inf. Serv.

58. McDonald, A., Cherry, N., Delorme, C., McDonald, J. D. 1986. Visual dis-

play units and pregnancy: evidence from the Montreal survey. *J. Occup. Med.* 28:1126–31

59. McDowall, M. E. 1986. Mortality of persons resident in the vicinity of electricity transmission facilities. *Br. J. Cancer* 53:271–79

60. McLeod, B. R., Liboff, A. R. 1986. Dynamic characteristics of membrane ions in multifield configurations of low-frequency electromagnetic radiation. *Bioelectromagnetics* 7:177–89

61. Milham, S. Jr. 1985. Mortality in workers exposed to electromagnetic fields. *Environ. Health Perspect.* 62:297–300

62. Mills, C. J. 1977. The electromagnetic flowmeter. *Med. Instrum.* 11:136–38

63. Myers, A., Cartwright, R. A., Bonnell, J. A., Male, J. C., Cartwright, S. C. 1985. Overhead power lines and childhood cancer. In *Abstr. Int. Conf. Electr. Magn. Fields Med. Biol.*, 4–5 Dec. London

64. Nair, I., Morgan, M. G., Florig, H. K. 1989. *Biological Effects of Power Frequency Electric and Magnetic Fields.* Rep. No. OTA-BP-E-53, Off. Technol. Assess. Washington, DC:GPO

65. Natl. Radiol. Prot. Board. 1986. *Advice on the Protection of Workers and Members of the Public from the Possible Hazards of Electric and Magnetic Fields with Frequencies Below 300 GHz: A Consultative Document.* Chilton, Oxon, UK

66. Neilsen, C. V., Brandt, L., Helsborg, L., Waldstrom, B., Neilsen, L. T. 1989. *Effects of VDT Work on Pregnancy: A Reproductive Epidemiological Investigation.* Rep. from Socialmed. Inst., Univ. Aarhus, Denmark

67. Nurminen, T., Kurppa, K. 1988. Office equipment, work with video display terminals, and course of pregnancy: Reference mothers' experience from a Finnish case-referent study of birth defects. *Scand. J. Work Environ. Health* 14:293–98

68. Öberg, P. A. 1973. Magnetic stimulation of nerve tissue. *Med. Biol. Eng.* 11:55–64

69. Parkinson, W. C., Hanks, C. T. 1989. Search for cyclotron resonance in cells in vitro. *Bioelectromagnetics* 10:129–45

70. Pavlicek, W., Geisinger, M., Castle, L., Borkowski, G. P., Meaney, T. F., et al. 1983. The effects of nuclear magnetic resonance on patients with cardiac pacemakers. *Radiology* 147:149–53

71. Preston-Martin, S., Peters, J. M., Yu, M. C., Garabrant, D. H., Bowman, J. D. 1988. Myelogenous leukemia and

electric blanket use. *Bioelectromagnetics* 9:207–13

72. Polk, C. 1974. Sources, propagation, amplitude and temporal variation of extremely low frequency (0-100 Hz) electromagnetic fields. In *Biological and Clinical Effects of Low Frequency Magnetic and Electric Fields,* ed. J. C. Llaurado, A. Sauces Jr., pp. 21–48. Springfield, Ill: Thomas

73. Polson, M. J. R., Barker, A. T., Freeston, I. L. 1982. Stimulation of nerve trunks with time-varying magnetic fields. *Med. Biol. Eng. Comput.* 20:243–44

74. Reese, J. A., Frazier, M. E., Morris, J. E., Buschbom, R. L., Miller, D. L. 1991. Evaluation of changes in diatom mobility after exposure to 16-Hz electromagnetic fields. *Bioelectromagnetics* 12:21–25

75. Reese, J. A., Jostes, R. F., Frazier, M. E. 1988. Exposure of mammalian cells to 60-Hz magnetic or electric fields: Analysis for DNA single-strand breaks. *Bioelectromagnetics* 9:237–47

76. Reilly, J. P. 1989. Peripheral nerve stimulation by induced electric currents: exposure to time-varying magnetic fields. *Med. Biol. Eng. Comp.* 27:101–10

77. Ross, S. M. 1990. Combined DC and ELF magnetic fields can alter cell proliferation. *Bioelectromagnetics* 11:27–36

78. Sander, R., Brinkmann, J., Kuhne, B. 1982. Laboratory studies on animals and human beings exposed to 50 Hz electric and magnetic fields. In *Proc. Int. Conf. on Large High Voltage Electr. Sys.*, No. 36-01, 1–9 Sept., Paris

79. Sandweiss, J. 1990. On the cyclotron resonance model of ion transport. *Bioelectromagnetics* 11:203–5

80. Savitz, D. A. 1986. Human health effects of extremely low frequency electromagnetic fields: Critical review of clinical and epidemiological studies. In *Biological Effects of Power Frequency Electric and Magnetic Fields,* ed. W. E. Feero, pp. 49–64. IEEE Spec. Publ. No. 86TH0139-6-PWR. Piscataway, NJ: Inst. Electr. Electron. Eng.

81. Savitz, D. A., Baron, A. E. 1989. Estimating and correcting for confounder misclassification. *Am. J. Epidemiol.* 129:1062–71

82. Savitz, D. A., Calle, E. E. 1987. Leukemia and occupational exposure to electromagnetic fields: Review of epidemiologic surveys. *J. Occup. Med.* 29:47–51

83. Savitz, D. A., Feingold, L. 1989. Association of childhood cancer with residential traffic density. *Scand. J. Work Environ. Health* 15:360–63

84. Savitz, D. A., John, E. M., Kleckner, R. C. 1990. Magnetic field exposure from electric appliances and childhood cancer. *Am. J. Epidemiol.* 131:763–73

85. Savitz, D. A., Wachtel, H., Barnes, F. A., John, E. M., Tvrdik, J. G. 1988. Case-control study of childhood cancer and exposure to 60-Hz magnetic fields. *Am. J. Epidemiol.* 128:21–38

86. Schnorr, T. M., Grajewski, B. A., Hornung, R. W., Thun, M. J., Egeland, G. M., et al. 1991. Video display terminals and the risk of spontaneous abortion. *N. Engl. J. Med.* 324:727–33

87. Scott-Walton, B., Clark, K. M., Holt, B. R., Jones, D. C., Kaplan, S. D., et al. 1979. *Potential Environmental Effects of 765-kV Transmission Lines: Views Before the New York State Public Service Commission, Cases 26529 and 26559, 1976–1978.* DOE/EV-0056, pp. II–7. Springfield, Va: Natl. Tech. Inf. Serv.

88. Severson, R. K., Stevens, R. G., Kaune, W. T., Thomas, D. B., Henser, L., et al. 1988. Acute nonlymphocytic leukemia and residential exposure to power frequency magnetic fields. *Am. J. Epidemiol.* 128:10–20

89. Silny, J. 1986. The influence threshold of a time-varying magnetic field in the human organism. In *Biological Effects of Static and Extremely Low Frequency Magnetic Fields,* ed. J. H. Bernhardt, pp. 105–12. München: MMV Medizin Verlag

90. Silva, M., Hummon, N., Rutter, D., Hooper, C. 1989. Power frequency magnetic fields in the home. *IEEE Trans. Power Deliv.* 4:465–77

91. Smith, S. D., McLeod, B. R., Liboff, A. R., Cooksey, K. 1987. Calcium cyclotron resonance and diatom mobility. *Bioelectromagnetics* 8:215–27

92. Speers, M. A., Dobbins, J. G., Miller, V. S. 1988. Occupational exposures and brain cancer mortality: a preliminary study of East Texas residents. *Am. J. Ind. Med.* 13:629–38

93. Stuchly, M. A., Lecuyer, D. W., Mann, R. D. 1983. Extremely low frequency electromagnetic emissions from video display terminals and other devices. *Health Phys.* 45:713–22

94. Stark, D. D., Bradley, W. G. Jr. 1988. *Magnetic Resonance Imaging.* St. Louis, Mo: Mosby

95. Taylor, L. S. 1981. The mechanisms of athermal microwave biological effects. *Bioelectromagnetics* 2:259–67

96. Tenforde, T. S. 1991. Biological interactions of extremely-low-frequency electric and magnetic fields. *Bioelectrochem. Bioenerget.* 25:1–17

97. Tenforde, T. S. 1990. Biological interactions and human health effects of extremely low frequency magnetic fields. In *Extremely Low Frequency Electromagnetic Fields: The Question of Cancer,* ed. B. W. Wilson, R. G. Stevens, L. E. Anderson, pp. 291–315. Columbus, Ohio: Battelle Press

98. Tenforde, T. S. 1989. Biological responses to static and time-varying magnetic fields. In *Interaction of Electromagnetic Waves in Biological Systems,* ed. J. C. Lin, pp. 83–107. New York: Plenum

99. Tenforde, T. S. 1988. Interaction mechanisms, biological effects and biomedical applications of static and extremely-low-frequency magnetic fields. In *Proc. of the 22nd Annu. Meet. of the Natl. Counc. on Radiat. Prot. and Meas.: Nonionizing Electromagn. Radiat. and Ultrasound,* pp. 181–217. Bethesda, Md: Natl. Counc. Radiat. Prot. Meas.

100. Tenforde, T. S. 1986. Interaction of ELF magnetic fields with living matter. In *Handbook of Biological Effects of Electromagnetic Radiation,* ed. C. Polk, E. Postow, pp. 197–225. Boca Raton, Fla: CRC

101. Tenforde, T. S., Budinger, T. F. 1986. Biological effects and physical safety aspects of NMR imaging and in vivo spectroscopy. In *NMR in Medicine: Instrumentation and Clinical Applications,* ed. S. R. Thomas, R. L. Dixon, pp. 493–548. New York: Am. Assoc. of Phys. Med.

102. Tenforde, T. S., Kaune, W. T. 1987. Interaction of extremely-low-frequency electric and magnetic fields with humans. *Health Phys.* 53:585–606

103. Tenforde, T. S., Liburdy, R. P. 1988. Magnetic deformation of phospholipid bilayers: Effects on liposome shape and solute permeability at prephase transition temperatures. *J. Theor. Biol.* 133:385–96

104. Thériault, G. 1991. *Health Effects of Electromagnetic Radiation on Workers: Epidemiologic Studies.* Prep. for Sci. Workshop on the Health Effects of Electromagn. Radiat. on Workers, spons. by US Dep. Health Hum. Serv. Natl. Inst. Occup. Safe. Health, Cincinnati, Jan. 30–31

105. Thomas, J. R., Schrot, J., Liboff, A. R.

1986. Low-intensity magnetic fields alter operant behavior in rats. *Bioelectromagnetics* 7:349–57

106. Thomas, T. L., Stolley, P. D., Stemhagen, A., Fontham, E. T. H., Bleecker, M. L., et al. 1987. Brain tumor mortality risk among men with electrical and electronics jobs: a case-control study. *J. Natl. Cancer Inst.* 79:233–38

107. Tofani, S., D'Amore, G. 1991. Extremely-low-frequency and very-low-frequency magnetic fields emitted by video display units. *Bioelectromagnetics* 12:35–45

108. Tomenius, L. 1986. 50-Hz electromagnetic environment and the incidence of childhood tumors in Stockholm County. *Bioelectromagnetics* 7:191–207

109. Ueno, S., Harada, K., Ji, C., Oomura, Y. 1984. Magnetic nerve stimulation without interlinkage between nerve and magnetic flux. *IEEE Trans. Mag.* MAG-20:1660–62

110. Ueno, S., Lövsund, P., Öberg, P. Å. 1978. Capacitive stimulatory effect in magnetic stimulation of nerve tissue. *IEEE Trans. Mag.* MAG-14:958–60

111. US Environ. Prot. Agency. 1990. *Evaluation of the Potential Carcinogenicity of Electromagnetic Fields.* Washington, DC: USEPA Doc. No. EPA/600/6-90/005B

112. Walleczek, J., Liburdy, R. P. 1990. Nonthermal 60-Hz sinusoidal magnetic-field exposure enhances $^{45}Ca^{2+}$ uptake in rat thymocytes: Dependence on mitogen activation. *FEBS Lett.* 271:157–60

113. Watson, J., Downes, E. M. 1978. The application of pulsed magnetic fields to the stimulation of bone healing in humans. *Jpn. J. Appl. Phys.* 17:215–17

114. Weaver, J. C., Astumian, R. D. 1990. The response of cells to very weak electric fields: The thermal noise limit. *Science* 247:459–62

115. Wei, L.-X., Goodman, R., Henderson, A. 1990. Changes in c-*myc* and histone H2B following exposure of cells to low-frequency sinusoidal electromagnetic fields: Evidence for a window effect. *Bioelectromagnetics* 11:269–72

116. Wertheimer, N., Leeper, E. 1986. Possible effects of electric blankets and heated waterbeds on fetal development. *Bioelectromagnetics* 7:13–22

117. Wertheimer, N., Leeper, E. 1982. Adult cancer related to electrical wires near the home. *Int. J. Epidemiol.* 11:345–55

118. Wertheimer, N., Leeper, E. 1980. RE: Electrical wiring configurations and childhood leukemia in Rhode Island. *Am. J. Epidemiol.* 111:461–62

119. Wertheimer, N., Leeper, E. 1979. Electrical wiring configurations and childhood cancer. *Am. J. Epidemiol.* 109:273–84

120. Wilson, B. W., Wright, C. W., Morris, J. E., Buschbom, R. L., Brown, D. P., et al. 1990. Evidence for an effect of ELF electromagnetic fields on pineal gland function. *J. Pineal Res.* 9:259–69

Annu. Rev. Publ. Health 1992. 13:197–221

WORKSITE DRUG TESTING

Diana Chapman Walsh

Department of Health and Social Behavior, Harvard School of Public Health, Boston, Massachusetts 02115

Lynn Elinson

Medical and Occupational Disease Policy Branch, Ontario Workers' Compensation Board, Toronto, Ontario, Canada M4W 3C3

Lawrence Gostin

American Society of Law and Medicine, Boston, Massachusetts 02115

KEY WORDS: drug abuse, urine screening for drugs, employee assistance programs

INTRODUCTION

Drug testing in the workplace presents a striking case of a policy instrument that has penetrated fast and far, accompanied by almost no credible scientific warrant of effectiveness. In just a decade, worksite drug testing programs have made their way through the entire military and all other federal employment, into many of the nation's largest and most prestigious private corporations, and all the way to the United States Supreme Court. Meanwhile, solid research has focused almost entirely on the efficacy of the testing procedures themselves, to the virtual exclusion of deeper questions of sound social policy. The most fundamental assumptions on competing sides of unresolved debates over the merits and demerits of screening workers' urine for traces of drugs are untested and untestable, knowing what we currently know. In fact, the gap between science and policy is so wide as to occasion real confusion about which goals are really being served by drug testing programs at work.

0163-7525/92/0501-0197$02.00

197

Goals and Types of Testing Programs

Ostensibly, employers test workers' urine for drugs to ensure the safety and productivity of their own labor force and to reduce the likelihood that their employees will report to work impaired by drugs, will use drugs while at work, will buy and sell them there, or will engage in other drug-related activities that might endanger themselves or others. Employers are also concerned that drug use will result in time away from work, distress coworkers or customers, or intrude in any other way on the safe and satisfactory conduct of whatever commerce the work entails.

As a matter of public policy, government encourages, facilitates, and partially subsidizes private-sector drug testing programs to reduce national consumption and traffic in illicit drugs, and the negative social consequences of these problems. Worksite testing presumably creates a sentinel effect and aids in the identification of drug abusers who could perhaps be helped by effective treatment. To what extent these objectives are actually being served has yet to be asked, except superficially.

Testing is generally conducted under three broad rubrics: at preemployment; "for cause"; and randomly, without cause or suspicion. Each situation has its own supporting logic and set of complexities. Employers have long conducted preemployment or preplacement tests of various kinds to establish fitness for duty (70). Drug testing continues in this tradition. A succession of state and federal handicap laws and regulations has narrowed the employer's discretion in hiring, but obligations to job applicants are still less compelling and constraining than those to employees on the payroll. Preemployment testing is, therefore, the most common and least contested form of drug testing at work.

Testing "for cause" extends an established tradition of investigating injuries and other incidents. Sometimes, such testing monitors compliance with a mandatory program of rehabilitation for a substance-abusing employee whose unsatisfactory performance has prompted a referral to an employee assistance program (EAP) (70). The purported link with safety, in a postincident investigation and with both safety and therapeutic intent in EAPs, renders this class of testing relatively less controversial and more common than testing without grounds for suspicion. However, the objection is raised that drug testing may preempt other accident investigation, which could lead to the abatement of hazards, and that the link between safety risk and a positive urine test is far from clear. Grievance processes provide some formal protection for union-represented employees. How frequently this testing results in employee dismissal, or in successful rehabilitation, is a question for future research.

Periodic, unannounced testing of employees picked at random, either from a sample of workers who perform "safety-sensitive" tasks or from a larger pool (extending occasionally to a firm's total labor force), is the most novel and least common form of worksite drug testing—and the form that civil libertarians find most objectionable. The further a random testing program strays from a convincing safety rationale, and the less attention it pays to procedural safeguards of the employee's perceived right to privacy and fair play, the wider it is open to critique.

From a public health perspective, the overriding question is whether and, if so, how drug testing programs prevent or postpone any death, disease, disability, or dysfunction associated with psychoactive drugs. Here, several important assumptions underlying worksite drug testing bear examination. The first is that a sufficiently serious problem exists to justify a response that may violate deeply felt norms. The second is that the response produces more benefits than harm. The third is that preferable solutions are unavailable or unaffordable.

Coverage of this Review and of the Available Literature

In this review, we seek to clarify what is and is not known about drug testing, by drawing on a sizeable descriptive and prescriptive literature that emanates chiefly from the National Institute on Drug Abuse (NIDA), as well as on other practitioner-directed sources.[1] In addition, the literature includes extensive discussion, often in special issues of law reviews, of ethical and legal ramifications, many of which are cited below.

The current literature lacks studies that would provide empirical grounding for the assumptions enumerated above: convincing studies documenting that drug abuse at work is, in fact, a serious threat (and, specifically, where and how the harms are manifest); evaluations demonstrating the effectiveness of drug testing strategies; and studies comparing drug testing with alternative policies and programs aimed at reducing worksite inefficiencies or malfunctions related to drug abuse, such as EAPs, or comparing EAPs with and without a drug testing component.

Several descriptive studies have discussed results of drug screening programs, but without adequate designs to test hypotheses regarding effectiveness (12, 48, 52, 64). Three electronic literature searches of bibliographic data bases in medicine, sociology, psychology, health administration, and government uncovered only six studies designed to test the hypothesis that drug screening is an effective strategy to ensure the safety and/or productive capacity of any employee group (5, 16, 50, 54, 61, 77). Three of these studies were published in peer-reviewed journals, and one evaluated costs versus benefits (50). Of the remaining three studies, two also analyzed costs and

---

[1]Course materials from the American College of Occupational Medicine, newsletters, loose-leaf services and reports from information management firms, such as the Bureau of National Affairs, Business Research Publications, and the Conference Board, as well as a few reports from the popular press and some unpublished results of opinion polls.

benefits (16, 61), and one of these (16) appeared in an NIDA monograph, thus not subject to peer review.

If the shortage of evaluative research is a problem, the lack of information on rudimentary questions—beginning with the extent and distribution of different types of drug testing—is more handicapping still. Many surveys have been done, but few well enough to inspire confidence in their validity; we cite the better ones, with caveats. Also, although debates regarding drug testing as a policy vehicle rely on the support (or opposition) of public opinion, most summary statistics withstand little scientific scrutiny, a point we elaborate.

Before reviewing the scientific literature on the extent of drug abuse in the workplace, the effectiveness of testing programs, and the feasibility of alternative approaches, we set the context with a brief overview of the emergence and apparently rapid diffusion of this technology, including the evolving legal doctrine and regulatory directive that shape its application.

EVOLUTION OF DRUG TESTING AS PUBLIC POLICY

Technological advances made drug testing practical on a mass scale, and much subsequent thinking has centered on "technique" (21). The seeds were sown some 16 years ago, when NIDA began supporting research on problems associated with drugs, including a line of work on methods to detect drug traces in urine and other bodily fluids. Originally, the technology was primarily used to monitor heroin and methadone use in drug treatment centers. Patients were forewarned that they would have to submit to drug testing as a condition of participation. In 1978, NIDA entered into a cooperative agreement with Syntex Corporation to develop a relatively inexpensive, rapid assay to detect marijuana use. Similar assays for amphetamine and opiate use were already available. By the end of 1981, new, portable assay machines were brought to market, under the trade name EMIT (enzyme-multiplied immunoassay test). Hoffman-LaRoche Company also came to market in the early 1980s with a test kit ("Abuscreen") that used radioactive immunoassay.

At about this time, Congress was pressing the Department of Defense to do something about drug abuse in the military, which was perceived to be a growing problem that could compromise national security. A Department of Defense survey, conducted in November 1980, found that 47% of Navy and Marine personnel, age 25 or under, reported having used marijuana, and 26% reported having been under the influence of drugs while on duty (10). The following May, a Navy plane crashed off the Florida Atlantic coast into the aircraft carrier US Nimitz, injuring 42 sailors and killing 14, six of whom were found on autopsy to have had traces of marijuana in their blood (10, 39). Soon thereafter, Naval Admiral Hayward announced a policy of "zero tolerance" of drugs, and instituted a Navy-wide testing program. By the end of 1982, the Navy had portable testing machines in most ships in the fleet; more than 2 million urine specimens are now tested annually by the US Navy (10).

Although the Navy's program was and is the most extensive in the armed forces, all branches were testing for drugs by 1981. The military crack-down attracted media attention, which, in turn, began to stimulate the interest of private-sector employers. IBM Corporation announced a job applicant drug testing program in 1984 (57), and American Airlines and Alabama Power Company soon followed suit. By 1986, many large private-sector firms were testing job applicants, as well as some current employees, for traces of drugs. Typically, drug screening in these large firms was placed in the context and under the aegis of long-established programs of occupational health surveillance, employee assistance, and/or health promotion, such as those at E. I. DuPont de Nemours, the General Electric Company, Eastman Kodak Company, and Exxon Corporation.

Federal Regulatory Initiatives

Rather than await spontaneous diffusion into the private sector, however, the government continued to promote urine screening through regulatory initiatives. At first, the program only covered federal employees; later, it was expanded to encompass private-sector employees engaged in specified types of governmental work. Executive Order 12564 (56) was a watershed. Signed on September 15, 1986, by President Ronald Reagan, the order required each executive agency to establish a program to test for use of illegal drugs by federal employees in "sensitive positions" (broadly defined),[2] and to offer voluntary testing. The order also authorized testing for cause, as follow-up to counseling or rehabilitation, and at preemployment.

The immediate stimulus for Executive Order 12564 was the final report of the President's Commission on Organized Crime in March 1986 (24), which recommended mandatory drug testing as part of an overall strategy shift. Resources would be diverted from the "supply-side" effort to a "demand-reduction" approach aimed at drying up the market in illicit drugs (24). The agencies were left latitude to shape their own programs' requirements and circumstances for testing, but overarching rules of procedure were specified in the order.

In 1987, Congress appropriated funds to implement the executive order (9), and the Department of Health and Human Services (DHHS) drew up technical and scientific guidelines, published in the Federal Register on April 11, 1988 (19). "At a minimum," marijuana and cocaine were to be included in govern-

---

[2]Sensitive jobs" were defined as any requiring a high degree of trust and confidence. Positions involving national security, handling sensitive documents or serving the President, enforcing the law, or protecting life, property, public health, and safety met this definition, which is believed to encompass 400,000–500,000 jobs (R. Harwood 1991, personal communication).

ment testing programs; opiates, amphetamines, and phencyclidine (PCPs) were optional; and testing for other drugs listed in Schedule I or II of the Controlled Substance Act required permission of DHHS. The five drugs for which testing was mandated and/or authorized came to be known as "the NIDA five." Alcohol—the most widely used of all psychoactive drugs, and by far the most costly from a social and health perspective—was not mentioned, although it has appeared on some (but not all) subsequent lists.

The Content of Federal Regulations and Guidelines

The DHHS guidelines also outlined collection protocols to discourage adulteration of urine specimens, procedures on "chain-of-custody" to protect against misidentification of specimens or results, and measures to assure the quality of laboratory testing. In addition, they created a new title and role for physicians: "Medical Review Officers." These physicians would review positive urinalysis test results, interpret their significance, and explore mitigating medical circumstances that might exonerate the employee in question.

Much of the administrative apparatus developed in connection with testing of government workers was later extended and elaborated in regulations from the Departments of Defense (18) and Transportation, (20) which required testing of employees of companies with defense contracts or those involved in transportation and employees of the Nuclear Regulatory Commission (NRC) (51), which stipulates fitness for duty requirements in nuclear reactor work. The various federal regulations are far from uniform, though, thus creating compliance headaches for large companies with diverse operations that fall within the ambit of multiple regulatory agencies.

The Drug-Free Workplace Act of 1988

These provisions were consolidated and extended when Congress enacted the Drug-Free Workplace Act of 1988. The act covered all federal grantees (including universities) and most federal contractors (including defense contractors), so that employees "providing services or products to the government should not be held to a lower standard than federal employees with whom the contractors work side-by-side" (9, p. 512). Although it does not require drug testing, the act does lend legitimacy to tougher approaches to drugs and provides a specific rationale for drug testing, as well as for strictly sanctioning employees convicted of drug infractions at work.

This cursory review of the emergence of drug testing as public policy shows how decisive a role the federal government has played. Early problems that surfaced because of invalid and unreliable drug testing procedures led the Executive Branch to devote much of its energy to developing a tight administrative system of quality controls. This effort has been quite successful, but has not spoken to more fundamental questions of social benefits and costs. It has taken a succession of court challenges to begin enlarging the terms of the public debate.

The Unfolding Legal Framework

Since the guarantees of the US Constitution constrain principally actions by the state, the legal battleground over drug testing has centered on government agencies, as well as private employers acting on federal or state rules that require or authorize drug testing (62). The primary constitutional impediment to drug testing is the Fourth Amendment's prohibition on unreasonable searches and seizures. The Supreme Court has long recognized that the collection and subsequent analysis of biological samples are "searches" under the Fourth Amendment (59). The question is whether the analysis of blood, urine, or breath for illicit substances is "unreasonable" within the meaning of the Fourth Amendment. What is reasonable "depends on all the circumstances surrounding the search or seizure and the nature of the search or seizure itself" (65). Thus, the permissibility of a particular search "is judged by balancing its intrusion on the individual's Fourth Amendment interests against its promotion of legitimate governmental interests" (17). Minimally, the courts have required "reasonable suspicion" that the illicit substance or contraband to be searched for will, in fact, be found.

The Supreme Court in the drug testing cases held that when the state has "special needs beyond the normal need for law enforcement," the warrant and probable or reasonable cause requirements may become impracticable. In *Skinner v. Railway Labor Executive Association* (62), the Supreme Court upheld a regulation that required drug and alcohol tests following major train accidents or incidents and authorized these tests for covered employees who violate certain safety rules, even without reasonable suspicion that any particular employee may be impaired. The Court viewed the government's interest in safety of the traveling public as "compelling." An individualized suspicion requirement would "impede the railroad's ability to obtain valuable information about the causes of accidents or incidents and how to protect the public . . ." (62, p. 1406).

The Court held that when balanced against the state's compelling interest, the drug tests represented a minimal imposition on the workers' privacy and bodily integrity, in part because the samples were furnished in a medical environment without direct observation. The workers' expectations of privacy, moreover, were diminished by their participation in an industry regulated pervasively to ensure safety. The Court also rejected the argument that the testing program was unreasonable because it could not measure current impairments; drug tests are "designed not only to discern impairment but to deter it" (62, p. 1407).

The Supreme Court followed a similar approach in *National Treasury*

Employees Union v. Von Raab (46), in which it upheld the constitutionality of suspicionless drug testing by the US Customs Service. The government's "compelling" interest in safeguarding borders and public safety outweighed the diminished privacy expectations of employees who are directly involved in interdiction or who are required to carry firearms. No evidence was presented to the Court that a drug problem existed in the Customs Service, that a preannounced suspicionless drug testing program was effective in detecting or deterring drug use, or that drug use impugned the integrity or interfered with the judgment of officers.

The question that emerges from the Supreme Court drug testing cases is how will the courts in the future balance the employee's interest in privacy with "compelling" state interests? The Supreme Court in *Von Raab* identified specific factors that minimize the program's intrusion on privacy, such as nonrandom tests, advance notice of a sample collection, and confirmatory tests. Court decisions subsequent to *Von Raab* have not used any single privacy factor as conclusive. The fact that a testing program is random has not persuaded the courts to undertake a fundamentally different analysis from that pursued by the Supreme Court (28).

Legal Constraints on Private Sector Employers

Private employers without significant government contracts or regulated lines of business enjoy greater freedom in their design and implementation of drug testing programs. However, they do face legal restraints embodied in state constitutions, federal and state statutes, common law, and collective bargaining agreements. Some state constitutions (California's, for example) constrain even the purely private sector.

Federal and state laws prohibit employment discrimination against persons with disabilities. The Americans with Disabilities Act of 1990 specifically excludes from protection any employee or applicant "who is currently engaging in the illegal use of drugs . . ." (2, Secs. 104, 510). Although the Act generally prohibits medical testing and examination of employees, if such testing is not job related and consistent with business necessity, the Act does not include drug testing. Indeed, the Act does nothing to encourage, prohibit, or authorize drug testing of job applicants or employees. The Federal Rehabilitation Act of 1973 (which prohibits discrimination against persons with disabilities only if an employer is in receipt of federal funds) also excludes current drug users from its protection, but does not have the same explicit exclusion of drug testing.

Many states and a few municipalities have enacted statutes or ordinances to regulate drug testing. The legislation varies in application and approach. Most statutes cover all drug testing, but a few protect only public employees, and most stress procedural fairness, privacy, and fair use of positive test results.

In summary, worksite drug screening has advanced rapidly in the last decade. Beginning as an isolated policy in the military, it has been expanded by increments into many areas of federal employment, then into government contractors, and finally into the private sector. The 1989 Supreme Court cases may limit future testing by federal and state agencies and their contractors to specific safety and security oriented jobs. Similar limitations on most of the private sector are likely to rest on state legislative and judicial initiatives, if they develop.

HOW SERIOUS IS THE PROBLEM OF DRUG ABUSE AT WORK?

If the nation's drug drama is being played out mostly in the shadow economy, outside of conventional places of work, then screening workers for drugs may be tantamount to looking under the lighted street lamp for the key that was lost somewhere else in the dark. To what extent this is the case is unknown. Overall rates of illicit drug use have been decreasing in recent years (33), despite pockets of problems in inner cities depicted in popular films and almost daily in metropolitan newspapers. But, empirical data on rates of drug use on or around the job are limited. If there are concentrations of serious drug problems in places of work, they have yet to be well characterized in systematic research.

Research on drug use at work is scarce and difficult. Employers have much to lose if they develop a reputation as a place where workers are abusing drugs. And, for a worker to admit using an illicit drug is to confess to an offense that could result in job loss or even arrest. Cross-sectional surveys can be conducted successfully with strong guarantees of anonymity, but even they require elaborate negotiations and a slow process of building trust. Reported rates of drug use among workers are low enough that samples have to be large to support multivariate analyses and meaningful statistical inferences (68). Most data on drug abuse come from national surveys, not from studies anchored in places of work, and few even differentiate workers from nonworkers, much less delve into which workers doing what kinds of work use drugs, and who uses drugs in the context of work, when, and with what effects.

National Trends in Drug Use

Since 1972, NIDA has been conducting a national survey on drug abuse. Well before President Reagan's 1986 executive order initiated drug testing of federal workers, such national surveys began to pick up signals that rates of illicit drug use were starting to decline. Between 1979 and 1988, rates of reported use among 18- to 25-year-olds in the household survey dropped from 37.1% to 25.7% (a 31% decrease) (45).

At the same time, drugs continue to be implicated in festering problems in the nation's inner cities: drug-related homicides, felony convictions, bystander deaths in shootings, domestic violence, emergency room admissions, HIV transmission, low birth weight, and multiply complicated deliveries (74). But, the 1988 NIDA household survey revealed that overall per capita consumption of cocaine (especially "crack") has declined in every age group, and that crack users are twice as likely to be unemployed as to be full-time employees (45).

Another NIDA-funded national study's annual survey and follow-up of high school seniors, conducted since 1976, has been corroborating the impression of declining rates of drug abuse in the general population (33). The implications for the workplace, however, are not well understood.

Drug Use Among Workers

A simple way to begin asking about workplace effects is to examine the employment status of respondents in national surveys. Voss (66) conducted a secondary analysis of data from the 1985 NIDA household survey and ascertained that marijuana use in the past month was reported by 11.7% of respondents who were employed full-time, and by 10.2% of part-time employees. It was the unemployed who reported the highest rates (21.5%) of marijuana use. Comparable rates of cocaine use among full- and part-time employees were 4% and 2.2%, respectively, compared with 6% among the unemployed. Data on the employment status of drug users still leave unanswered the question of drug use on the job or the effect of drug use on the conduct of work (49).

The limited data suggest that we actually know almost nothing about the impact of drug abuse in particular worksites. That being the case, we need to look elsewhere for the underpinnings of drug testing programs at work.

Public Perceptions of the "Drug Problem" and Attitudes Toward Worksite Testing

Americans are frequently told that the drug problem is among the most serious that society faces. These conclusions are derived from public opinion polls that are widely quoted in the lay press. Methodological limitations tend to be glossed over, and the strong impression is left that the general public, management, workers, and selected working groups are very worried about drugs.

Furthermore, we are told, employees and managers perceive drug use at work to be a real concern (3, 8, 42) and are generally supportive of drug testing, particularly for cause and for safety-sensitive positions (31, 32, 36). Flaws in the sampling and data collection procedures of many of these surveys cast doubt on their reliability, validity, and especially their generalizability.

Although a few representative national polls have been done, it is still unclear how broad, deep, and stable the support for drug testing really is.

For example, organizations like the Institute for a Drug-Free Workplace and the American Productivity and Quality Center commission and quote the results of surveys that purport to show that American workers and managers are very concerned about the drug problem and quite willing to be tested for drugs. In 1990, the Institute (32) reported that 28% of employees interviewed said that drugs were the greatest problem facing the United States today, 49% said that illegal drug use occurs in their own workplaces, 22% called illegal drug use at least "somewhat widespread" where they work, and 41% said drug use by employees "seriously affects" getting the job done. A full 97% of respondents were said to favor drug testing under some circumstances: 75% for cause, 68% at preemployment, and 53% on a random basis.

These findings tend to be reported with little or no contextual information on basic methodological issues: how the questions were posed, how the samples were drawn, what the response rates were, and so on. The organizations sponsoring the polls often have vested interests that are not immediately evident. The Institute for a Drug-Free Workplace, for example, comprises representatives of large corporations, many already with drug testing programs firmly in place. Hoffman-La Roche, a major competitor in the drug testing market, is an especially active member.

This is not to say that the public opposes drug testing at work, only to raise concerns about the quality or strength of the evidence. Several news organizations have released more reliable opinion polls that do tend to support findings in favor of drug testing. A CBS/*New York Times* survey, conducted in September 1989, found that 61% of respondents would favor a policy that required "workers in general to be tested to determine whether they have used illegal drugs recently . . ." (58). A May 1986 poll (Decision/Making/ Information for *Populus, Inc.*) found that 88% of respondents supported mandatory testing among airline pilots, 85% among police and law enforcement agents, and 74% among teachers (58). Other, more limited surveys have reported similar results (3, 36).

What seems to be operative here is a tendency that historians and students of the social construction of reality have observed in the cyclical nature of public attitudes toward various kinds of drug use. Tolerance of drugs seems to be shaped as much by larger social and economic forces, and by conservative or liberal strains in the general social mood, as by the objective reality of the prevalence or impact of the problem itself (27, 44, 71). An historical perspective suggests that the United States had already begun to enter a new period of public reaction against drug use before testing became widespread in the workplace. With or without testing programs, if history is an accurate guide, those trends would likely continue (44, 72). To believe that drug testing has played a significant role in promoting or accelerating this process, we would need convincing evidence of direct impacts that these testing programs are having.

HOW WIDESPREAD ARE DRUG TESTING PROGRAMS?

Data on the prevalence and distribution of drug testing programs in public- and private-sector employment are thin. Most available surveys have been weak; federal requirements are complex and require no formal reporting; and drug testing programs are diverse, protean, and sometimes different on paper than in practice. The evidence suggests the following tentative conclusions: much (but not all) of drug testing has been precipitated by federal regulation; testing is much more common in large, rather than small, companies; preemployment screening of job applicants is the most common form of testing; testing of current employees is conducted mostly for cause; and random, unannounced testing not based on suspicion is still relatively rare.

Coverage of federal mandates for drug testing ought to provide some sense of the number of employees who are subject to testing, but no one data base currently exists to provide actual numbers on how many workers are covered by the Departments of Transportation and Defense and NRC regulations, how many actually are tested, and under which circumstances. In principle, the Drug-Free Workplace Act has sweeping ramifications for private-sector employment, but the extent and nature of responses to date is undocumented.

Growth in the numbers of commercial drug testing laboratories or in their volume of sales might be an objective indicator of the diffusion of testing programs, but no unified accounting system provides access to such data. Federal guidelines have been established for all laboratories that test federal employees (23), and NIDA conducts a program to certify laboratory quality. As of 1990, 73 laboratories had been certified (D. Bush 1991, personal communication). Also, the College of American Pathologists (CAP) instituted a private-sector, voluntary accreditation program in 1987. The number of accredited laboratories now stands at 82, up from 36 in 1988, with eight more under review (G. Hopewell 1991, personal communication). The extent of overlap between the NIDA and CAP programs is unclear, and there is no way to know how many nonaccredited laboratories have been attracted into the drug testing business as the market has expanded.

Surveys are another way to assess the extent of drug testing in the workplace (3, 7, 22, 25, 29, 42). Most have been highly selective in their sampling frames, insufficiently alert to bias associated with low response rates, and elliptical in their reports of methodological detail. An exception is the 1988 Bureau of Labor Statistics (BLS) survey (7), which has been recently updated (29). This is the most authoritative source of data on the extent of drug testing programs in private employment.

Of "establishments" (contiguous worksites) surveyed in the BLS study (1988 data; published in 1989), 3.2% had a drug testing program, and the prevalence increased with employment size: Among establishments with 1000 or more employees, 43% had drug testing programs, but only 2.7% of those with less than 50 workers at the reporting site had programs. This has important implications for the reach of drug testing programs, as large establishments (with more than 1000 employees) account for almost 16% of the workforce, but more than 90% of the nation's establishments have fewer than 50 workers, which accounts for more than one third of all American workers (7).

The BLS survey underscored that testing is most commonly conducted on job applicants. Of establishments with programs, 85.2% (or 123,881) tested job applicants (usually applicants for all jobs), whereas 63.5% (92,000) tested current employees. Two thirds of companies who tested current employees did so only "for cause," not on a regular or random basis. All together, the establishments with programs tested under 1 million employees, or 1% of the private workforce, in the year before the survey.

The 1990 BLS update involved a random sample of close to 800 respondents to the 1988 survey; 749 were still in business (29). Overall, drug testing had increased insignificantly, from 3.2% to 4.4%. In larger establishments, which employ 250 or more workers, the increase in rates of drug screening (from 31.9% to 45.9%) was substantial and statistically significant (29). In addition, almost one third of programs reported in 1988 had been discontinued by 1990, more often in small and medium establishments than in those with 250 or more workers.

Some published accounts have estimated much higher rates of testing than those found by the BLS (for example, see Ref. 30). Operational definitions are often unspecified, so that the reader cannot tell, for example, whether drug tests on military and government employees are included in estimates, the types of testing they include, whether they refer to numbers of employees eligible or to those actually tested, and whether the unit of analysis is numbers of tests or numbers of employees tested. Considering all of this, it seems safe to conclude that as a proportion of the entire American labor force, the number of workers who have been asked to submit a urine sample for a worksite drug test is small. The actual number is unknown, as is the rate of increase.

HOW EFFECTIVE ARE DRUG SCREENING PROGRAMS?

The effort expended to date on assessing the effectiveness of drug testing programs has centered on the accuracy of systems to collect and analyze urine samples and to report and interpret subsequent results. A more complete assessment of the effectiveness of drug testing as policy would take account of probabilities all the way down a longer (and messier) decision chain: the likelihood of false-positives and false-negatives in various laboratories; the chance of errors along the chain-of-custody; the danger of misinterpreting (technically correct) laboratory test results; the even more complex questions about the impact of testing programs on subsequent drug abuse; the correlation between a positive drug test and future fitness to perform on the job; and, finally, larger unanswered questions about whether drug testing programs actually identify the drug users most likely to experience serious problems on the job.

The Accuracy of Laboratory Drug Tests

The National Institute on Drug Abuse's effort to develop a hierarchical system of quality controls has been successful. The full system includes an initial, inexpensive screen, which uses chain-of-custody control procedures, followed by more costly confirmatory testing of all positives and a medical review of the few remaining confirmed-positive cases. When the system is implemented correctly, the general consensus now seems to be that sensitivity and specificity are very high. Procedural shortcomings and human error can always reduce accuracy, and private-sector testing programs not conducted under federal regulation still have enough discretion to omit crucial elements in NIDA's ideal system of checks and balances.

Without confirmatory testing and medical review, the predictive validity of drug screening is unacceptably low. Positive predictive validity refers to the percentage of those individuals who tested positive who truly had traces of drugs in their urine. This is an especially important consideration in the workplace, as a false-positive error can trigger serious harm, including damage to reputation and denial or loss of a job. Predictive validity is affected by the prevalence of the condition in a particular population. The prevalence of drug use in samples of workers is low, so caution is needed (13).

Because predictive validity depends on specificity and prevalence (27, 73), the most commonly used drugs are most likely to be identified in drug testing programs. Therefore, tests for these drugs should have relatively high accuracy. Unfortunately, the predictive validity for marijuana is approximately 38%, because the sensitivity and specificity of its tests are not high. With a 3% prevalence of cocaine, the predictive value is approximately 35%. Even with a sensitivity and specificity of 95% for cocaine testing (an accuracy rate not always achieved by all laboratories), in a population with a prevalence rate of 3%, the positive predictive value would be less than 50%: Of four positive samples, two or more would be false-positives, if proper confirmatory steps were not taken.

False-positive results usually reflect cross-reactivity or human error, or both (6, 53). Cross-reactivity occurs when chemicals other than the ones of interest provide the same reaction in a drug test (e.g. the analgesic ibuprofen and some nonsteroidal inflammatory agents may mimic illicit drugs) (6). Confirmatory tests, which use gas chromatography/mass spectroscopy (GC/MS) techniques, can rule out cross-reactions with near-perfect accuracy (38). All federally regulated drug testing programs are required to use back-up GC/MS, but how widely these expensive tests are run in private sector programs, especially at preemployment, is not known. The same is true of the chain-of-custody and medical review procedures built into federal programs. The Navy, according to one estimate, allocates a full 20% of the total costs of its testing program to quality controls as a hedge against the inevitable human errors (38). To what extent employers in the private sector ensure test accuracy is unclear.

Some states have passed legislation to anticipate potential problems that inaccurate testing can create. According to a survey conducted by the US General Accounting Office in 1988 (23), 11 states had specific statutes and regulations to govern laboratories that do employment drug testing. These statutes and regulations vary considerably. Ten require confirmation of positive tests, and seven specifically require GC/MS. Eight require chain-of-custody procedures on all urine specimens to reduce the likelihood of human error.

Federal guidelines have been established for all laboratories that do drug testing of federal employees (23), and NIDA conducts its laboratory certification program. However, many small laboratories scattered throughout the United States elude the scrutiny of NIDA and other certifying agencies, and some employers apparently do their own drug screening on-site. One estimate placed the number of drug screening reagent sales to nonlaboratory customers at more than $11 million in 1987 (4), which accounts for an estimated 15% of the drug screening market, the accuracy of which is unlikely to be high. Two pieces of pending federal legislation have recently been introduced in Congress, in the hope of setting minimum federal standards for all drug testing programs (D. Crouch 1991, personal communication).

Likelihood of Detection

Even when tests are technically accurate, it is generally felt that drug users can find ways to subvert the tightest system. If the testing is preannounced, casual users can avoid drugs in anticipation of a job interview or a testing program at work (26). Random, unannounced drug testing adds an element of surprise, but is generally conducted so infrequently that the odds of identifying any one drug user remain low (26). Testing for cause may be the only circumstance in which the likelihood of discovery is high (26), but the discovery occurs after something has already gone wrong.

Reports of adulterated urine specimens make good copy; whether they are exaggerated is hard to know. Drug screening is said to select for the less experienced drug users (1, 63). Powdered drug-free urine is available for sale (1, 63), as are guidebooks with practical hints on how to outmaneuver an employer's drug detection screen (14, 37).

Interpretation of Test Results

A laboratory report is marked positive when the urine specimen has been found to contain an amount of drug equal to a certain threshold concentration, or cutoff level (14), usually set higher than the detection limit of the drug test to avoid false-positives (14). The Department of Health and Human Services has standard cutoff levels for employers governed by the mandatory guidelines. On their own, employers often establish different cutoffs: In a six-state survey of union workplaces in the mid-South, only 24% of private companies that do drug testing used the federal cutoff guidelines (40).

The most important conceptual distinction, however, is between a positive test and evidence of functional impairment. A positive result indicates exposure, but not a pharmacological effect, and many of the metabolites that are traceable in urine are still detectable long after psychoactive effects have abated (40). Marijuana metabolites, for example, may still be detectable in the urine of frequent users for as many as 21 days after the last use; the dwell time for PCPs is roughly eight days and for cocaine, two to three days. Further, there is no definitive evidence that illicit drugs impair job performance more than do other exigencies or distractions, such as lack of sleep, chronic conditions, or emotional distress.

Many laboratory experiments and simulations have shown that alcohol and other drugs do impair coordination and performance, but how these findings translate to work situations is less well understood (43). It is generally acknowledged that alcohol, marijuana, and certain other drugs can seriously impair judgment and reaction time and should be avoided while doing anything (on or off the job) that cannot be done safely without concentration or coordination.

However, two post-mortem studies of industrial fatalities found no convincing evidence of excess drug involvement, although the studies were methodologically weak. One examined case files of a Florida county medical examiner (15). In 147 instances of fatal industrial injuries, 50% were tested on autopsy for traces of drugs. Of those, only 15% had a positive drug test, which suggested possible drug impairment. The other autopsy study (35) found that only 7% of 172 workers killed on the job had detectable levels of drugs that might have impaired their physiologic functioning. In both studies, the offending substances were more often alcohol and prescription drugs, rather than the illicit drugs that most worksite screening programs emphasize.

In studies of performance per se, the evidence is again equivocal. In one study, simulated performance of complex tasks by airline pilots was affected by smoking marijuana a full 24 hours before the experiment (76); but, in another study, women smoked as many as a dozen marijuana cigarettes every day for three weeks, with no measurable effect on their output of work (41).

Does Drug Testing Affect Drug Use or Related Problems at Work?

When the evaluative questions shift from the mechanics of testing to the impact of overall programs, the literature consists primarily of descriptive reports from the field (12, 48, 52, 64). Often, these reports include rates of positive tests over time, but rarely have adequate historical or comparative controls to inspire confidence that observed changes might have been partly produced by a drug testing program.

A report from the Southern Pacific Railroad Company went a step further and examined outcome data (64). In 1984, the company instituted preemployment drug screening, regular testing at the time of a periodic physical examination, and "for cause" testing of urine samples for drugs and alcohol. Between 1983 and 1988, the number of train accidents per million miles traveled declined from 22.2 to approximately 2.2, and total accidents dropped from 2234 to 322. The percentage of employees who tested positive for drugs or alcohol in these programs declined substantially, from approximately 23% in 1984 to around 5% in 1988. Marijuana was the most commonly detected drug over the five years; in 1984, 53.8% of positive results were marijuana. Positive alcohol tests jumped from 12% of all positive results in 1984 to 24% by the first half of 1988. What, if any, role the drug testing program played in the changes observed (and the meaning of the alcohol finding) are a matter of conjecture without a comparison group.

Does Drug Testing Predict Subsequent Job Performance?

To believe that preemployment screening programs effectively select out potential employees who would otherwise be impaired by drugs, we need evidence that a positive drug test is a good predictor of future job performance. A total of six studies (three peer-reviewed) have obliquely addressed this question. Again, the overall results have been mixed.

Blank & Fenton (5) conducted an unmatched comparison study of 500 male Navy recruits who tested positive for marijuana and 500 who tested negative. The study compared demographic characteristics and attrition patterns in the two groups 2.5 years after intake and found no significant differences in age, marital status, and home of origin. Significant differences were found in education level, score on a Navy qualification test, and race; the marijuana users had lower education and qualification scores and they were also more likely to be nonwhite. In terms of retention, 81% of the negative-test group, but only 57% of positive-test recruits, were still in the Navy after 2.5 years. To what extent the different retention rates were a function of the history of marijuana use, other preexisting differences in the two groups, subsequent surveillance of recruits who tested positive, negative labeling at the time of enrollment, and/or other combinations of factors is impossible to unravel.

Parish (54) conducted a blind prospective study of 180 hospital employees to assess how well a preemployment drug test result correlated with performance after 12 months on the job. All employees hired over a six-month period were screened for ten substances; all positive tests were confirmed, but none were used in hiring decisions. Potential employees were aware that their urine would be tested, and there was no observation of specimen collection. Researchers who were blind to drug test results extracted from personnel files information on job evaluations, disciplinary actions, promotions, commendations, terminations, and absenteeism.

The analysis compared those employees who tested positive and negative. No differences were found in job retention, supervisor evaluations, and reasons for termination. Eleven employees who were drug free at intake were fired from their jobs, whereas none were fired from the test-positive group, a challenging finding. The numbers were small (12%, or 22 employees tested positive), so the statistical power was low, and a Type II error (the inability to detect a true difference) could have occurred.

Zwerling et al (77) conducted another prospective blind study of preemployment drug testing among postal workers, who provided a larger sample (N=2537). EMIT was used as the screen, followed by confirmation by GC/MS. A quality control test of spiked samples indicated 90–100% sensitivity and 100% specificity of the laboratory tests. Employees, hiring officials, medical personnel, and management were all blinded to the results of the urine tests. No significant association was found between the decision whether to hire applicants and the (undisclosed) results of their urine tests. The prevalence of drug positives was 7.8% for marijuana, 2.2% for cocaine, and 2.2% for other or multiple drugs.

At follow-up more than one year later, the two groups were compared after controlling for age, sex, smoking and exercise status, race, and job classification. Employees who had tested positive for marijuana at preemployment were significantly more likely to have been terminated from their jobs [relative risk (RR), 2.07]. The test-positive group had a higher rate of absence (RR, 1.56) and time to first injury (RR, 1.85), as well as earlier time to first accident (RR, 1.55) and to disciplinary action (RR, 1.55). Cocaine-positive workers had significantly greater risk of earlier first injury (RR, 1.85) and absence rate (RR, 2.37), but cocaine did not predict termination, time to first accident, or time to first disciplinary action.

Normand et al (50) conducted the most thorough evaluation of drug testing to date, a follow-up of 4396 new postal service employees who had provided urine samples at preemployment interviews. The samples were tested for eight classes of drugs (amphetamines, barbiturates, benzodiazepines, cannabinoids, cocaine, methadone, opiates, and PCPs), and all positive EMIT readings were confirmed by GC/MS. The results were withheld from everyone except the research staff.

In contrast to the Zwerling study, this one found that job applicants who tested positive were less often hired (81% of test-negative applicants were hired, compared with 73% of test-positive, even though the information on their testing status was unavailable for the hiring decision). Of applicants who were hired, 5.7% tested positive for marijuana, 2.2% tested positive for cocaine, and 0.9% tested positive for all other drugs combined.

Workers who did and did not test positive at preemployment were compared on absenteeism, voluntary and involuntary separation, and injury and accident rates after just over one year of employment. Postal workers who tested positive for both cocaine and marijuana were placed in the cocaine-positive group for purposes of analysis.

Compared with the group of workers who tested negative for any drug, the marijuana-positive group was 1.5 times more likely and the cocaine-positive group 4.29 times more likely to exhibit heavy absenteeism over the 1.3 years of follow-up. These were odds ratios, which were statistically significant at the 0.01 level. The odds of voluntary separation were the same irrespective of testing status, but involuntary separation was 1.55 times as likely (and statistically significant at the 0.01 level) in the group testing positive for any drug and 2.4 times as likely in the cocaine-positive group (again, statistically significant).

A logistic regression analysis controlling for age, sex, and job category revealed that a positive test result significantly predicted absenteeism. After controlling for job category, the analysis predicted involuntary separation. The investigators speculated that the associations probably underestimated the true relationships between drug use and job performance indicators, owing to misclassification, measurement error, construct invalidity, and other factors.

After assessing the predictive capability of a preemployment testing program, Normand et al (50) also conducted an analysis of costs versus benefits. This analysis produced an estimated cost savings for the drug testing program (through absenteeism and turnover costs) of $52,750,000 for one (annual) cohort of new employees, a figure the investigators considered an underestimate of all the potential savings. The authors were careful to note that their study did not purport to establish a causal link from drug use to absenteeism and the other performance indicators. They argued that a positive drug test may stand as a proxy for a whole complex of factors, including personal characteristics and lifestyles, that combine to produce a worker who is significantly less likely to perform well, whatever the proximal cause. Work by Kandel & Yamaguchi (34) would tend to support this assumption as it relates to job separation in young adults.

Among the indicators of performance used as outcome measures in these studies, absenteeism may be more objective and reliable than job termination or supervisor assessment because the latter measures include an element of subjectivity. Absenteeism, however, is not often documented as well and operationalized as carefully as it needs to be to support rigorous evaluation research (67). As an outcome, it does tend to yield greater statistical power than some alternatives (e.g. injuries or job terminations) that occur less frequently. Only two of the evaluations of drug testing in the workplace (50, 77) had sufficient statistical power and they both found significantly higher absenteeism rates among the groups of employees who tested positive for drugs in the preemployment screen.

Do the Benefits of a Drug Testing Program Outweigh the Costs?

Other than in the postal worker studies, information on the costs of drug testing programs is thin. The Navy is believed to spend approximately $90–$100 per specimen on drug testing (including collection, transportation, and analysis) (10), which, at 2 million tests a year, would sum to approximately $190 million, just in test handling costs. Private companies pay $15–$30 per specimen for EMIT or radioimmunoassay, depending on volume and location (40). A GC/MS confirmation costs $35–$100 per specimen (40). In addition, there are initial start up costs, costs of staff time, legal fees, and time off from work, as well as difficult-to-quantify indirect costs. Whether these costs are justified depends on the benefits achieved.

Too little valid evaluation research has been conducted to date to support cost-benefit analyses of drug screening programs. Two studies are widely quoted, one conducted at the Utah Power and Light Company (16), the other at Georgia Power and Light (unpublished). In both cases, selection bias and insufficient attention to competing explanations for presumed program effects cast doubt on positive returns on investment both studies purported to show.

None of the cost-benefit analyses conducted to date compares drug testing with alternative methods for deterring employees from using drugs, or alternative methods for screening out workers who may be unfit for duty on any given day. As just one example, a California-based company, Performance Factors, manufactures and markets a computerized job performance testing machine called "Factor 1000" (55). When employees in safety-sensitive jobs report to work daily, they are required to perform tasks on a computer that tracks their hand-eye coordination and reaction time (but not critical activity or judgment) against their own baseline, which is constantly updated in the computer file as their skill improves. The company asserts that Factor 1000 can detect impairment, irrespective of cause (prescription or illicit drug use, alcohol, severe stress, fatigue, or illness). Customers include the National Highway Traffic Safety Administration and several private firms. A serious study of Factor 1000, and/or similar devices, might compare their performance with that of a drug testing program in a randomized controlled trial.

For policy analysis, an adequate cost-benefit framework should encompass a variety of alternative expenditures designed to address a given problem. No studies have compared the relative costs and benefits of worksite drug screening with more investment (for example) in primary prevention, health promotion, or employee assistance in the workplace or in fuller coverage for treatment of drug-abusing employees. No analyses have widened the framework to ask (as one of many examples) whether an equivalent expenditure in treatment for pregnant cocaine addicts would yield a greater social payoff, all things considered. These are the kinds of questions that need thoughtful consideration.

QUESTIONS FOR THE FUTURE

Technological advances and administrative innovations have made worksite drug screening almost perfectly accurate, when structured according to protocol. The protocol virtually removes from consideration the danger of falsely accusing a worker of having used an illicit drug. More surveillance is needed to ensure that the protocol is being followed wherever employers are testing for drugs, but most of the technical questions have been addressed and can be resolved.

What remain now are questions about what it means to learn that an employee has a trace of an illicit drug in his or her urine, what the social costs and benefits are of expending the resources to find that out, and what subsequent actions are justified if the goal is to enhance the health and productive capacity of the American labor force. We know almost nothing about what happens to applicants denied employment because of a positive drug test, or even whether they are told why they were not selected for the job. We have no information on how many (if any) employees have lost their jobs because of drug testing and what has been their fate. We have no information on how workers have been affected by drug testing programs. If some have been referred for treatment, we have no knowledge of how they have fared and whether the drug test helped or hindered their recovery. If some were not referred to treatment, we do not know if they are still employed.

We have only unsubstantiated assertions that worksite drug testing programs have changed beliefs, attitudes, and values concerning drugs and work. We have no knowledge of their impact on labor relations and other aspects of the employment relationship. No one has gauged whether they have had an impact on other health, safety, and mental health programs in the workplace; whether they have further complicated delicate relationships between occupational physicians and employees (69); and whether they have strengthened or shackled EAPs. If drug screening programs have had a beneficial or adverse effect on employees' motivation, trust, or morale, we have no way to know, although we have reason to care, in light of growing concern about American competitiveness in world markets. Policymakers and lawmakers have no way to know how often, to what extent, and in which ways drug screening programs may be violating rights of privacy and due process of law. Nor do they know if these programs support or undermine general feelings of autonomy, community, good faith, and decency in places of work. Legislative and regulatory restrictions may or may not have their desired effect. Employees in large firms are often protected by multiple layers of law and regulation, whereas those in smaller and nonunion shops and plants may have little such protection.

The most important gap in knowledge about drug testing programs pertains to their effectiveness. We have little cogent evidence to support the supposition that these programs reduce drug use in the workplace, improve performance and productivity, or produce other positive results. In the absence of such evidence, civil libertarians and labor leaders are asking whether these programs are anything more than symbolic politics, whether they are an implicit statement by the federal government that responsibility for health and productivity resides with workers themselves, and whether they deflect attention from structural problems in the macroeconomy by implying that American industry's competitive problems are the fault of workers who use drugs.

A rule of thumb in the clinical management of substance abuse could profitably be applied to the evaluation of drug testing at work: The least intensive, intrusive, and coercive approaches should be given a fair trial first, before ratcheting up to treatments with greater potential for harm. More invasive interventions should carry a heavier burden of proof that they hold genuine promise of doing more good than harm. Such tests have yet to be applied objectively to drug testing at work.

ACKNOWLEDGMENTS

We are indebted to Buck Cameron, Jonathan E. Fielding, Leonard Glantz, Steven Gust, Vernon MacDougall, and Jacques Normand, for insightful and helpful comments on an earlier draft of the manuscript, and to Kent Peterson, Steven Gust, M. Beth Grigson Babecki, and George Baldwin for assistance with the literature search.

Literature Cited

1. Am. Coll. Occup. Med. 1990. *Medical Review Officer Information Handbook.* Houston: Am. Coll. Occup. Med.
2. *Americans with Disabilities Act of 1990.* Public Law 101–336, 104 Stat. 327, 42 USC 12101
3. Axel, H. 1990. *Corporate Experiences with Drug Testing Programs. Res. Rep. No. 941.* New York: The Conference Board. 37 pp.
4. Baer, D. M., Belsey, R. E., Skeels, M. R. 1990. A survey of state regulation of testing for drugs of abuse outside of licensed (accredited) clinical laboratories. *Am. J. Public Health* 80(6):713–15
5. Blank, D. L., Fenton, J. W. 1989. Early employment testing for marijuana: Demographic and employee retention patterns. See Ref. 27a, pp. 139–50
6. Blanke, R. V. 1986. Accuracy in urinalysis. In *Drugs in the Workplace. Research and Evaluation Data NIDA Research Monograph 73,* ed. S. W. Gust, J. M. Walsh, pp. 43–53. Rockville, Md: Natl. Inst. Drug Abuse. 121 pp.
7. Bur. Labor Stat. US Dep. Labor. 1989. *Survey of Employer Anti-Drug Programs. Report 760.* Washington, DC: GPO
8. Bur. Natl. Aff. 1988. Managers favor drug screens of present, potential workers. *Natl. Rep. Subst. Abuse. Biwkly. Newsl.* 2(23):6
9. Cairns, S. S., Grady, C. V. 1990. Drug testing in the workplace: A reasoned approach for private employers. Drug Testing in the Workplace: Status and Prospects. *George Mason Law Rev.* 12(4):491–544
10. Cangianelli, L. A. 1989. The effects of a drug testing program in the Navy. See Ref. 28a, pp. 211–17
11. Deleted in proof
12. Cent. Dis. Control. 1989. Drug use among applicants for military service–United States, June—December 1988. *Morbid. Mortal. Wkly. Rep.* 38(33):580–83
13. Chiang, L. N., Hawks, R. L. 1986. Implications of drug levels in body fluids: Basic concepts. In *Urine Testing for Drugs of Abuse. NIDA Res. Monograph 73,* ed. R. L. Hawks, C. N. Chiang, pp. 62–83. Rockville, Md: Natl. Inst. Drug Abuse. 121 pp.
14. Clark, H. W. 1990. The role of physicians as medical review officers in workplace drug testing programs: In pursuit of the last nanogram. *West. J. Med.* 152(5):514–24
15. Copeland, A. R. 1985. Fatal occupational accidents—the five-year Metro Dade County Experience, 1979–1983. *J. Forensic Sci.* 30(2):494–503
16. Crouch, D. J., Webb, D. O., Peterson, L. V., Buller, P. F., Rollins, D. E. 1989. A critical evaluation of the Utah Power and Light Company's substance abuse management program: Absenteeism, accidents and costs. See Ref. 27a, pp. 169–93
17. *Delaware v. Prouse.* 1979. 99 S.Ct. 1391
18. Dep. Defense. 1988. Department of Defense Federal Acquisition Regulation Supplement: Drug-Free Workforce. 53 *Fed. Regist.* 53(188):37, 763–65
19. Dep. Health Hum. Serv. 1988. Mandatory Guidelines for Federal Workplace Drug Testing Programs. *Fed. Regist.* 53(69):11979–89
20. Dep. Transp. 1989. Procedures for Transportation Workplace Drug Testing Program; Final Rule and Notice of Conference. *Fed. Regist.* 54(230):49854–84
21. Ellul, J. 1964. *The Technology Society.* New York: Vintage Books. 449 pp.
22. Gen. Account. Off. 1988. Employee Drug Testing. Information on Private Sector Programs. Washington, DC: US Gen. Account. Off.
23. Gen. Account. Off. 1988. Employee Drug Testing Regulation of Drug Testing Laboratories. Washington, DC: US Gen. Account. Off.
24. Glantz, L. 1989. A nation of suspects. Drug testing and the Fourth Amendment. *Am. J. Public Health* 79 (10):1427–31
25. Godefroi, R., McCunney, R. J. 1988. Drug screening practices in small businesses: A survey. *J. Occup. Med.* 30:300–2
26. Grabowski, J., Silverman, P. B. 1989. Drug screening in the workplace: Use, abuse and implications. See Ref. 28a, pp. 225–31
27. Gusfield, J. R. 1987. Passage to play: Rituals of drinking time in American society. In *Constructive Drinking: Perspectives on Drinking from Anthropology,* ed. M. Douglas, pp. 73–90. New York: University Press. 291 pp.
27a. Gust, S. W., Walsh, J. M., eds. 1989. *Drugs in the Workplace. Research and Evaluation Data NIDA Res. Monograph 91.* Rockville, Md: Natl. Inst. Drug Abuse. 340 pp.
28. *Harmon v. Thornburgh.* 1989. 878 F.2d 484 (DC Cir. 1989)
28a. Harris, L. S., ed. 1989. *Proc. 51st. Annu. Sci. Meeting. NIDA Res. Mono-*

graph 95. Rockville, Md: Natl. Inst. Drug Abuse. 727 pp.
29. Hayghe, H. V. 1991. Anti-drug programs in the workplace. *Month. Lab. Rev.* 114(4):26–29
30. Horgan, R. W. 1990. Test negative: A look at the evidence justifying illicit drug tests. *Sci. Am.* 262(13):18, 22
31. Inst. Drug-Free Workplace. 1990. The Drug-Free Workplace Report 2(1):1–16
32. Institute for a Drug-Free Workplace. 1990. *What Employees Think About Drug Abuse. Special Report.* Washington, DC: Inst. Drug-Free Workplace
33. Johnston, L. D., O'Malley, P. M., Bachman, J. G. 1989. *Drug Use, Drinking, and Smoking: National Survey Results from High School, College, and Young Adults Populations.* Rockville, Md: Natl. Inst. Drug Abuse. 339 pp.
34. Kandel, D. B., Yamaguchi, K. 1987. Job mobility and drug use: An event history analysis. *Am. J. Sociol.* 992(4):836–78
35. Lewis, R. J., Cooper, S. P. 1989. Alcohol, other drugs, and fatal work-related injuries. *J. Occup. Med.* 31(1):23–28
36. Linn, L. S., Yager, J., Leake, B. 1990. Physicians' attitudes toward substance abuse and drug testing. *Int. J. Addict.* 25(4):427–44
37. Lundberg, G. D. 1986. Mandatory unindicated urine drug screening: Still chemical McCarthyism. Editorials. *J. Am. Med. Assoc.* 256(21):3003–5
38. Marshall, E. 1988. Testing urine for drugs. News and comments. *Science* 241(4862):150–52
39. Marwick, C., Gunby, P. 1989. Like other segments of culture, military has had to come to grips with drug abuse problems. Medical News and Perspectives. *J. Am. Med. Assoc.* 261 (19):2784
40. McMillan, D. E. 1989. Urine screening: What does it mean? See Ref. 28a, pp. 206–10
41. Mello, N. K., Mendelson, J. H. 1985. Operant acquisition of marihuana by women. *J. Pharmacol. Exp. Ther.* 235(1):162–71
42. Mercer Meidinger Hansen Inc. 1988. *Substance Abuse in the Workforce.* A survey of employers conducted for Marsh & McLennan Co., Inc. 13 pp.
43. Moskowitz, H. 1985. Adverse effects of alcohol and other drugs on human performance. *Alcohol Health Res. World* 9(4):11–15, 64–65
44. Musto, D. F. 1989. The history of American drug control. *Update Law-Relat. Educ.* 13(2):3–6, 47, 54–56
45. Natl. Inst. Drug Abuse. 1989. *National Household Survey on Drug Abuse: Main Findings 1988.* Washington, DC: Natl. Inst. Drug Abuse
46. *Natl. Treas. Empl. Union v. Von Raab.* 1989. 109 S.Ct. 1384
47. Deleted in proof
48. Needleman, S. B., Romberg, R. W. 1989. Comparison of drug abuse in different military populations. *J. Forensic Sci.* 34(4):848–57
49. Newcomb, M. D. 1989. *Drug Use in the Workplace: Risk Factors for Disruptive Substance Use Among Young Adults.* Dover. Mass: Auburn. 254 pp.
50. Normand, J., Salyards, S., Mahoney, J. J. 1990. An evaluation of preemployment drug testing. *J. Appl. Psychol.* 75(6):629–39
51. Nucl. Regul. Comm. 1989. Fitness-for-Duty Programs. Final Rule and Statement of Policy. *Fed Regist.* 54 (108):24468–24508
52. Osborn, C. E., Sokolov, J. J. 1989. Drug use trends in a nuclear power company: Cumulative data from an ongoing testing program. See Ref. 27a, pp. 69–80
53. Osterloh, H., Becker, C. 1990. Chemical dependency and drug testing in the workplace. *West. J. Med.* 152(5):506–13
54. Parish, D. C. 1989. Relation of the preemployment drug testing result to employment status: A one-year follow-up. *J. Gen. Intern. Med.* 4:44–47
55. Performance Factors. Factor 1000. Innovating for Accident-Free and Error-Free Performance. 3 pp.
56. The President. 1986. Executive Order 12564 of September 15, 1986. Drug-Free Federal Workplace. *Fed. Regist.* 51(180):32889–93
57. Regan, M. A. 1989. Performance appraisal: An antidote for substance abuse? *Bull. NY Acad. Med.* 65(2): 202
58. Roper, B. W., Ladd, E. C. 1989. Drugs: The public's response to a national crisis. *Public Perspect. Roper Cent. Rev. Public Opinion Polling* 1(1):31–40
59. *Schmerber v. California.* 1966. 86 S.Ct. 1826
60. Deleted in proof
61. Sheridan, J. R., Winkler, H. 1989. An evaluation of drug testing in the workplace. See Ref. 27a, pp. 81–96
62. *Skinner v. Railway Labor Exec. Assoc.* 1989. 109 S.Ct. 1402
63. Sonnenstuhl, W. J., Trice, H. M., Staudenmeir, W. J. Jr., Steele, P. 1987. Employee assistance and drug testing:

Fairness and injustice in the workplace. Testing for Drug Use in the American Workplace. A Symposium. *Nova Law Rev.* 11(2):709–31

64. Taggart. R. W. 1989. Results of the drug testing program at Southern Pacific Railroad. See Ref. 27a, pp. 97–108

65. *US v. Montoya de Hernandez.* 1985. 105 S.Ct. 3304

66. Voss, H. L. 1989. Patterns of drug use: Data from the 1985 National Household Survey. See Ref. 27a, pp. 33–46

67. Walsh, D. C. 1991. Costs of illness in the workplace. In *Managing for Health and Productivity,* ed. G. Green, F. Baker, pp. 217–41. New York: Oxford

68. Walsh, D. C. 1991. Explorations and experiments in large corporations. Reflections on opportunities and barriers associated with worksite research. In *Research Methods in Workplace Settings. NIDA Technical Review Meeting, September 27, 1991.* In press

69. Walsh, D. C. 1987. *Corporate Physicians: Between Medicine and Management.* New York: Springer-Verlag. 267 pp.

70. Walsh, D. C. 1982. Employee assistance programs. *Milb. Mem. Fund Q. Health Soc.* 60(3):492–517

71. Walsh, D. C., Hingson, R. 1986. Epidemiology and alcohol policy. In *Epidemiology and Health Policy,* ed. S. Levine, A. M. Lilienfeld, pp. 265–91. London: Tavistock. 301 pp.

72. Weiss, C., Millman, R. B. 1989. Alcohol and drug abuse in the workplace in broad perspective. *Bull. NY Acad. Med.* 65(2):173–84

73. Wells, V. E., Halperin, W., Thum, M. 1988. The estimated predictive value of screening for illicit drugs in the workplace. *Am. J. Public Health* 78(7):817–19

74. The White House. 1989. *National Drug Control Strategy.* Washington, DC:GPO

75. Deleted in proof

76. Yesavage, J. A., Leirer, V. O., Denari, M., Hollister, L. E. 1985. *Am. J. Psychiatr.* 142:1325–29

77. Zwerling, C., Ryan, J., Endel, J. O. 1990. The efficacy of pre-employment drug screening for marijuana and cocaine in predicting employment outcome. *J. Am. Med. Assoc.* 264 (20):2639–43

Annu. Rev. Publ. Health 1992. 13:223-37

GLOBAL IMMUNIZATION

R. Kim-Farley and the Expanded Programme on Immunization Team

Expanded Programme on Immunization, World Health Organization, Geneva 27, Switzerland

KEY WORDS: Expanded Programme on Immunization, poliomyelitis eradication, measles reduction, neonatal tetanus elimination, vaccination

INTRODUCTION

Immunization programs are recognized as one of the most cost-effective interventions of public health. However, even as late as the mid-1970s, it was estimated that less than 5% of children in developing countries were adequately immunized against diphtheria, tetanus, pertussis, measles, poliomyelitis, and tuberculosis.

In response to the tragic numbers of deaths due to these vaccine-preventable diseases, the World Health Assembly (WHA) of the World Health Organization (WHO) initiated the Expanded Programme on Immunization (EPI) in 1974. The EPI forms the basis of a global effort to reduce morbidity and mortality from these six diseases by providing immunization services for all children and women of the world.

In this article, we document the significant progress, the lessons learned, and the challenges facing global immunization efforts in the 1990s. And, we discuss many of the recommendations of the EPI Global Advisory Group (13).

OVERVIEW OF PROGRESS

For the first time, reported immunization coverage is surpassing the 80% mark for a third dose of polio or DPT vaccines for children in their first year of life (Figure 1). This represents a milestone towards universal childhood

223

0163-7525/92/0501-0223$02.00

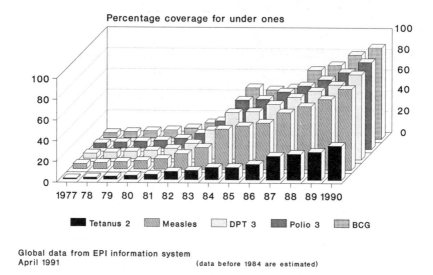

Percentage coverage for under ones

1977 78 79 80 81 82 83 84 85 86 87 88 89 1990

■ Tetanus 2   ▨ Measles   □ DPT 3   ▨ Polio 3   ▨ BCG

Global data from EPI information system
April 1991   (data before 1984 are estimated)

Figure 1   Expanded Programme on Immunization, immunization coverage 1977 to 1990.

immunization. However, the percentage of pregnant women who receive tetanus toxoid immunization to protect their newborns from neonatal tetanus is much lower. In developing countries, only 38% of pregnant women receive the two-dose primary series or a booster dose. It is also important to note that global statistics mask disparities among regions (Figure 2), countries, provinces/states, and districts (6). These immunization coverage levels, which reflect the varied development of the primary health care infrastructure, are one of the measures of the degree of equity and social justice that communities have achieved.

The progress in global immunization is directly attributable to the efforts of national governments, WHO, the United Nations Children's Fund (UNICEF) and other UN agencies, bilateral development agencies, and nongovernmental organizations. The development of the capacity to achieve these levels of coverage of infants represents a major public health triumph for the 1980s.

At the present levels of immunization coverage, an estimated 3.2 million deaths due to measles, neonatal tetanus, and pertussis are prevented annually. And, some 450,000 cases of paralytic poliomyelitis are also prevented (Figure 3). The urgency to raise immunization coverage levels and focus on disease

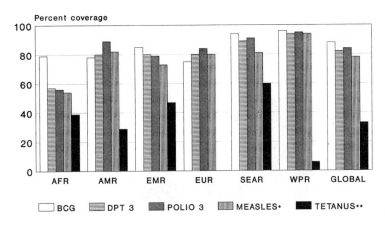

Figure 2   Immunization coverage of children less than 12 months of age by WHO region, April 1991.

control is underlined by the occurrence of an estimated 1.8 million deaths each year due to these diseases and some 120,000 cases of paralytic poliomyelitis—all of which are preventable through immunization (6).

LESSONS LEARNED

Over the last 15 years, the global immunization effort has demonstrated that a global coalition, which shares common goals, can create an unprecedented degree of cooperation among a wide spectrum of national governments and international, national, and local organizations.

The development of the EPI over these years has taught specific lessons that will continue to guide immunization programs in the 1990s:

1. Goals endorsed by the WHA help galvanize the international community to action;
2. Policies and strategies recommended by the EPI Global Advisory Group provide a common direction for immunization efforts (13);
3. Personal involvement of heads of state and the political, religious, and social leadership at all levels generates political will, creates demand for immunization services, and mobilizes communities to meet that demand;
4. Nearly all mothers and children of the world can be reached with immunization services, and significant reductions in morbidity, disability, and mortality can be achieved;
5. Research and development in logistics, cold chain, injection equipment,

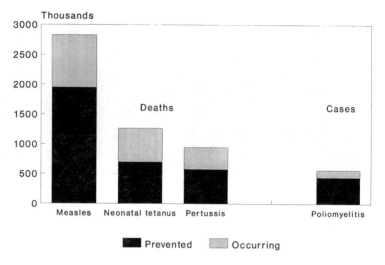

EPI Information system - April 1991

Figure 3   Cases and deaths occurring and prevented in developing countries only.

new and improved vaccines, delivery strategies, immunization schedules, and monitoring and evaluation methodologies (11) provide a technical basis for advancing program policies and strategies;
6. Emphasis on training in technical skills, planning, and management develop the needed human resources at senior, middle, and peripheral levels; and
7. Some diseases can be eradicated from the face of the earth; the cost of such an effort ultimately saves money by halting the need to immunize against the diseases or treat its victims.

The progress and lessons learned provide optimism that the new challenges set by the WHA for global immunization programs in the 1990s will be met.

GOALS

In May 1989, the Forty-Second World Health Assembly set the 1990s agenda for the EPI in resolution WHA42.32 (16). Six major challenges to be addressed during the decade were cited:

1. Achieving and sustaining in all countries full immunization coverage with all the vaccines used by the EPI;
2. Controlling the target diseases, including reduction of measles by 90% compared with pre-immunization levels by 1995, elimination of neonatal

tetanus by 1995, and global eradication of poliomyelitis by the year 2000;

3. Improving disease surveillance to provide accurate assessment of the progress of the program;

4. Introducing within routine national immunization services new or improved vaccines as these become available for public health use;

5. Promoting other primary health care practices that are appropriate for the program's delivery system and target populations; and

6. Conducting research and development in support of the above.

These challenges, among others, were dramatically reinforced in the Declaration on the Survival, Protection, and Development of Children, which was enunciated at the World Summit for Children held at the UN in September 1990 (19). The plan of action associated with the Declaration brings the goals for children and development to the highest levels of political visibility. The international community must now move forward rapidly to use the momentum of this summit to translate the Declaration into the actions necessary to achieve these goals.

PLANNING

Development of immunization and disease control plans of action at global, regional, national, state/province, and local levels, with periodic review and revision, are necessary to set priorities on activities to meet the above challenges. Plans for achieving specific immunization coverage and disease reduction, elimination, and eradication targets should be part of an overall immunization plan of action, which, in turn, should be part of a primary health care plan.

The establishment and effective functioning of interagency coordinating committees, which improve the coordination of donors in support of regional and national immunization programs, are useful in planning and integrating activities aimed at sustaining immunization programs. In many countries, most notably in the region of the Americas, interagency coordinating committees have elaborated detailed financial plans that outline the commitments of the national governments and their donor partners over a medium-term period. These committees review program performance at country level through periodic meetings and make adjustments to plans and their funding. This coordination benefits both receiving countries and donor agencies by promoting effective use of available resources and by providing individual donors with the accountability and visibility needed for continuing support. Interagency coordinating committees, although perhaps initially formed for immunization programs, should ultimately have a broader mandate for coordination of primary health care activities in general.

The planning process provides the opportunity for regions, governments, and donors to balance global targets with regional and national priorities. Each region and country sets its own priorities based on the magnitude of the disease burden, available resources, expected outcome, and fit within the overall health care goals. The WHA resolutions represent the combined will of all the WHO member states. The WHA has stated that EPI goals and targets "should be pursued in ways which strengthen the development of the Expanded Programme on Immunization as a whole, fostering its contribution, in turn, to the development of the health infrastructure and of primary health care" (16, 17).

ACHIEVING AND SUSTAINING FULL IMMUNIZATION COVERAGE

A major goal of the EPI continues to be raising and sustaining immunization coverage. High levels of immunization coverage provide the foundation on which specific efforts at disease control can be mounted and ensure that disease control, once achieved, can be maintained. The WHA has urged all countries to continue their vigorous pursuit of providing immunization services for all children and women of the world. Immunization coverage levels of 90% for all vaccines, including tetanus toxoid in women of childbearing age, can be achieved in all countries by the year 2000. This will require increased emphasis on directing program resources to achieve and sustain high immunization coverage levels in all districts/municipalities and, ultimately, in all communities. The separate analysis of immunization coverage data by district or community helps identify low coverage areas.

Immunization schedules need to be simple, effective, and epidemiologically appropriate. The EPI Global Advisory Group periodically reviews recommendations for immunization schedules. The current schedule endorsed by the EPI Global Advisory Group is designed to provide protection at the earliest possible age (Table 1, see also Ref. 12).

Priority activities to raise immunization coverage include:

1. Improving the management of health services: Decentralizing responsibilities and providing training and supportive supervision to the health workers who provide immunizations.

2. Making primary health care services more accessible: Increasing the frequency and range of outreach activities to extend immunization services to populations currently without access.

3. Informing and motivating the public: Creating demand for immunization services by specifically recognizing that fathers, as well as mothers, play important health roles.

4. Immunizing at every opportunity: Providing immunization services as frequently as feasible at all health facilities attended by women and children,

Table 1 Recommended immunization schedule for providing protection at the earliest possible age

Age	Vaccine
Birth	TOPV[a], BCG[b]
6 weeks	TOPV, DPT[c]
10 weeks	TOPV, DPT
14 weeks	TOPV, DPT
6–9 months	Measles (high titer Edmonston-Zagreb strain of measles vaccine has been recommended at 6 months of age in countries in which measles before the age of 9 months is a significant cause of death)
	Yellow fever (in endemic countries)

[a] TOPV = trivalent oral polio vaccine (the dose at birth or first contact is recommended in countries where poliomyelitis has not been controlled)
[b] BCG = vaccine against tuberculosis
[c] DPT = diphtheria, tetanus, and pertussis vaccine

reviewing the immunization needs of both mother and child at the time of immunization of the child, and avoiding false contraindications so that immunizations are not withheld unnecessarily.

5. Reducing drop-out rates: Providing courteous services at times and places convenient for the users, informing parents of the importance of returning to complete the immunization schedule, and identifying women and children who are eligible for immunization and actively following up those who default.

6. Using special immunization activities: Including one or more of the following activities in high risk areas where routine coverage remains significantly below average or where there is continuing transmission of disease: employing mass media to encourage the use of existing services; increasing immunization outreach activities; utilizing national, state/province, or local immunization days, weeks, or months (18); and performing "mopping-up" operations (providing oral polio vaccine to all children of an epidemiologically appropriate age group, as well as all other needed EPI vaccines to women and infants on a house-to-house basis).

Priority actions to ensure sustainability of high levels of immunization coverage include:

1. Coordinating donor support: Establishing interagency coordinating committees, thus recognizing that, in many developing countries, donor support of immunization activities must continue for the foreseeable future.

2. Monitoring quality of services: Implementing such quality of service indicators as acceptability of immunization services provided to the community, appropriateness of health education messages, adequacy of cold chain, sterility of injection equipment, reports of adverse events following immunization, and field evaluation of vaccine efficacy.

3. Costing, budgeting, and financing: Determining costs and developing

budgets for immunization programs help governments mobilize internal and external resources. Reduction of recurrent and hard currency costs can be achieved through reduced vaccine wastage, vehicle whole life contracts, sale of solar energy, and financing alternatives that use local currency revolving funds for the critical recurrent cost of vaccines.

4. Transferring technology: Producing vaccine or packaging from bulk may be appropriate for some countries. To transfer technology, the National Control Authority must be sufficiently developed to certify that the final vaccine product meets WHO requirements.

5. Providing relief in situations of armed conflict: Establishing "days of tranquility" and "special relief corridors" for the benefit of children and women in situations of armed conflict that endanger sustainability of immunization services.

IMPROVING DISEASE SURVEILLANCE

As immunization coverage levels rise, there is an increasing focus on disease surveillance as an indicator of program impact. Surveillance as "information for action" helps direct immunization activities to areas of greatest need and is a prerequisite to achieve the specific disease control targets.

Surveillance for the EPI target diseases is ideally improved through strengthening a national surveillance system that reports only a selected number of high priority infectious diseases. A properly functioning system of surveillance includes the following: an appropriate mix of routine, sentinel, active, and laboratory-based surveillance activities; monthly or weekly reports submitted in a timely manner from all health units, including reports of zero cases; neonatal tetanus reported separately from other forms of tetanus; a mechanism for following up late or absent reports; and immediate reporting of rare, notifiable diseases of high importance, including poliomyelitis, in areas where this disease is close to eradication.

Actions based on surveillance, including outbreak investigation, outbreak control measures, assessment of vaccine efficacy, and review of immunization policies and strategies, become increasingly important with higher levels of immunization coverage. Disease surveillance also serves as an indicator of program quality by identifying areas of low immunization coverage and detecting vaccine failure caused by inadequate vaccine quality, transport, storage, or administration.

Managers responsible for disease surveillance should use indicators, such as timeliness and completeness of reporting and promptness in taking necessary action, to assess progress in surveillance. Computerized surveillance information systems are excellent management tools for disease surveillance and for monitoring surveillance indicators and immunization coverage.

CONTROLLING THE TARGET DISEASES

The measles reduction, neonatal tetanus elimination, and poliomyelitis eradication initiatives were formulated to strengthen a sustainable health infrastructure that can deliver immunization and other primary health care services. Many of the strategies of the disease control initiatives, such as the following, are common to all: raising and sustaining high levels of immunization coverage, improving disease surveillance, creating and maintaining public awareness to sustain political and financial commitment, and providing information and education to parents and other community members to increase immunization coverage and improve detection of cases.

The following three sections provide information on the objectives, current status, and special strategies unique to each of these initiatives.

Measles Reduction

The objectives of this reduction initiative are to achieve, by 1995, a reduction by 90% in measles cases and 95% in measles deaths compared with pre-immunization levels. These morbidity and mortality reduction targets are a major step toward global eradication of measles in the longer run.

Currently, 78% of infants have reportedly received measles vaccine. The global immunization program prevents an estimated 84 million measles cases and 2 million measles deaths in developing countries each year. This represents a 74% decrease in measles cases and a 69% decrease in measles deaths compared with estimates of cases and deaths that would occur annually in the absence of immunization programs at pre-immunization rates of disease. The continuing significant disease burden due to measles is recognized by the estimated 29 million cases and 900,000 deaths that occur in developing countries each year (6).

The 95% reduction in measles deaths will be achieved through such strategies as directing program resources to areas of highest mortality rates, immunizing at the most vulnerable early ages, supplementing and treating with vitamin A in areas of severe vitamin A deficiency, and improving treatment and management of complications through acute respiratory infection and diarrheal disease control programs. Measles before the age of nine months continues to be a major cause of mortality in many developing countries. The EPI Global Advisory Group recommends that high titer Edmonston-Zagreb measles vaccine be administered, as it becomes available, at six months of age or as soon thereafter as possible in these countries.

Measles outbreaks must be expected even in programs with relatively high coverage. A temporary period of low incidence usually follows accelerated measles control activities, but outbreaks are still likely to occur because of the accumulation of susceptibles (2). Outbreaks should be analyzed to ensure that there is high vaccine efficacy and that immunization schedules and delivery strategies are epidemiologically appropriate. Such outbreaks may identify high risk areas that are suitable for special immunization activities and may provide an opportunity to secure additional resources for immunization programs from political leaders.

Neonatal Tetanus Elimination

The objective of this elimination initiative is to reach a stage at which there are no cases of neonatal tetanus in the world by 1995. However, the term "elimination" recognizes that it is not feasible to remove the causative tetanus organism from the environment. Given the awareness of the importance of clean delivery practices and the availability of effective vaccines, the continuing occurrence of maternal and neonatal tetanus represents a major failure of public health practice.

Currently, only 38% of pregnant women in developing countries have received the two-dose primary series or a booster dose of tetanus toxoid to protect their newborns from neonatal tetanus. The global immunization program prevents an estimated 700,000 neonatal tetanus deaths in developing countries each year. This is an estimated 55% decrease in neonatal tetanus deaths compared with estimates of deaths that would occur annually in the absence of immunization programs at pre-immunization rates of disease. The percentage of prevented deaths is greater than the global percentage of immunization coverage because coverage levels are higher than the global average in some larger countries that have the highest pre-immunization neonatal tetanus mortality rates. Neonatal tetanus, however, remains a significant cause of neonatal deaths, as an estimated 600,000 deaths occur each year (6). The 1995 target date has helped emphasize that neonatal tetanus is a major killer of the world's children.

The goal of elimination of neonatal tetanus is being pursued in ways that foster the development of maternal and child health services. The global plan of action for neonatal tetanus elimination emphasizes a twofold strategy (9): achieving high levels of immunization coverage in women of childbearing age with tetanus toxoid, and raising the proportion of clean deliveries (clean hands, clean delivery surface, and clean cutting and care of the umbilical cord). The priority for all countries in which neonatal tetanus remains endemic is to increase tetanus toxoid protection in women of childbearing age rapidly, especially in high risk areas. The number of neonatal tetanus deaths could be dramatically reduced if all women were screened and appropriately immunized when they brought their children for immunization and if all antenatal care clinics offered tetanus toxoid to their clients.

Poliomyelitis Eradication

In May 1988, the WHA committed WHO to the goal of the global eradication of poliomyelitis by the year 2000 (17). The term "eradication" means that the final objective of this initiative is to reach a stage in which there is no circulation of wild poliovirus. In practical terms, this means that no cases of clinical poliomyelitis are associated with wild poliovirus and no wild poliovirus can be identified through sampling of the environment.

A reported 84% of children in the world have received a full course of polio vaccine before their first birthday. More than 400,000 cases of paralytic poliomyelitis are prevented in developing countries each year. This represents an estimated 79% decrease in paralytic poliomyelitis cases, compared with estimates of cases that would occur annually in the absence of immunization programs at pre-immunization rates of disease. However, an estimated 120,000 paralytic poliomyelitis cases still occur each year (6).

Much has been learned from the experience of poliomyelitis eradication in the Americas, which began a regional eradication initiative in 1985. The number of cases in the Americas has been so dramatically reduced that transmission of wild poliovirus may be completely interrupted in the region in 1991 (see Ref. 3). This experience has permitted the rapid development of poliomyelitis eradication plans of action at global, regional, and country levels. The global plan of action for poliomyelitis eradication emphasizes the following strategies in addition to those common to all of the disease control initiatives (10):

1. Surveillance for acute flaccid paralysis and the development of capabilities for outbreak control;
2. Development of a laboratory network of global, regional, and national reference laboratories through strengthening laboratory capabilities, including training of laboratory personnel, for the isolation and characterization of polioviruses, vaccine quality control, and environmental surveillance for the presence of wild poliovirus;
3. Improvement of poliomyelitis rehabilitation services, particularly through community-based programs; and
4. Promotion of research to develop better eradication strategies, including improved poliomyelitis vaccines, and reliable, rapid diagnostic methods.

The EPI Global Advisory Group recommends trivalent oral poliomyelitis vaccine (TOPV) as the vaccine of choice for poliomyelitis eradication. Routine immunization with TOPV provides individual protection for most recipients and, if high coverage is achieved, markedly reduces the incidence of acute poliomyelitis. However, in many countries, special immunization activities, such as mopping-up operations with the mass administration of TOPV in high risk areas over a short space of time, will be required to displace wild poliovirus and reliably achieve eradication by the year 2000.

Intensified international assistance is required to eradicate poliomyelitis from areas in which transmission remains endemic and local resources are insufficient. This assistance will increasingly be recognized as beneficial to the international community through future savings because of the cessation of production, storage, and administration of poliomyelitis vaccines; the treatment of the disease and its complications; and the avoidance of any adverse reactions to immunization.

INTRODUCTION OF NEW AND IMPROVED VACCINES

There is a large list of additional vaccines, either in existence or under development, that are suitable for widespread use in developing countries. Finding ways to make these vaccines affordable for developing countries is a major challenge. The Children's Vaccine Initiative, enunciated in the Declaration of New York in September 1990, states: "universal immunization will be facilitated by accelerating the application of current science to make new and better vaccines, benefiting children in all countries. These include vaccines which: require one or two rather than multiple doses; can be given earlier in life; can be combined in novel ways, reducing the number of injections or visits required; are more heat stable . . .; are effective against a wide variety of diseases . . . and are affordable."

To date, the main cost of national immunization programs has been the salaries of health staff to give the vaccines, rather than the cost of the vaccines themselves. The cost to immunize a child fully is approximately US$5 to US$15; the cost of the vaccines is less than US$1. Vaccine costs will increase as more expensive new and improved vaccines are introduced.

Hepatitis B vaccine is currently serving as an example of how a relatively expensive vaccine might be introduced. As a means of long-term control of hepatitis B infection, the EPI Global Advisory Group has recommended that all infants be immunized through complete integration of hepatitis B vaccine into routine childhood immunization programs (1, 13). The World Health Organization, UNICEF, and others in the international community are using the Children's Vaccine Initiative to bring such vaccines into general use in developing countries. It will be a great tragedy if hepatitis B and other vaccines, which could have their greatest impact in developing countries, cannot be used in these countries because of cost.

SUPPORT OF OTHER PRIMARY HEALTH CARE PRACTICES

Some 500 million contacts with infants and their mothers occur each year through immunization programs. These contacts can be used to provide other primary health care practices that target infants and women of childbearing age. One example is the assistance of immunization programs in vitamin A and iodine supplementation activities in areas in which deficiencies remain serious problems. The EPI is seeking simplified ways to implement and monitor the provision of such supplements through the contacts afforded by immunization services.

Another example is the teaching module on birth spacing, which was developed jointly by the WHO Divisions of Family Health and Diarrheal and Acute Respiratory Disease Control and the EPI. This teaching module can be introduced into training courses. Other examples of EPI contributions to general primary heatlh care include the development of management skills, problem-solving approaches, logistics systems, training and survey methodologies, and evaluation tools suitable for primary health care use (4).

RESEARCH AND DEVELOPMENT

Research and development activities are a prominent feature of global immunization programs. Such activities have resulted in accomplishments that include improved and alternative energy refrigeration equipment, cold chain monitors, field steam sterilizers, plastic reusable and autodestruct syringes, immunization coverage and missed opportunity survey methodologies, and successful field trials of new vaccines (7, 8, 14, 15).

Continued research and development activities directed at solving operational problems are an important aspect of immunization programs at all levels. High priority areas of research include:

1. Improved disease control strategies: Refining immunization strategies, developing and introducing new or improved vaccines, studying the acceptability of immunization, and studying the delivery of immunization-related services through the primary health care infrastructure.

2. Improved methods and materials for diagnosis of the EPI target diseases and environmental sampling: Making full use of available technology for rapid and simplified diagnosis at field level and identification of wild polioviruses in the environment.

3. Improved surveillance and program monitoring tools: Testing the ability of surveillance system indicators to improve routine surveillance of preventable infectious diseases; developing methods for improving surveillance for

acute flaccid paralysis, neonatal deaths, and rash illness; and determining methods of assessing the effectiveness of mopping up and outbreak response activities.

4. Improved methods and materials for the cold chain and logistic support: Developing and testing refrigeration and injection equipment; conducting and refining studies and surveys on the quality of the cold chain; and investigating technologies and methodologies for improving logistics and transport (including computerized logistics management tools, vehicle maintenance, and driver safety). This research relies extensively on TECHNET, a global network of cold chain and logistic experts who plan and conduct such research (7).

A complete list of priority research needs is periodically reviewed by the EPI Research and Development Group, which meets every six months to monitor progress in immunization program related research (5).

CONCLUSION

The EPI promotes extremely cost effective interventions. The investment in immunization services makes sound economical, epidemiological, and political sense. Disease prevention through immunization reduces not only deaths, but also the need for expensive curative and rehabilitative care. Immunization programs can contribute to building up the health infrastructure from which many other health interventions are more effectively and efficiently promoted. This infrastructure helps provide the health contribution to national development.

Immunization, in both industrialized and developing countries, will continue to be an important element of national health programs as new and improved vaccines become available. Each dollar invested will result in an even greater return in prevented medical care costs, disability, and death.

To these direct benefits are added important indirect benefits: Immunization provides a means of helping break the vicious cycle of high infant and childhood mortality rates. It acts in strong synergy with family planning activities to reduce the total number of births to that which is desired by the family and safe for the mother. This reduction in births further reduces infant and child mortality, as well as maternal mortality. These benefits make the further expansion of immunization services one of the best bargains available for primary health care and national development.

Immunization programs have entered into a new decade filled with exciting challenges. The continued commitment of the international community to help countries meet these challenges will move us all closer to the ultimate vision of a world free of suffering, disability, and death caused by vaccine-preventable diseases.

ACKNOWLEDGEMENTS

The EPI acknowledges the extrabudgetary support of the following donors: the Governments of Australia, Canada, China, Denmark, Finland, Italy, Japan, the Netherlands, Norway, Sweden, Switzerland, the United Kingdom, and the United States of America; the nongovernmental organizations of the Rockefeller Foundation, Rotary International, and Sight and Life; and the international organizations of the United Nations Development Program, UNICEF, and the World Bank.

The author would also like to acknowledge the members of the EPI team who helped prepare this paper: A. Batson, L. Belgharbi, K. Bergstrom, J. Cheyne, C. J. Clements, N. Cohen, P. Evans, A. Galazka, F. Gasse, H. Hull, S. Kingma, T. Kobayakawa, J. Lloyd, V. Mattei, B. Poulsen, S. Robertson, A. Savinykh, R. Scott, C. Torel, C. Voumard, N. Ward, C. Whitman, M. Zaffran, and H. Zoffmann.

Literature Cited

1. Beasley, R. P. 1988. *Hepatitis B Immunization Strategies.* Geneva: WHO
2. Cutts, F. T., Henderson, R. H., Clements, C. J., Chen, R. T., Patriarca, P. A. 1991. Principles of measles control. *Bull. WHO* 69:1–7
3. de Quadros, C. 1991. Polio eradication from the Western Hemisphere. *Annu. Rev. Public Health* 13:239–52
4. Expand. Programme Immun. 1991. *List of Articles in the Weekly Epidemiological Record.* Geneva: WHO
5. Expand. Programme Immun. 1991. *List of EPI Research Topics.* Geneva: WHO
6. Expand. Programme Immun. 1991. *Statistics.* Geneva: WHO
7. Expand. Programme Immun. 1990. *Report of 1990 TECHNET Consultation.* Geneva: WHO
8. Expand. Programme Immun. 1989. *EPI Product Information Sheets.* Geneva: WHO
9. Expand. Programme Immun. 1989. *A Vision for the World: Global Elimination of Neonatal Tetanus by the Year 1995.* Geneva: WHO
10. Expand. Programme Immun. 1988. *Global Poliomyelitis Eradication by the Year 2000.* Geneva: WHO
11. Expand. Programme Immun. 1986. *Evaluation and Monitoring of National Immunization Programmes.* Geneva: WHO
12. Expand. Programme Immun. 1986. *Immunization Policy.* Geneva: WHO
13. Global Advisory Group. 1991. *Report of the Expanded Programme on Immunization Global Advisory Group Meeting.* Geneva: WHO
14. Markowitz, L. 1990. *Measles Control in the 1990s: Immunization Before 9 Months of Age.* Geneva: WHO
15. Patriarca, P. A., Wright, P. F., John, T. J. 1991. Factors affecting the immunogenicity of oral polio vaccine in developing countries: A review. *Rev. Infect. Dis.* In press
16. World Health Assem. 1989. *Resolution 42.32.* Geneva: WHO
17. World Health Assem. 1988. *Resolution 41.28.* Geneva: WHO
18. World Health Organ. and United Nations Child. Fund. 1985. *Joint Statement on Planning Principles for Accelerated Immunization Activities.* Geneva: WHO
19. World Summit Child. 1990. *World Declaration on the Survival, Protection, and Development of Children and Plan of Action for Implementing the World Declaration on the Survival, Protection, and Development of Children in the 1990s.* New York: United Nations

Annu. Rev. Publ. Health 1992. 13:239–52

POLIO ERADICATION FROM THE WESTERN HEMISPHERE[1]

Ciro A. de Quadros, Jon K. Andrus, Jean-Marc Olive, and Carlyle Guerra de Macedo

Pan American Health Organization, Washington, DC 20037

Donald A. Henderson

Office of Science and Technology Policy, Executive Office of the President of the USA; Technical Advisory Group, Expanded Programme on Immunization, Pan American Health Organization, Washington, DC 20037

KEY WORDS: immunization campaign, surveillance, poliomyelitis, paralysis, vaccine

INTRODUCTION

Paralytic poliomyelitis, once so greatly feared, is on the verge of being eliminated from the Western Hemisphere. A 1985 eradication program has helped guide a more recently launched global eradication effort. In addition, oral polio vaccine (OPV), given in large-scale programs, has been essential to this success.

Before 1955, and the licensure of inactivated polio vaccine (IPV), poliomyelitis was a continuing major cause of permanent disability across the world. In the United States alone, more than 20,000 cases of paralytic polio cases were annually reported during the early 1950s (32). From 1955 to 1961, more than 300 million doses of the newly licensed IPV were administered, with a resultant decrease of 90% in the incidence of polio (Figure 1). However, because of the occurrence of induced polio in the spring of 1955,

[1]The US Government has the right to retain a nonexclusive royalty-free license in and to any copyright covering this paper.

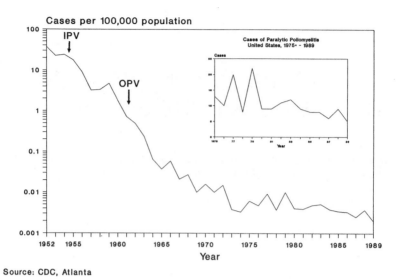

Figure 1   Reported paralytic poliomyelitis in the United States, 1952–1989.

the process of vaccine manufacture had to be changed, thus resulting in a vaccine of substantially lower potency than that which had been used in prelicensure trials (19). Not surprisingly, there was an increase in polio incidence during 1958 and 1959, partly because of the use of low potency vaccine (12). This occurrence gave added impetus to the development of a live, oral polio vaccine, which was introduced in 1961. The OPV was initially a monovalent preparation, but, within three years, a trivalent preparation was substituted. The formulation was based on successful programs in Canada, where investigators used a trivalent OPV preparation comprised, respectively, of 1,000,000, 100,000, and 300,000 TCID50 of the poliovirus types 1, 2, and 3 (36). By 1965, trivalent OPV had completely replaced the monovalent antecedents in the US (40). Since 1965, approximately 20 million doses of trivalent OPV have been administered each year in the US. Since 1968, only 0.5% of the polio vaccine doses applied in the US have been IPV (12).

In 1974, nearly 20 years after polio vaccine was first introduced, the World Health Organization (WHO) established the Expanded Programme on Immunization (EPI) (42). Thereafter, several vaccines were increasingly used. In addition to OPV, there are vaccines against measles and tuberculosis, as well as the familiar diphtheria-pertussis-tetanus vaccine.

This review describes the experience of the program coordinated by the Pan American Health Organization (PAHO) in the Americas. We focus on the OPV, which was first used to control, and then to interrupt, the indigenous transmission of wild poliovirus. In addition, we discuss the choice of vaccine, the polio eradication initiative, the strategies for vaccine delivery, important problems that have been encountered, and the progress achieved thus far.

THE POLIO ERADICATION INITIATIVE

In 1985, 11 years after the EPI was launched, PAHO adopted the goal of polio eradication (8, 29). The stated objective was to interrupt the transmission of wild poliovirus in the Americas by the end of 1990, thereby eradicating the disease. Many public health experts were skeptical that this goal was realistic. Several factors, however, encouraged this decision. Most important was the situation with smallpox (9), which proved that an infectious disease could be eradicated. By 1985, polio incidence had decreased sharply in most countries (Figure 2), and the number of countries reporting cases of poliomyelitis in the Americas had decreased from 19 to 11 (7). Moreover, vaccine coverage levels for polio had reached all-time highs in many countries.

PROGRAM STRATEGIES

General

The overall program called for a three-part strategy: achievement and maintenance of high immunization levels by using OPV, from the smallest geopolitical level, the municipality or county, to the national level; effective surveillance and accurate diagnosis of all cases of acute flaccid paralysis

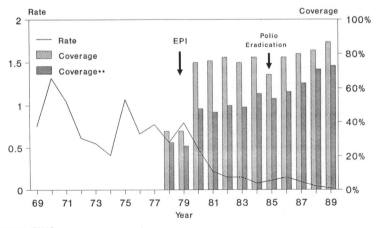

Source: PAHO
•• Excludes Brazil, Mexico, Paraguay,
and Cuba since they use only two doses.

Figure 2 Rate per 100,000 population of reported paralytic poliomyelitis and OPV coverage in children one year of age.

among those individuals under 15 years of age; and area-wide vaccination around all new cases. During the four years since funding became available, this strategy, which uses OPV as the vaccine of choice, has been remarkably successful.

For technical guidance and to provide recommendations crucial for program management, PAHO has established the EPI Technical Advisory Group (TAG), which is composed of five international experts. They meet every six to nine months to review progress and to alter, as necessary, program strategies. The TAG also promotes the understanding and support for program goals among bilateral, multilateral, and private agencies, technical institutions, and political leaders.

To address the financial support issues for implementation of EPI and the polio eradication effort, an Inter-Agency Coordinating Committee (ICC) was created at the regional level. The ICC has representatives from PAHO, UNICEF, the United States Agency for International Development, Inter-American Development Bank, Rotary International, and the Canadian Public Health Association, and the committee has been replicated in each country where representatives from the governments were included. The ICC has demonstrated that diverse organizations can work together to achieve important public health objectives.

Oral Poliovirus Vaccine

The success of OPV in the US, Canada, most European countries, and the USSR, made it a logical choice for use in the Americas (31). Other important reasons to use OPV included the substantially lower cost of OPV compared with IPV; the ability of OPV to induce intestinal immunity, thus facilitating the interruption of wild poliovirus transmission; the capacity of OPV viruses to spread and immunize close contacts; the demonstrated efficacy of OPV in controlling outbreaks; the ease of administration of OPV, a significant advantage in mass campaigns; and the potential ability of OPV viruses to displace the circulation of wild poliovirus in the environment (13, 18, 39).

Investigators recognized that two factors could potentially reduce the effectiveness of OPV programs and that these factors needed special attention. Oral polio vaccine is more heat sensitive than IPV and must be preserved at 0–8° Celsius or lower almost to the time of administration. This required the development and operation of a cold chain for vaccine distribution, which has been achieved. Also, unlike IPV, OPV can cause vaccine-associated paralysis. Studies show, however, that this occurs so infrequently that OPV is a very safe product by any pharmaceutical standards.

The question of the vaccine of choice was explicitly addressed in 1977, and again in 1988, by a select committee of the Institute of Medicine of the National Academy of Sciences, which reaffirmed the validity of the PAHO policy (13, 14). The committee considered the polio immunization policy for the US to determine whether a change to routine use of IPV or IPV followed by OPV was warranted to reduce vaccine-associated paralysis without affecting achievements of the program. Their review showed that, during 1975–1986 in the US, the risk of vaccine-associated acute flaccid paralysis was about one case for every 2.7 million doses of OPV administered. Most cases were associated with the administration of the first dose (20), a risk estimated to be one case for every 560,000 first doses of vaccine. To assess the risks and benefits of each vaccine, a mathematical modeling analysis was performed to estimate risks and benefits over a 30-year period for two cohorts of 3.5 million children each; one cohort would have received OPV, and the other IPV (12). The model assumed periodic importations of wild poliovirus, a coverage rate of 95%, and an efficacy of 98% for both vaccines. The model predicted seven times as many cases of paralytic disease if IPV, rather than OPV, were used. Because of these and other considerations, the committee recommended no change in current US policy (13). However, the committee did recommend that after enhanced IPV combined with diphtheria-tetanus-pertussis (DPT-E-IPV) was licensed, consideration should be given to a regimen of two or more doses of DPT-E-IPV (in place of DPT alone) followed by successive doses of OPV.

Delivery of OPV

When the eradication program began, alternative vaccine delivery strategies were weighed (38). A review was undertaken of the experience of countries in which wild poliovirus transmission appeared to have been interrupted.

Cuba was the first country to undertake organized mass campaigns (37) and the first populous country to interrupt wild poliovirus transmission. Annual campaigns began in 1962, and shortly thereafter paralytic poliomyelitis disappeared (Figure 3). In Cuba, OPV is distributed only during two one-week periods each year with a two-month interval between them. During these periods, OPV is given to all children aged 0–10 years (more recently, 0–5 years), irrespective of immunization status.

Before 1980, the Brazilian Ministry of Health found it impossible to eliminate polio by using a distribution system that relied solely on immunization in the existing health services units (35). Because of the negligible impact on disease incidence in many states, the Ministry decided to inaugurate National Vaccination Days (Figure 4). As in Cuba, the Vaccination Days were organized twice each year with a two-month interval between them. During these days, every child less than five years of age was offered vaccination, regardless of immunization status. Similar strategies were implemented in Chile and Costa Rica where, as in Brazil, the impact on disease incidence was similar to that observed in Cuba (7, 16).

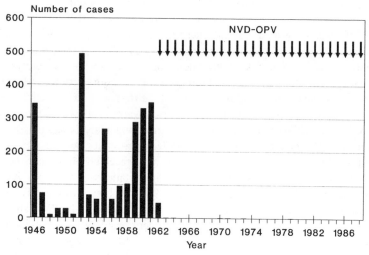

Source: Country Reports to PAHO

Figure 3   Poliomyelitis in Cuba, 1946–1988.

Similar delivery strategies had been previously used by industrialized countries. In the early days of oral polio immunization, the US likewise held campaigns, which were referred to as "Polio Sundays" (32). Through the first three years after OPV licensure, almost all vaccine was utilized in mass vaccination campaigns (3, 5). Subsequently, vaccine was administered as a

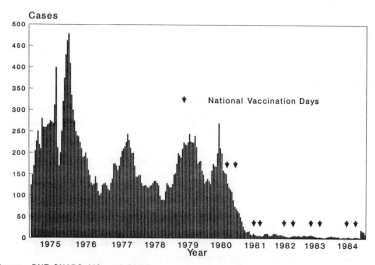

Source: DNE–SNABS, MS, and, PAHO

Figure 4   Polio cases by four-week period in Brazil, 1975–1984.

routine service by health care providers. The transmission of indigenous wild poliovirus appears to have been interrupted in the early 1970s (Figure 5) (15). Only three outbreaks of polio have occurred in the US during the last 15 years. All three outbreaks followed importations, and a total of 40 cases were reported (4). The last case caused by wild poliovirus occurred in 1979 among a religious sect that had refused immunization services. Since 1980, six to ten cases of vaccine-associated polio have occurred each year (Figure 5).

These experiences led PAHO in 1983, two years before its decision to undertake eradication, to state in a position paper that National Vaccination Days should be an integral part of the EPI strategy and that these days should not be a substitute for immunizations offered during routine health care visits (28). The paper recognized that because of existing health care infrastructures in Latin America, the eradication of polio would be impossible, as would satisfactory levels of coverage with the other antigens. The managerial skills acquired in the course of these programs greatly enhanced the capacity of the health service staff to deal with other infectious diseases.

Surveillance

From the inception of the eradication program, surveillance has been a critical strategy for its success (7). Uniform case definitions (Table 1) were adopted by all countries. Surveillance indicators of program performance, especially those relating to the completion and timeliness of case investigations, were established and incorporated as an integral part of the surveillance system (27). By the end of 1989, after the system had been computerized (Polio

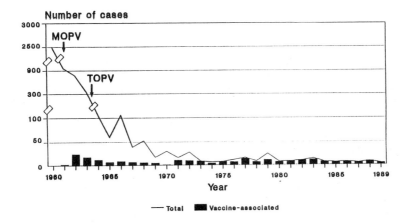

Source: CDC, Atlanta

Figure 5 Reported paralytic polio cases (total, excluding imported cases, and vaccine-associated cases), in the United States, 1960–1989.

Table 1   Case definitions for paralytic poliomyelitis used by PAHO for the Americas, 1985–1989

Suspected case:	Any acute onset of paralysis in a person less than 15 years of age for any reason other than severe trauma, or paralytic illness in a person of any age in whom polio is suspected. This classification is temporary, and within 48 hours the case should be reclassified as probable polio or discarded.
Probable case:	Suspected case with acute flaccid paralysis for which no other cause can be immediately identified. Within ten weeks of onset of paralysis, this case should be reclassified as confirmed polio or discarded.
Confirmed case:	A probable case is classified as confirmed if there is wild-type poliovirus isolated in the stool; epidemiologic linkage to a probable or confirmed case; residual paralysis 60 days after onset; death; or lack of follow-up of a case.

Eradication Surveillance System), analysis of data could be performed at various levels of the health system. The information gained from the analysis of these data has been used to adjust program strategies.

Analysis of the cases throughout the Americas that occurred in 1989 [and subsequently repeated in 1991 (unpublished data)], suggested that some of the 128 polio cases confirmed that year had almost certainly been erroneously classified as confirmed polio, particularly those cases lost to follow-up or who died (1). Compared with wild polio cases, patients who died or were lost to follow-up were likely to be more than five years of age and to be afebrile at the time of onset of paralysis. These patients were also less likely to have had adequate stool specimens taken for virus culture. To increase the specificity of diagnosis, a revised case definition of confirmed polio was decided upon and implemented in 1990: acute flaccid paralysis associated with isolation of wild poliovirus. A separate category, termed "compatible" polio case, included those patients with paralytic illness from whom no wild poliovirus was isolated, but who had clinically compatible residual paralysis at 60 days, had died, or had been lost to follow-up and from whom two adequate stool specimens had not been obtained within two weeks after onset of paralysis. The definition for vaccine-associated cases remained the same, but these cases were separately reported and tabulated.

Accelerated Strategies: The Final Stages

As polio incidence declined to low levels, another strategy, "Operation Mop-up," was incorporated into the eradication program in 1989 (24, 25). Based on the genomic sequencing of strains of wild polioviruses, different wild poliovirus strains apparently occupied distinct geographic areas, and these areas were steadily shrinking in size (6, 34). Moreover, sustained transmission, as with smallpox, appeared to require crowded, lower socioeconomic populations. Accordingly, special house-to-house campaigns were mounted to vaccinate all children less than five years of age who lived in areas considered to be at risk for transmission of disease. Areas at risk were determined by using information on vaccination coverage, previous occurrence of polio cases, population density, and size of migrant population. This special intervention was expected to be a final blow for the interruption of transmission of virus in the few remaining loci.

OTHER ISSUES ENCOUNTERED

The surveillance program, which was greatly strengthened after eradication began, almost immediately identified problems with the vaccine. This was shown in outbreaks of type 3 polio in Brazil in 1986 and in Mexico in 1989. Before the outbreak in Brazil, the formulation of the OPV used was 10^6, 10^5, and $10^{5.5}$ for types 1, 2, and 3 (a 10/1/3 ratio of amounts of types 1, 2, and 3 components in the vaccine), as recommended by WHO (41). The choice for global utilization of the 10/1/3 formulation was based on the results of the original Canadian field trial performed in 1961 (36) and on the subsequent success of programs that used the 10/1/3 formulation ratio, such as those in Canada and the US. However, as pointed out in an extensive review of the subject (31), the reason for choosing such a relatively low dosage of the type 3 component, as compared with the type 1 component, appears questionable, as the infectivity of both types 1 and 3 is almost the same (33). Investigators of the 1986 Brazilian outbreak noted that many of the children who contracted type 3 poliovirus had previously been fully immunized with OPV (30). Because of concern about the vaccine, a field trial was conducted to compare the immunogenicity of different formulations of OPV. This study revealed that children receiving vaccine with a 10/1/6 formulation were almost three times more likely to have a serological response to the type 3 component than children receiving vaccine with the 10/1/3 formulation. As a consequence, PAHO promptly recommended the use of 10^6, 10^5, $10^{5.8}$ for types 1, 2, and 3, a ratio of 10/1/6 formulation, and WHO subsequently followed suit (26).

In Mexico, the 1989 outbreak of 17 cases of polio was also caused by wild type 3 poliovirus, apparently because of vaccine failure. The OPV used in Mexico for routine vaccination is made locally, whereas that customarily used for campaigns is imported. Because many children in the outbreak had previously received more than three doses of vaccine from health service units, this vaccine was tested and found to be of low potency for all three components (unpublished data). Immediate steps were taken to assure that OPV with the 10/1/6 formulation was routinely used throughout Mexico.

As noted previously, it would not be possible to replace OPV with IPV alone. Other strategies propose combining OPV and IPV use (17). Presumably, this would prevent or reduce the frequency of vaccine-associated paralysis (10). Because the greatest risk of vaccine-associated polio occurs after the first dose of OPV (20), investigators have proposed that IPV be given as the first dose of a series, with OPV given subsequently to insure the desired intestinal immunity.

Any change in strategy must not disrupt existing immunization schedules. To assure this, IPV would need to be administered coincident with DPT. To avert multiple injections, the antigens should be incorporated into a single DPT-IPV injection. Such a preparation is available commercially, but, so far, DPT-IPV has been cost prohibitive in the Americas. One dose each of DPT and OPV costs PAHO less than US$0.05, compared with more than US$0.60 for one dose of DPT-IPV. Most countries of the Americas are not currently prepared to assume the burden of a tenfold increase in the cost of vaccines.

PROGRESS OF ERADICATION

In 1989, 128 cases of confirmed poliomyelitis were reported in the Americas, an 86% decline from the 930 confirmed cases reported in 1986. This decline occurred despite better surveillance and a twofold increase in the number of reported cases of acute flaccid paralysis, from about 1000 in 1985 to 2000 in 1989.

As the program progresses, fewer cases of acute flaccid paralysis are determined to be confirmed poliomyelitis. In 1990, over 50% of cases of acute flaccid paralysis 1990 were diagnosed as Guillain-Barré syndrome. Other, less frequent causes were transverse myelitis, tumors, and traumatic neuritis.

The decline in the incidence of paralytic polio was also coincident with greatly improved OPV coverage in young children. In 1978, regional estimates of coverage with three doses of OPV in one-year-old children was 38%. In 1988, coverage estimates were greater than 70%; in 1989, estimated coverage reached 73%. By the end of 1990, immunization coverage for all the EPI vaccines had reached an all-time high: No vaccine was at less than 70%, and levels of 80% were recorded in several subregions, such as the English speaking Caribbean countries and the countries of the Southern Cone (Argentina, Chile, Paraguay, and Uruguay) (21). Although polio vaccination levels should be interpreted with caution, because of changes over time in the methodology for assessing coverage, results such as these are encouraging for the rest of the world.

The 128 confirmed polio cases that occurred in 1989 were located in 99 (0.7%) of the 14,372 counties in Latin America. Of the 128 confirmed cases,

24 were associated with wild poliovirus isolation (7). The cases associated with isolation of wild poliovirus were located in three areas: 13 (all with type 3 isolates) in northwestern Mexico; three with type 3 and six with type 1 isolates in the northern Andean subregion; and two with type 1 isolates in northeastern Brazil. Of the remaining 128 confirmed cases, seven were vaccine associated, 19 were lost to follow-up, ten died, and 60 had clinically compatible residual paralysis, but no poliovirus isolation.

In 1990, there were 18 confirmed cases of poliomyelitis, a 25% decline from the 24 cases with wild virus isolates that occurred in 1989, and a 44% decline from 32 such cases in 1988. The 1990 confirmed cases were located in only two geographic regions: seven in western Mexico and three in neighboring Guatemala; and eight in the northern Andean subregion in the countries of Colombia, Ecuador, and Peru (2, 21, 23). Poliovirus isolates from Mexico and Guatemala were wild type 3, and genomic sequencing indicated that they were genetically linked to one common ancestral focus of infection. The poliovirus isolates from the northern Andean subregion were all type 1 and, unlike the type 3 isolates from Mexico and Guatemala, were genetically unrelated. Apparently, there are separate foci of wild virus transmission in the northern Andean area, which will require more intensive efforts for interruption of transmission. Of the 75 compatible cases that occurred in 1990, 21 were lost to follow-up, 13 died, and 41 had clinically compatible residual paralysis.

Thus far in 1991, there has been six confirmed polio cases with wild type 1 isolated (onset last case April 8) in Colombia. Extensive immunization campaigns have been undertaken in all areas with cases in 1990 and 1991 and in other areas at risk.

In brief, despite progressively improved reporting, as exemplified by yearly increases in the number of cases of acute flaccid paralysis reported, there has been a rapid decline in confirmed cases of polio, reaching record lows each year from 1986 to 1990. By using mass campaigns with OPV as its primary strategy, the program is on the verge of achieving the eradication of polio in the Western Hemisphere.

In July 1990, the International Commission for the Certification of Eradication of Poliomyelitis in the Americas met for the first time to discuss certification procedures (22). The Commission recommended that not only would countries need to document the absence of wild poliovirus circulation by using conventional surveillance procedures, but environmental studies would also be needed. Encouraging results have been reported by utilizing the polymerase chain reaction technique for the direct detection and characterization of polioviruses in sewage samples collected from high risk areas in Brazil. This will be an important new tool for wild poliovirus surveillance in the Americas (unpublished data).

CONCLUSIONS

Although OPV is not a perfect vaccine, it remains one of the cheapest, safest, and easiest of all vaccines to administer. New candidate vaccines derived from existing Sabin strains may potentially improve on safety and immunogenicity (43). Regardless, barring extensive civil disorder or other unforeseen difficulties, the eradication of polio will soon be achieved in the Americas. Progress in the Americas precipitated the May 1988 decision by the 41st World Health Assembly to decide on a goal of global eradication by the year 2000 (11–42, 44). To that end, WHO is recommending the same strategies used in the Americas, including the use of OPV in mass campaigns.

However, several critical questions remain to be answered for the global initiative. Although adequate for the Americas, is the current level of antigenicity of OPV capable of eradicating wild poliovirus transmission in the rest of the world, notably Africa? Is there sufficient political and social will to accomplish such a task? Are the financial and technical resources available to develop and maintain the necessary surveillance and laboratory support systems? How we respond to these questions will decide whether we leave our children the legacy of the eradication of polio.

Literature Cited

1. Andrus, J. K., de Quadros, C. A., Olive, J.-M., Silviera, C. M., Eikhof, R. M., et al. 1990. *Classification and Characteristics of Confirmed Polio Cases, the Americas 1989.* Vlll Meet. of the Tech. Adv. Group on EPI on the Erad. of Polio. in the Americas, (Ref. doc.:EPI/TAG8/90–10. Oral Present.). Mexico City: Pan Am. Health Organ.
2. Cent. for Dis. Control. 1990. Update: Progress toward eradicating poliomyelitis from the Americas. *Morbid. Mortal. Wkly. Rep.* 39:557–61
3. Cent. for Dis. Control. 1982. *Poliomyelitis Surveillance Summary 1980–1981.* Atlanta: Cent. for Dis. Control
4. Cent. for Dis. Control. 1981. *Poliomyelitis Surveillance Summary 1979.* Atlanta: Cent. for Dis. Control
5. Commun. Dis. Cent. 1964. *Poliomyelitis Surveillance.* Rep. no. 283. Washington, DC: US Dep. of Health, Educ., and Welf.
6. da Silva, E. E., Pallansch, M. A., Holloway, B. P., Oliviera, M. J. C., Schatzmayr, H. G., et al. 1991. Oligonucleotide probes for specific detection of wild poliovirus types 1 and 3 endemic to Brazil. *Intervirology*. In press
7. de Quadros, C. A., Andrus, J. K., Olive, J.-M., Silviera, C. M., Eikhof, R. M., et al. 1991. The eradication of poliomyelitis: Progress in the Americas. *Pediatr. Infect. Dis. J.* 10:222–29
8. de Quadros, C. A., de Macedo, C. G. 1989. *The Americas Take the Lead.* Geneva: World Health Organ.
9. Fenner, F., Henderson, D. A., Arita, L., Ježek, Z., Ladnyi, I. D. 1988. *Smallpox and Its Eradication*, pp. 593–625. Geneva: World Health Organ. 1st ed.
10. Henderson, D. A., Witte, J. J., Morris, L., Langmuir, A. D. 1964. Paralytic disease associated with oral polio vaccines. *J. Am. Med. Assoc.* 190:41
11. Hinman, A. R., Foege, W. H., de Quadros, C. A., Patriarca, P. A., Orenstein, W. A., et al. 1987. The case for global eradication of poliomyelitis. *Bull. WHO* 65:835–40
12. Hinman, A. R., Koplan, J. P., Orenstein, W. A., Brink, E. W., Nkowane, B. M. 1988. Live or inactivated poliomyelitis vaccine: An analysis of the benefits and risks. *Am. J. Public Health* 78:291–95
13. Inst. of Med. 1988. *An Evaluation of Poliomyelitis Vaccine Policy options.* IOM Publ. 88-04., pp. 1–50. Washington, DC: Natl. Acad. Sci.

14. Inst. of Med. 1977. *Evaluation of Poliomyelitis Vaccines,* Univ. Microfilms #2004357, pp. 1–75. Washington, DC: Natl. Acad. Sci.

15. Kim-Farley, R. J., Bart, K. J., Schonberger, L. B., Orenstein, W. A., Nkowane, B. M., et al. 1984. Poliomyelitis in the USA. Virtual elimination of disease caused by wild virus. *Lancet* 2:1315–17

16. Leon de Coto, E. M. 1984. Evolution of the poliomyelitis vaccination program in Costa Rica. *Rev. Infect. Dis.* 6(Suppl. 2):S442–43

17. McBean, A. M., Modlin, J. F. 1987. Rationale for the sequential use of inactivated poliovirus vaccine and live attenuated poliovirus vaccine for routine poliomyelitis immunization in the United States. *Pediatr. Infect. Dis. J.* 6:881–87

18. Melnick, J. L. 1978. Advantages and disadvantages of killed and live poliomyelitis vaccines. *Bull. WHO* 56: 21–38

19. Nathanson, N., Langmuir, A. D. 1963. The Cutter incident. Poliomyelitis following the formaldehyde-inactivated poliovirus vaccination in the United States during the spring of 1955. I. Background. II. Relationship of poliomyelitis to Cutter vaccine. III. Comparison of the clinical character of vaccinated and contact cases occurring after use of high rate lots of Cutter vaccine. *Am. J. Hyg.* 78:16–81

20. Nkowane, B. M., Wassilak, S. G. F., Orenstein, W. A., Bart, K. J., Schonberger, L. B., et al. 1987. Vaccine-associated paralytic poliomyelitis, United States: 1973 through 1984. *J. Am. Med. Assoc.* 257:1335–40

21. Pan Am. Health Organ. 1991. *Final Report.* 9th Tech. Adv. Group Meet. in Vaccine-Prev. Dis. Guatemala City, Pan Am. Health Organ.

22. Pan Am. Health Organ. 1990. *Final Report.* 1st Meet. of the Int. Comm. for the Certif. of the Erad. of Polio. in the Americas., Ref. doc: EPI/TAG9/91-REF#4. Washington, DC: Pan Am. Health Organ.

23. Pan Am. Health Organ. 1990. Surveillance of wild poliovirus in the Americas. *EPI Newsl.* 12:1–3

24. Pan Am. Health Organ. 1989. Mop-up operation. *EPI Newsl.* 11(3):3

25. Pan Am. Health Organ. 1989. Operation mop-up. *EPI Newsl.* 11(1):6

26. Pan Am. Health Organ. 1988. *Final Report.* 5th Meet. of the Tech. Adv. Group on Polio Erad. in the Americas. Lima: Pan Am. Health Organ.

27. Pan Am., Health Organ. 1988. *Polio Eradication Field Guide,* Tech. paper No. 6, pp. 1–53. Washington, DC: Pan Am. Health Organ. 2nd ed.

28. Pan Am. Health Organ. Oct. 1987. *EPI Policy and Strategic Approaches in the Americas: A Joint Statement by ICC Member Agencies.* Joint ICC Commun., Ref. doc:HPM/EPI/14100

29. Pan Am. Health Organ. 1985. Director announces campaign to eradicate poliomyelitis from the Americas by 1990. *Bull. Pan Am. Health Organ.* 19:213–15

30. Patriarca, P. A., Laender, F., Palmeira, G., Oliviera, M. J. C., Filho, J. L., et al. 1988. Randomized trial of alternative formulations of oral poliovaccine in Brazil. *Lancet* 1:429–33

31. Patriarca, P. A., Wright, P. F., John, T. J. 1991. Factors affecting the immunogenicity of oral polio vaccine in developing countries: A review. *Rev. Infect. Dis.* 13:926–39

32. Paul, J. R. 1971. *A History of Poliomyelitis.* New Haven: Yale Univ. Press

33. Payne, A. M. M. 1961. Field safety and efficacy of live attenuated poliovirus vaccines. In *Papers and Discussions Presented at the 5th International Poliomyelitis Conference, Copenhagen, Denmark,* ed. M. Fishbein, pp. 257–61. Philadelphia: Lippincott

34. Rico-Hesse, R., Pallansch, M. A., Nottay, B. K., Kew, O. M. 1987. Geographic distribution of wild poliovirus type 1 genotypes. *Virology* 160:311–22

35. Risi, J. B. 1984. The control of poliomyelitis in Brazil. *Rev. Infect. Dis.* 6(Suppl. 2):S400–3

36. Robertson, H. E., Acker, M. S., Dillenberg, H. O., Woodrow, R., Wilson, R. J., et al. 1962. Community-wide use of a "balanced" trivalent oral poliovirus vaccine (Sabin). *Can. J. Public Health* 53:179–91

37. Rodriquez Cruz, R. 1984. Cuba: Mass polio vaccination program. *Rev. Infect. Dis.* 6(Suppl. 2):S408–12

38. Sabin, A. B. 1984. Strategies for elimination of poliomyelitis in different parts of the world with use of oral poliovirus vaccine. *Rev. Infect. Dis.* 6(Suppl. 2):S391–96

39. Sabin, A. B. 1980. Vaccination against poliomyelitis in economically underdeveloped countries. *Bull. WHO* 58:141–57

40. Sutter, R. W., Brink, E. W., Cochi, S. L., Kew, D. M., Orenstein, W. A., et al. 1989. A new epidemiologic and laboratory classification system for paraly-

tic poliomyelitis cases. *Am. J. Public Health* 79:495–98

41. WHO Expert Comm. on Biol. Stand. 1988. *Requirements for Poliomyelitis Vaccine*, 38th Rep. (oral) WHO Tech. Rep. Ser. No. 771. Geneva: World Health Organ.

42. World Health Assem. 1977. *Expanded Programme on Immunization (EPI) in the Americas*, Resolut. WHA30.53. Geneva: World Health Organ.

43. World Health Organ. 1990. Potential use of new poliomyelitis vaccines: Memorandum from a WHO meeting. *Bull. WHO* 68:545–48

44. World Health Organ. 1988. Global eradication of poliomyelitis by the year 2000. *Wkly. Epidemiol. Rec.* 63:161–62

Annu. Rev. Publ. Health 1992. 13:253–68
Copyright © 1992 by Annual Reviews Inc. All rights reserved

HEALTH ISSUES FOR COLLEGE STUDENTS

Kevin Patrick,[1,2] Ted W. Grace,[1] and Chris Y. Lovato[1,3]

[1]Student Health Services, Division of Student Affairs; [2]The University of California, San Diego-San Diego State University General Preventive Medicine Residency Program; and [3]Graduate School of Public Health, Division of Health Promotion, San Diego State University, San Diego, California 92182

KEY WORDS: student health, adolescent health, school health, higher education

INTRODUCTION

This paper addresses issues pertinent to the health of, and health care systems for, college students. We describe characteristics of the college student population, including important subgroups of students with unique health problems. After briefly reviewing the history and current practice of college health services, we address specific health problems and current and future issues for college student health.

INSTITUTIONS OF HIGHER EDUCATION

In 1990, there were more than 3500 colleges and universities in the United States (49), which range in size from the smallest technical and trade schools to comprehensive research universities with enrollments that exceed 50,000 students. Generalizations are difficult, because of the remarkable diversity of institutional morphology, which arises from variations in public or private governance and accountability; student population size, gender, ethnic characteristics, and residential versus commuter status; number and type of graduate, professional, and/or research programs; and the overall financial resource base of the institution.

253

0163-7525/92/0501-0253$02.00

From a public health standpoint, these institutions may be viewed as complex combinations of schools and workplaces in which social, environmental, behavioral, political, economic, legal, philosophical, and cultural issues conspire to create unique and difficult challenges for health promotion, disease prevention, and medical care. In part, this is because of the traditionally open nature of college communities. Colleges and universities are unlike primary and secondary schools, in which the local school district and parents share authority. They are also distinct from traditional workplaces, in which employer-employee relationships, management structures, collective bargaining rules, and other hierarchical processes define issues of authority, accountability, and responsibility.

Post-secondary students come and go. They commonly shift geopolitical jurisdictions because of their education. Although they often need them, students typically are ineligible for public social and human services, the eligibility for which is usually based upon complicated residence, income, and working status requirements. Universities vary tremendously with respect to how much, if at all, they attend to their students' nonacademic needs. Thus, college and university environments exist as extraordinarily complex social systems with nonuniform policies, unstable populations, and a wide range of relationships to the communities in which they are located.

THE COLLEGE STUDENT POPULATION

In the fall of 1988, 13,043,118 students attended colleges and universities in the US (50). Only 57% of these students were 24 years of age or younger, thus dispelling the common misperception that college students are 18–22 years old. Nearly 30% were aged 30 years or older. Overall, 54.6% were female. With regard to ethnicity, 81% were non-Hispanic whites, 9% were blacks, 5% were Hispanics, 4% were Asian/Pacific Islands, and 1% were American Indian; 20% lived in school-owned housing, 50% off-campus, and 30% with parents. Some 38% described themselves as independent.

It is common for college health practitioners to define and characterize subpopulations of students (57). Grouping may be based upon preexisting health status or other shared characteristics on entry, or upon participation, while at the university, in environments associated with risk for health problems. Four important groups are as follows:

Disabled Students

Of the 12.5 million college students enrolled in the fall of 1986, 1,319,229 (10.5%) had at least one disability (51). In 1988, 6% of full-time college freshmen were reported as having at least one disability, which more than doubles the figure for 1978 (47). Over half of these students have "hidden" disabilities, such as learning disorders (27). According to Section 504 of the Rehabilitation Act of 1973, a student qualifies as having a disability if he or she "has a physical or mental impairment which substantially limits one or more major life activity; has a record of such impairment; or is regarded as having such impairment." Common disabilities seen among college students include visual handicaps; deafness and hearing impairment; speech impairment; neurologic and orthopedic handicaps; chronic diseases and conditions, such as asthma, arthritis, lupus, diabetes, and cystic fibrosis; and chronic psychiatric disorders.

International Students

In 1989–1990, there were more than 385,000 international college students (66). The majority came from Asian nations, with China, Taiwan, Japan, and Korea leading the list. Latin America, Europe, the Middle East, and Africa accounted for 11.9%, 9.7%, 6.4%, and 4.8%, respectively, of the international student population. An estimated 35,000 additional students are enrolled in intensive English language programs, which are often attended before official enrollment in a college or university. Although most international students come to the US alone, some bring spouses and children. International students, who have unique ethnic and culture-specific beliefs, present special health needs (6). It is common to have only a few fellow nationals on a given campus at any one time. The sense of isolation felt by such students contributes to, and is often made worse by, illness and its concomitant dependency.

Health Professions Students

The health and health-related professions, such as medicine, nursing, dentistry, dental hygiene, physical therapy, and many of the biologic sciences, account for almost 450,000 students (26). Characterized by learning environments that require either direct patient contact or exposure to blood and patient tissue, such students are unique in their needs and demands for health services. Routine health problems found in this age group may be exaggerated in their incidence and importance because of heightened awareness brought about through study. The prevention and management of communicable diseases, such as tuberculosis, hepatitis B, and human immunodeficiency virus (HIV) infection present major challenges for student health practitioners.

Nontraditional Students

"Nontraditional student" is a term used often and imprecisely, which generally denotes older, part-time, and working students. On some campuses, particularly commuter campuses, they comprise more than half of all students.

However, one must not assume that all students over a certain age, for example 28 or 35, fit into this category. Many older students are full-time students who have left a job, the military, or some other environment to pursue one or more years of study, or they are graduate students in extended length programs. We reserve the term nontraditional student for those students whose primary sphere of activity is away from the campus environment. Depending upon their age and health status, nontraditional students may substantially broaden the range and complexity of health problems seen in a campus health center.

HISTORICAL ASPECTS OF COLLEGE HEALTH

The history of college health practice has been addressed in numerous publications over the past several decades (7, 8, 33, 34, 38, 40). Some historical aspects of college health are of particular relevance to the field of public health. For example, of the many early influences on college health, physical activity and health education were among the most important. This was represented in the early 1800s, through an effort to import the *mens sana in corpore sano* model of fitness from European higher education. Coupled with curricula in what was popularly called "hygiene," at Williams College in 1851 and later in the same year at the City College of New York, students were educated on "the active duties of operative life, rather than those more particularly regarded as necessary for the pulpit, bar, or medical profession" (41).

During the latter half of the 1800s, several colleges and universities opened health centers based upon the sentiment expressed in 1856 by President Stearns of Amherst who noted that "the breaking down of health of students, especially in the spring of the year, which is exceedingly common, involving the necessity of leaving college in many instances, and crippling the energies and destroying the prospects of not a few who remain, is in my opinion wholly unnecessary if proper measures could be taken to prevent it" (22). In 1859, Amherst established a Department of Physical Education and Hygiene, generally regarded as the first college health service. Mount Holyoke and Vassar followed suit in 1861 and 1865, respectively. The health physician at each of these colleges had both clinical and teaching duties. The first "comprehensive" student health care services were probably offered at these two women's colleges. Combining medical services, infirmary care, nursing services, and health promotion activities, these centers carried out almost all aspects of current-day student health services.

The ascendency of public health knowledge and practice from the turn of the century through World War I contributed to college health practice. The federal government turned to Dr. Thomas Storey, Professor and Director of

Hygiene at the City College of New York, to head an agency aimed at allocating federal resources for venereal disease control. Because of his view of the importance of university environments to the control of this problem, Dr. Storey ensured that some of these resources were spent to improve college health practice (7). After World War I, Dr. Storey's influence on college health continued with his 1927 publication, *The Status of Hygiene Programs in Institutions of Higher Education in the United States* (44), which stimulated the development of the first set of recommended practices for college health centers. With an expanding economy and growth in size and number of institutions of higher education, almost 85% of colleges offered some sort of student health service by the early 1950s (34).

COLLEGE HEALTH PRACTICE

Approximately 1500 institutions of higher education, which enroll 80% of the nation's college students, provide some form of organized student health care (39). Student health centers (SHCs) range in size and scope of activity from small, nurse-directed facilities, which provide limited nursing and health educational services to comprehensive health facilities that resemble multi-specialty group practices, some with their own Joint Commission on Accreditation of Healthcare Organizations-accredited hospitals. Three areas of emphasis predominate for SHCs: medical, psychological, and health promotion.

Medical services range from those that address acute problems only to full-spectrum care, including the management of chronic disease (15). Facilitating access to primary medical care is a central rationale for the existence of SHCs. High rates of uninsurance, unfamiliarity with the local community resources and/or how to get to them, and lack of understanding about whom to see if a medical problem develops are traits common to college students. Resource-poor SHCs often give only advice and assistance with access to community providers. On large campuses, the predominant model of SHC medical service is a primary care setting staffed by physicians, nurse practitioners, physician assistants, nurses, medical assistants, and various supporting laboratory, pharmacy and radiologic personnel. Immunization clinics and family planning clinics are common. Some campuses provide dental services, and a few provide optometric care.

Psychological services are an important part of college health practice. These services range from small campuses, which might employ a masters level counselor for crisis intervention and minimal, short-term counseling duties, to large-scale operations staffed by psychologists, psychiatrists, and other mental health personnel. Services might include short-term, individual patient counseling, extended psychotherapy, crisis intervention, rape and sexual assault counseling, initiation and maintenance of psychopharmacologic agents, group therapy, and facilitation for such groups as Alcoholics Anonymous and Adult Children of Alcoholics (59).

Health promotion and health educational services are the third "mainstay" of traditional college health practice. Zapka & Love (65) have stated that there is no arena in which health educational services plays a relatively greater role than in college health settings. Small SHCs usually dispense health education through the nursing staff. In larger SHCs, departments of health education or health promotion exist, staffed by masters or doctoral trained health promotion or health education professionals.

College students visit an SHC an average of two to three times during a school year (39). This level of utilization is somewhat lower than the 3.5 medical visits per year for individuals aged 19–24 noted in the National Health Care Expenditures Survey (60). The lower average number of visits estimated for SHC utilization may result because students are only on campus part of the year, and many have conditions treated electively during the summer or other breaks from school.

Although this paper concentrates on student health issues, it is important to recognize that some institutions extend campus health services to serve staff and/or faculty and occasionally student, staff, or faculty dependents. This becomes important when considering health education and health promotion programing. Smoking and alcohol policies, sexual harassment, and injury control are just a few areas in which comprehensive approaches aimed at the entire membership of the campus community are common.

Student health centers are funded through a combination of fee-for-service, identified (prepaid) health fees, insurance reimbursement, and general university support (39). Some SHCs augment these sources through creative arrangements with state or local health departments, research dollars, or other fund-raising activities. Private colleges are more likely than public institutions to require proof of health insurance before entry. This is also true of health professions schools.

Health services, like most other components of universities, exist as a result of university policy. These policies are extremely important to the day to day operation of health centers, as they dictate everything from health center resource base to hiring policies. Policies and standards, which ultimately govern SHC activities, vary in proportion to the heterogeneity of colleges and universities themselves. Even in states with centrally managed, multisite university systems, such as the California State University or the State University of New York, the actual manifestations of uniform student health service policies may differ. The reasons for this difference include the proximity of the campus to other medical or health resources, academic offerings of the campus (e.g. nursing or medical schools), local financial and programatic interpretation of central policy, administrative recognition and support of student health needs, and advocacy on the part of students themselves for health care.

Since 1964, the American College Health Association has offered recommended standards for SHCs to use to develop externally valid and consistent programs. Revised on a periodic basis, most recently in 1991, these standards address clinical, mental health, health promotion, environmental health, and support services, as well as ethical and professional issues (2).

HEALTH PROBLEMS OF COLLEGE STUDENTS

Only one study in the recent medical or public health literature examines the types of problems encountered in student health centers (19), although some studies do address issues in specific subpopulations (18, 63). The lack of such data is an important public health problem, because its absence can lead medical and public health professionals to the conclusion that relatively few, and only minor, health needs occur among college students. Lack of information can also lead to poor planning for health services delivery. A wide range of acute and chronic health problems, which represents a substantial burden of morbidity and mortality, does occur among college students.

Acute health problems include genitourinary, respiratory, or gastrointestinal infections. Outbreaks of vaccine-preventable diseases, such as measles, mumps, and rubella, continue on college campuses (61, 62). Nearly two thirds of sexually transmitted disease cases occur among persons under 25 years of age (13), many among college students. Sexual assault of college students is common: One study suggests that one of six female college students were victimized by rape or attempted rape within the preceeding year (30). Dermatologic conditions, musculoskeletal problems, and minor trauma, including sprains, fractures, and lacerations, are commonly seen in student health centers.

Injuries account for up to half of all deaths for those aged 10 to 24 years (53, 64), although with respect to college and university populations these statistics can be misleading. As stated earlier, only about 57% of the current college population fall into the "typical" 18–24 age range. Also, certain causes of death, such as homicide, are clearly more common in nonstudent groups.

Some chronic medical problems begin as a new event in the 18–24 age group, whereas others carry over from childhood. Seizure disorders, migraine headaches, bronchial asthma and other atopic disorders, type I insulin-dependent diabetes, arthritis, inflammatory bowel disease, and peptic ulcer disease are just a few of the diseases encountered on a regular basis in student health facilities. Some cancers occur more frequently in college-age populations. Acute leukemias, Hodgkin's disease, testicular neoplasms, and malignant bone tumors, such as osteogenic sarcomas, are more common in adolescents and young adults. More than 50% of all cases of acquired immunodeficiency syndrome (AIDS) are diagnosed in persons aged 25 to 39. A seroprevalence survey among university students reported one positive result per 500 students tested, or 0.2% (21).

Student health centers serve a growing number of students with serious physical and psychological disabilities, such as patients with Down's syndrome, muscular dystrophy, cerebral palsy, trauma-induced neurologic deficits, and cystic fibrosis. Mental health problems, including stress and situational reactions, anxiety and panic disorders, sexual identity and dysfunctional problems, personality disorders, schizophrenia, and major depressive disorders, often begin during the college years.

HEALTH RISK BEHAVIORS

A series of behavioral, developmental, and environmental issues, which recur throughout the above set of health problems and concerns for college students, contribute to premature morbidity and mortality and reduced quality of life for college youth. From a public health and preventive medical perspective, these factors may be enumerated and addressed. Although they may be considered separately, it is essential to understand their interrelated nature.

Alcohol Use

Alcohol use is the single most important public health problem for college students. Alcohol intoxication may be associated with up to 25% of all deaths in college-aged students (42). Heavy drinking episodes (five or more drinks) are more prevalent among college youth than their same age peers (54). Of injury-related deaths among persons aged 15–24, 75% are caused by motor vehicle accidents, and nearly half of all motor vehicle accidents involve alcohol (14). Besides motor vehicle accidents, alcohol abuse is closely related to other social and health problems of college students. On college campuses, alcohol consumption is related to two thirds of all violent behavior, almost half of all physical injuries, a third of all emotional difficulties, and 30% of all academic problems (25).

Tobacco and Other Drugs

Although the rate of daily cigarette use among college students is lower than among the general population (13% versus 26%), nearly one in four college students smokes at least one cigarette per month (54), which suggests that they are experimenting with the substance and are at risk of addiction. Daily smoking rates are estimated at 9% for men and 15% for women (54). The concurrent use of tobacco and oral contraceptives among many women in this age group places them at higher risk of developing heart disease and cancer, in addition to the other negative health consequences of tobacco consumption.

College students have an annual prevalence rate for marijuana use equal to their noncollege-age peers (35%), and a lower rate of daily marijuana use (1.8% versus 4.8%, respectively). Although other drug use among college students tends to be lower than among their same-age peers, the difference varies according to type of drug. Annual prevalence rates for any illicit drug other than marijuana is 19% for those enrolled in college versus 24% for high school graduates in the same age group (54).

Sexual Behavior

Reportedly, 78% of adolescent girls and 86% of adolescent boys have engaged in sexual intercourse by age 20 (52). The relationships of sexual behaviors to alcohol and drug use, stress, and developmental and cultural issues are a Gordian knot for researchers and practitioners in the field of college health. Sexually transmitted diseases, unintended pregnancy, and worry over these problems are the daily fare of college health centers.

An assessment of the prevalence and risk factors for HIV among college students suggests that, although the overall prevalence of infection is low and confined to high-risk groups, the occurrence of behaviors that facilitate sexual transmission of HIV is high (31). Although college students appear to be knowledgeable about HIV infection, they have not adequately adopted preventive behaviors (28). One survey of college students found that only 25% of men and 16% of women always used a condom during sexual intercourse (32). However, condom use does appear to have increased minimally among college students in recent years (17).

Unintended pregnancy continues to be a serious, and often life-changing, problem among college women, although a review of the recent medical and public health literature reveals no reports of pregnancy rates specific to college student populations. Cumulative evidence suggests that a substantial proportion of sexually active college students do not use contraceptives (17, 46). Alcohol and drug use has been associated with unprotected/unsafe sexual practices. A recent survey of freshman at 14 US colleges indicated that one of six students reported engaging in unplanned sexual activity after drinking alcoholic beverages (58).

Suicide and Stress

Suicide is the third leading cause of death among youth aged 15–24, and the second leading cause of death among young white men in the same age group. Young women attempt suicide unsuccessfully approximately three times more often than their male counterparts (52). The causes of suicide are multiple and complex; however, substance abuse and severe stress in school or social life have been linked to suicide among youth (55). The college years represent a time of transition from adolescence to adulthood, and from more structured environments to independent living situations. Coping and adapting to this transition coincides with emotional and often psychologically traumatic experiences, as well as life-style changes that can have lifetime consequences.

Nutrition and Physical Activity

During the college years, adolescents and young adults develop health habits that put them at greater risk for the development of many chronic diseases, including cardiovascular disease, cancer, and osteoporosis. Dietary habits and physical activity are primary risk factor areas subject to change during the college years. Stephens et al (43) have suggested that the most dramatic reduction in physical activity levels occurs between the ages of 18 and 24. There is increasing epidemiologic evidence to support a positive relationship between physical activity and physical health, and a similar relationship apparently exists between physical activity and mental health (9).

Diet is linked to heart disease and cancer, yet American eating habits do not reflect our current level of knowledge (16). The college years represent a time during which there are likely to be unique barriers (e.g. resources, skills, and facilities) that limit college students' ability to maintain healthful eating habits. The intense academic and social pressures of campus life may increase the risk for development of an eating disorder, such as binge-eating, purging, and dieting (45).

UNIQUE ISSUES FOR THE FIELD OF COLLEGE HEALTH

To complete the picture of college health in this country, we address some final issues.

Nonstandard Age Definitions for Adolescence and Youth

One of the most important barriers to the development of coherent health programs for college-age youth is that of differing definitions of "adolescence" and "youth." Without commonly agreed upon standards for these terms, it is virtually impossible to collect meaningful morbidity and mortality data; develop, compare, and evaluate programs aimed at addressing health issues of adolescents and youth; or even create appropriate policies aimed at health promotion, disease prevention, and medical care. Age grouping permeates everything in medicine and public health, from medical practice arrangements to research agendas to journal publications. Some age groupings for adolescence end at 17 or 18 years (48). Others extend to 24 years. For example, the United Nations' definition of "youth" or "young people" encompasses the age limits 15 to 24 years (4). Similarly, the World Health Organization's definition of adolescence has raised the upper age limit to 24 years, or about the time of total socioeconomic independence (4).

Three recent reports on adolescent health have avoided addressing the health issues of college-age youth. The Congressional Office of Technology Assessment's April 1991 report on adolescents limited its scope to those aged 10 through 18 years (48). The American Medical Association acknowledged the importance of barriers to health care access faced by those aged 19 to 24, but excluded them from its report (20). Finally, preliminary data from the National Center for Health Statistics on the health care utilization patterns of adolescents covers only those aged 11 to 20 years (35). It is difficult not to conjecture that the reason young adults were ignored in these reports is that unique data for them is sparse and confusing. In an environment in which information on adolescents and young adults is either not collected at all, or collected in nonstandard ways, it can easily appear that few problems exist.

Responsibility, Accountability, and Perceptual Issues

One of the largest "cracks" in the way our society handles health problems is that confronted by adolescents and young adults as they transit from the sphere of authority and responsibility of their family-of-origin and move into that of their own family and workplace. Who is responsible for the health of the 22-year-old emancipated college student with a part-time job in the service industry: the student, his/her parents, the college, the student's employer, the community in which the student lives, or some combination of these?

The "structure" of our health care system does not yield an answer to this question. Our discipline-bound perspectives in public health and medicine only confound the issue. Organized medicine has overlooked the college student population in the past, probably because of the limited economic incentives in such a traditionally "healthy" group. This has contributed to the rising concern over the competency of health care professionals to meet the health needs of young people (5). School health, a traditional area of public health practice, is almost always considered to address only those issues relevant to preschool through 12th grade students. Public health practice, on the other hand, tends to focus upon defined disadvantaged and underserved populations in governmental jurisdictions. College students are not included when planning these services, even in the face of profound shifts in their social and demographic characteristics.

Students covered by their parents' insurance policies are usually only eligible through age 22 or 23, and many lack insurance (37). A recent survey in California found that up to 30% of students had no medical insurance (10). Experience on our campus suggests that another 30% have only partial health insurance coverage. Temporary status in low-skilled labor positions does not provide insurance for self-supporting students. Also, even though most adolescents and young adults do not incur great expenses for health care during any given year, average expenditure data can be misleading. One study found that 10% of adolescents with the highest expenses accounted for 65% of all out-of-pocket expenses (36). Given that college is now commonly a five- to seven-year undertaking, with variable amounts of time "off" to either join the temporary workplace or to pursue individual interests, questions of responsibility are very complicated indeed.

DIRECTIONS FOR THE FUTURE OF COLLEGE HEALTH

Several current, anticipated, and necessary developments are likely to shape the future of college health theory and practice.

Healthy People 2000

Healthy People 2000: National Health Promotion and Disease Prevention Objectives for the Year 2000 specifically addresses college student health as follows: "Increase to at least 50% the proportion of postsecondary institutions with institution-wide health promotion programs for students, faculty, and staff" (52). Postsecondary institutions, including two- and four-year community colleges, private colleges, universities, and trade and technical schools, have been identified as settings in which many 18- to 24-year-olds can be reached. Currently, there are no reliable national estimates of the proportion of postsecondary schools that offer institution-wide health promotion programs. A survey of 3000 postsecondary institutions conducted by the American College Health Association in 1989–1990 suggests that at least 20% of the institutions surveyed offered health promotion activities for students (1). It is encouraging that *Healthy People 2000* recognizes young people as a special population that, in many cases, experiences higher rates of morbidity, disability, and mortality than the general population (3).

Comprehensive College Health and the Integration of School Health, College Health, Worksite Health, and Public Health Promotion

A comprehensive approach to college health requires the integration of programs and services similar to that which is now advocated for school health. College communities share many characteristics with K–12 schools. Traditional school health, including only health instruction and clinical health services, is expanding to incorporate five additional areas: integrated school and community health promotion efforts, physical education, food service, counseling, and health promotion programs for faculty and staff (29). College health practice is likely to expand similarly. A framework for the development of campus-based health programs would include environmental, biomedical, behavioral, and organizational interventions (23). However, as we noted earlier, the unique, independent, and often balkanized nature of college campuses will make such logical and coherent approaches difficult.

The first step should be measurable success in community health promotion—combined educational, social, and environmental actions aimed at a population in a geographically defined area (23). In college communities, these actions may be directed at high-risk students, special interest groups, faculty and staff, and/or the entire campus community. Models of comprehensive college health must be developed and tested. Because the college community plays an essential role in the day-to-day lives of students and because it is oftentimes the only stable environment to which a college student relates, the college community is uniquely situated to accomplish this.

To complement the development and implementation of comprehensive college health practice, it is essential to coordinate and articulate college health promotion, disease prevention, and medical service activities with similar activities in schools, worksites, and the public health sector. Outcomes desired from each enterprise are the same. We are a long way, however, from a common vision, which unifies theory or clear policies that provide for meaningful working relationships among all of these sectors.

Increased Recognition and Understanding of College Student Health Issues

The most critical step in attaining appropriate recognition for college student health needs is the development of a common language for data relevant to adolescents and young adults. This must be a joint undertaking of representatives from the college health community; representatives from adolescent health, public health, pediatrics, internal medicine, family practice, school health, psychiatry, psychology, nursing, other health care sciences; and representatives from governmental health, education, and welfare agencies. A set of agreed-upon age groupings, definitions, and terms must be developed so that uniform data on morbidity, mortality, health, social, and economic status of adolescents and young adults can be collected, aggregated, and reported.

The development of a common language will facilitate research into the determinants of health and illness in college students, including the creation and maintenance of surveillance systems aimed at tracking important health risk behaviors. This should become standard practice for public health professionals.

Finally, research into the relationships between health and academic performance is needed. In one study of a university that had an 8.5% overall attrition rate, and a 25% loss of freshmen after the first year, health-related problems were found to be a leading cause of school drop-out (12). At the University of California, Berkeley, over 25% of the students who withdraw list health as a reason for doing so (56). These reports notwithstanding, there is a dearth of quality research on the relationships between health status, academic performance, undergraduate or graduate education completion rates, and ultimate career success.

CONCLUSION

Public health professionals should become familiar with the unique health problems of college students and the potential that college communities have as environments for health promotion and disease prevention. In addition, the question of responsibility for the health of college students must be addressed, as they are among the most likely groups to be uninsured. President Nils Hasselmo of the University of Minnesota has proposed a seventh principle to be added to six principles for campus life, which was recently published by the Carnegie Foundation for the Advancement of Teaching (11): "A college or university is a healthy community, one in which personal and public health is an accepted institutional commitment, backed by policies and programs that apply the knowledge we have acquired" (24). This statement is an extremely productive starting point. However, continued dialogue must occur among representatives of higher education, public health, the medical community, local, state, and federal government, and other sectors of society with a stake in the health of youth.

Literature Cited

1. Am. Coll. Health Assoc. 1991. *Health Promotion on Campus: Resource & Referral Directory.* Rockville, Md: Am. Coll. Health Assoc.
2. Am. Coll. Health Assoc. 1991. *Recommended Standards for a College Health Program.* Rockville, Md: Am. Coll. Health Assoc. 5th ed.
3. Am. Med. Assoc. 1990. *Healthy Youth 2000: National Health Promotion and Disease Prevention Objectives for Adolescents* Excerpted from the US Public Health Service's *Healthy People 2000: National Health Promotion and Disease Prevention Objectives.* Chicago: Am. Med. Assoc.
4. Bennett, D. L. 1985. Young people and their health needs. A global perspective. *Semin. Adolesc. Med.* 1:1–14
5. Blum, R. W., Bearinger, L. H. 1990. Knowledge and attitudes of health pro-fessionals toward adolescent health care. *J. Adolesc. Health Care* 11:289–94
6. Bowen, P. A., DeArmond, M. 1991. College health care for international students. See Ref. 57. In press
7. Boynton, R. E. 1971. The first fifty years: A history of the American college health association. *J. Am. Coll. Health* 19:269–85
8. Boynton, R. E. 1962. Historical development of college health services. *Stud. Med.* 10(3):294–305
9. Brown, D. R. 1990. Exercise, fitness, and mental health. In *Exercise, Fitness and Health: A Concensus of Current Knowledge,* ed. C. Bouchard, R. J. Shepard, T. Stephens, J. R. Sutton, B. D. McPherson, pp. 607–26. Champaign, Ill: Human Kinetics
10. Brown, R. E., Valdez, R. B., Morgan-stern, H., Bradley, T., Hafner, C. 1987.

Californians Without Health Insurance: A Report to the California Legislature. Berkeley: Univ. Calif.

11. Carnegie Found. for the Adv. of Teach. 1990. *Campus Life: In Search of Community.* Lawrenceville, NJ: Princeton Univ. Press

12. Cavendish, J. M., Morgan, E. J. 1990. Health service utilization by non-returning freshman. Abstract of a scientific program. *J. Am. Coll. Health* 39:38

13. Cent. for Dis. Control. 1990. Div. of STD/HIV Prev. *Sexually Transmitted Disease Surveillance 1989,* Atlanta: US Dept. Health Hum. Serv., Public Health Serv.

14. Cent. for Dis. Control. 1984. Temporal patterns of motor vehicle-related fatalities associated with young drinking drivers: United States, 1983. *Morbid. Mortal. Wkly. Rep.* 33:699–701

15. Christmas, W. 1991. Medical services for college health. See Ref. 57. In press

16. Crawford, P. 1988. The nutrition connection: Why doesn't the public know? *Am. J. Public Health* 78(9):1147–48

17. DeBuono, B. A., Zinner, S. H., Daamen, M., McCormack, W. M. 1990. Sexual behavior of college women in 1975, 1986 and 1989. *N. Engl. J. Med.* 322(12):821–25

18. Ebben, A. J., Blankenship, E. S. 1986. A longitudinal health care study: International versus domestic students. *J. Am. Coll. Health* 34:177–82

19. Fingar, A. R. 1989. Patient problems encountered at a student health service. *J. Am. Coll. Health* 38:142–44

20. Gans, J. E., McManue, M. A., Newacheck, P. W. 1991. *Adolescent Health Care: Use, Costs, and Problems of Access.* Chicago: Am. Med. Assoc.

21. Gayle, H. D., Keeling, R. P., Garcia-Tunon, M., Kilbourne, B. W., Narkunas, J. P., et al. 1990. Prevalence of the human immunodeficiency virus among university students. *N. Engl. J. Med.* 323:1538–41

22. Ginsburg, E. L. 1955. *The College and Student Health.* New York: Natl. Tuberc. Assoc. From Allen, N. 1869. *Physical Culture in Amherst College,* Lowell, Mass: Stone & Huse

23. Green, L. W. 1991. *Community Health.* Boston: Mosby. 6th ed.

24. Hasselmo, N., Robb, G. M. 1991. A university president's perspective on college health. See Ref. 57. In press

25. Held, S. E., Black, D. R., Tappe, M. K., Babrow, A. S., Tiffany, S. T., et al. 1990. *Alcohol Consumption on a University Campus: A Public Health Con-*

cern. Presented at the annu. meet. Soc. of Behav. Med., Chicago

26. Hembrie, W. C. 1991. Unique health care needs of health science students. See Ref. 57. In press

27. Hidden Disabil: Inf. from HEATH (Higher Education and Adult Training for People with Handicaps). Spring 1989. 8(1):7

28. Keeling, R. 1991. Human immunodeficiency virus disease in the college population. See Ref. 57. In press

29. Kolbe, L. J. 1986. Increasing the impact of school health promotion programs: Emerging research perspectives. *Health Educ.* 17(5):47–52

30. Koss, M. P., Gidycz, C. A., Wisniewski, N. 1987. The scope of rape: incidence and prevalence of sexual aggression and victimization in a national sample of higher education students. *J. Clin. Consult. Psychol.* 55:162–70

31. Kotloff, K. L., Tacket, C. O., Clemens, J. D., Wasserman, S. S., Cowan, J. E., et al. 1991. Assessment of the prevalence and risk factors for human immunodeficiency virus Type 1 (HIV-1) infection among college students using three survey methods. *Am. J. Epidemiol.* 133(1):2–8

32. MacDonald, N. E., Wells, G. A., Fisher, W. A., Warren, W. K., King, M. A., et al. 1990. High-risk STD/HIV behavior among college students. *J. Am. Med. Assoc.* 263:3155–59

33. Means, R. K. 1975. *Historical Perspectives on School Health.* Thorofare, NJ: Slack

34. Moore, N. S., Summerskill, J. 1954. *Health Services in American Colleges and Universities, 1953: Findings of the American College Health Association Survey.* Ithaca, NY: Cornell Univ. Press

35. Nelson, C. 1991. *Office Visits by Adolescents.* Adv. data from vital and health stat: No. 196. Hyattsville, Md: Natl. Cent. for Health Stat.

36. Newacheck, P. W., McManus, M. A. 1990. Health care expenditure patterns for adolescents. *J. Adolesc. Health Care* 11:133–40

37. Newacheck, P. W., McManus, M. A., Brindis, C. 1990. Financing health care for adolescents: Problems, prospects, and proposals. *J. Adolesc. Health Care* 11:398–403

38. Patrick, K. 1991. The history and current status of college health. See Ref. 57. In press

39. Patrick, K. 1988. Student health: Medical care within institutions of higher education. *J. Am. Med. Assoc.* 260 (22):3301–5

40. Raycroft, J. E. 1940. *History and Development of Student Health Programs in Colleges and Universities.* Proc. 21st Annu. Meet., Am. Stud. Health Assoc., Ann Arbor, Mich.

41. Rogers, J. F. 1936. *Instruction in Hygiene in Institutions of Higher Education.* Washington, DC: US Dep. of the Inter., Off. Educ., p. 3.

42. Schwartz, R. H. 1989. Alcohol-related injuries and objective screening tests. *J. Am. Coll. Health* 38:49–53

43. Stephens, T., Jacobs, D. R., White, C. C. 1985. A descriptive epidemiology of leisure-time physical activity. *Public Health Rep.* 100(2):147–58

44. Storey, T. E. 1927. *The Status of Hygiene Programs in Institutions of Higher Education in the United States.* Stanford: Stanford Univ. Press

45. Striegel-Moore, R. H., Silberstein, L. R., Frensch, P., Rodin, J. 1989. A prospective study of disordered eating among college students. *Int. J. Eating Disord.* 8(5):499–509

46. Swinford, P. 1991. Pregnancy, contraception, and issues of sexuality for college students. See Ref. 57. In press

47. Am. Counc. of Educ. 1989. *The American Freshman: National Norms for Fall, 1988.* Los Angeles: Univ. of Calif.

48. US Congr. Off. of Technol. Assess. 1991. *Adolescent Health, Vol. 1: Summary and Policy Options,* p. 2, OTA-H-468. Washington, DC: GPO

49. US Dep. Educ., Natl. Cent. for Educ. Stat. 1991. *Digest of Education Statistics, 1990,* Table 218, p. 230. Washington, DC: GPO

50. US Dep. Educ. 1990. See Ref. 49, Table 174, p. 183

51. US Dep. Educ. 1990. See Ref. 49, Table 193, p. 202

52. US Dep. Health Hum. Serv., Public Health Serv. 1991. *Healthy People 2000: National Health Promotion and Disease Prevention Objectives.* (PHS) 91-50213. Washington, DC: GPO

53. US Dep. Health Hum. Serv., Public Health Serv. 1988. *Disease Prevention/ Health Promotion: The Facts.* Palo Alto, Calif: Bull Publishing

54. US Dep. Health Hum. Serv., Public Health Serv. Alcohol, Drug Abuse and Mental Health Adm. 1989. *Drug Use, Drinking, and Smoking: National Survey Results from High School, College, and Young Adult Populations 1975–1988.* DHHS 89-1638. Washington, DC: GPO

55. US Dep. Health Hum. Serv., Public Health Serv. Alcohol, Drug Abuse and Mental Health Adm. 1989. *Report of the Secretary's Task Force on Youth Suicide.* (ADM) 89–1624. Washington, DC: GPO

56. Univ. Calif. at Berkeley. 1991. *Promoting Student Success at Berkeley: Guidelines for the Future.* Berkeley: Univ. of Calif. Press

57. Wallace, H. M., Patrick, K., Parcel, G. S., Igoe, J., eds. 1991. *Principles and Practices of Student Health.* Oakland, Calif: Third Party Publishing. In press

58. Wechsler, H., Isaac, N. 1991. *Alcohol and the College Freshman: "Binge" Drinking and Associated Problems.* Rep. to the AAA Found. for Traffic Safe. Boston: Harvard Sch. Public Health

59. Whittaker, L. 1991. Mental health services for college health. See Ref. 57. In press

60. Wilensky, G. R., Bernstein, A. 1983. *Contacts With Physicians in Ambulatory Settings: Rates of Use, Expenditures, and Sources of Payment: National Health Care Expenditures Survey.* PHS 83-3361. Washington, DC: US Dep. Health Hum. Serv.

61. Williams, W. W., Markowitz, L. E., Cochi, S. L., Hawkins, C. E., Rovira, E. Z., et al. 1987. Immunizations in college health: The remaining tasks. *J. Am. Coll. Health* 35:252–60

62. Williams, W. W., Sosin, D. M., Kaplan, K. M., Hersh, B. S., Preblud, S. R. 1989. Vaccine-preventable diseases on college campuses: The emergence of mumps. *J. Am. Coll. Health* 37:197–203

63. Winer, J. A., Dorus, W. 1972. Complaints patients bring to a student mental health clinic. *J. Am. Coll. Health* 21:134–39

64. World Health Organ. 1989. *The Health of Youth. Technical discussions,* A42. Geneva: WHO

65. Zapka, J. G., Love, M. B. 1986. College health services: Setting for community, organizational, and individual change. *J. Am. Coll. Health* 35:81–91

66. Zikopoulos, M., ed. 1990. *Open Doors: 1989/90, Report on International Educational Exchange.* New York: Inst. Int. Educ.

Annu. Rev. Publ. Health. 1992. 13:269–85

MORTALITY OF AMERICAN INDIAN AND ALASKA NATIVE INFANTS[1]

Everett R. Rhoades, George Brenneman[2], Jerry Lyle[3], and Aaron Handler[4]

Indian Health Service, Rockville, Maryland 20857

KEY WORDS: Native Americans, Indian Health Service, fetal alcohol syndrome, sudden infant death syndrome

INTRODUCTION

The incidence rates and patterns of certain diseases and conditions in American Indians and Alaska Natives often prove useful in understanding the nature of these conditions (5, 37, 42, 45, 52). This may also be true for infant mortality. In this review, we examine infant mortality data for American Indians and Alaska Natives and compare these data with those for the general US population. In some instances, comparisons between Indian groups are made. Because excellent general discussions of infant mortality are available (7, 28, 29, 53), in most instances we cite only references to American Indians and Alaska Natives. For convenience, we use the term "Indian" to denote those persons commonly identified as American Indians and Alaska Natives. The Indian Health Service (IHS), its relationship with the various tribes, the sovereign nature of the tribes, and the changing health conditions of Indians have recently been described (16, 38–40).

[1]The views expressed are the views of the authors and are not intended to represent official US Public Health Service policy. The US Government has the right to retain a nonexclusive royalty-free license in and to any copyright covering this paper.
[2]Maternal and Child Health Branch
[3]Programs for Children with Special Needs
[4]Demographic Statistics Branch

DIFFICULTIES IN CALCULATING INDIAN DEATH AND DISEASE RATES

Confounding factors that accompany enumerations of vital events relating to Indians dictate caution in drawing conclusions. For example, the heterogeneity and complexity of tribal groups and organizations, and the small size of many tribes, make accurate data collection difficult and expensive and often limit general conclusions. On the other hand, many differences are sufficiently large that errors of sampling are less important. For example, death rates for certain conditions are severalfold greater for Indians than for the general population (18); thus, conclusions can be made with sufficient confidence to permit program planning and design. When intergroup differences are not so great, however, considerable caution is advised and special care is required to avoid erroneous conclusions. To compensate for the small numbers in many communities, the IHS averages vital event rates for three years centered in the year being studied. Other problems arise from identification and reporting variations, which in some instances are quite large. *Trends in Indian Health* (18), an annual publication, presents the sources of IHS vital event and health data and discusses the care to be taken in their interpretation.

To establish baseline denominator numbers, estimates of the total US Indian population are made during the decennial censuses, which enumerate individuals who identify their race as American Indian, Eskimo, or Aleut. From these data, and from annual birth and death counts reported on state vital records, the IHS projects the number of Indians who are eligible for IHS services. For this purpose, the IHS utilizes the number of self-identified Indians who reside in counties "on or near" federal Indian reservations in the 33 "reservation states" in which the IHS has health care responsibilities. These counties make up the IHS service area and contain the Indian population thought to most nearly approximate the population that utilizes IHS services. This IHS service area population differs from both statewide (reservation states) and national Indian populations, and failure to distinguish between these populations can lead to confusion. The number of both counties and reservation states continually changes as Indian tribes receive federal recognition and as tribes add members to their rolls. As a result of such changes, Connecticut, Rhode Island, and Texas in 1983, and Alabama in 1984, were designated as reservation states. Between 1980 and 1990, the IHS added 58 counties to the IHS service area. Of the 3150 counties and independent cities in the United States, 505, or 16%, now make up the IHS service area. As of October 1989, there were an estimated 1,780,000 Indians residing in the United States. Of these, 1,642,000, or 92%, resided in the reservation states and 1,105,000, or 62.1%, resided in the IHS service area. As a result, there are more than 500,000 Indians who may be included in tabulations of state or national data, but are not included in analyses of those living in the IHS service area. Also, estimates include all persons reported as American Indian and Alaska Native, not just those eligible for IHS services by virtue of belonging to tribes that have federal recognition. Only statewide vital event data are available before 1972, so the IHS utilizes this data base to project trends back to 1955.

The accuracy of the decennial census in enumerating certain groups has often been questioned. Passel (33) found that the 1970 census estimates of the number of American Indians under 20 years of age could have been as much as 6.9% too low. However, for all ages there was a net "overcount" by as much as 67,000 between the 1960 and 1970 censuses. Some of this variation arose from differences in racial self-identification, which suggests that many Indians were reported as white on their birth certificates and on the 1960 census, but their designation was changed to Indian during the 1960s. In addition, racial designation was completed by enumerators in most rural areas of the US during the 1960 census, whereas self-identification was used to report race during the 1970 census. Recent trends suggest that the number of persons identifying themselves as Indian is increasing, and the 1990 census is expected to add a substantial number of newly identified Indians. This will increase the denominator, thus adding another confounding factor to an already difficult field of study.

For most routine vital event analyses, the IHS utilizes data for Indians compiled by the National Center for Health Statistics (NCHS) from state birth and death records (18). Norris & Shipley (31), who examined California data, found considerable variation in the identification of race between the birth and death certificates of Indian infants. Of 148 Indian infants identified by race of either parent on birth records, 90, or 60.8%, were coded as white on the death certificate. Use of the birth cohort method caused an increase in the calculated rate for Indians from 13.9/1000 to 29/1000. Staub and coworkers (46), who examined data for the Cattaraugus Reservation in New York, found that Indian children were often registered at birth as Caucasian and that the recorded number of Indian births for the reservation might actually be falsely low, which possibly caused a falsely high mortality rate. Examination of every tenth state birth record of a group of 84 Cattaraugus children disclosed that of the nine records studied, five newborns were recorded as American Indian and two as white; no record could be found for the other two. Similar results were reported for Indians in Washington State by Frost & Shy (6) and in Oklahoma by Kennedy & Deapen (20).

In summary, Indians are a heterogeneous population that is organized into small groups; live in arbitrarily defined geopolitical areas; and comprise several subsets of populations that identify themselves, or are variously identified, as Indian. The lack of congruence between the several population subsets, including those receiving services from the IHS, is not surprising.

These reporting and identification variations influence the size of both the numerator and the denominator, with obvious effects on calculated vital event rates.

EFFORTS TO IMPROVE CALCULATIONS OF INFANT MORTALITY

To provide more detailed characteristics of infant deaths and more accurate estimates of infant mortality rates among ethnic minorities, the NCHS began to match birth and infant death files, beginning with the national 1983 birth cohort. Kleinman (21), who used 1983 and 1984 cohort data, found that differences in classification of race on birth and death certificates were less than 2% for whites and blacks, but 25–40% for Indians and Asians. By calculating infant mortality rates according to race of mother, he found that, throughout the US, Indians had a mortality rate of 14.3/1000 and a relatively low neonatal mortality rate of 6.9/1000; but, they had the highest postneonatal mortality rate (7.4/1000) of all racial groups studied. Handler & Macken (9) reviewed the race of parents on reservation state birth certificates of newborns who had at least one parent reported as Indian for calendar years 1972–1987. They calculated the 1987 Indian infant mortality rate for reservation states to be 12.3/1000 if only the mother's race were used to identify Indian births, compared with 9.8/1000 if both parents' race were used. Because the latter cohort group most nearly resembles the IHS service area population, the IHS proposes to use linked data, when available, thus considering the identification of race of both parents for most program purposes. In the future, the IHS intends to publish Indian infant mortality data by using two criteria for identifying Indian births: race of the mother only (the NCHS criteria) and race of either parent reported as Indian.

INDIAN INFANT MORTALITY

Table 1 shows the aggregate infant mortality rates for Indians within the IHS service area for 1976 to 1987 from unlinked death records. Each year's rates represent a three-year average centered on the year shown. In 1976, the Indian infant mortality rate was 20.1/1000 live births. By 1987, it had fallen to 11.1/1000, a decrease of 45%. During this interval, the infant mortality rate for US all races declined from 15.2/1000 to 10.1/1000, a decrease of 34%. The Indian neonatal death rate fell from 9.8/1000 to 5.1/1000, a decrease of 48%; the postneonatal death rate fell from 10.3/1000 to 6.0/1000, a decrease of 42%.

Figure 1 illustrates the leading causes of Indian infant deaths, compared with US all races. The first six leading causes of Indian infant deaths under one year of age are the same as those experienced by US all races, although in a slightly different order of ranking.

Table 1 Number and rate of American Indian and Alaska Native infant deaths by age. IHS service areas, 1976–1987 (unlinked birth/death records)[a]

Twelve IHS Areas for mid year of 3-year period	Births[b]	Infant Deaths[b]			Infant Death Rate		
		Total	Neonatal	Postneonatal	Total	Neonatal	Postneonatal
1987	91,903	1017	469	548	11.1	5.1	6.0
1986	89,534	1007	475	532	11.2	5.3	5.9
1985	87,575	967	440	527	11.0	5.0	6.0
1984	86,404	966	444	522	11.2	5.1	6.0
1983	84,811	983	436	547	11.6	5.1	6.4
1982	79,712	994	428	566	12.5	5.4	7.1
1981	74,407	965	421	544	13.0	5.7	7.3
1980	67,583	999	464	535	14.8	6.9	7.9
1979	63,591	997	488	509	15.7	7.7	8.0
1978	59,022	1009	507	502	17.1	8.6	8.5
1977	55,553	1016	495	521	18.3	8.9	9.4
1976	51,729	1041	509	532	20.1	9.8	10.3

[a] Source: Division of Program Statistics, OPEL, IHS.
[b] Three-year totals.

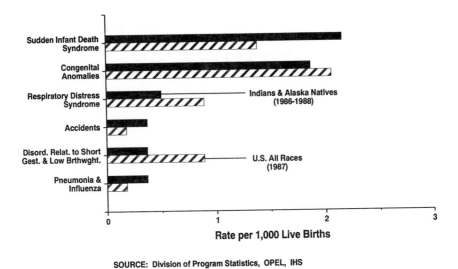

SOURCE: Division of Program Statistics, OPEL, IHS

Figure 1   Leading causes of Indian infant deaths under one year of age compared with US all races, 1987 (unlinked data from "Reservation States").

The leading causes of Indian neonatal deaths are congenital anomalies, disorders relating to short gestation and low birthweight, respiratory distress syndrome, sudden infant death syndrome (SIDS), effects of maternal complications of pregnancy, and infections specific to the perinatal period (Figure 2). Although there are differences between Indians and US all races in the rates of each cause, the rank order is the same, except for the higher ranking of SIDS for Indians. The distribution of leading causes of postneonatal deaths is quite different between the Indian and the US all races population, as shown in Figure 3. The significance of SIDS for both Indians and the US all races is striking, followed by congenital anomalies, accidents and adverse effects, pneumonia and influenza, meningitis, and septicemia. The conditions in which there is an "excess" of Indian deaths compared with the US all races are SIDS, accidents and adverse effects, pneumonia and influenza, and meningitis. In 1987, SIDS was responsible for more than 39% of all postneonatal Indian infant deaths, and the Indian rate was 1.5 times than that for US all races.

INFANT MORTALITY RATES BY IHS AREA

Not surprisingly, considerable variation in infant mortality rates exists between IHS areas (17), with a low of 8.3/1000 in the Albuquerque area to a high of 19.8/1000 in Aberdeen (Table 2). In California and Oklahoma, where reporting differences are known to be large, the rates are considered unreli-

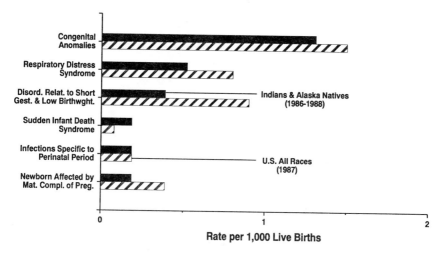

Rate per 1,000 Live Births

SOURCE: Division of Program Statistics, OPEL, IHS

Figure 2 Leading causes of Indian deaths under 28 days compared with US all races, 1987 (unlinked data from "Reservation States").

ably low. The differences between the low rates in the Southwest, compared with the Central Plains and Northwest, are striking. For example, the 1987 average infant mortality rate of the Albuquerque, Phoenix, Tucson, and Navajo areas was 11.0/1000, compared with an average of 17.2/1000 for Billings and Aberdeen. The mortality rate of the latter two areas even exceeds that of 14.7/1000 for the Alaska area.

Similar differences exist in neonatal death rates: The highest is 7.9/1000 in the Aberdeen area, compared with 4.6/1000 in the Navajo area. In 1987, the average postneonatal death rate for the Navajo, Albuquerque, Tucson, and Phoenix areas was 5.3/1000, compared with 10.5/1000 for Aberdeen and Billings. Thus, the excess mortality experienced in the Northern Plains is especially marked in the postneonatal period, and the single most important cause is SIDS. Again, neonatal and postneonatal data for California and Oklahoma are considered unreliable.

The infant mortality experience for Navajos has not always been favorable. In 1970, Brenner and coworkers (3) reported that the infant mortality rate for Navajos born on the reservation was 31.5/1000. Almost one-half occurred in the neonatal period. These authors found that hospital records were superior to death certificates for identifying the cause of death. They state that "there were numerous instances in which the primary cause of death listed on the death certificate was grossly inconsistent with hospital chart observations." In 1969, Van Duzen and coworkers (49) reported that 616 children were suffering from malnutrition at the Tuba City, Arizona, facility. Of these children,

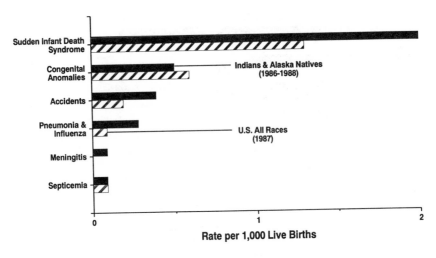

SOURCE: Division of Program Statistics, OPEL, IHS

Figure 3   Leading causes of Indian deaths 28 days to under one year compared with US all races, 1987 (unlinked data from "Reservation States").

15 were diagnosed as having kwashiorkor, and 29 had marasmus. The authors concluded that malnutrition contributed to the mortality of these Navajo children.

In recent years, the development of a strong maternal and child health (MCH) program has greatly increased the accuracy of reporting Navajo infant deaths. Ross (41) found that both prenatal and postpartum visits increased after the 1969 institution of a nurse midwife program. This program seemed to be associated with a decrease in length of hospitalization and improved infant mortality rates.

FACTORS CONTRIBUTING TO INDIAN INFANT MORTALITY

Historical Review

In 1970, Hill & Spector (11) found that about 8% of liveborn Indian infants weighed 2500 g or less, compared with 7% for whites and 14% for nonwhites. The 1967 infant mortality rate was 32.2/1000 for Indians, 19.7 for whites, and 35.9 for nonwhites. The authors reported that the infant mortality of Indians had declined nearly 50% since 1955, compared with a decline of 16% for both whites and nonwhites. Neonatal death rates of Indians were about the same as for whites, but Indian postneonatal death rates were four times higher than that for whites. Wallace (51) reported that the 1967 Indian infant mortality rate was 34.5% higher, and the postneonatal rate three times

Table 2 Number and rate of American Indian and Alaska Native infant deaths by IHS area, 1987 (unlinked birth/death records)[a]

	Infant Deaths[b]			Infant Death Rate		
	Total	Neonatal	Postneonatal	Total	Neonatal	Postneonatal
All IHS areas	1017	469	548	11.1	5.1	6.0
Aberdeen, SD	158	63	95	19.8	7.9	11.9
Alaska	122	59	63	14.7	7.1	7.6
Albuquerque, NM	36	24	12	8.3	5.5	2.8
Bemidji, Minn.	63	27	36	12.8	5.5	7.3
Billings, Mont.	67	25	42	14.6	5.4	9.1
California	40	14	26	7.1	2.5	4.6
Nashville, Tenn.	28	16	12	11.9	6.8	5.1
Navajo	173	79	94	10.1	4.6	5.5
Oklahoma City	98	53	45	6.0	3.2	2.8
Phoenix, Ariz.	108	53	55	10.8	5.3	5.5
Portland, Ore.	98	43	55	11.6	5.1	6.5
Tucson, Ariz.	26	13	13	14.9	7.4	7.4

[a] Source: Division of Program Statistics, OPEL, IHS.
[b] Total number of deaths, 1986–1988.

higher, than that of the US general population. By using data from the National Infant Mortality Surveillance, Vanlandingham and coworkers (50) compared relative risks of mortality between Native Americans and white infants in Alaska, Arizona, Montana, New Mexico, North Dakota, and South Dakota, where the major proportion of nonwhite, nonblack infants were Native American. The infant mortality rate among Native Americans was 15.3/1000 live births, compared with 8.7/1000 among whites. These authors confirm the variations that exist in different surveys and reporting systems. They also confirm the importance of infections and SIDS in postneonatal deaths of Indians. Hirschhorn & Spivey (12), who examined data from 1965 through 1971, found that the infant mortality rate of White Mountain Apaches was 76/1000 live births, compared with 32/1000 for all Indians and 22/1000 for US all races. The proportion of low birthweight for Apaches was approximately 10%, compared with 8% for the general population. Given the low socioeconomic conditions prevailing in many Indian communities, one might expect a higher infant mortality rate than has been found by either the IHS or the NCHS. In 1983, Sullivan & Beeman (47) reported that Indians in Arizona experienced less prenatal care, higher incidence of newborn problems, a higher rate of communication problems with providers, and considerably less satisfaction with the care received. Honigfeld & Kaplan (14) pointed out that several factors contribute to the excess Indian postneonatal deaths, and essentially all of them related to the low socioeconomic conditions in which many Indians live. The authors recommended that programs to lower postneonatal mortality should focus on promoting prompt health care and preventing accidents and other postneonatal health problems. However, Nutting et al (32), who studied the effect of the establishment of a MCH program on the Papago reservation in Arizona, found that the greatest effect of the program was on the group "who sought and received reasonably good care prior to the program" and that the group most at risk did not derive the expected benefits of the program.

Low Birthweight and Prematurity

Comparisons of low birthweight between Indians and US all races are shown in Figure 4. Of births to Indians under the age of 15, 7.4% are low birthweight, compared with nearly 14% of births to the same age group for US all races. This predisposition to larger babies continues until age 25–29, during which the occurrence of low birthweight babies is almost the same for both groups. The ratios are reversed after age 30–34, when US all races mothers slightly exceed Indian women in producing "normal" weight newborns. This difference is offset by the greater number of Indian births in mothers under age 24. Of Indian births in reservation states in 1987, 19% occurred among women under age 20, compared with only 12.4% of the US all races births in

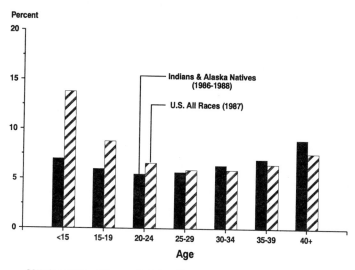

SOURCE: Division of Program Statistics, OPEL, IHS

Figure 4   Incidence of low birthweight (<2500 g) Indian newborns as a percent of total live births, by age of mother, compared with US all races, 1987 (unlinked data from "Reservation States").

this age group (18). This difference was not present in the linked birth/death calculations of Kleinman (21), who found that Indians had a low birthweight rate of 62/1000 live births, compared with 56/1000 for whites and 127/1000 for blacks.

Iba et al (15) confirmed the importance of genetic and environmental factors in low birthweight babies; when these factors were considered, lack of prenatal care was significantly associated with low birthweights and newborn deaths. Adams and coworkers (1) identified two different populations of low birthweight Indian infants: those who were part of a "normal" distribution and those who belonged to a group that they termed "deviant" low birthweight. They pointed out sharp tribal differences in the makeup of each group.

Congenital Anomalies

Indian Health Service data suggest that congenital anomalies play a slightly smaller role in Indian infant mortality than in US all races infant mortality. However, Lynberg & Khoury (26), who used linked birth/infant death data, found that infant deaths associated with birth defects were highest for American Indians (2.9/1000), compared with Asians and Hispanics (2.6/1000) and blacks (2.5/1000). American Indians also had the highest incidence rate of major defects: 22.0/1000 compared with 18.0/1000 for blacks and 19.0/1000 for whites. Lowry and coworkers (25), on the other hand, found a lower frequency of congenital defects in British Columbia Indians than in the general population. Niswander and coworkers (30) reported that Indians experienced more cleft lip and palate and polydactyly and a lower frequency of clubfoot and central nervous system malformations compared with Caucasians. They also found considerable variation in the rates of congenital malformations between Indian groups.

Although data are incomplete, there is a strong suggestion that fetal alcohol syndrome (FAS) contributes to infant mortality (24, 48). This syndrome, which is defined as a pattern of mental retardation, facial deformities, and growth failure that occurs in fetuses and infants who were exposed to alcohol in utero, results in a higher than expected number of fetal deaths during pregnancies of alcohol-abusing women (35). Estimates of the incidence of FAS in the general population vary greatly, ranging from one to three cases per 1000 live births (35). Among Indians of the Southwest, the incidence is reported to vary from 1.3/1000 to 10.3/1000 live births (27). Fetal alcohol syndrome is an important issue because it is currently the most common preventable cause of congenital anomalies.

Sudden Infant Death Syndrome

The cause of this prominent contributor to infant mortality, especially in the postneonatal period, is not known, and many aspects are incompletely understood (43). Among Indians, SIDS causes 40% of postneonatal deaths and may currently be considered the most significant cause of Indian infant mortality. In Kleinman's (21) linked studies, the SIDS rate for Indians was nearly three times higher than for whites. SIDS is also differentially distributed among Indian populations, as it is especially prevalent in the northern parts of the US. Recent suggestions of a possible relationship to tobacco smoking (2, 4, 8, 13, 22) are of special interest in view of the known high rates of smoking in the same IHS areas where SIDS is most prevalent (23, 34, 44). Shannon & Kelly (43) describe several epidemiologic factors that increase the risk of SIDS: "If the mother is less than 20 years of age, unmarried, poor, if she has delayed or failed to seek prenatal care, had a short interval between pregnancies, been ill during pregnancy, or had previous fetal loss, or if she has smoked cigarettes, or abused narcotics. The risk is also increased if the father is less than 20 years old or of low social or economic level. . . . In the United States, where the overall risk is about 2.0 cases per thousand, Asians have the lowest risk, and American Indians, Alaska Natives, and poor Blacks have the highest." Kraus and coworkers (23) found that variables with a high degree of discriminatory power for sudden unexplained death were age of the mother, total number of children born alive, birthweight, multiple birth, duration of prenatal care, and sex of the infant. For Indians, the most important discriminating variable was birthweight, but for whites it was the age of the mother. Kaplan and coworkers (19) were unable to confirm a significantly greater incidence of SIDS among Oklahoma Indians compared with the non-Indian population.

Injuries

In 1987, accidents constituted the fourth leading cause of death among Indians under one year of age in the reservation states. The death rate (0.4/1000) is twice that for US all races infants, with differences especially noticeable in the postneonatal period. Indian male infants are more likely to die of injuries than are Indian females, a situation somewhat at variance with that for US all races infants, among whom gender differences are less striking. The mortality rate of Indian male infants associated with motor vehicle injuries is more than four times greater than that for US all races male infants (22.6/100,000 compared with 5/100,000) (18).

Homicide

In 1987, the homicide rate for those less than one year of age was 12.2/ 100,000, with males affected approximately three times more often than females (18.8/100,000 compared with 5.6/100,000, respectively). Comparable rates for US all races (both sexes) were 7.4/100,000 (males, 7.9; females, 6.4/100,000). The rate of homicides among male Indian infants is more than two times greater than that for US all races males (18). The estimates of Indian infant death rates from injuries and homicide would undoubtedly be higher if linked birth/death records were employed.

IHS MATERNAL AND CHILD HEALTH PROGRAM

From its inception in 1955, the IHS has emphasized attention to maternal and child health as the most efficient way to deal with general Indian health. The specific goal is to provide a wide range of health promotion services that relate to childbearing and to the female reproductive cycle, including family planning, in comprehensive, community-oriented programs carried out through both the general program and certain special MCH activities. Programs include well-child surveillance, special programs for the developmentally disabled, and services for chronically and acutely ill patients. Emphasis is placed on early prenatal and postpartum care. Health education and prevention activities, such as immunizations, are stressed, and immunization levels of Indian children regularly exceed those for the general population.

In 1991, the IHS will expend an estimated $218,000,000 for all services related to maternal and child care, including prevention of infant mortality. This is approximately 17% of the $1,275,000,000 appropriated for IHS clinical services and includes $2,100,000 for special projects aimed at defining the problem of FAS and implementing programs to decrease its incidence. Another special program is the utilization of bacterial polysaccharide immune globulin combined with vaccine to control the unusually high prevalence of invasive *Hemophilus influenzae* type b infections in certain Alaskan and southwestern United States communities.

In December 1989, in response to amendments to PL 94-437, the Indian Health Care Improvement Act (36), the IHS developed a plan to further reduce infant mortality (G. Brenneman and J. Lyle 1989, unpublished data). This multidisciplinary plan is being updated and will focus on the objectives in *Healthy People 2000* (10). The plan places primary responsibility in each IHS area office to strengthen existing MCH programs, cooperate with the Bureau of Indian Affairs in efforts to deal with FAS, and reduce the number of teen pregnancies. The beneficial collaboration with the Indian Health Committees of the American Academy of Pediatrics and the American College of Obstetrics and Gynecology will be continued. Each IHS area office will establish multidisciplinary and interagency infant and maternal mortality review teams. Information and recommendations from the American Academy of Pediatrics Postneonatal Infant Mortality Project will be incorporated into the program as appropriate. Because of both the importance of injuries as a cause of death among Indians and advances in injury prevention, the IHS formalized a Community Injury Prevention program in the early 1980s, which is located in the IHS Office of Environmental Health and Engineering. A full-time coordinator was appointed with authority to oversee the development of multidisciplinary approaches to decrease the number of injuries among American Indians. Several elements of this program have already been successful. In 1990, approximately 30,000 students participated in an annual safety poster contest. In 1987, a unique training fellowship, in conjunction with Yale University, was established to provide training for selected field employees. This training includes special epidemiologic projects and the design of prevention programs, which are then implemented by the fellows. A memorandum of agreement with the Centers for Disease Control provides funding for competitive grants to support innovative community injury control programs. An active education program is coupled with distribution of car restraints for infants in virtually all service units.

The improvement in infant mortality since 1955 represents a major achievement and remains impressive, regardless of the techniques used to calculate infant mortality (9, 18). Unfortunately, the previously steady downward trend in infant mortality slowed by 1981 and, by 1983, had leveled off. An important unanswered question is whether there is a difference in the infant mortality rates of Indians who receive care in the IHS compared with those who do not. Such a comparison would be extremely difficult and costly with present data systems.

SUMMARY

Accurate determination of infant mortality rates among Indians is seriously hampered by variations in the identification of Indian persons and use of different subsets of the Indian population for various purposes. Lack of consistency in the reporting of racial origin on birth and death records is a source of substantial error. Because of these factors, more than the usual care must attend comparisons and inferences drawn from data in which these differences are present. At present, it would seem prudent to regard all data about American Indians as provisional. Even though Indian infant mortality remains higher than that for US all races, regardless of techniques used for estimates, the decline of Indian infant mortality by more than 80% since the establishment of the IHS is a truly remarkable achievement. This success has been ascribed to a combination of activities, including the provision of safe drinking water, especially as an integral part of the IHS program; the nearly universal immunization of Indian children; and emphasis upon comprehensive, community-oriented programs focused on maternal and child care. These successes have contributed to changes in the distribution of the leading causes of Indian infant mortality, so that the most prominent causes now are SIDS, congenital anomalies, injuries, and various infections. Because of these changes and advances in knowledge, the IHS has recently revised its five-year plan for dealing with infant mortality to provide greater attention to injuries and infections and has embarked upon a series of discussions with the American Academy of Pediatrics to address postneonatal deaths and the difficult problem of SIDS. Low socioeconomic conditions, so important in influencing mortality rates (7, 14, 29), have thus far proved to be intractable. In the meantime, success will depend upon ensuring optimal prenatal care, reducing those risk factors amenable to correction, and solving the problem of SIDS.

ACKNOWLEDGMENTS

We are grateful to the late Dr. Joel Kleinman for his review and helpful advice.

Literature Cited

1. Adams, M. S., MacLean, C. J., Niswander, J. D. 1968. Discrimination between deviant and ordinary low birth weight: American Indian infants. *Growth* 32:153–61

2. Bergman, A. B., Wiesner, L. A. 1976. Relationship of passive cigarette-smoking to sudden infant death syndrome. *Pediatrics* 58:665–68

3. Brenner, C., Reisinger, K. S., Rogers, K. D. 1974. Navajo infant mortality, 1970. *HSMHA Health Rep* 89:353–59

4. Bulterys, M., Kraus, J. F., Greenland, S., Nourjah, P. 1987. A nested case-control study of maternal cigarette smoking during pregnancy and sudden infant death syndrome. *Am. J. Epidemiol.* 126:744–45 (Abstr)

5. Freeman, W. L., Hosey, G. M., Diehr, P., Gohdes, D. 1989. Diabetes in American Indians of Washington, Oregon, and Idaho. *Diabetes Care* 12:282–88

6. Frost, F., Shy, K. K. 1980. Racial differences between linked birth and infant

death records in Washington State. *Am. J. Public Health* 70:974–76

7. Graham, G. G. 1985. Poverty, hunger, malnutrition, prematurity, and infant mortality in the United States. *Pediatrics* 75:117–25

8. Haglund, B., Cnattingius, S. 1990. Cigarette smoking as a risk factor for sudden infant death syndrome: A population-based study. *Am. J. Public Health* 80:29–32

9. Handler, A., Macken, C. 1990. *The Impact of the Decision by NCHS to Revise Its Presentation of Natality Data by Race on American Indian and Alaska Native Natality and Infant Mortality Rates.* US Dep. HHS, Public Health Serv., IHS

10. *Healthy People-Goals for the Nation for the Year 2000.* 1991. US Dep. HHS, Public Health Serv. Washington, DC: GPO (PHS) 91-50212

11. Hill, C. A. Jr., Spector, M. I. 1971. Natality and mortality of American Indians compared with US whites and nonwhites. *HSMHA Health Rep.* 86:229–46

12. Hirschhorn, N., Spivey, G. H. 1972. Health and the White Mountain Apache. *J. Infect. Dis.* 126:348–50

13. Hoffman, H. J., Damus, K., Hillman, L., Krongrad, E. 1988. Risk factors for SIDS. Results of the National Institute of Child Health and Human Development SIDS Cooperative Epidemiological Study. *Ann. NY Acad. Sci.* 533:13–30

14. Honigfeld, L. S., Kaplan, D. W. 1987. Native American postneonatal mortality. *Pediatrics* 80:575–78

15. Iba, B. Y., Niswander, J. D., Woodville, L. 1973. Relation of prenatal care to birth weights, major malformations, and newborn deaths of American Indians. *HSA Health Serv. Rep.* 88:697–701

16. Indian Health Serv. 1989. *A Comprehensive Health Care Program for American Indians and Alaska Natives.* US Dep. HHS, Public Health Serv. 650-884/09008. Washington, DC: GPO

17. Indian Health Serv. 1990. *Regional Differences in Indian Health—1990.* US Dep. HHS, Public Health Serv., IHS

18. Indian Health Serv. 1991. *Trends in Indian Health.* US Dep. HHS, Public Health Serv., IHS

19. Kaplan, D. W., Bauman, A. E., Krous, H. F. 1984. Epidemiology of sudden infant death syndrome in American Indians. *Pediatrics* 74:1041–46

20. Kennedy, R. D., Deapen, R. E. 1991. Differences between Oklahoma Indian infant mortality and other races. *Public Health Rep.* 106:97–99

21. Kleinman, J. C. 1990. Infant mortality among racial/ethnic minority groups, 1983–1984. *Morb. Mortal. Wkly. Rep.* 39:31–39

22. Kleinman, J. C., Pierre, M. B. Jr., Madans, J. H., Land, G. H., Schramm, W. F. 1988. The effects of maternal smoking on fetal and infant mortality. *Am. J. Epidemiol.* 127:274–82

23. Kraus, J. F., Franti, C. E., Borhani, N. O. 1972. Discriminatory risk factors in post-neonatal sudden unexplained death. *Am. J. Epidemiol.* 96:328–33

24. LaDrague, P. 1901. Alcoolisme et enfants. These pour le doctorat en medicine, ed. G. Steinheil, Paris. Cited in Petrakis, P. L. 1987. Alcohol and Birth Defects: The Fetal Alcohol Syndrome and Related Disorders. *DHHS Publ. No. ADM 87-1531.* Washington, DC: GPO

25. Lowry, R. B., Thunem, N. Y., Silver, M. 1986. Congenital anomalies in American Indians of British Columbia. *Genet. Epidemiol.* 3:455–67

26. Lynberg, M. C., Khoury, M. J. 1990. Contribution of birth defects to infant mortality among racial/ethnic minority groups, United States, 1983. *Morb. Mortal. Wkly. Rep.* 39:1–12

27. May, P. A., Hymbaugh, K. J., Aase, J. M., Samet, J. M. 1983. Epidemiology of fetal alcohol syndrome among American Indians of the Southwest. *Soc. Biol.* 30:374–87

28. Morb. Mortal. Wkly. Rep. 1989. National Infant Mortality Surveillance (NIMS). US Dep. HHS, Public Health Serv. Cent. Dis. Control 38:1–46

29. Nersesian, W. S. 1988. Infant mortality in socially vulnerable populations. *Annu. Rev. Public. Health* 9:361–77

30. Niswander, J. D., Barrow, M. V., Bingle, G. J. 1975. Congenital malformations in the American Indian. *Soc. Biol.* 22:203–15

31. Norris, F. D., Shipley, P. W. 1971. A closer look at race differentials in California's infant mortality, 1965–1967. *HSMHA Health Rep.* 86:810–14

32. Nutting, P. A., Barrick, J. E., Logue, S. C. 1979. The impact of a maternal and child health care program on the quality of prenatal care: An analysis by risk group. *J. Community Health* 4:267–79

33. Passel, J. S. 1976. Provisional evaluation of the 1970 census count of American Indians. *Demography* 13:397–409

34. Peterson, L. P., Leonardson, G., Wingert, R. I., Stanage, W., Gergen, J., Gilmore, H. T. 1984. Pregnancy com-

plications in Sioux Indians. *Obstet. Gynecol.* 64:519–23

35. Petrakis, P. L. 1987. *Alcohol and Birth Defects: The Fetal Alcohol Syndrome and Related Disorders.* DHHS Publ. No. ADM 87-1531. Washington, DC: GPO

36. PL 94-437, The Indian Health Care Improvement Act (25 U.S.C. 1601 et seq), as amended by PL 100-713, The Indian Health Care Amendments of 1988

37. Rhoades, E. R. 1990. The major respiratory diseases of Ameican Indians. *Am. Rev. Respir. Dis.* 141:595–600

38. Rhoades, E. R., D'Angelo, A. J., Hurlburt, W. B. 1987. The Indian Health Service record of achievement. *Public Health Rep.* 102:356–60

39. Rhoades, E. R., Hammond, J., Welty, T. K., Handler, A. O., Amler, R. W. 1987. The Indian burden of illness and future health interventions. *Public Health Rep.* 102:361–68

40. Rhoades, E. R., Reyes, L. L., Buzzard, G. D. 1987. The organization of health services for Indian people. *Public Health Rep.* 102:352–56

41. Ross, M. G. 1981. Health impact of a nurse midwife program. *Nurs. Res.* 30:363–66

42. Samet, J. M., Key, C. R., Hunt, W. C., Goodwin, J. S. 1987. Survival of American Indian and Hispanic cancer patients in New Mexico and Arizona, 1969–82. *J. Natl. Cancer Inst.* 79:457–63

43. Shannon, D. C., Kelly, D. H. 1982. SIDS and Near SIDS. *New Engl. J. Med.* 306:959–65, 1022–28

44. Sievers, M. L. 1968. Cigarette and alcohol usage by southwestern American Indians. *Am. J. Public Health* 58:74–83

45. Sievers, M. L., Fisher, J. R. 1981. Diseases of North American Indians. In *Biocultural Aspects of Disease,* ed. H. R. Rothchild, pp. 191–252. New York: Academic. 653 pp.

46. Staub, H. P., Hoekelman, R. A., Bien, S. J., Drazek, G. A. 1976. Health supervision of infants on the Cattaraugus Indian Reservation, New York. *Clin. Pediatr.* 15:44–52

47. Sullivan, D. A., Beeman, R. 1983. Utilization and evaluation of maternity care by American Indians in Arizona. *J. Community Health* 9:18–29

48. Sullivan, W. C. 1899. A note on the influence of maternal inebriety on the offspring. *J. Ment. Sci.* 45:489–503

49. Van Duzen, J., Carter, J. P., Secondi, J. Federspiel, C. 1969. Protein and calorie malnutrition among preschool Navajo Indian children. *Am. J. Clin. Nutr.* 22:1362–70

50. Vanlandingham, M. J., Buehler, J. W., Hogue, C. J. R., Strauss, L. T. 1988. Birthweight-specific infant mortality for Native Americans compared with whites, six states, 1980. *Am. J. Public Health* 78:499–503

51. Wallace, H. M. 1973. The health of American Indian children. *Am. J. Dis. Child.* 125:449–54

52. West, K. M. 1978. *Epidemiology of Diabetes and Its Vascular Lesions.* New York: Elsevier

53. Yankauer, A. 1990. Editorial: What infant mortality tells us. *Am. J. Public Health* 80:653–54

Annu. Rev. Publ. Health 1992. 13:287–318

THE PUBLIC HEALTH PRACTICE
OF TOBACCO CONTROL:
Lessons Learned and Directions
for the States in the 1990s[1]

Thomas E. Novotny

Public Health Practice Program Office, Centers for Disease Control, University of California, Berkeley, School of Public Health, Berkeley, California 94720

Rosemary A. Romano

Health Resources and Services Administration, Rockville, Maryland 20857

Ronald M. Davis

Michigan Department of Public Health, Lansing, Michigan 48909

Sherry L. Mills

Investigator-Initiated Research Section, Prevention and Control Extramural Research Branch, Division of Cancer Prevention and Control, National Cancer Institute, National Institutes of Health, Bethesda, Maryland 20892

KEY WORDS: smoking and health, preventing smoking, behavioral risks, smoking, health departments

INTRODUCTION

The public health practice of tobacco control in the United States has evolved considerably since the publication of the US Surgeon General's 1964 advisory

[1]The US Government has the right to retain a nonexclusive royalty-free license in and to any copyright covering this paper.

287

committee report on the health consequences of smoking (84). The report initially provided the scientific information needed to launch an effective, sustained national public health campaign against tobacco (76). As a result of this campaign and other healthy lifestyle changes among Americans, the prevalence of smoking among adults has declined from 40.4% in 1965 to 29.1% in 1987 (32). Mortality rates for chronic diseases, such as ischemic heart disease, lung cancer, and chronic obstructive lung disease, were greatly affected by the increase in tobacco consumption after World War I to the mid-1960s. Subsequently, mortality rates for cardiovascular disease have declined since the 1960s, and lung cancer mortality rates among men have declined since 1985 (2, 66). The antitobacco campaign has successfully reduced tobacco use since 1964. Because of this reduction, an estimated 789,000 deaths due to tobacco use were avoided or postponed during the period 1964–1985 (84). Further progress against tobacco-related diseases depends on systematically incorporating effective public health programs at the state and local levels.

In September 1990, the Secretary of Health and Human Services released the Year 2000 Objectives for the nation. Tobacco use was prominently featured in these objectives (80), which provide realistic goals for states and the nation in the public health practice of tobacco control. The objectives include six specific tobacco-related risk reduction goals and seven services and protection goals (Appendix). Periodic evaluation reports on progress toward achieving the objectives will be developed by different agencies to monitor the nation's progress.

As the national effort against tobacco matures, the actions of state and local health departments become more important. The states have well-defined public health powers and functions in relation to personal health services, environmental health, health resources, laboratory services, general administration and services, and support of local health departments (46). *The Future of Public Health,* a recent report by the Institute of Medicine, emphasized that states are and must be the central force in public health (44). Tobacco use is a public health problem that needs to be strongly addressed by these agencies. The essential elements of health department tobacco prevention and control programs have not yet been fully implemented or evaluated. This paper describes some of these elements and provides examples from the national effort that can be applied in the states. Future tobacco-control initiatives geared toward states are outlined.

ESSENTIAL ELEMENTS OF TOBACCO PREVENTION AND CONTROL

Effective strategies for tobacco control derive from those that have proved effective in reducing the population burden of communicable diseases: surveillance; increases in host resistance through immunization and improvement in general health; breaking the chain of transmission through case detection, containment, clinical treatment, control of vectors of transmission, environmental control, and support of personal measures to avoid exposure to the infectious agent; inactivation of the infectious agent through physical methods and treatment; and planning, implementation, and evaluation of control programs (20). Many of these strategies can be applied to the control of chronic diseases caused by tobacco use.

In 1989, the Association of State and Territorial Health Officials (ASTHO) conducted a survey of state health departments on programs, policies, and public health systems to prevent and control tobacco. The survey provided detailed data on components of state tobacco control programs, including budgets, planning activities, community activities, legislation, educational activities, and health department policies. The results showed that states varied widely in the strength and breadth of tobacco-control programs (21).

Surveillance

Communicable disease surveillance has been defined by the World Health Organization (WHO) as " . . . the exercise of continuous scrutiny of, and watchfulness over, the distribution and spread of infections and factors related thereto, of sufficient accuracy and completeness to be pertinent to effective control" (20). Tobacco-related surveillance systems must also be simple, informative, uniform, and sensitive to changes in behavior, especially among target groups for whom interventions are planned. Such surveillance is critical in evaluating the long-term effects of tobacco control measures.

ADULT SURVEILLANCE   On the national level, several different surveys have provided extensive information on trends in tobacco-related knowledge, attitudes, beliefs, and behavior (Table 1).

The Office on Smoking and Health's Adult Use of Tobacco Surveys (AUTS) have provided detailed information on tobacco-related behavior, beliefs, and attitudes. In assessing public knowledge about the harmful effects of tobacco, these surveys found that beliefs about health consequences of smoking increased significantly between 1964 and 1986 (Table 2) (54).

Data from the National Health Interview Survey (NHIS) have helped identify high-risk groups for targeting in the Year 2000 Objectives. For example, educational attainment has been found to be the single most important predictor for changes in the prevalence of current smoking (60). Those persons with the least educational attainment have not shown the same rapid decline in prevalence as those with the highest educational attainment. Current smoking prevalence declined among both men and women between 1973 and 1987, but the rate of decline was greater among men (Figure 1) (32).

Table 1 Surveys of adult smoking behavior in the United States

Survey Name	Years of Survey	Sample Size	Age Groups
Adult Use of Tobacco Survey (AUTS)	1964, 1966, 1970, 1975, 1986	range 4000 in 1964 and 1966 to 13,000 in 1986	≥17 years
Behavioral Risk Factor Surveillance System (BRFSS)	1981–1991	1100 to 3200 persons/state in 1989[a]	≥18 years
Current Population Surveys (CPS)[b]	1955, 1966–1968, 1985, 1989	114,342 persons (1989)	≥16 years
National Health Interview Surveys (NHIS)	1965, 1966, 1970, 1974, 1976–1980 (inclusive), 1983, 1985, 1987, 1989	range 10,000 households in 1978–1980; 49,000 households in 1989	≥18 years
National Health and Nutrition Examination Survey (NHANES)	1971, 1976, 1984	approximately 28,000 persons	6 months–74 years
Hispanic Health and Nutrition Examination Survey (HHANES)	1982–1984	15,924 persons[c]	6 months–74 years
National Institute on Drug Abuse (NIDA) National Household Surveys on Drug Abuse	1979, 1982, 1985, 1988	approximately 8000 persons	≥12 years

[a] Began in 1981–1983 and included 28 states and the District of Columbia conducting one time telephone surveys with a representative sample for the remaining states. Since 1984, continuous monthly surveys by state with over 40 states and the District of Columbia currently participating.
[b] Allows state specific estimates.
[c] Combined population of Cuban Americans, Mexican Americans, and mainland Puerto Ricans.

Table 2 Percentage of US adults who believed smoking causes disease, 1964 and 1986[a]

Year and smoking status	Lung cancer	Heart disease	Chronic Lung disease
Smokers			
1964	53	32	42
1986	85	71	85
Nonsmokers			
1964	74	41	55
1986	95	83	91

[a]From Ref. 54.

Epidemiologists predict that smoking will be more common among women than among men in the US by the late 1990s (61).

Beginning in 1985, a sufficient number of blacks were sampled by the NHIS to analyze smoking trends and race differences in behavior. The diffusion rate for the decline in smoking prevalence among blacks is similar to that among whites, even though the prevalence of smoking among blacks is higher than among whites in every survey year (32). When the 1985 NHIS data were adjusted for sociodemographic factors, blacks were found to have lower rates of quitting, but no differences were observed among blacks and whites in ever-smoking rates (56).

The 1982–1984 Hispanic Health and Nutrition Survey (HHANES) found a higher prevalence of current smoking among men (40%) and women (26%) than in the general population. The HHANES also revealed a remarkable prevalence of smoking among Cuban-American men aged 20–34 years (50.1%) (42).

State-specific data from the Centers for Disease Control (CDC) Behavioral Risk Factor Surveillance System (BRFSS) and the two Current Population Surveys (CPS) for 1985 and 1989 indicate that the prevalence of smoking is highest in the South and East (50; Office on Smoking and Health 1991, unpublished tabulations). State-specific progress toward the Year 2000 Objectives, with respect to current smoking prevalence (Appendix), can be measured by using these data (Table 3). By using the 1985 CPS data, with an estimated −0.5 percentage point change per year in adult smoking prevalence, Remington et al (64) predicted that only nine states would reach the 1990 Objective of 25%. By using the 1989 CPS and the national rate of change for projection of the state-specific adult prevalence of smoking to the Year 2000 [−0.58 percentage points change per year (84)], we found that only four states would meet the objective of 15% prevalence (Table 3).

In addition to adult smoking prevalence, the BRFSS can now describe a

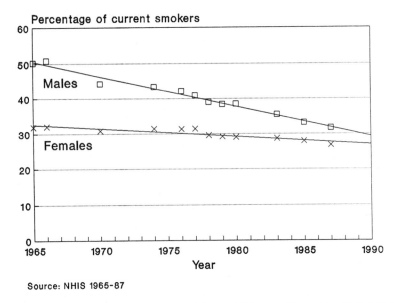

Figure 1 Prevalence of smoking among adults aged 20 years old or older, United States, 1965–1987.

dynamic model in smoking cessation at the state level. Quitting smoking is a continuum, with attempts lasting days, months, or years before relapses and repeated efforts to quit. In 1990, the BRFSS questionnaire was modified to include questions on when, for how long, and how many quit attempts were made in the last year. A quit attempt was defined as one day of abstinence; a major quit attempt was defined as at least seven days of abstinence; short-term quitting was defined as abstinence for less than three months; and long-term quitting was defined as abstinence for 3–12 months. Data based on these questions will enable states to evaluate recent changes in intentions and serious quitting attempts in response to programs at the state level. National data on this "quitting continuum" from the AUTS show that 34% of persons who smoked in the last year quit for at least one day and that 22.5% of the attempts resulted in abstinence for at least three months (41).

Data from several different surveys suggest that the prevalence of smoking among pregnant women remains an area of concern. For the 42 states participating in the 1988 BRFSS, the collective prevalence of smoking among 500 pregnant respondents was 18% (9). In the Year 2000 Objectives, the baseline estimate of current smoking prevalence for pregnant women was 25% in 1987 (80). Small sample sizes for the BRFSS do not permit state-specific assessment of smoking prevalence among pregnant women.

Table 3 State-specific prevalence of cigarette smoking among adults aged 20 years and older, 1989 and projected for the year 2000[a]

State	1989	Projected for Year 2000
Alabama	29.3	22.9
Alaska	28.6	22.2
Arizona	25.5	19.1
Arkansas	28.6	22.2
California	20.0	13.6
Colorado	26.2	19.8
Connecticut	28.8	22.4
Delaware	29.9	23.5
District of Columbia	21.3	14.9
Florida	25.0	18.6
Georgia	27.0	20.6
Hawaii	22.1	15.7
Idaho	23.0	16.6
Illinois	25.9	19.5
Indiana	25.1	18.7
Iowa	25.0	18.6
Kansas	23.4	17.0
Kentucky	31.2	24.8
Louisiana	27.5	21.1
Maine	27.0	20.6
Maryland	27.0	20.6
Massachusetts	24.7	18.3
Michigan	29.4	23.0
Minnesota	23.1	16.7
Mississippi	24.9	18.5
Missouri	30.4	24.0
Montana	24.8	18.4
Nebraska	23.0	16.6
Nevada	31.4	25.0
New Hampshire	27.4	21.0
New Jersey	24.5	18.1
New Mexico	25.6	19.2
New York	23.5	17.1
North Carolina	28.2	21.8
North Dakota	21.3	14.9
Ohio	27.7	21.3
Oklahoma	29.2	22.8
Oregon	22.6	16.2
Pennsylvania	26.0	19.6
Rhode Island	23.7	17.3
South Carolina	28.4	22.0
South Dakota	22.1	15.7
Tennessee	30.8	24.4
Texas	25.6	19.2
Utah	14.9	8.5

Table 3   (Continued)

State	1989	Projected for Year 2000
Vermont	25.6	19.2
Virginia	25.6	19.2
Washington	23.0	16.6
West Virginia	32.4	27.8
Wisconsin	24.0	17.6
Wyoming	27.1	20.7
United States	25.5	19.1

[a] From Office on Smoking and Health. 1989 Current Population Survey, US Bureau of the Census, unpublished tabulations.

Another important surveillance system for states may be the use of data from birth certificates. These will include information on maternal smoking status in all states (33). The data will assist states in tracking possible smoking-associated infant mortality caused by Sudden Infant Death Syndrome, low birthweight, and respiratory conditions. One study using data on more than 300,000 births in Missouri found that approximately 10% of infant mortality was attributable to smoking (49). This system does not account for exposure of the newborn to smoking by household members other than the mother.

The 1989 ASTHO survey reported that only ten states collected data on specific target populations, primarily women of reproductive age (21). Thus, standardized surveillance of high-risk groups should be strengthened to monitor progress toward the Year 2000 Objectives.

ADOLESCENTS   In the US, about 90% of smokers begin to use tobacco before age 21 (84). Useful trend data have been provided by the National Institute on Drug Abuse (NIDA) High School Seniors yearly survey (45). The prevalence of daily cigarette smoking among high school seniors decreased from 29% in 1975 to 21% in 1980. After 1980, the prevalence leveled off at 18% to 21% (Figure 2). Since 1976, prevalence of daily cigarette smoking among females has consistently exceeded that of males.

The CDC's 1989 Teenage Attitudes and Practices Survey (TAPS) will permit detailed national analyses of all forms of tobacco use and of the predictors of tobacco use among young persons. Preliminary data from this survey suggest that the national prevalence of smoking (any cigarette in the last 30 days) among persons aged 12–17 years is 15% (11). The CDC has also recently released the Youth Risk Behavior Survey (YRBS), a standard questionnaire to be used in school surveys. This survey contains be-

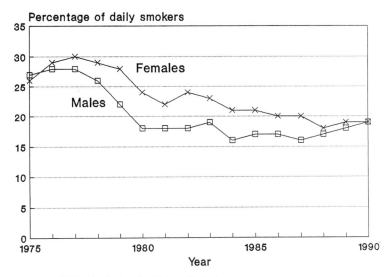

Source: NIDA, Monitoring the Future Project

Figure 2   Percentage of high school seniors reporting daily cigarette smoking, United States, 1975–1990.

havioral questions standardized to the national TAPS (39) and can provide state-specific information on tobacco use by school children. In addition, CDC used the YRBS to survey a national sample of 11,631 students in 50 states and the District of Columbia in 1990. These data may be compared with state data when available. In 1990, more than one third (36.0%) of school-aged youths (grades 9–12) reported that they had smoked at some time in the 30 days before the survey, and 13% reported that they had used cigarettes "frequently" (12). Assessing the smoking behavior among school dropouts, a high-risk group, is problematic for the YRBS and all other school-based surveys.

One other source of data for smoking behavior among young persons is the CPS. This survey collects state-specific information on persons aged 16–19 years, whether or not they are in school. No reported analyses have used these data, and it is not known how many of the small sample of 16–19-year-olds in each state are dropouts.

The ASTHO survey reported that 34 states collected information on the prevalence of tobacco use among adolescents, but none of the states' surveys covered all the standard questions included in the YRBS (21). These questions cover experimentation, current use of tobacco, age of initiation, and smokeless tobacco use. Thus, by using the YRBS, standardized surveillance of youth will be strengthened so that states can evaluate programs and progress toward specific Year 2000 Objectives. Core questions will be used in both national and state-based surveys to assure comparability (80).

PUBLIC OPINION POLLS   Information from such sources as the Gallup Organization Surveys provides some idea of the coverage of public information campaigns and important ongoing information about public beliefs and attitudes toward tobacco. These data may be important in formulating public policy. For example, in 1988, the Gallup Survey reported that 60% (75% of smokers and 26% of nonsmokers) favored a total ban on smoking in public places, and 55% (64% of nonsmokers and 34% of smokers) favored restrictions or a ban on cigarette advertising. In addition, NHIS and AUTS data show that attitudes among adults toward environmental tobacco smoke support additional restrictions on smoking in public places (16, 26). This type of information supports the enactment of health-policy interventions by informing legislators about the true public sentiment toward controversial bills (84). Such surveys also help evaluate the effect of public information campaigns through questions that ask about the recognition of material presented in a targeted community (62). The analysis of data from public information surveys is a useful method of identifying "high-risk" groups in which antitobacco campaign messages have not been fully received.

PROCESS MEASURES   The ASTHO survey compares state health department's current activities in tobacco prevention and control and establishes a baseline for measuring future progress toward Year 2000 Objectives 3.10, 3.11, 3.12, 3.13, 3.14 (Appendix) (21).

Data on worksite policies are not available on a state-specific basis, but national data can be obtained from various national sources, such as business groups and unions (8, 30). States may collect worksite data from local resources, such as business groups, chambers of commerce, or specific worksite surveys.

If schools are targeted to be tobacco-free, state departments of education should establish surveillance systems so that progress towards this goal can be measured. The National School Boards Association has conducted two national surveys of school boards to evaluate smoking policies. In 1989, 78% of all responding school boards had antismoking programs, and 95% had a written policy on smoking in schools (17). Antitobacco educational programs in schools may be considered "immunization" for students against cues that encourage tobacco use. Assurance of the application of this education is necessary to provide youth with resistance skills needed to meet Year 2000 Objectives. The National Cancer Institute (NCI) has developed guidelines for antitobacco education in schools (34).

EXCISE TAX DATA AND TOBACCO CONSUMPTION   Measurement of state-specific tobacco consumption is possible by using data on excise taxes collected on tobacco products (73). These data are usually expressed in terms of per capita cigarette consumption for adults aged 18 years and older. A recent report demonstrated that for 1974–1985, self-reported consumption (including data from surveys of youth, recent quitters, and current smokers) was about 30% lower than consumption based on cigarette sales. The report concluded that a consistent bias has remained between self-reported consumption data and actual tobacco sales data over time. Thus, the validity and reliability of survey data on smoking behavior have not changed in recent years (40). A correlation between significant social and health information events and national per capita consumption has been observed over several decades (Figure 3). Similar tracking of significant state-level events, such as increases in excise tax, may be used by states to monitor changes in consumption. In California, the total number of cigarettes purchased per month is used to track tobacco sales in response to implementation of an additional excise tax on cigarettes that took effect in January 1989 (43, 74) (Figure 4).

Because of year-to-year fluctuation in inventory at the wholesale level (at which excise taxes are collected), these data are best reported as three-year moving averages, or as 12-month averages for monthly changes.

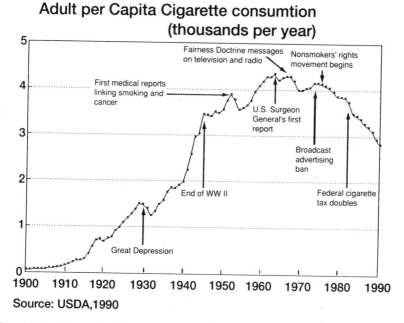

Figure 3 Adult per capita cigarette consumption and major smoking and health events, United States, 1900–1985.

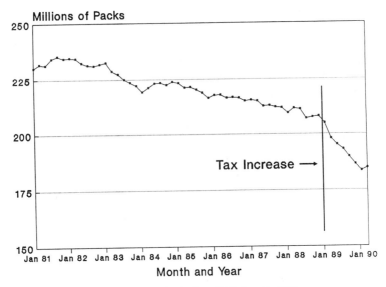

Figure 4   Total cigarettes sold in California from 1980 through 1990.

Problem Assessment

The second element of tobacco control activities in the US is problem assessment. This process consists of a detailed analysis of current smoking behavior, tobacco consumption, current program capabilities, and disease impact of smoking (smoking-attributable morbidity, mortality, and economic costs). We described the first three aspects of this analysis in the first section of this report.

The analysis of the disease impact of smoking in the US includes both standard epidemiologic concepts (attributable risk calculations based on prevalence and relative risk), as well as economic cost estimates based on prevalence of risk factors and relative rates of medical care utilization and disability. The critical calculation in prevalence-based disease impact estimation is the attributable fraction formula:

$$\text{Smoking-attributable fraction} = \frac{p(RR-1)}{p(RR-1) + 1}$$

where p is the prevalence of smoking and RR is the relative risk of death from a particular disease for smokers compared with never-smokers (87). The relative risks for 14 smoking-associated conditions were reported in the

Surgeon General's 1989 report (84). These risk estimates and 1988 smoking prevalence and national mortality data indicate that an estimated 434,000 deaths were attributable to smoking in 1988 in the US (10). Economic estimates based on direct medical care costs and indirect losses attributable to disability and premature mortality have also been made. One national estimate is approximately $65 billion in smoking-attributable economic costs for 1985 (86).

Each state may individualize its smoking-attributable disease impact estimate by using software [Smoking Attributable Mortality, Morbidity, and Economic Costs (SAMMEC, and its successor SAMMEC II)] specifically designed for this purpose (69). State-specific mortality, 1985 CPS prevalence data, and economic data from the Health Care Financing Administration were used to compile a 50-state estimate of smoking-attributable morbidity, mortality, and economic costs for the National Status Report on Tobacco and Health (81). In this report, the number of smoking-attributable deaths for 1985 ranged from 271 in Alaska to 28,533 in California. The range of direct and indirect prevalence-based economic costs of smoking was $82.3 million in Alaska to $5.8 billion in California in 1985. By performing disease impact estimation at several-year intervals, behavioral surveillance information from CPS or BRFSS may be utilized to demonstrate state-specific patterns of tobacco-related mortality over time. These data are useful in reinforcing the importance of the tobacco-related disease burden (compared with other risks) to policymakers (88). The Institute of Medicine's report stressed the federal capacity-building role in disseminating data and information useful to states. SAMMEC II software is an example of such public health capacity building.

Another source of information about the mortality impact of smoking for states may be death certificates. Tobacco-use disorder is a specific category in the *International Classification of Diseases,* ninth revision; some researchers recommend that this diagnostic category (405.1) be used more frequently by physicians in the assignation of cause of death (63). In 1989, five states recorded smoking history on death certificates (21). Few analyses of these data have been reported, but researchers in Oregon have used follow-back surveys of physicians to compile detailed data on the listing of smoking as a cause of death certificates. The researchers found that smoking was recorded as a contributing or underlying cause on death for 77.1% of lung cancer deaths (37). This is remarkably close to the mathematically derived national smoking-attributable fraction (87%) of lung cancer deaths reported by the Surgeon General (84).

Legislation and Policies

Policies and legislative actions are essential to state and local public health efforts in meeting the Year 2000 Objectives. They refocus tobacco use as a

community public health concern, rather than as simply an individual behavior problem. In 1983, WHO's Expert Committee on Smoking Control
stated:

> It may be tempting to try introducing smoking control programmes without a legislative
> component, in the hope that relatively inoffensive activity of this nature will placate those
> concerned with public health, while generating no real opposition from cigarette man-
> ufacturers. This approach, however, is not likely to succeed. A genuine broadly defined
> education programme, aimed at reducing smoking must be complemented by legislation
> and restrictive measures . . . (90)

Policies and laws that regulate smoking in public places, the access to tobacco
by children and youths, and tobacco product advertising (at least on public
property) are within the jurisdiction of state and local governments.

CLEAN-INDOOR-AIR POLICIES   The Year 2000 Objectives call for comprehensive laws on clean indoor air in all states, for 75% of all worksites to
have a formal smoking policy that prohibits or restricts smoking, and for all
schools to have tobacco-free environments (80). In the US, state clean-
indoor-air laws have become more widespread and stronger over the last two
decades because of concerns about the health consequences of environmental
tobacco smoke and a growing "nonsmokers rights" movement. Nominal laws
regulate smoking in one to three public places, excluding restaurants and
private worksites; basic laws regulate smoking in four or more different public
places, excluding restaurants and private worksites; and moderate laws regulate smoking in restaurants, but not private worksites. Laws that cover private
workplaces (as opposed to those only covering public-sector worksites) are
considered "extensive" laws by the Surgeon General (84), because it is
difficult to enact policies in the private sector. Preemptive laws, which
appeared first in 1990, are state laws that prohibit local jurisdictions from
enacting restrictions more stringent than the state law.

Before the mid-1970s, minimal state legislation restricted smoking in
public places. As of 1990, 45 states and the District of Columbia have laws
that restrict smoking in public places (Figure 5); in 16 of these states and the
District of Columbia, the restrictions also apply to private-sector workplaces
(21). States in tobacco growing areas are the least likely to have extensive
clean-indoor-air legislation. However, a trend has begun that may help con-
vince states to strengthen and enforce their laws as part of a larger national
effort.

Another trend, evident since 1990, is the inclusion of preemption clauses in
state laws. These clauses effectively prohibit local governments from enacting
stronger clean-indoor-air restrictions than found in the state law. Preemption
clauses usually signal a victory for the protobacco interests, because they

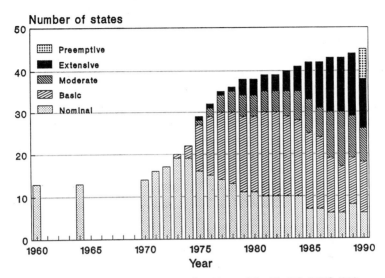

Source: Unpublished data, Office on Smoking and Health, U.S. DHHS 1989

Figure 5   Number of states with laws regulating smoking in public places, by year, United States, 1960–1990.

effectively weaken local efforts that are usually more restrictive on smoking in public places than the state laws. As of October 1990, clean-indoor-air legislation has included preemption clauses in seven states (72) (Figure 5).

Local ordinances restricting smoking in a wide range of public areas (e.g. restaurants, elevators, hotels, libraries) are found in more than 450 communities (3). As a result of these local ordinances, 23% of the US population (57 million persons) is covered by specific local regulations (21). When the state laws are included in this calculation, over 90% of the US population is covered by some kind of clean-indoor-air regulation.

An increasing proportion (from 36% in 1986 to 57% in 1987) of businesses have adopted their own restrictions (8), but most businesses report that the presence of laws or regulations lead to the adoption or extension of smoking policies at worksites (29). Many laws regulating smoking at the worksite exclude smaller establishments from coverage; however, small companies employ a large proportion of the national workforce (80). One spin-off of widespread worksite restrictions on smoking is that worksites with restrictive policies are more likely to offer cessation programs (64%) than are companies without such policies (38%) (8).

Governors or municipal administrators may also impose restrictions on those offices controlled by the executive branch. The governors of Colorado and North Dakota have completely banned smoking in executive-controlled offices. These actions avoid the competing political agendas often encountered in legislative actions, but require strong support from state health departments in developing and implementing the directives (21).

Restrictive policies on tobacco in state health department buildings may be important in demonstrating official commitment to tobacco control activities. The 1989 ASTHO survey reported that all state health departments, with the exception of North Carolina and Virginia, had a written policy on smoking in state health department buildings (Virginia has since passed a clean-indoor-air law that covers public workplaces). However, only 23 of these departments completely ban smoking in all health department facilities. Thirty-one states permit the sale of tobacco products in health department buildings (21).

In 1991, the Environmental Protection Agency's Scientific Advisory Board drafted a report that designated environmental tobacco smoke as a Class A (human) carcinogen, a substance to which there is no completely safe exposure level (85). The increasing trend in strength and coverage of restrictions on smoking in public will probably be supported by this finding (29) when and if the report is officially released.

RESTRICTIONS ON ACCESS TO TOBACCO BY MINORS   Few states have ever enforced restrictions on the purchase of tobacco products by minors (14). Although 45 states and the District of Columbia prohibit the sale of tobacco products to underage persons, only 21 states and the District of Columbia require a retail vendor's license to sell tobacco, and only eight states' laws had clear enforcement provisions. A report by the Inspector General of the US Public Health Service concluded that only 32 violations were cited in the five states that collected such data in 1990 (82).

Additional strengthening and enforcement of these restrictions have been encouraged by the US Department of Health and Human Services. In May 1990, the Secretary of Health and Human Services released model legislation that would improve the enforcement and coverage of laws restricting minors' access to tobacco (71). Seven essential elements are covered in this model legislation:

1. Create a licensing system similar to that used to control the sale of alcoholic beverages.
2. Set the minimum age of legal purchase at 19 years.
3. Set forth a graduated schedule of penalties for illegal sales to minors (fines and license suspensions).
4. Provide separate penalties for failure to post warning signs about the illegality of sales to minors.
5. Place primary responsibility for enforcement with a designated state agency.

6. Rely primarily on civil penalties, rather than on the court system, to punish offenders.
7. Ban the use of vending machines to dispense tobacco products.

RESTRICTIONS ON ADVERTISING   Cigarettes are the most heavily advertised consumer product (25). In the infectious disease control model cited above, advertising may be thought of as a critical vector in the "chain of transmission" of the tobacco epidemic. Thus, vector control may require restrictions on advertising to prevent initiation of tobacco use by susceptible persons. The preemption clause of the 1969 Public Health Cigarette Smoking Act prevents state governments from regulating most cigarette advertising (84). However, states and localities can and do regulate some local advertising. In Utah, tobacco advertising is banned by law from any billboard, public transport facility, or any other object of display. Six other states (Arizona, California, Colorado, Massachusetts, Hawaii, and Nebraska) have communities that restrict tobacco advertising through local legislation on public properties, such as sports stadiums and transit facilities. Cities and states can also restrict or ban the free distribution of tobacco product samples, and at least 14 cities in the US have done so (84).

INCREASING TAXES   Another legislative effort that may effectively inhibit young persons from smoking is increasing the excise tax on cigarettes. Currently, all states impose a tax on each package of cigarettes. These taxes, which range from three cents (North Carolina) to 41 cents (Texas) per pack, are generally lowest in the tobacco-producing states (21, 73). According to econometric studies by Lewit & Coate (48), the negative price elasticity of demand observed for such consumer goods as tobacco is most effective in reducing consumption for those who have the least amount of disposable income. These authors found that the overall price elasticity of demand was -0.42 for cigarettes, but that the value for youths aged 12–17 years was more than three times as high (-1.40). Thus, an increase in the price of cigarettes through taxation will particularly inhibit the initiation of smoking by teenagers, although it will also suppress the per capita consumption of cigarettes for the population in general.

Two correlation studies using state-specific consumption data have been reported. Changes in excise taxes over time appear to be more closely correlated longitudinally with changes in consumption than the enactment of clean-indoor-air legislation (59). However, those states with the strongest clean-indoor-air acts appear to have the lowest per capita consumption (28). In 1981, Warner (89) suggested that the dramatic correlation between diffusion of clean-indoor-air legislation and cigarette consumption was best interpreted as parallel changes in social attitudes toward smoking. The same principle probably holds true in 1991. Besides the economic effects of increasing cigarette prices, portions of the revenue from excise taxes have been earmarked by some states to fund tobacco-control programs (6, 84).

In 1988, California voters passed Proposition 99, which increased the state excise tax on cigarettes from 10 to 35 cents per package of 20 cigarettes; one fifth of the revenues from this tax initiative were directed to tobacco-related public education (more than $100 million per year). The imposition of a 25 cent/pack tax increase, combined with a large intervention program, was associated with a sharp (15%) decline in tobacco sales in California (Figure 4) (74). Hu et al (43) estimated that this decline was 1.22 packs less per person (aged 15 years or older), i.e. the effect of the tax is to suppress consumption by 1.22 packs over that which would be predicted without the tax. By December 1990, however, the effect of the tax had dwindled to 0.64 packs less than predicted before the tax. Without constant adjustments for inflation or an *ad valorem* tax, the effect of tax increases diminishes over time. In California, the effect of the 1989 tax will be negligible by 1993, if not increased.

The health benefits of increases in cigarette taxes are substantial. One report estimated that over 800,000 premature deaths in a 1984 cohort of Americans 12 years and older would have been averted if the federal excise tax on cigarettes had been maintained at its real value in 1951 (38). The positive health effects of increasing cigarette taxes may also be appreciated by the states, but because of the long lag periods characteristic of smoking-attributable chronic diseases, the benefits may not be observed for several years.

Health Department and Community-Based Programs

ASTHO TOBACCO PREVENTION AND CONTROL NETWORK   In 1989, ASTHO developed a network of state health department personnel concerned with tobacco issues in each state. These persons generally represented the health education or health promotion divisions within the departments, but they were also epidemiologists and chronic disease specialists. This network now acts as a conduit for information, the dissemination of new technology, and communications between states. National meetings, as well as special projects of the network, are supported through funding from the NCI, the CDC, and the National Heart, Lung, and Blood Institute (4).

A unique effort supported through the ASTHO network to increase community involvement in tobacco control has been established by the governors of eight western states through the Rocky Mountain Tobacco-Free Challenge. This challenge has a goal to achieve significant (50%) reductions in tobacco use and tobacco-related disease by the year 2000 (18). Over the first three years of this effort, the participating states have increased funding, surveillance activities, community interventions, and other program components that may contribute to an accelerated decline in tobacco use in the region (55, 57). Such regional efforts help strengthen states' capacity through collegial relationships among states who have similar geography, target populations, and political climate.

NCI INTERVENTION TRIALS   In 1988, Cullen (22) articulated the NCI strategies for reducing smoking in the US, so that the NCI goal of reducing the cancer mortality rate 50% by the Year 2000 could be met. A key component in these strategies was the ambitious community-based intervention trial for smoking cessation among smokers in 22 different sites (COMMIT) (52). This trial, the largest in the NCI repertoire, will involve almost 2 million persons in the application of smoking cessation strategies through community organizations and social institutions. Heavy smokers ($\geq$ 25 cigarettes per day) are prime targets of these interventions. The rationale for the intervention is based on data from community heart disease prevention trials in the US. These data emphasize that multiple interventions should be incorporated into natural educational channels and social structures that have the potential to reach large segments of the smoking population (52). For instance, worksite promotion of cessation through presentations, cessation programs, development of audiovisual materials, and consultations are a major focus of COMMIT activities. The COMMIT approach is based on previous NCI community-based research. The overall intervention goals of the project are the following:

1. Increase the priority of smoking as a public health issue.
2. Improve the community's ability to modify smoking behavior.
3. Increase the influence of existing policy and economic factors that discourage smoking.
4. Increase social norms and values supporting nonsmoking.

Results from the COMMIT project are not yet available.

Besides COMMIT, NCI has funded individual interventions in eight specific problem areas. More than 10 million individuals in 25 states and over 299 cities are affected by these efforts. The interventions include the following:

1. School-based programs. These comprehensive programs teach social pressure resistance to students, involve parents and peer leaders in the education, call for schoolwide support of nonsmoking norms, and emphasize longitudinal follow-up. Curricula, which have been developed to target high-risk youths, include an emphasis on the stages of change model (infrequent use leading to addiction) (34). In 1989, the National School Boards Association found that 95% of school districts in the US had a written policy on

smoking in schools and that 17% of schools banned smoking on school premises or at school functions (17). The ASTHO survey found that 26 states and the District of Columbia ban smoking for students, and only eight states completely ban smoking in schools for both students and staff. However, only 23 states and the District of Columbia are able to report information on policies and education activities in school districts, which are basically autonomous units within their jurisdictions.

2. Minimal interventions. Self-help programs are the most cost-effective method of delivering cessation messages (35). These can be supported through telephone hot lines, social support groups, worksites, newsletters, community groups, manuals, and health care providers (23).

3. Health care providers. Approximately 700 providers and more than 40,000 smokers were originally expected to be targeted by this intervention (22). Through wide dissemination of an NCI "Train the Trainer" program, cosponsored by the American Medical Association and the American Dental Association, over 100,000 physicians and dentists will be trained to counsel smokers (36). The Year 2000 Objectives for the nation call for 75% of primary care and oral health care providers to advise cessation routinely and provide assistance and follow-up for all tobacco-using patients (80). Over 70% of smokers visit a health care provider once a year, which may be considered a "teachable moment" in a time of vulnerability. According to the 1986 AUTS, only 45% of smokers reported that a physician had ever advised them to stop smoking (24).

4. Mass media. Mass media reaches the largest number of smokers (an estimated 5 million) in NCI intervention trials. A more detailed description of media and communications efforts is presented later.

5–7. High-risk groups. Blacks, Hispanics, and women are targeted through NCI programs that use multiple channels. These high-risk groups may be at a lower point in the classic diffusion of innovations curve (in this case, nonsmoking is the innovation) than others (65). Their smoking patterns may be unique. Thus, targeted interventions are included in the NCI community intervention protocols to improve the diffusion of the nonsmoking norm among these groups.

8. Smokeless tobacco. These NCI intervention efforts concentrate on identifying patterns of use and channels through which users may be influenced. Channels include 4-H clubs, dental health maintenance organizations, Little League, and Native American organizations.

Overall, the NCI goal is to integrate effective cancer control technology into existing health care delivery systems, health promotion efforts, or cancer control programs (22). Several consensus documents have been published that deal with this integration. They include consensus reports on health maintenance organizations, pregnant women, self-help programs for smoking cessation, and school-based programs (70).

State health departments are the focus for the next stage (Phase V research) in the demonstration of NCI COMMIT and other program results. In 1991, the NCI mounted the world's largest demonstration project for tobacco control and health promotion. The American Stop Smoking Intervention Study (ASSIST) is sponsored by both the NCI and the American Cancer Society. Almost $120 million will be spent in 17 states to support this project between 1991 and 1999, and it will include an extensive evaluation by using data from future Current Population Surveys (51).

CESSATION PROGRAMS   Smoking cessation programs (the clinical treatment component of the disease control model) are essential in the multiple channel approach to tobacco control. These are provided by many private voluntary health organizations, state and local health departments, for-profit companies, hospitals, and schools. Although the majority (90%) of successful quitters do not use formal programs (31), heavier (more than 25 cigarettes per day), more addicted smokers tend to use programs more frequently than lighter smokers, thus demonstrating a need for these programs within broad-based tobacco control activities (31, 79).

The average success of cessation programs depends on their clientele, the methods used, the definition of "success," and other factors, but most programs that report follow-up evaluation studies show about 20–40% success rates at one-year of follow-up (68). Rates for voluntary participation in cessation programs are low (31). Moreover, medical insurance does not, as a rule, cover payment for such programs, and cessation programs are often not appropriately designed for, nor accessible to, the most hard-to-reach populations. Thus, the recent proliferation of smoking cessation services may not be associated with widespread behavioral changes. In 1989, 34 states and the District of Columbia offered smoking cessation programs to state health department employees, and 26 states offered such programs to members of the community (21).

Economic incentives and deterrents may be effective in supporting cessation. The state governments of Colorado, Kansas, and Washington offer differential health insurance rates to smokers and nonsmokers (21). The impact of these programs may be widespread, because the state government is the largest or one of the largest employers in many states. Once again, the state can act as a change agent in setting an example for other providers of health insurance.

HIGH-RISK GROUPS   The NCI has placed emphasis on special populations, including blacks, Hispanics, and women, in their individual community trials (70). These trials focus on late adaptors of the nonsmoking norm and on those for whom the health consequences of smoking are of particular concern, such as heavy smokers. In 1989, most states ($n = 38$) had programs that included education and information for some or all of these groups (21). Most states (*n* = 37) addressed women of reproductive age, and fewer states had programs for the other groups: youths (20 states), blacks (14 states), Hispanics (11 states), Native Americans (eight states), Asian/Pacific Islanders (three states), and elderly adults (three states). The CDC has also supported the Smoking Cessation in Pregnancy Project in three states (Missouri, Colorado, Maryland), which will be disseminated to others through existing state resources. In Colorado, preliminary data suggested that an intensive intervention directed toward pregnant women who attend public clinics can produce a 50% improvement in quitting (13.9% of women in the experimental group and 9.3% of women in the control group quit in response to the intervention) (91).

Public Information Campaigns

The effect of past media campaigns has been seen in the decline in tobacco consumption associated with public service announcements in the early 1970s (Figure 3). Over the past 25 years, media campaigns have been developed for specific groups (minorities, pregnant women, and adolescents) and have contributed to the reduction in tobacco use by these groups. Unfortunately, the tobacco industry has also systematically targeted many of these same groups (12, 25).

At first, communications campaigns were "passive," in that information was provided to the public so that personal decisions could be made based on accurate health information. Now, media also serves to change attitudes, reinforce and maintain interest, provide cues to simple action, set a social agenda, and demonstrate simple skills (53). Media messages are now likely to provide a stimulus to positive behavior change because of a changed social milieu and a "conditioned" target audience that supports nonsmoking (27). The recent competitive and complex media environment and the increase in intense counterefforts of the industry have resulted in a need for increased communication capacity in tobacco control by state and local health departments. The NCI has published a consensus document on media and tobacco control that is particularly applicable to state and local health departments (53).

Social marketing is a technique for creating a need for a particular product or service (7). Social marketing can also create a milieu in which tobacco use is no longer the norm, thus facilitating change among users and discouraging young persons from beginning to use tobacco (27). Public information campaigns are the cornerstone of social marketing efforts.

Training constituency groups (in particular, health department personnel) in media relations is another key component of successful public health communications efforts (27). These groups can then disseminate scientific information to the public about tobacco-related disease and the need for tobacco-control programs. State involvement in media now calls for a combined, systematic approach that uses media relations to build a media constituency for the issue; public information that can craft appropriate prevention and cessation messages for target audiences through appropriate channels; and media advocacy to focus media attention on tobacco issues. The 1989 ASTHO survey indicated strong public information activities by states. Thirty-one states and the District of Columbia originated public information campaigns within the last three years. All but seven states made use of public service announcements produced by such federal agencies as the NCI and CDC (21).

An increasing number of states, including California, Michigan, and Minnesota, are appropriating public funds to buy media time for nonsmoking advertisements. In California, $28.6 million were dedicated to the media campaign alone in 1989–1990. Because paid advertising allows for more control over the message, these messages can have more of an impact than those that use free time. However, the costs for paid advertising can be prohibitive (27). The NCI has recently published guidelines on the use of paid media in tobacco control (58).

Computer networks permit the rapid dissemination of information and exchange of ideas. An electronic bulletin board specifically dedicated to tobacco, the Smoking Control Advocacy Resource Center Network (SCARC-Net), has been developed by the Advocacy Institute in Washington, DC (1). To date, 13 states participate in this service (Advocacy Institute 1991, personal communication), which includes daily news briefings, information exchange, and issue updates. With complete participation in this service, coordinated responses by health departments to constantly changing tobacco-related issues would be possible.

Technical Information Collection and Dissemination

More than 60,000 articles have been written about tobacco and health issues (84). The database of information on tobacco use is expanding daily; the scientific community and the public need to be kept informed about progress in controlling tobacco use. Thus, the maintenance and dissemination of technical information about tobacco is a major component of the public health practice of tobacco control. The Office on Smoking and Health's Technical Information Center maintains the database by using inhouse library software (STAR) and a standard database for medical literature (DIALOG, File 160). New publications are included in the quarterly *Bibliography on Smoking and Health* (78). This document covers about 2000 citations and abstracts each year in the field of tobacco and health. All of these resources are directly accessible to states.

Brief, clear, technical information that has local relevance is an important tool for state and local health departments in efforts to reduce tobacco use among their constituents. A wealth of factual resources, as well as cessation and prevention materials, exists for both the public and health professionals. An important function of state tobacco control programs is to provide access to these products and apply them at the local level.

Coalition Building, Community Planning, and Evaluation

COALITIONS   Coalitions are an integral part of tobacco-control activities in the US. The more a coalition extends beyond the health community, the more ownership the entire community exerts over tobacco-control initiatives. Coalitions may represent public health officials, health care providers, advocacy groups, voluntary health organizations, business groups, religious groups, government officials, the insurance industry, the legal profession, the military, labor organizations, economists, educators, advertisers, and communications specialists. Activities of coalitions include advising the state health department, lobbying for antitobacco legislation, developing and implementing tobacco-control plans, conducting research and evaluation, and providing public and professional education. Based on data from the ASTHO survey, 49 states and the District of Columbia have tobacco-related coalitions, with membership including an average of 13 disciplines (13, 21). Their most important activities included public education (82%), legislative efforts (71%), professional education (47%), planning for tobacco control (45%), and research and evaluation (26%). In North Dakota, a well-organized coalition sought and received block grant funds from the Maternal and Child Health Program. Even small amounts of funding, such as $10,000, can be effective in supporting coalition activities (57), but most state-level coalitions are unfunded (21).

PLANNING   State health departments have created plans to solve specific health problems, such as tuberculosis, sexually transmitted diseases, and measles. The Year 2000 Objectives call for all states and territories to create, implement, and monitor tobacco prevention and control plans (80). Planning articulates the process of public health practice, unites the disparate change agents, and focuses public health programs on the spectrum of tobacco control activities.

According to the ASTHO survey, nine states had separate public health plans for tobacco use in 1989, and 16 states addressed tobacco use as part of another program plan (15). To assist states with tobacco-control plans, ASTHO analyzed existing plans and published a guide for developing control plans (5). The steps for developing a tobacco-control plan include the following:

1. Utilize national expertise and resources and establish a coalition or advisory group.
2. Assess the tobacco problem.
3. Develop the mission, goals, and objectives of the plan.
4. Analyze existing tobacco-control potentials.
5. Package and market the plan.
6. Evaluate and revise the plan.

To date, no formal evaluations of state tobacco control plans have been published.

EVALUATION   Evaluation studies of state-based tobacco-control programs are still rather rudimentary. The data from COMMIT are not yet available, but these will only cover 11 intervention and 11 control sites. ASSIST will not even begin until 1993 and will only cover 17 states. However, some data for use in evaluating states' progress provide preliminary information about overall state activities on tobacco control. In this review, all state activities, including NCI trials, state and local legislation, coalitions, and tobacco control plans are part of the state-based effort. Comparisons of outcome data, such as changes in prevalence, quit rates, per capita cigarette consumption, and smoking-attributable mortality for different states and regions, are possible by using currently available data sources. The outcomes change slowly in response to state antitobacco efforts. For example, the overall prevalence of adult smoking is decreasing at only 0.58 percentage points per year in the US (32).

Changes in state-specific current smoking prevalence, quit rates, and per capita cigarette consumption have not yet been linked to data on the various state tobacco-control interventions. In addition, it is very difficult to differentiate between cause and effect of these interventions. For example, a state in which there is a large change in current smoking prevalence will have a population sympathetic to a very restrictive law on smoking in public places. The presence of the law is thus the effect, rather than the cause, of favorable changes in behavior. However, several community-based cardiovascular risk reduction projects have demonstrated that multipronged interventions can have significant effects in reducing cardiovascular disease risk factors in targeted populations; the evidence for effective intervention is particularly strong for smoking. In North Karelia, Finland, significant reductions in smoking prevalence among men aged 30–59 years (28%) were achieved over ten years of intervention. In the Stanford Three Community Study, the number of cigarettes smoked per day decreased after two years of intervention. The most important aspect in the evaluation of these interventions is that reduction of risk factor scores produced significant reduction in cardiovascular disease outcomes (67).

It is also important to evaluate behavioral change in response to specific policies, such as those restricting smoking in public places. In places where evaluation studies have been carried out (e.g. worksites), some policy changes have resulted in no changes in overall cigarette consumption, some have been associated with a decrease in the daily consumption of cigarettes, and some have been associated with a decline in the prevalence of smoking (29, 84). Yet, such policies contribute to an overall social norm of not smoking. This change may be thought of as an "environmental" intervention similar to one that may be effective as part of the infectious disease control model.

The overall goal for the education campaign funded by the recent tax increase in California is to reduce the smoking prevalence by 75% by the year 1999. Preliminary evaluation data on consumption and cigarette smoking prevalence indicate that there may be 750,000 fewer smokers in California since the application of the tax and education campaign (47). The prevalence of smoking declined to 21.2% in 1990 (following the tax increase and institution of the educational campaign) from a 1987 baseline of 26.3% (74). Six months after the campaign began, preliminary results from the California media campaign evaluation showed that the awareness of the campaign was 86.9% among in-school youths and 78.3% among adults. The proportion of adults who think about quitting increased from 38.6% to 41.8%, and the proportion of nonsmoking youths who think about starting decreased from 24.6% to 21.4% during this period (IOX Associates 1991, personal communication).

Additional evaluations of the effect of cigarette excise taxes have shown that these policies discourage smoking, particularly among teenagers (48, 84). On a state basis, cigarette excise taxes have contributed to significant changes in consumption. Between 1955 and 1988, enactment of state cigarette tax increases were associated with an average 3% greater decline in state cigarette sales than in years without tax increases (59).

The effect of laws restricting minors access to tobacco can be evaluated through several sources, which include survey data on adolescent smoking behavior (such as the YRBS), as well as data from law enforcement sources charged with enforcing these laws. Vendors' compliance with laws will not ensure behavior changes among adolescents, but the community nonsmoking norm will be supported through visible enforcement of these laws. The CDC is conducting an evaluation of a law restricting minor's access to tobacco in Marquette, Michigan (A. Trontell 1991, personal communication).

THE FUTURE OF STATE TOBACCO-USE PREVENTION AND CONTROL PROGRAMS

Tobacco-control activities in the US will increase as state and local programs are further developed. ASSIST will begin in 1993, just as COMMIT is finishing. This multistate program will coordinate, provide training for, and evaluate tobacco-use prevention and control efforts in 17 states through 1998 (51). It will use the technology and resources developed through COMMIT and the other eight individual intervention trials sponsored by NCI over the last several years (70).

The Program Directions of the Department of Health and Human Services (in particular, Program Direction 3, Objective 2), calls for a reduction in the incidence of smoking among high-risk and other groups. Tobacco control interventions for minorities, women, youth, and the federal work force are called for by these directions. The directions also call for strengthening the capacity of the public health infrastructure to reduce smoking, especially among high-risk groups. Because so much of the public health practice of tobacco control is state-based, the National Institutes of Health and CDC will provide increased assistance to states as part of their responsibility to implement these objectives (77).

The successful tax initiative in California may similarly encourage other states to fund tobacco control programs. Despite reductions in the second round of legislative appropriations for Proposition 99, a substantial portion of the program funds will still be directed to the media campaign. Here and in other states, media campaigns will continue to expand in importance if financial resources are available.

The Rocky Mountain Tobacco-Free Challenge will continue until the year 2000 (18). Key elements of this program include increased community interest, strengthened interstate and intrastate collaboration, promotion of state activities for reducing tobacco use, and long-term evaluation of tobacco-related policies. As additional resources become available, other regions of the country may adopt this innovative, competitive approach.

Additional coordination of state and local health department activities will be supported by ASTHO through the Tobacco Prevention and Control Network. These health professionals will serve as the opinion leaders for the diffusion of public health practice activities in tobacco prevention and control at the state and local levels. The public health practice of tobacco control continues to evolve, and evaluation methodologies for tobacco-control activities need further development. No single intervention will stop the tobacco epidemic. Multifaceted public health activities for controlling tobacco use need continuous assessment and evaluation; as successful strategies emerge, they should be adapted to different cultural and social environments.

Finally, it is important to note the efforts of the tobacco industry in opposition to tobacco control programs and policies. About $3.3 billion is spent yearly on cigarette advertising—cigarettes are the second most common subject of advertising in magazines and the most common in the outdoor media (mostly billboards) (12, 25). Each state and nearly every local jurisdiction considering tobacco-related public health legislation gains the attention of protobacco lobbyists. Therefore, the effects of major efforts to control tobacco use in state and local jurisdictions may be masked by the well-funded, and often successful, efforts of the tobacco industry in defeating antitobacco initiatives.

APPENDIX: YEAR 2000 OBJECTIVES FOR THE NATION ON TOBACCO AND HEALTH

3.1. Reduce coronary heart disease deaths to no more than 100 per 100,000 people.

3.2. Slow the rise in lung cancer deaths to achieve a rate of no more than 42 per 100,000.

3.3. Slow the rise in deaths from chronic obstructive pulmonary disease to achieve a rate of no more than 25 per 100,000.

3.4. Reduce cigarette smoking to a prevalence of no more than 15% among people aged 20 and older. (Several special population targets are specified.)

3.5. Reduce the initiation of cigarette smoking by children and youth so that no more than 15% have become regular cigarette smokers by age 20.

3.6. Increase to at least 50% the proportion of cigarette smokers aged 18 and older who stopped smoking cigarettes for at least one day during the preceding year.

3.7. Increase smoking cessation during pregnancy so that at least 60% of women who are cigarette smokers at the time they become pregnant quit smoking early in pregnancy and maintain abstinence for the remainder of their pregnancy.

3.8. Reduce to no more than 20% the proportion of children aged 6 and younger who are regularly exposed to tobacco smoke at home.

3.9. Reduce smokeless tobacco use by males aged 12–24 to a prevalence of no more than 4%.

3.10. Establish tobacco-free environments and include tobacco use prevention in the curricula of all elementary, middle, and secondary schools, preferably as part of comprehensive school health education.

3.11. Increase to at least 75% the proportion of worksites with a formal smoking policy that prohibits or severely restricts smoking at the workplace.

3.12. Enact in 50 states comprehensive laws on clean indoor air that prohibit or strictly limit smoking in the workplace and enclosed public places.

3.13. Enact and enforce in 50 states laws prohibiting the sale and distribution of tobacco products to youth younger than age 19.

3.14. Increase to 50 the number of states with plans to reduce tobacco use, especially among youth.

3.15. Eliminate or severely restrict all forms of tobacco product advertising and promotion to which youth younger than age 18 are likely to be exposed.

3.16. Increase to at least 75% the proportion of primary care and oral health care providers who routinely advise cessation and provide assistance and follow-up for all of their tobacco-using patients.

Literature Cited

1. Advocacy Inst. 1990. *SCARCNET Handbook,* Version 1.0. Washington, DC: Advocacy Inst.

2. Am. Cancer Soc. 1990. *Cancer Facts and Figures—1990.* Atlanta: Am. Cancer Soc.

3. Am. Nonsmokers Rights. 1990. *Major Local Smoking Ordinances in the United States. A Detailed Matrix of the Provisions of Workplace, Restaurant, and Public Places Smoking Ordinances.* DHHS Publ. No. (NIH) 90-479. Bethesda: US Dep. Health Hum. Serv., Public Health Serv., Natl. Inst. Health

4. Assoc. State Territ. Health Off. 1990. *Conf. on the Public Health Practice of Tobacco Prevention and Control,* Proc., Mar. 8–9, Houston, Tex. Rockville, Md: Cent. Dis. Control, Cent. Chron. Dis. Prev. Health Promot., Off. Smoking Health

5. Assoc. State Territ. Health Off. and Natl. Cancer Inst. 1989. *Guide to Public Health Practice: State Health Agency Tobacco Prevention and Control Plans.* McLean, Va: Assoc. State Territ. Health Off.

6. Bal, D. G., Kizer, K. W., Gelten, P. G., Mozar, H. N., Niemeyer, D. 1990. Reducing tobacco consumption in California: development of a statewide antitobacco use campaign. *J. Am. Med. Assoc.* 264:1570–74

7. Bandura, A. 1986. *Social Foundations of Thought and Action: A Social Cognitive Theory.* Englewood Cliffs, NJ: Prentice-Hall

8. Bur. Natl. Aff. 1987. *Where There's Smoke: Problems and Policies Concerning Smoking in the Workplace. A BNA Special Report.* Rockville, Md: Bur. Natl. Aff. 2nd ed.

9. Cent. Dis. Control. 1991. Cigarette smoking among reproductive aged women—Behavioral Risk Factor Surveillance System, 1989. *Morbid. Mortal. Wkly. Rep.* 40:719–23

10. Cent. Dis. Control. 1991. Smoking-attributable mortality and YPLL—United States, 1988. *Morbid. Mortal. Wkly. Rep.* 40:60–71

11. Cent. Dis. Control. 1991. Cigarette smoking among youth, United States-1989. *Morbid. Moral. Wkly. Rep.* 40: 712–15.

12. Cent. Dis. Control. 1990. Cigarette advertising—United States, 1988. *Morbid. Mortal. Wkly. Rep.* 39:261–65

13. Cent. Dis. Control. 1990. State coalitions for prevention and control of tobacco use. *Morbid. Mortal. Wkly. Rep.* 39:476–85

14. Cent. Dis. Control. 1990. State laws restricting minors' access to tobacco. *Morbid. Mortal. Wkly. Rep.* 39:349–53

15. Cent. Dis. Control. 1990. State tobacco-use prevention and control plans. *Morbid. Mortal. Wkly. Rep.* 39:133–36

16. Cent. Dis. Control. 1989. Passive smoking: attitudes and exposure in the United States. *Morbid. Mortal. Wkly. Rep.* 37: 239–41

17. Cent. Dis. Control. 1989. School policies and programs on smoking and health—United States, 1988. *Morbid. Mortal. Wkly. Rep.* 38:202–3

18. Cent. Dis. Control. 1989. State-based

chronic disease control: the Rocky Mountain Tobacco-Free Challenge. *Morbid. Mortal. Wkly. Rep.* 38:749–52

19. Cent. Dis. Control. 1991. Current tobacco, alcohol, marijuana, and cocaine use among high school students—United States, 1990. *Morbid. Mortal. Wkly. Rep.* 40(38):659–63

20. Chin, J. 1986. Communicable disease control. In *Public Health and Preventive Medicine*, ed. J. M. Last, pp. 103–4. Norwalk, Conn: Appleton-Century-Crofts

21. Choi, W. S., Novotny, T. E., Davis, R. M., Silver, J. 1991. State tobacco prevention and control activities: results of the 1989–1990 ASTHO Survey —Final Report. *Morbid. Mortal. Wkly. Rep.* (Rep. Recomm.) 40(RR-11): Aug. 16

22. Cullen, J. W. 1988. The National Cancer Institute's intervention trials. *Cancer* 62:1851–64

23. Davis, A. L., Faust, R., Ordentlich, M. 1984. Self-help smoking cessation and maintenance programs: A comparative study with 12-month follow-up by the American Lung Association. *Am. J. Public Health* 74:1212–17

24. Davis, R. M. 1988. Uniting physicians against smoking: The need for a coordinated national strategy. *J. Am. Med. Assoc.* 259:2900–1

25. Davis, R. M. 1987. Current trends in cigarette advertising and marketing. *N. Engl. J. Med.* 316:725–32

26. Davis, R. M., Boyd, G. M., Schoenborn, C. A. 1990. 'Common courtesy' and the elimination of passive smoking: results of the 1987 National Health Interview Survey. *J. Am. Med. Assoc.* 263:2208–10

27. Erickson, A. C., McKenna, J. W., Romano, R. M. 1990. Past lessons and new uses of the mass media in reducing tobacco consumption. *Public Health Rep.* 105:239–44

28. Emont, S. L., Choi, W., Novotny, T., Giovino, G., Davis, R. 1991. Statewide legislation, taxation, and smoking behavior. *Epidemic Intell. Serv.*, 40th Conf., Atlanta. Atlanta: Cent. Dis. Control

29. Fielding, J. E. 1991. Smoking control at the workplace. *Annu. Rev. Public Health.* 12:209–34

30. Fielding, J. E. 1990. Worksite health promotion survey: smoking control activities. *Prev. Med.* 19:402–13

31. Fiore, M. C., Novotny, T. E., Pierce, J. P., Giovino, G. A., Hatziandreu, E. J., et al. 1990. Methods used to quit smoking in the United States: do cessation programs help? *J. Am. Med. Assoc.* 263:2760–65

32. Fiore, M. C., Novotny, T. E., Pierce, J. P., Hatziandreu, E. J., Patel, K. M., Davis, R. M. 1989. Trends in cigarette smoking in the United States: the changing influence of gender and race. *J. Am. Med. Assoc.* 261:49–55

33. Freedman, M. A., Gay, G. A., Brockert, J. E., Patrzeboxski, P. W., Rothwell, C. J. 1988. The 1989 revisions of the US standard certificates of live birth and death and the US standard report of fetal death. *Am. J. Public Health* 78:168–72

34. Glynn, T. J. 1989. Essential elements of school-based smoking prevention programs. *J. Sch. Health* 59:181–88

35. Glynn, T. J., Boyd, G. M., Gruman, J. C. 1990. Essential elements of self-help/minimal intervention strategies for smoking cessation. *Health Educ. Qt.* 17:329–45

36. Glynn, T. J., Manley, M. W. 1989. *How To Help Your Patients Stop Smoking: A National Cancer Institute Manual for Physicians.* Bethesda: Natl. Cancer Inst.

37. Grant-Worley, J. 1990. State use of death certificates to report smoking-attributable mortality. *5th Natl. Conf. Chron. Dis. Prev. Control: From 1990 to 2000, Detroit.* Atlanta: Cent. Dis. Control

38. Grossman, M. 1989. Health benefits of increases in alcohol and cigarette taxes. *Br. J. Addict.* 84:1193–1204

39. Harel, Y., Kann, L., Collins, J., Kolbe, L. 1990. Implementing the youth risk behavior surveillance system: a progress report. *5th Natl. Conf. Chron. Dis. Prev. Control: From 1990 to 2000, Detroit.* Atlanta: Cent. Dis. Control

40. Hatziandreu, E. J., Pierce, J. P., Fiore, M. C., Grise, V., Novotny, T. E., Davis, R. M. 1989. The reliability of self-reported cigarette consumption in the United States. *Am. J. Public Health* 79:1020–23

41. Hatziandreu, E. J., Pierce, J. P., Lefkopoulou, M., Fiore, M. C., Mills, S. L., et al. 1990. Quitting smoking in the United States in 1986. *J. Natl. Cancer Inst.* 2:1402–6

42. Haynes, S. G., Harvey, C., Montes, H., Nickens, H., Cohen, B. H. 1990. Patterns of cigarette smoking among Hispanics in the United States: results from HHANES 1982–84. *Am. J. Public Health* 80(Suppl.):47–54

43. Hu, T., Bai, J., Keeler, T. E., Barnett, P. G. 1991. The impact of a large tax

increase on cigarette consumption: the case of California. Work. Pap. No. 91–174. Univ. of Calif. Berkeley, Dep. of Econ., July

44. Inst. Med. 1988. *The Future of Public Health.* Washington, DC: Natl. Acad. Press

45. Johnston, L. D., O'Malley, P. M., Bachman, J. G. 1987. *National Trends in Drug Use and Related Factors Among American High School Students and Young Adults, 1975–1986.* Rockville, Md: Natl. Inst. Drug Abuse

46. Jonas, S. 1986. Provision of public health services. In *Public Health and Preventive Medicine,* ed. J. M. Last, pp. 1628–29. Norwalk, Conn: Appleton-Century-Crofts

47. Kizer, K. W., Honig, B. 1990. *Toward a Tobacco-Free California: A Status Report to the California Legislature on the First Fifteen Months of California's Tobacco Control Program.* Sacramento: Calif. Dep. Health Serv.

48. Lewit, E. M., Coate, D. 1982. The potential for using excise taxes to reduce smoking. *J. Health Econ.* 1:121–45

49. Malloy, M. H., Kleinman, J. C., Land, G. H., Schramm, W. F. 1988. The association of maternal smoking with age and cause of infant death. *Am. J. Epidemiol.* 128(1):46–55

50. Marcus, A. C., Shopland, D. R., Crane, L. A., Lynn, W. R. 1989. Prevalence of cigarette smoking in the United States: Estimates from the 1985 current population survey. *J. Natl. Cancer Inst.* 1:409–14

51. McKenna, J., Carbone, E. 1989. Huge tobacco control project begun by NCI, ACS. *J. Natl. Cancer Inst.* 81:93–94

52. Natl. Cancer Inst. 1988. *COMMIT Protocol Summary.* Bethesda: Natl. Cancer Inst., Natl. Inst. Health, US Dep. Health Hum. Serv.

53. Natl. Cancer Inst. 1988. *Media Strategies for Smoking Control—Guidelines.* Consensus workshop conducted by the Advocacy Inst. for Natl. Cancer Inst. Jan. 14–15. Bethesda: US Dep. Health Hum. Serv., Public Health Serv., Natl. Inst. Health, Natl. Cancer Inst.

54. Novotny, T. E. 1991. Passive smoking—beliefs, attitudes, and exposures in the United States. In *Compendium of Technical Information on Environmental Tobacco Smoke.* Washington, DC: Environ. Prot. Agency. In press

55. Novotny, T. E., Thomas, W. I. 1990. *The Rocky Mountain Tobacco-Free Challenge Evaluation Report 1990.* Rockville, Md: US Dep. Health Hum.

Serv., Public Health Serv., Cent. Dis. Control, Cent. Chron. Dis. Prev. Health Promot., Off. Smoking Health

56. Novotny, T. E., Warner, K. E., Kendrick, J. S., Remington, P. M. 1988. Socioeconomic factors and racial smoking differences. *Am. J. Public Health* 79:1416–19

57. Off. Smoking Health Program Serv. Act. 1991. *The Rocky Mountain Tobacco Free Challenge—Evaluation Report 1991.* Atlanta: Off. Smoking Health, Natl. Cent. Chron. Dis. Prev. Health Promot., Cent. Dis. Control. In press

58. O'Keefe, A. M. 1991. *Guidelines for the Use of Paid Media in Tobacco Control.* Bethesda: US Dep. Health Hum. Serv., Natl. Cancer Inst., Div. Cancer Prev. Control. In press

59. Peterson, D. E., Remington, P. L., Anderson, H. A. 1990. Price, taxes, and trends in cigarette sales in the United States, 1979–88. In *Epidemic Intell. Serv.,* 39th Annu. Conf., Atlanta. Atlanta: Cent. Dis. Control

60. Pierce, J. P., Fiore, M. C., Novotny, T. E., Hatziandreu, E. J., Davis, R. M. 1989. Trends in cigarette smoking in the United States: educational differences are increasing. *J. Am. Med. Assoc.* 261:56–60

61. Pierce, J. P., Fiore, M. C., Novotny, T. E., Hatziandreu, E. J., Davis, R. M. 1989. Trends in cigarette smoking in the United States: projections to the year 2000. *J. Am. Med. Assoc.* 261:61–65

62. Pierce, J. P., Macaskill, P., Hill, D. 1990. Long-term effectiveness of mass media led antismoking campaigns in Australia. *Am. J. Public Health* 80:565–69

63. Ravenholt, R. T. 1985. Tobacco's impact on twentieth-century US mortality patterns. *Am. J. Prev. Med.* 1:4–17

64. Remington, P. L., Novotny, T. E., Williamson, D. F., Anda, R. F. 1989. State-specific progress toward the 1990 Objective for the Nation for cigarette smoking prevalence. *Am. J. Public Health* 79:1416–19

65. Rogers, E. M. 1983. *Diffusion of Innovations.* New York: Free Press. 3rd ed.

66. Rothenberg, R. B., Koplan, J. P. 1990. Chronic disease in the 1990s. *Annu. Rev. Public Health* 11:267–96

67. Shea, S., Basch, C. E. 1990. A review of five major community-based cardiovascular disease prevention programs. Part II: intervention strategies, evaluation methods, and results. *Am. J. Health Promot.* 4(4):279–87

68. Schwartz, J. L. 1987. *Review and Evaluation of Smoking Cessation*

Methods: The United States and Canada, 1978–1985. NIH Publ. No. 87-2940. Bethesda: Natl. Cancer Inst.

69. Shultz, J. M., Novotny, T. E., Rice, D. P. 1991. Quantifying the disease impact of cigarette smoking with SAMMEC II software. *Public Health Rep.* 106:326–32

70. Smoking, Tobacco, Cancer Program. 1990. *1985–1989 Status Report.* DHHS Publ. No. (NIH) 90-3107. Bethesda: US Dep. Health Hum. Serv., Public Health Serv., Natl. Inst. Health, Natl. Cancer Inst.

71. Sullivan, L. W. 1990. Statement of Louis W. Sullivan, M. D., Secr. Health Hum. Serv., before the Comm. on Finance, US Senate, May 24

72. Tobacco-Free Am. 1990. *State Legislated Actions on Tobacco Issues.* Washington, DC: Tobacco-Free Am., Legis. Clearinghouse

73. Tobacco Inst. 1988. *The Tax Burden on Tobacco. Historical Compilation,* Vol. 22. Washington, DC: Tobacco Inst.

74. Univ. of Calif., San Diego. 1990. *Tobacco Use in California—1990.* Sacramento: Calif. Dep. Health Serv.

75. Deleted in proof

76. US Dep. Health, Educ., Welf. 1964. *Smoking and Health. Report of the Advisory Committee to the Surgeon General of the Public Health Service.* PHS Publ. No. (HEW) 1103. Washington, DC: US Dep. Health, Educ., Welf., Public Health Serv., Cent. Dis. Control

77. US Dep. Health Hum. Serv. 1991. *Secretary's Program Direction Plans—Fiscal Years 1991 and 1992.* Washington, DC: US Dep. Health Hum. Serv.

78. US Dep. Health Hum. Serv. 1990. *Bibliography on Smoking and Health.* DHHS Publ. No. (CDC) 90-8399. Rockville, Md: US Dep. Health Hum. Serv., Public Health Serv., Cent. Dis. Control, Cent. Chron. Dis. Prev. Health Promot., Off. Smoking Health

79. US Dep. Health Hum. Serv. 1990. *The Health Benefits of Smoking Cessation—A Report of the Surgeon General.* DHHS Publ. No. (CDC) 90-8416. Rockville, Md: US Dep. Health Hum. Serv., Public Health Serv., Cent. Dis. Control, Cent. Chron. Dis. Prev. Health Promot., Off. Smoking Health

80. US Dep. Health Hum. Serv. 1990. *Healthy People 2000: National Health Promotion and Disease Prevention Objectives.* (Conf. Ed.) Washington, DC: US Dep. Health Hum. Serv.

81. US Dep. Health Hum. Serv. 1990. *Smoking and Health: A National Status Report. A Report to Congress,* 2nd ed. DHHS Publ. No. (CDC)87-8396. Rockville, Md: US Dep. Health Hum. Serv., Public Health Serv., Cent. Chron. Dis. Prev. Health Promot., Cent. Dis. Control, Off. Smoking Health

82. US Dep. Health Hum. Serv. 1990. *Youth Access to Cigarettes.* Off. Inspect. Gen., Off. Eval. Inspect. Publ. No. OEI-02-90-02310. New York: US Dep. Health Hum. Serv.

83. US Dep. Health Hum. Serv. 1989. *Making Health Communication Programs Work: A Planner's Guide.* DHHS Publ. No. (NIH) 89-1493. Bethesda: US Dep. Health Hum. Serv. Public Health Serv., Natl. Inst. Health, Natl. Cancer Inst., Off. Cancer Commun.

84. US Dep. Health Hum. Serv. 1989. *Reducing the Health Consequences of Smoking: 25 Years of Progress. A Report of the Surgeon General.* DHHS Publ. No. (CDC)89-8411. Rockville, Md: US Dep. Health Hum. Serv., Public Health Serv., Cent. Dis. Control, Cent. Chron. Dis. Prev. Health Promot., Off. Smoking Health

85. US Environ. Prot. Agency. 1990. *Health Effects of Passive Smoking: Assessment of Lung Cancer in Adults and Respiratory Disorders in Children.* EPA/600/6-90/006A. Washington, DC: Off. Health Environ. Assess., Off. Res. Dev. Indoor Air Div., Off. Atmospheric Indoor Air Programs, Off. Air Radiat., US Environ. Prot. Agency

86. US Off. Technol. Assess. 1985. *Smoking-Related Deaths and Financial Costs.* Washington, DC: Off. Technol. Assess. US Congr., Health Program

87. Walter, S. D. 1976. The estimation and interpretation of attributable risk in health research. *Biometrics* 32:829–49

88. Warner, K. E. 1987. Health and economic implications of a tobacco-free society. *J. Am. Med. Assoc.* 258:2080–86

89. Warner, K. E. 1981. State legislation on smoking and health: a comparison of two policies. *Policy Sci.* 13:139–52

90. World Health Organ. WHO Expert Comm. 1983. *Smoking Control Strategies in Developing Countries: Report of a WHO Expert Committee.* WHO Tech. Rep. Ser. No. 695. Geneva: WHO

91. Zahniser, S. C., Floyd, R. L., Salas, N., Miller, N., Kendrick, J., et al. 1989. Integrating smoking cessation into public prenatal clinics. (Poster) In *Am. Public Health Assoc. 117th Annu. Meet.* Chicago, Oct. 23. Washington, DC: Am. Public Health Assoc.

Annu. Rev. Publ. Health. 1992. 13:319–39
Copyright © 1992 by Annual Reviews Inc. All rights reserved

DEPRESSION: Current Understanding and Changing Trends

Myrna M. Weissman

College of Physicians and Surgeons of Columbia University; Department of Clinical and Genetic Epidemiology, New York State Psychiatric Institute, New York, NY 10032

Gerald L. Klerman

Department of Psychiatry, Cornell University Medical Center, Payne Whitney Psychiatric Clinic, New York, NY 10021

KEY WORDS: psychiatric epidemiology, age-period-cohort, psychiatric diagnosis, treatment of depression, genetic epidemiology

INTRODUCTION

In the last decade, our understanding of the epidemiology of mood disorders, including bipolar disorder, major depression, and dysthymia, has accelerated. There is also clearer understanding of the rates and risk factors, comorbidity and social morbidity, and the changing patterns of these disorders, both nationally and cross-nationally. Notions about the age of onset of these disorders have changed considerably (1). Investigators now recognize that depression can occur prepubertally and often begins in adolescence and that family history (i.e. the presence of a mood disorder in a first degree biological relative) is one of the most important risk factors. Considerable data, based on controlled clinical trials, are now available on the efficacy of a broad range of pharmacologic and psychotherapeutic treatments, for both acute and maintenance treatment for the various types of the mood disorders. This chapter reviews these relatively recent advances in understanding the epidemiology, familial nature, treatment, and morbidity of mood disorders.

319

0163-7525/92/0501-0319$02.00

DIAGNOSIS AND CLASSIFICATION

Mood disorder refers to a group of clinical conditions, whose common feature is the patient's disturbed mood, either depression or elation. This distinction does not imply a common etiology. Mood disorders are probably biologically heterogeneous, comparable to the situation for mental retardation or jaundice. The major distinction in mood disorders is between bipolar and the depressive disorders and, within the depressive disorders, major depression and dysthymia.

The concept of a mood disorder (sometimes called affective disorder) itself is noteworthy. This chapter could not have been written two decades ago. The conditions that are today grouped together as mood disorders were treated separately in the American Psychiatric Association's *Diagnostic and Statistical Manual of Mental Disorders,* second edition (DSM-II) as part of either psychosis or neurosis, the two predominant psychiatric categories in the 1960s.

Over the last decade, diagnostic criteria have been specified for the major mental disorders. These criteria are based on type, number, frequency, and duration of symptoms, as well as on exclusions, and were codified in 1980 in DSM-III (2). In 1987, minor revisions were made in the classification and published as DSM-IIIR. The DSM-IV will appear in 1994.

The DSM-III abolished the distinction between psychotic and neurotic conditions and brought together several depressive conditions, which were first called affective disorders and, later, mood disorders in DSM-IIIR. The separation of depressions into bipolar and major depression is widely accepted because of differences in family patterns, effective treatment, and natural course.

Table 1 lists the broad outline of the DSM-IIIR classification of the mood disorders. Each disorder can be further classified by severity, whether it is in remission, or whether psychotic features are present. Each disorder also has a category [Not Otherwise Specified (NOS)] for patients who typically do not fit the criteria for subclassification. Each diagnosis has specified criteria. The specified criteria for the major categories follow.

Bipolar Disorder

The presence of mania defines bipolar disorder. Mania is a distinct period during which the predominant mood is either elevated, expansive, or irritable and there are associated symptoms, including hyperactivity, pressure of speech, racing thoughts, inflated self-esteem, decreased need for sleep, distractibility, and excessive involvement in activities that have high potential for painful consequences.

Mania without major depression, sometimes called "unipolar mania," is

Table 1 DSM-IIIR classification of mood disorders

Bipolar Disorder	Depressive Disorders
Mixed	Major Depression
Manic	single episode
Depressed	recurrent
Cyclothymia	Dysthymia
Bipolar Disorder (NOS)[a]	primary or secondary
	early or late onset
	Depressive Disorder (NOS)

[a] Not Otherwise Specified.

uncommon, but does occur. Bipolar disorder can present as either a manic or a depressive state. Cyclothymia, which is a mild chronic form of mood swings, is interesting because of its aggregation in the biological relatives of patients with bipolar disorder. For this reason, cyclothymia is considered part of the spectrum of bipolar disorder. However, it is often difficult to differentiate the boundaries between cyclothymia and normal moods.

Depressive Disorders

MAJOR DEPRESSION   The essential feature is either a dysphoric mood or a loss of interest or pleasure in all or almost all of usual activities and pastimes. The disturbance is prominent, relatively persistent, and associated with other symptoms, including appetite disturbance, change in weight, sleep disturbance, psychomotor agitation or retardation, decreased energy, feelings of worthlessness or guilt, difficulty concentrating or thinking, and thoughts of death or suicide or suicidal attempts. Major depression is only diagnosed in the absence of current or past manic symptoms. Although there is general agreement that major depression is a heterogenous disorder, there is no consensus or little empirical basis for most of the subtypes used clinically, such as endogenous, seasonal, or melancholic depression.

DYSTHYMIA   The essential feature is a chronic disturbance in mood, involving either depressed mood or loss of interest or pleasure in all or almost all usual activities and pastimes, and associated symptoms, but not of sufficient severity or duration to meet the criteria for major depression. The primary distinction between dysthymia and major depression is that the former is chronic, but symptomatically less severe, and must persist for at least two years to meet the criteria. Whether dysthymia is an independent disorder or a variant of major depression is controversial. At least some dysthymias are probably prodromal of major depression or the residual of untreated major depression. At this point, these issues have not been resolved, and the

DSM-IIIR divides dysthymia by whether it occurs primary or secondary to another disorder and by age of onset, with age 21 being the division. Many patients have depressive symptoms, but do not meet the criteria for either dysthymia or major depression and do not have manic episodes. These patients often appear in primary care and medical clinics and are important from the public health point of view, because of their high prevalence and disability. These depressive symptoms that do not meet criteria do not appear in the official DSM-III nomenclature or may be classified as an adjustment disorder that persists for more than six months secondary to major identifiable psychosocial stresses.

EPIDEMIOLOGY

With the exception of a few European studies, epidemiologic approaches were infrequently applied to the study of psychiatric disorders in the community until the 1970s. The major obstacles were the lack of specification of the diagnostic criteria and the difficulty in obtaining reliable diagnoses.

In the US, the period after World War II was one of considerable activity in the epidemiology of mental impairment and health. Several classic epidemiologic studies of this period were completed, including studies that showed the relationship between social class and mental illness, the effects of changing traditions and values in a small town, and the effects of urban life. These studies demonstrated the importance of poverty, urban social stress, and social change in the development of impairment. The investigators used sophisticated statistical and sampling techniques. However, symptom or impairment scales that did not generate rates of specific psychiatric disorders were used. The findings from these studies did not have a major impact on clinical psychiatry (3, 4).

Psychiatric epidemiology, clinical psychiatry, and clinical research did not begin to converge until the mid-1970s. The introduction into psychiatry of specified diagnostic criteria, which had standardized methods of assessing signs and symptoms of psychiatric disorders necessary to make the criteria, provided the technology for systematic diagnoses in epidemiologic studies. Epidemiologic researchers were skeptical about the ability to use these methods in community studies. The methods, which were first applied in 1975 in a small community study of 500 subjects who lived in New Haven, Connecticut, were shown to be feasible and reliable (5). In the late 1970s, President Carter's Commission on Mental Health request for data on the magnitude of psychiatric illness in the community for planning mental health programs gave impetus to the next phase of studies.

In 1980, the National Institute of Mental Health (NIMH) Epidemiologic Catchment Area (ECA) study was initiated by using the Diagnostic Interview

Schedule (DIS), a new instrument developed specifically for large-scale epidemiologic studies of psychiatric disorders (6). The purpose was to collect data on the rates, risk factors, and treatment patterns of the major mental illnesses in the community. The study, which is based on over 18,000 persons living in five communities in the US (New Haven, St. Louis, Baltimore, Durham, and Los Angeles), forms the basis of our current understanding of the epidemiology of the major psychiatric disorders (7).

Parallel developments were being undertaken in England (8, 9, 10). As knowledge of ECA grew, similar studies that used identical methodology were undertaken in different parts of the world (see Table 2). In many cases, the staff in other countries were trained in the use of the DIS by Robins and colleagues in St. Louis. Thus, for the first time, independent, cross-national comparisons of epidemiologic rates, which use data obtained with similar methods, is now possible. The findings from these studies for the mood disorders are summarized below.

Bipolar Disorder

The community-based lifetime rates in the US for bipolar disorder are about 1% (range .7–1.6%). The rates are lower (about .5%) in Edmonton, Canada;

Table 2   Lifetime prevalence rates/100 in adults aged 18+ for bipolar disorder, major depression, and dysthymia, based on community surveys using DIS and DSM-III diagnosis

	Time	N	Bipolar	Major Depression	Dysthymia
USA-ECA	1980–1983	18572	1.2	4.4	3.0[55]
New Haven	1980	5034	1.6	5.8	3.2
Baltimore	1981	3481	1.2	2.9	2.1
St. Louis	1981	3004	1.6	4.4	3.8
Durham	1982	3921	.7	3.5	2.3
Los Angeles	1983	3132	1.1	5.6	4.2
Edmonton	1983	3258	.6	8.6	3.7[56]
Puerto Rico	1984	1551	.5	4.6	4.7[57]
Florence[b]	1985	1000	1.3	6.2	2.6[58]
Seoul	1984	5100	.4	3.4	2.2[59]
Taiwan	1982	11004	—[60]		
Urban		5005	.16	0.9	0.9
Small towns		3004	.07	1.7	1.5
Rural area		2995	.10	1.0	0.9
New Zeland	1986	1498	—	12.6	—[61]

[a] Rates rounded off to one decimal in most cases.
[b] Only annual prevalence rates reported.

Puerto Rico; and Seoul, Korea. Only annual rates have been reported in Florence, Italy, and these rates (1.3%) are similar to the US lifetime rates. The similarity in lifetime US and annual Florence rates may result because physicians are used as interviewers in Florence or because bipolar disorder is a chronic illness. The similarities, rather than the differences, in cross-national rates are notable, with the exception of Taiwan (about .1 and .6%). However, the rates for most psychiatric disorders, and particularly the mood disorders, are lower in Taiwan and in the limited unpublished data available from Shanghai (W. Lui 1990, personal communication). Without data from Chinese who live outside of the Republic of China (Taiwan) or the Peoples Republic of China, it is not possible to determine if this finding is unique to the Chinese.

The rates of bipolar disorder are similar in men and women. There is a trend for increased risk in urban areas. The mean age of onset is the late teens and early 20s, with many onsets occurring in adolescence. There is suggestion of temporal changes of the rates of bipolar disorder with an increase of rates and an earlier age of onset in the cohorts born since 1940 (11, 12). Family history, although not assessed in the community surveys, remains one of the most important risk factors for bipolar disorder, as we discuss later.

Marital problems and depression are often closely associated, although the specific type of depression has usually not been specified. For bipolar disorder, the rates are highest for persons who are cohabitating, but not married; have a history of divorce, regardless of their current marital status; or who have never married. The rates are lowest in married or widowed persons without a history of divorce. However, assumptions about any causal relationship require caution. A break-up of a marriage may be a response by the well spouse to the stress of living with a depressed person, or may be brought about by the affected person who attributes the distress to failings in the spouse (13).

Major Depression

Major depression is considerably more prevelant than bipolar disorder and, unlike bipolar disorder, has higher prevalence in women than in men. There is also more variability in the rates by site. The lifetime rates vary between 3.5% and 5.8% in the US sites, including Puerto Rico (Table 2). The higher rates in New Haven are undoubtedly due to the use of slightly broader criteria for major depression of one, rather than two, weeks duration. The rates are highest in Edmonton and New Zealand. Again, Taiwan has low rates of .9%–1.7%.

Unlike Taiwan, Korea is a more westernized country, and the lifetime prevalence rate of major depression is 3.4%, comparable to the lower end of the ECA five-site range. Most non-US studies sampled more homogenous communities than did the ECA five-study, which by design had diverse ethnic, racial, and socioeconomic sampled. Puerto Rico's data resembled the ECA results, with a lifetime prevalence of 4.6%.

Several risk factors in major depression have emerged from community studies. Female sex continues to be the clearest and most consistent risk factor in all sites listed on Table 2, as well as in family studies (14). Positive family history of major depression, although not assessed in community studies, is also a risk factor and is discussed later. The ECA found few black-white differences in rates of major depression, once social class and education were controlled. However, as noted before, the Chinese appear to have substantially lower rates of major depression than US whites or blacks, as reflected in the rate in Taiwan, as well as unpublished rates from an epidemiologic study in Shanghai, China. Unfortunately, there are no data from Japan.

There are higher rates in urban rather than rural areas (15), but not a strong effect for social class. As with bipolar disorder, a history of divorce or separation had a profound effect on increasing rates of major depression. More specifically, continuously married and never married people had the lowest rate, and divorced people the highest.

Dysthymia

Dysthymia is slightly less prevalent over a lifetime than major depression. In both Puerto Rico and Taiwan, however, lifetime risk for major depression and dysthymia are about equal. Dysthymia in the US, including Puerto Rico, ranges from 2.1% to 4.7%. The rates are considered lower in Taiwan (.9–1.5%). In all countries, the rate is about twice as high in females than in males.

With dysthymia, the variations found with race, marital status, and urban/rural areas are similar to those found for major depression. However, for dysthymia, unlike major depression, there is a significant inverse relationship with income, especially in young persons. Unlike major depression or bipolar disorder, the rate begins to decrease around age 45. The similarity in rates, risk factors, and high comorbidity between major depression and dysthymia (termed double depression) has raised questions about whether these are distinct disorders. This issue is still unresolved.

Changing Rates of Depression

There is reasonably consistent evidence for a change in the rates of major depression, with higher rates in more recent birth cohorts and an earlier age of onset (14). This observation was first made in the 1960s and 1970s, based on the following: admission at hospitals for affective illness had increased between 1950 and 1970, as compared with the previous three decades; the average age of onset for major depression in clinical samples was considerably younger than had been reported before World War II; childhood depression was seen in increasing frequency in pediatric and psychiatric settings; an increase in suicide attempts and deaths among adolescents was noted; and the rates of major depression based on community studies in the elderly were low (16). However, investigations of temporal changes in the rates of depression and other psychiatric disorders before the mid-1980s were hampered, because of lack of large systematic studies that used standardized diagnostic criteria. Thus, it was not possible to tell whether the differences observed in rates were real or caused by changing methodology, treatments, or concepts.

The ECA study in the US, as well as several large family studies of relatives of depressed patients that used diagnostic methods comparable to the ECA, suggested the following temporal changes in the rates of major depression: an increase in the rates of the cohorts born after 1940; a decrease in the age of onset, with an increase in the teenage and early adult years (see Figure 1); an increase in rates for the cohorts born between 1960 and 1975, with an increase in the rates of depression for all ages, but particularly among younger age groups in that period; a persistent gender effect with the risk of major depression consistently two or three times higher among women than in men; a persistent family effect with the risk of major depression about two to three times higher in the first-degree relatives of depressed patients, as compared with controls; and a possible narrowing of the differential risk to men and

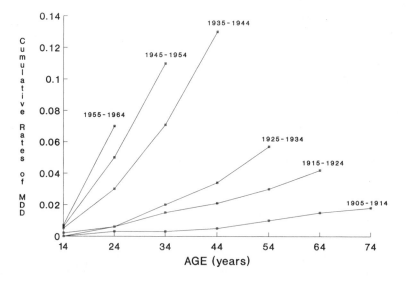

Figure 1 The temporal trends (period-cohort effects) and lifetime prevalence of major depression, from the ECA study at five sites. Includes both sexes, white only.

women because of a greater increase in the risk of major depression among young men (14, 17–20).

These trends were noted in epidemiologic studies, as previously described, in the US, Germany, Canada, and New Zealand, but they were not found to the same extent in studies conducted in Korea or Puerto Rico.

Various efforts have been undertaken to explain the findings and whether they could be artifact, because of selective mortality and/or institutionalization, selective migration, changing diagnostic criteria, threshold changes in reporting among mental health professionals and/or society at large, reporting bias of interviewers, and recall problems among the elderly (14).

In disorders with familial aggregation, exclusive genetic interpretations are ruled out by observations of temporal changes, because genes are unlikely to change in a relatively short time. The environmental risk factors for depression that have also been suggested include changes in the ratio of males to females; increased urbanization; greater geographic mobility, which results in loss of attachments; increasing social anomie; changes in family structure; alteration in the role of women, especially the increased number of women in the labor force; and shifts in occupational patterns.

Thus far, the increase in the rate over time and by birth cohort have been best established for major depression. However, two independent studies show that the same increase may occur for bipolar disorder (11, 12).

Future Directions in Epidemiologic Studies

The American system of DSM-III, or its forthcoming DSM-IV, is not universally used. A new diagnostic method, Schedules for Clinical Assessment in Neuropsychiatry (SCAN) is being field tested in 20 centers in 11 countries (21). The aim is to develop a comprehensive procedure for clinical examination that is also capable of generating many of the categories of the *International Classification of Disease*, 10th edition (ICD-10), as well as the DSM-III and IV. The Composite International Diagnostic Interview (CIDI), based on the DSM-III and the ICD, has also been developed (22). The two instruments are complementary, as the CIDI is designed for use in large community surveys that necessitate the employment of lay interviewers, whereas SCAN can only be used in its full form by clinically trained professionals. The availability of two diagnostic methods that bridge the major classification systems will facilitate future cross-national comparative studies.

Lastly, none of the epidemiologic studies mentioned included children, even though mood disorders, as well as many of the major mental illnesses, often first occur in adolescence and, to a lesser extent, in childhood. Currently, there is field testing of diagnostic methods applicable to epidemiologic studies of children at Columbia, Yale, and Emory Universities and the University of Puerto Rico in preparation for a multisite epidemiologic study of children comparable to the ECA study for adults. By the year 2000, we can expect that information on the epidemiology of childhood psychiatric disorders will become available.

GENETICS

Evidence for the role of genetic factors in bipolar disorder and, to a lesser extent, major depression has accumulated over the past two decades, based on twin, adoption, and family studies. The interest in the genetics of bipolar disorder has recently been stimulated by the findings of linkage between bipolar disorder and markers on chromosome 11 and the X chromosome (23). The failure to replicate these findings has been a disappointment and highlights the scientific problems in applying the new genetic approaches to complex disorders.

In 1990, the NIMH launched a multisite collaborative program to study the genetics of bipolar disorder, as well as schizophrenia and Alzheimer's disease. Their goal is to establish a national resource of immortalized cell lines and psychiatric histories in reliably diagnosed pedigrees and to collect sufficiently large samples to detect any linkage. The focus in the first year has been on standardizing the assessment procedures across sites. The recent report in *Nature* of a pinpoint mutation in a single gene on chromosome 21 for some forms of Alzheimer's disease makes this collaborative project timely (24).

Bipolar Disorder

The selection of bipolar disorder for this first NIMH collaborative genetics initiative derives from the reasonably strong evidence from twin, adoption, and family studies for the genetic transmission of bipolar disorder. The mode of transmission, the spectrum of bipolar disorder, and the relationship between bipolar disorder and major depression are unclear (11, 25, 26). With increasing chromosome markers to map the entire genome, perhaps more definitive information will become available on linkage by using restriction fragment length polymorphisms. The findings of linkage could well call for additional family and epidemiologic work to identify other factors, both genetic and nongenetic, that may modify the expression of a disorder. The concordance in monozygotic twins for bipolar disorder is much below 100%; thus, other factors may be operating. The findings of possible temporal changes in the rates of bipolar disorder imply that there are environmental factors in the expression of the disorder.

Major Depression

The phenotypic heterogeneity of major depression presents a problem for recombinant DNA approaches, and the search in family and clinical studies has been for subtype(s) of major depression that might be homogeneous and possibly genetic. Twin data generally support the role of genetic factors in some of the depressions, particularly psychotic depression (27). These findings do not extend to all subtypes of major depression and seem less likely with dysthymia. However, the twin studies completed by using modern diagnostic criteria have been based on very small samples, so that conclusions about concordance cannot be drawn. A large twin study by Kendler at the University of Virginia, which may clarify these issues, is under way.

Over the past decade, there have been several, well designed family studies, which indicates clearly that major depression is highly familial (see Table 3) (28). The lifetime rate of major depression in the first-degree relative ranges from 8.6% to 34.9%, which is usually about two- to threefold higher than in relatives of matched comparison groups and higher than the population rates. The Bland et al (29) study that had the lowest rate of major depression in relatives also had the oldest patients with later ages of onset. No substantial increase of bipolar disorder is found in the relatives of patients with major depression.

There is a long history of searching for specific homogeneous subtypes of major depression. Some of the subtypes suggested as possibly homogeneous and more biological, such as endogenous or melancholic depression, have not been shown to have a higher familial aggregation than the nonendogenous, nonmelancholic subtypes. However, an increased familial aggregation and specificity transmission of early onset (<20 yrs.) of major depression has been demonstrated (30).

Adoption studies have been inconclusive for major depression. A recent

Table 3   Morbid risk of depression in first-degree relatives of unipolar depressive probands[a]

Reference	% (N) at Risk
Winokur et al 1982 (62)	11.2 (305)
Gershon et al 1982 (63)	16.6 (133)
Baron et al 1982 (64)	17.7 (143.5)
Weissman et al 1984 (65)	18.4 (287)
Bland et al 1986 (66)	8.6 (763*)
Stancer et al 1987 (67)	24.4 (282)
Rice 1987[b] (68)	28.6 (1176)
Giles et al 1988[b] (69)	34.9 (43)
McGuffin et al 1988 (70)	
Outpatient treatment only	24.6 (199.5)
Inpatient + outpatient treatment	11.8 (187)
Kupfer et al 1989 (71)	
Recurrent depressive probands	20.7 (725)

[a] From Ref. 61a, with permission.
[b] Unadjusted number and morbid risk.

adoption study from Stockholm did not find a higher rate of depression in the biological parent of adopted-away depressed offspring (31). The lack of an association may be due to their reliance on hospital records. Moreover, these data are at variance with other adoption studies of major depression (32).

Dysthymia

There are several family studies of dysthymia under way, and information will be forthcoming in the next few years. The family studies of patients with major depression find that dysthymia aggregates in their first-degree relatives, thus suggesting that dysthymia is on the spectrum of major depression.

CHILDREN

Whether or not a precise genetic etiology of the mood disorders is determined, the findings on familial aggregation have public health implications for children. Until recently, the conventional wisdom was that children were not capable of becoming depressed. In fact, before 1972, there were no textbooks of psychiatry that mentioned depression in children. With the increased use of systematic diagnostic assessments of children over the last decade, it has become clear that depression does occur in prepubertal children and is common in adolescence. Moreover, the offspring of depressed parents are at increased risk for depression, as well as a variety of other types of social, school, and health problems. Several research efforts are under way to understand the clinical characteristics, familial aggregation, treatment, and course of depression in children. Although most of the studies have been on the children of parents with major depression (33–37), there have been some studies of the children of bipolar parents (38).

In general, the findings show that major depression in a parent increases the risk for psychiatric disorders in children, particularly for major depression and anxiety disorders. In addition, the children of depressed parents, as compared with children of nondepressed parents, are more impaired in school and with peers and have higher rates of developmental and medical problems.

Although the children of parents without psychiatric disorder also develop major depression, their rate is significantly lower and the age of onset may be later, most commonly in the midteens, and rarely prepubertally. In the one study that found specificity of transmission of age of onset of major depression between parent and child, all the prepubertal depression occurred in the offspring of parents who had a first onset of major depression before age 20 (33). A two-year follow-up study of the same cohort suggested that depressions that occur in the children of nondepressed parents tend to be more transient and milder (39).

Based on a limited number of studies, the children of bipolar parents appear to be at increased risk for psychiatric disorders and possibly cyclothymia. Because bipolar disorder is less common than major depression, large samples of children may be required to show an effect. However, if the proband is defined as the adolescent with bipolar illness, and the rates of illness are assessed in the adolescent's first-degree relatives (i.e. siblings and parents), then an increased risk for both major depression and bipolar illness in the relatives is found (40, 41). It is unclear if bipolar disorder occurs prepubertally and, if so, what the early signs are.

A related question regarding depressed children concerns the continuity between childhood and adult depression. To date, there is not one longitudinal study that has sampled groups of children who are depressed, by using modern diagnostic criteria, and has followed them into adulthood. The study that comes closest to having the ideal design (42) used a "catch-up longitudinal design" to assess adult psychiatric status and social adjustment of 52 depressed children and adolescents, compared with 52 individually matched controls. The authors' major findings were that the depressed children were at an increased risk for mood disorders in adult life and had elevated risk of psychiatric hospitalization and treatment. They were no more likely than the control group to have nondepressive adult psychiatric disorders. These findings strongly suggested that there was substantial specificity and continuity in mood disturbance between childhood and adult life.

Information from long-term follow-up of depressed children to determine the continuity between childhood and adult disorders may clarify two puzzling findings: depressed children do not have the same good response to the tricyclic antidepressants as seen in adults; and their sleep patterns and cortisol response during depression are somewhat different than adults, although the biologic studies on depressed children are limited. Better understanding of the nature of depression in childhood and its relationship to adult depression could have implications for treatment and earlier preventive intervention.

SOCIAL MORBIDITY AND QUALITY OF LIFE

The social morbidity and impairment of functioning in work and marriage in patients with major depression has been well documented for more than 20 years. However, it is unclear how their functioning compares with patients who have chronic medical conditions, or whether patients with depressive symptoms that do not meet criteria for DSM-III disorders are impaired. These latter patients represent a large number who are seen in primary care and medical clinics, but do not come to the attention of mental health professionals (43). The recent Rand Case medical Medical Outcome Study (44, 45) monitored the patterns of morbidity outcome in health care in patients with major depression, dysthymia, or depressive symptoms that do not meet full criterion of either. They compared chronic medical conditions, including hypertension, diabetes, coronary artery disease, angina, arthritis, back problems, lung problems, and gastrointestinal problems, as well as a sample of patients who had acute, but not chronic, medical problems (46). Of the 11,000 patients sampled, 466 had depressive symptoms that did not meet the criteria of disorder, and an additional 168 met the criteria for a depressive disorder. These patients were monitored over two years, and an assessment was made of the number of days in bed, self-perceived current health status, and extent of body pain in the past month.

The major finding was that, among the patients seen by medical clinicians, those with major depression had poorer current health status than those with depressive symptoms alone. Patients in the two depressive samples and the eight chronic medical samples were compared as to physical activities, such as sports, climbing stairs, walking, dressing, and bathing; normal social role performance at work or in the household; and social functioning with friends and relatives. Patients with depressive symptoms had significantly worse social functioning and reported significantly more days in bed than patients with six of the eight chronic medical conditions, the main exception being coronary artery disease. Depressive symptoms and current medical conditions had additive effects with regard to measures of patient functioning and well-being. The functioning of depressed patients was comparable to and, at times, worse than patients with several chronic medical conditions (47).

In a separate study, excessive mortality from multiple causes was found in a large community sample derived from the ECA of depressives over age 55 (48). Previous reports of mortality among depressed patients, also based on community samples, indicated an excess of death by suicide and accidents for younger depressed patients; in older age groups, suicide becomes less prominent, whereas chronic medical conditions, especially cardiovascular disease, provided the excess mortality.

TREATMENT

Pharmacologic

Since the 1960s, there have been advances in the treatment of depression, a decrease in hospitalization, reduction in the duration of an episode, and strategies developed for prevention of relapse and recurrence. Most treatment for all mood disorders is now ambulatory. The tricyclic antidepressants have been available for more than two decades, and their therapeutic value for major depression was seen in the early 1960s. Only recently has there been sufficient experience with the range of doses and with blood-level determinations. There is excellent evidence that the symptoms of depression can be reduced in two to four weeks with pharmacologic treatment, usually a tricyclic antidepressant. Soon after the antidepressants were introduced, however, investigators found that a high percentage of patients relapsed following short-term treatment; continuation therapy strategies were common in clinical practice and became the subject of several research studies. The goal of continuation treatments are to sustain the remission brought about by short-term treatment, to prevent relapse, and to facilitate social and economic functioning. There is no agreement as to the optimal duration of continuation drug treatment, although commonly six months to two years have been efficacious. Beyond one or two years, treatment is considered maintenance or prophylactic. The longest studies of drug therapy are of three years' duration. These studies show clearly that maintenance treatment of lithium for bipolar disorder and tricyclic antidepressants for major depression will markedly reduce relapse rates.

For many patients, mood disorders fit the model of chronic illness, with periods of remission and recurrence. For many, the need for treatment beyond the acute phase is increasingly supported by follow-up and treatment studies. Over the last decade, several newer antidepressants have appeared, with a wide variety of chemical structures and pharmacologic profile (49). These drugs have been aimed at counteracting or eliminating problems with the original generation of antidepressants by reducing the anticholinergic effects, i.e. dry mouth and urinary retention, lowering cardiac toxicity and seizure thresholds, and/or reducing weight gain. One new drug, fluoxetine, a compound with highly specific action on serotonin reuptake, has received considerable publicity in the lay press, partially because it has few anticholinergic side effects and does not produce weight gain. Whether its antidepressant effects are remarkably different than the other available compounds is not fully clear.

In regard to other new areas of pharmacologic treatment research, efforts are under way to test the efficacy of antidepressants in patients with dysthymia, a disorder primarily the domain of psychotherapy. The data on the efficacy of tricyclic antidepressants on depressed children and adolescents are limited and inconclusive. Data on the efficacy of tricyclic antidepressants in geriatric depressed patients, based on controlled clinical trials, are also limited. However, the data that are available suggest that the usual antidepressant drugs in lower doses are efficacious in this population and that the side effects are problematic. These populations—dysthymics, depressed children, adolescents, and the elderly—clearly need further study.

The full details for treatment of bipolar disorder, as well as our scientific understanding, has been recently summarized by Goodwin & Jamison (50). This book in itself is an achievement of this past decade, because of its reliance on and gleanings from empirical evidence.

Psychotherapy

Over the last ten years, there has been considerable improvement in the quality and quantity of information on the efficacy of psychotherapy treatment in comparison and in combination with pharmacotherapy of adults with major depression. Similar data on the efficacy of psychotherapy are not available for bipolar disorder or dysthymia or for adolescents with major depression, although several clinical trials are now in the planning phase. Several short-term psychotherapies developed specifically for depression, particularly cognitive therapy (CB), interpersonal psychotherapy (IPT), and some behavior approaches, have been specified in manuals. These manuals standardize the treatment and are used in the training of therapists who conduct the treatment in the clinical trials (51). Currently, about 20 clinical trials test the efficacy of these psychotherapies in homogenous samples of patients with major depression. Two recently published, large-scale treatment studies deserve attention: the NIMH Collaborative Treatment Study (52) and the Maintenance Treatment Study of Recurrent Depression (53).

NIMH COLLABORATIVE TREATMENT STUDY   In 1980, the results of several small clinical trials were sufficiently promising, so that the NIMH initiated the first multisite collaborative study of the treatment of depression to include psychotherapy. Based on the models used to test the efficacy of the new psychotropic drugs in the 1960s, this study was designed to test IPT and CB. In three university centers, 250 depressed patients were studied simultaneously. Overall, the findings showed that all active treatments were superior to placebo in the reduction of symptoms over a 16-week period. The overall degree of improvement was highly significant clinically. Over two thirds of the patients were symptom free at the end of treatment. More patients in the placebo-clinical management condition dropped out or were withdrawn, twice as many as in the IPT group, which had the lowest attrition rate. At the end of 12 weeks of treatment, the two psychotherapies and imipramine were equivalent in the reduction of depressive symptoms and in overall functioning. Imipramine had the most rapid initial onset of action and the most consistent positive effect on the various symptom measure. Although many of the less severely depressed patients improved with all treatment conditions, including the placebo group, the more severely depressed patients in the placebo condition did poorly. For the less severely depressed group, there were no differences among the treatments. The severely ill patients in the IPT and imipramine groups had significantly better response (less depressive symptoms) than the placebo group (52). There has been some controversy about the analytic approach used in this study. Reanalysis will soon be forthcoming, although it is unclear if the results will change.

THE MAINTENANCE TREATMENT STUDY OF RECURRENT MAJOR DE-PRESSION   Also in the early 1980s, the University of Pittsburgh group undertook a long-term clinical trial to determine the efficacy of drugs (imipramine) and/or IPT in the prevention of relapse for severe recurrent depression (53). The impetus for this study was the finding that many patients with multiple recurrent episodes were difficult to treat, had a high relapse rate, and were high utilizers of medical and social services. In this study, patients with recurrent depression, who had responded to imipramine plus interpersonal psychotherapy, were randomly assigned to one of five treatments for three years maintenance treatment: IPT alone; IPT and placebo; IPT and imipramine; clinical management; and imipramine, clinical management, and placebo. Contrary to previous experience, imipramine was administered in the highest doses (over 200 mg), and IPT was administered monthly, in the lowest dose ever used in the clinical trials. There were four major findings: high rate of recurrence in one year for untreated control groups; clinically meaningful and statistically significant prevention of relapse and recurrence by both imipramine and IPT; a nonsignificant trend towards value of combined treatment over either treatment alone; and the value of high dose imipramine (over 200 mg/day) (previously considerably lower maintenance doses had been recommended). This long-term study, along with several others that used drugs with and without psychotherapy, clearly established the value of maintenance treatment in the prevention of relapse and recurrence in unipolar depression.

Alternatives to medication as a treatment for depression are enormously important. For various reasons, many patients will not or cannot take drugs, e.g. women of child-bearing age and the elderly who often have concommitant medical problems (54).

The NIMH Depression Awareness, Recognition, and Treatment Program (DART)

Emerging epidemiologic findings on prevalence and morbidity of depression and available treatments and numerous studies of clinical practices in primary care and other general medical settings have indicated that only one half of patients diagnosed with depressive and other psychiatric conditions are detected by general and family practitioners. In 1989, the NIMH initiated DART, a program of secondary prevention of depression. This program is comparable to the one initiated by the Heart Institute to educate the public about the treatment of hypertension. Initial efforts have been on educating the public and professionals about the availability of effective treatments for severe disorders, particularly bipolar and recurrent unipolar depression. In the early policy discussions on the focus of the DART, relatively low priority was given to patients with milder depressions, including those with depressive symptoms seen in general medical health settings. It is still too early to know if the program will have an effect on improving detection and treatment of depression. A strong evaluation component has not been added to the program.

CONCLUSION

There has been considerable progress in understanding the epidemiology and familial patterns of the mood disorders and in testing new treatments. The challenge of the 1990s is to bridge the gap between our understanding of treatment efficacy and the delivery of service; to identify the genetic mechanism(s), particularly for bipolar disorder; and to learn more about the continuity between childhood and adult depression so that appropriate interventions can occur earlier. The opportunities for secondary and tertiary prevention have increased. With increased knowledge of risk factors, particularly familial risk factors suggestive of genetic contribution for some of the mood disorders, the opportunity for primary prevention now seems less remote.

ACKNOWLEDGEMENTS

Preparation of this chapter was supported in part by grants #MH43525, #MH28274, and #MH43077 from the NIMH and the John D. and Catherine T. MacArthur Foundation. Permission was obtained to reproduce the following: A portion from Weissman, M. M. "Epidemiology overview," in *American Psychiatric Association Annual Review, Vol. 6: Psychiatry Update;* and portions of Klerman, G. L., Weissman, M. M. "Increasing rates of depression," from *J. Am. Med. Assoc.* 261:2229–35.

Literature Cited

1. Christie, K. A., Burke, J. D., Regier, D. A., Rae, D. S., Boyd, J. H., et al. 1989. Epidemiologic evidence for early onset of mental disorders and higher risk of drug abuse in young adults. *Am. J. Psychiatry* 145:971–75
2. Am. Psychiatr. Assoc. 1987. *Diagnostic and Statistical Manual of Mental Disorders DSM-III*. Washington, DC: Am. Psychiatr. Assoc. Press. 3rd ed.
3. Weissman, M. M., Klerman, G. L. 1978. Epidemiology of Mental Disorders. *Arch. Gen. Psychiatry* 35:705–12
4. Weissman, M. M. 1987. Epidemiology overview. In *American Psychiatric Association Annual Review, Vol. 6: Psychiatry Update,* ed. R. E. Hales, A. J. Frances, pp. 574–88. Washington, DC: Am. Psychiatr. Assoc. Press

5. Weissman, M. M., Myers, J. K. 1978. Affective disorders in a US urban community. *Arch. Gen. Psychiatry* 35: 1304–11
6. Robins, L. N., Helzer, J. E., Croughan, J., Ratcliff, K. S. 1981. National Institute of Mental Health diagnostic interview schedule. *Arch. Gen. Psychiatry* 38:381–89
7. Robins, L. N., Regier, D. A., eds. 1991. *Psychiatric Disorders in America: The Epidemiologic Catchment Area Study*. New York: The Free Press. 449 pp.
8. Wing, J. K., Mann, S. A., Leff, J. P., Nixon, J. M. 1978. The concept of "case" in psychiatric population surveys. *Psychol. Med.* 8:203–17
9. Brown, G. W., Harris, T. O. 1978. *So-

cial Origins of Depression: A Study of Psychiatric Disorder in Women. London: Tavistock

10. Smith, A. L., Weissman, M. M. 1991. The epidemiology of affective disorders. In Handbook of Affective Disorders, ed. E. Paykel. Edinburgh: Churchill Livingston (Longman Group). 2nd ed. In press

11. Gershon, E. S., Hamovit, J., Gurroff, J. J., Nurnberger, J. N. 1987. Birth-cohort changes in manic and depressive disorders in relatives of bipolar and schizoaffective patients. Arch. Gen. Psychiatry 44:314–19

12. Lasch, K., Weissman, M. M., Wickramaratne, P. J., Bruce, M. L. 1990. Birth cohort changes in the rates of mania. Psychiatry Res. 33:31–37

13. Henderson, S., Duncan-Jones, P., Byrne, D. G., Scott, R., Adcock, S. 1979. Psychiatric disorder in Canberra: A standardized study of prevalence. Acta Psychiatr. Scand. 60:355–74

14. Klerman, G. L., Weissman, M. M. 1989. Increasing rates of depression. J. Am. Med. Assoc. 261:2229–35

15. Blazer, D. G., Crowell, B. A., George, L. K., Landerman, R. 1986. Urban-rural differences in depressive disorders: Does age make a difference: In Mental Disorders in the Community: Progress and Challenge, ed. J. Barrett, R. M. Rose, pp. 32–46. New York: Guilford

16. Klerman, G. L., Lavori, P. W., Rice, J., Reich, T., Endicott, J., et al. 1985. Birth-cohort trends in rates of major depressive disorder among relatives of patients with affective disorder. Arch. Gen. Psychiatry 42:689–93

17. Hagnell, O., Lanke, J., Rorsman, B., Ojesjo, L. 1982. Are we entering an age of melancholy? Psychol. Med. 12:279–89

18. Lavori, P. W., Klerman, G. L., Keller, M. B., Reich, T., Rice, J. 1987. Age-period-cohort analysis of secular trends in onset of major depression: Findings in siblings of patients with major affective disorder. J. Psychiatr. Res. 21:23–36

19. Wickramaratne, P. J., Weissman, M. M., Leaf, P. J., Holford, T. R. 1989. Age, period, and cohort effects on the risk of major depression: Results from five United States communities. J. Clin. Epidemiol. 42:333–43

20. Karno, M., Hough, R. L., Burnam, M. A., Escobar, J. I., Timbers, D. M., et al. 1987. Lifetime prevalence of specific psychiatric disorders among Mexican Americans and non-Hispanic whites in Los Angeles. Arch. Gen. Psychiatry 44:695–701

21. Wing, J. K., Babor, T., Brugha, T.,

Burke, J., Cooper, J. E. 1990. SCAN: Schedules for clinical assessment in neuropsychiatry. Arch. Gen. Psychiatry 47:589–92

22. Robins, L. N., Wing, J., Wittchen, H. U., Helzer, J. E., Babor, T. F., et al. 1988. The composite international diagnostic interview: An epidemiologic instrument suitable for use in conjunction with different diagnostic systems and in different cultures. Arch. Gen. Psychiatry 45:1069–77

23. Blehar, M. C., Weissman, M. M., Gershon, E. S., Hirschfeld, R. M. A. 1988. Family and genetic studies of affective disorders. Arch. Gen. Psychiatry 45: 289–92

24. Wright, A. F., Goeder, M., Hastie, N. D. 1991. Beta amyloid resurrected. Nature 349(6311):653–54

25. Weissman, M. M., Kidd, K. K., Prusoff, B. A. 1982. Variability in rates of affective disorders in relatives of depressed and normal probands. Arch. Gen. Psychiatry 39:1397–1403

26. Tsuang, M. T., Winokur, G., Crowe, R. R. 1980. Morbidity risks of schizophrenia and affective disorders among first degree relatives of patients with schizophrenia, mania, depression and surgical conditions. Br. J. Psychiatry 137:497–504

27. Torgersen, S. 1986. Genetic factors in moderately severe and mild affective disorders. Arch. Gen. Psychiatry 43: 222–26

28. Moldin, S. O., Reich, T., Rice, J. 1991. Current perspectives on the genetics of unipolar depression. Behav. Genetics 21(3):211–42

29. Bland, R. C., Newman, S. C., Orn, H. 1988. Age of onset of psychiatric disorders. Acta Psychiatr. Scand. 77:43–49

30. Weissman, M. M., Wickramaratne, P., Merikangas, K. R., Leckman, J. F., Prusoff, B. A., et al. 1984. Onset of major depression in early adulthood. Increased familial loading and specificity. Arch. Gen. Psychiatry 41:1136–43

31. von Knorring, A. L., Cloninger, C. R., Bohman, M., Sigvardsson, S. 1983. An adoption study of depressive disorders and substance abuse. Arch. Gen. Psychiatry 40:943–50

32. Wender, P. H., Kety, S. S., Rosenthal, D., Schulsinger, F., Ortmann, J., et al. 1986. Psychiatric disorders in the biological and adoptive families of adopted individuals with affective disorders. Arch. Gen. Psychiatry 43:923–29

33. Weissman, M. M., Gammon, G. D., John, K., Merikangas, K. R., Warner, V., et al. 1987. Children of depressed

parents. Increased psychopathology and early onset of major depression. *Arch. Gen. Psychiatry* 44:847–53

34. Beardslee, W. R., Keller, M. B., Klerman, G. L. 1985. Children of parents with affective disorder. *Int. J. Fam. Psychiatry* 6:283–99

35. Orvaschel, H., Walsh-Allis, G., Ye, W. 1988. Psychopathology in children of parents with recurrent depression. *J. Abnorm. Child Psychol.* 16:17–28

36. Hammen, C. 1990. Longitudinal study of diagnoses in children of women with unipolar and bipolar affective disorder. *Arch. Gen. Psychiatry* 47:1112–17

37. Keller, M. B., Beardslee, W. R., Dorer, D. J., Lavori, P. W., Samuelson, H., Klerman, G. L. 1986. Impact of severity and chronicity of parental affective illness on adaptive functioning and psychopathology in their children. *Arch. Gen. Psychiatry* 43:930–37

38. Anderson, C. E., Weissman, M. M. 1991. Family studies of affective disorders. In *Depression in Children and Adolescents*, ed. H. S. Koplewicz, E. Klass. London: Harwood Academic. In press

39. Fendrich, M., Weissman, M. M., Warner, V. 1991. Longitudinal assessment of major depression and anxiety disorders in children. *J. Am. Acad. Child Adolesc. Psychiatry* 30(1):67–74

40. Strober, M., Morrell, W., Burrough, J., Lampert, C., Danforth, H., Freeman, R. 1988. A family study of bipolar disorder in adolescence: Early onset of symptom linked to increased familial loading and lithium resistance. *J. Affect. Disord.* 15:255–68

41. Puig-Antich, J., Goetz, D., Davies, M., Kaplan, T., Davies, S., et al. 1989. A controlled family history study of prepubertal major depressive disorder. *Arch. Gen. Psychiatry* 46:406–18

42. Harrington, R., Fudge, H., Rutter, M., Pickles, A., Hill, J. 1990. Adult outcomes of childhood and adolescent depression. *Arch. Gen. Psychiatry* 47:465–73

43. Regier, D. A., Goldberg, I. D., Taube, C. A. 1978. The de facto US mental health services system. *Arch. Gen. Psychiatry* 35:685–93

44. Tarlov, A. R., Ware, J. E. Jr., Greenfield, S., Nelson, E. C., Perrin, E., et al. 1989. The Medical Outcomes Study: an application of methods for monitoring the results of medical care. *J. Am. Med. Assoc.* 262:925–30

45. Stewart, A. L., Greenfield, S., Hays, R. D., Wells, K., Rogers, W. H., et al. 1989. Functional status and well-being

of patients with chronic conditions: results from the Medical Outcomes Study. *J. Am. Med. Assoc.* 262:907–13

46. Wells, K. B., Stewart, A., Hays, R. D., Burnam, M. A., Rogers, W., et al. 1989. The functioning and well-being of depressed patients: results form the Medical Outcomes Study. *J. Am. Med. Assoc.* 262:914–19

47. Klerman, G. L. 1989. Depressive disorders: Further evidence for increased medical morbidity and impairment of social functioning. *Arch. Gen. Psychiatry* 46:856–60

48. Bruce, M. L., Leaf, P. J. 1989. Psychiatric disorders and 15-month mortality in a community sample of older adults. *Am. J. Public Health* 79:727–30

49. Blackwell, B. 1987. Newer antidepressant drugs. In *Psychopharmacology: The Third Generation of Progress*, ed. H. Y. Meltzer, pp. 1041–49. New York: Raven

50. Goodwin, F. K., Jamison, K. R. 1990. *Manic Depressive Illness*. New York: Oxford Univ. Press

51. Weissman, M. M., Jarrett, R. B., Rush, J. A. 1987. Psychotherapy and its relevance to the pharmacotherapy of major depression: A decade later (1976–1985). In *Psychopharmacology: The Third Generation of Progress*, ed. H. Y. Meltzer, pp. 1059–69. New York: Raven

52. Elkin, I., Shea, M. T., Watkins, J. T., Imber, S. D., Sotsky, S. M., et al. 1989. National Institute of Mental Health Treatment of Depression Collaborative Research Program: General effectiveness of treatments. *Arch. Gen. Psychiatry* 46:971–83

53. Frank, E., Kupfer, D. J., Perel, J. M., Cornes, C., Jarrett, D. B., et al. 1990. Three-year outcomes for maintenance therapies in recurrent depression. *Arch. Gen. Psychiatry* 47(12):1093–99

54. Klerman, G. L. 1990. Treatment of recurrent unipolar major depressive disorder: Commentary on the Pittsburgh study. *Arch. Gen. Psychiatry* 47:1158–62

55. Weissman, M. M., Leaf, P. J., Tischler, G. L., Blazer, D. G., Karno, M. 1988. Affective disorders in five United States communities. *Psychol. Med.* 18:141–53

56. Bland, R. C., Orn, H., Newman, S. C. 1988. Lifetime prevalence of psychiatric disorders in Edmonton. *Acta Psychiatr. Scand.* 77:24–32

57. Canino, G. J., Bird, H. R., Shrout, P. E., Rubio-Stipec, M., Bravo, M., et al. 1987. The prevalence of specific psy-

chiatric disorders in Puerto Rico. *Arch. Gen. Psychiatry* 44:727–35

58. Faravelli, C., Degl'Innocenti, G., Aiazzi, L., Incerpi, G., Pallanti, S. 1990. Epidemiology of mood disorders: A community survey in Florence. *J. Affect. Disord.* 20:135–41

59. Lee, C. K., Han, J. H., Choi, J. O. 1987. The epidemiological study of mental disorders in Korea (IX): Alcoholism, anxiety and depression. *Seoul J. Psychiatry* 12:183–91

60. Hwu, H. G., Yeh, E. K., Chang, L. Y. 1989. Prevalence of psychiatric disorders in Taiwan defined by the Chinese Diagnostic Interview Schedule. *Acta Psychiatr. Scand.* 79:136–47

61. Joyce, P. R., Oakley-Brown, M. A., Wells, J. E., Bushnell, J. A., Hornblow, A. R. 1990. Birth cohort trends in major depression: Increasing rates and earlier onset in New Zealand. *J. Affect. Disord.* 18:83–90

61a. Moldin, S., Reich, T., Rice, J. 1991. Current perspectives on the genetics of unipolar depression. *Behav. Genet.* 21(3):211–42

62. Winokur, G., Tsuang, M. T., Crowe, R. R. 1982. The Iowa 500: Affective disorder in relatives of manic and depressive patients. *Am. J. Psychiatry* 139:209–12

63. Gershon, E. S., Hamovit, J., Guroff, J. J., Dibble, E., Leckman, J. F., et al. 1982. A family study of schizoaffective, bipolar I, bipolar II, unipolar, and normal control probands. *Arch. Gen. Psychiatry* 39:1157–67

64. Baron, M., Gruen, R., Asnis, L., Kane, J. 1982. Schizoaffective illness, schizophrenia and affective disorders: morbidity risk and genetic transmission. *Acta Psychiatr. Scand.* 65:253–62

65. Weissman, M. M., Gershon, E. S., Kidd, K. K., Prusoff, B. A., Leckman, J. F., et al. 1984. Psychiatric disorders in the relatives of probands with affective disorders. *Arch. Gen. Psychiatry* 41:13–21

66. Bland, R. C., Newman, S. C., Orn, H. 1986. Recurrent and nonrecurrent depression. *Arch. Gen. Psychiatry* 43:1085–89

67. Stancer, H. C., Persad, E., Wagener, D. K., Jorna, T. 1987. Evidence for homogeneity of major depression and bipolar affective disorder. *J. Psychiatr. Res.* 1:37–53

68. Rice, J. P. 1987. Diagnostic error and linkage analysis. *Am. J. Hum. Genet.* 41:261

69. Giles, D. E., Biggs, M. M., Rush, A. J., Roffwarg, H. P. 1988. Risk factors in families of unipolar depression. I. Psychiatric illness and reduced REM latency. *J. Affect. Disord.* 14:51–59

70. McGuffin, P., Katz, R., Aldrich, J., Bebbington, P. 1988. The Camberwell Collaborative Depression Study. II. Investigation of family members. *Br. J. Psychiatry* 152:766–74

71. Kupfer, D. J., Frank, E., Carpenter, L. L., Neiswanger, K. 1989. Family history in recurrent depression. *J. Affect. Disord.* 17:113–19

Annu. Rev. Publ. Health. 1992. 13:341–62

SOCIAL MARKETING:
Its Place in Public Health

Jack C. Ling, Barbara A. K. Franklin, Janis F. Lindsteadt, and Susan A. N. Gearon

International Communication Enhancement Center, Tulane University School of Public Health and Tropical Medicine, New Orleans, Louisiana 70112

KEY WORDS: social mobilization, community education, health communication, health promotion, audience analysis

INTRODUCTION

Social marketing is often perceived as a contradiction in terms and an odd fit for the public health professional. For if marketing, the business of selling goods and services, is pursued singlemindedly—exclusive of all other considerations but profit—it will eventually clash with the social purpose of public health. Yet, in less than 20 years, social marketing for health has emerged as a recognized practice.

Multiple channels of mass communication and new methods of knowledge diffusion have touched all but the more remote and isolated communities. Messages aimed at influencing personal choices and decisions come from several sources at any given time, and often at cross purposes. Useful information reaches an ever larger number of people and improves prospects for good health. But, the same channels of information have also conveyed words and images harmful to health. The changing environment of communication provides an important backdrop for efforts to change attitude and behavior of which social marketing is an example. This article reviews the origin of social marketing, its practices, its strengths and weaknesses, and its place in the future of public health.

341

0163-7525/92/0501-0341$02.00

What Is Social Marketing?

Forty years ago, Wiebe (67) asked, "Why can't you sell brotherhood and rational thinking like you sell soap?" Few responded to his challenge at the time. The use of advertising media for a social purpose had existed for decades, and audiences were familiar with public service announcements (PSAs) and campaigns that popularized such slogans as "Uncle Sam Wants You." However, marketers did not consider social causes in terms of product, price, and place until the 1960s and 1970s (60). By the late 1960s, such marketers as Richard Manoff were applying the full range of marketing techniques to nutrition and other health education campaigns (49). The general heightened social consciousness at the time may well have helped initiate marketing's probe into the social arena. Some advocates of change learned and used marketing techniques to advance their causes.

In 1971, marketing professor Philip Kotler and his collaborator, Gerald Zaltman, called the application of marketing practices to nonprofit and social purposes "social marketing." They described it as a "a promising framework for planning and implementing social change" (31). Social marketing attempts to persuade a specific audience, mainly through various media, to adopt an idea, a practice, a product, or all three. It is a social change management strategy that translates scientific findings into action programs. It combines elements of traditional approaches and modern communication and education technologies in an integrated, planned framework.

Social marketing uses marketing's conceptual framework of the 4 Ps: Product, Price, Place, and Promotion. Social marketers adopted several methods of commercial marketing: audience analysis and segmentation; consumer research; product conceptualization and development; message development and testing; directed communication; facilitation; exchange theory; and the use of paid agents, volunteers, and incentives.

Audience analysis is needed to identify segments for specific approaches. Consumer research yields valuable data about the wants and needs of targeted segments and provides a basis for product design and message development. Testing sharpens the effectiveness of products and messages. Specific channels appropriate to the targeted segments are chosen for product distribution and message dissemination. Paid and voluntary agents reinforce and facilitate message dissemination and product distribution by face-to-face communication. Incentives are employed to motivate the sales force and stimulate consumer demand. Exchange theory illuminates the relationship between price and perceived benefit.

However, there is not a universally accepted definition of legitimate social marketing. Such lack of consensus has contributed to misconceptions about the role of social marketing in public health and has probably fueled skepticism and criticism. Although the American Marketing Association has been challenged to provide a standardized definition (45), the official definitive statement has yet to be written (36).

REVIEW OF THE LITERATURE AND EXPERIENCES

Literature

Social marketers have written many articles about their experiences. Besides discussing and arguing for their respective definitions, they have written about their successes, the difficulties encountered, and the lessons to be learned. In addition, theorists from various fields have explained and critiqued social marketing. The literature on social marketing now spans some 40 years, counting Wiebe's original challenge. But, the bulk of the written work is concentrated in the last 25 years and can be divided roughly into three periods: early theory, experiences evaluated, and increasing acceptance.

EARLY THEORY   In the late 1960s and early 1970s, theorists attempted to define and justify social marketing amid criticism from all sides. There were four central questions: What is social marketing? What is its role? Is it possible? Is it marketing?

Ironically, Wiebe has seldom been given credit for his own thoughtful answer to his challenge: "Advertising does not move people to unilateral action. It moves them into interaction with social mechanisms . . . It is the crucial importance of the retail store, viewed as a social mechanism which facilitates the desired behavior, that social scientists often seem to overlook when they yearn for behavioral changes comparable to those achieved by advertisers" (67). Although Wiebe uses the word advertising, his insistence on an adequate and compatible social mechanism and his concept of "distance" (the effort audience members believe the new product or behavior requires, compared with its benefit) indicate that he was talking about social marketing (the comprehensive use of marketing methods for a social cause), and not merely social advertising (the use of advertising media to publicize a social cause).

Debate on the role of marketing for social causes began in earnest in the late 1960s and accelerated in the 1970s, much of it in the marketing journals. Martin's "An Outlandish Idea: How a Marketing Man Would Save India" (50) led the way, followed by numerous discussions of how marketing should change or broaden its concept to meet the needs of society (2, 13, 25, 29, 34, 45). Lazer (35) proposed that marketing's responsibility was only partially fulfilled through economic processes, whereas Dawson (8) and Lavidge (34) predicted the new question for marketers would soon be whether the product or service should be sold at all. Kotler & Levy (28) proposed "demarketing" to reduce demand for certain products. Against this backdrop of questioning and redefinition within the marketing field, Kotler & Zaltman (31) proposed social marketing as an approach to planned social change and outlined its essential features.

Not everyone greeted marketing's expanded role with enthusiasm. Luck (45) objected that replacing a tangible product with a complex bundle of ideas and practices overextended the exchange-of-value concept, which even social marketing proponents agreed was at the heart of the marketing discipline. Takas (64) noted that the ongoing debate about social marketing was unknown or ignored by most of the business community, for whom the essential concern remained sales for profit. Nevertheless, the new ideas took hold, and, by 1973, several reports and case studies of social marketing projects began to appear in the literature (9, 36).

EXPERIENCES EVALUATED   In the late 1970s and early 1980s, while theorists wrangled, practitioners eagerly applied the new approach to several fields, notably family planning, and asked, Does it work? How does it work? What are the constraints?

During this period, many theorists turned their attention away from the debate over definitions and toward the growing mound of data from social marketing efforts (27, 43, 44, 55). Books and articles that explained the social marketing process and gave guidelines for the practitioner included Kotler's *Marketing for Nonprofit Organizations* (26); Manoff's *Social Marketing: A New Imperative for Public Health* (49); applications to specific fields, such as nutrition (24); and studies of strategy mix, channels, and evaluation (1, 4, 59).

In 1980, Fox & Kotler (15) described the evolution of social advertising into social communication and social marketing. Social marketing added four elements to social communication: marketing research, product development, use of incentives, and facilitation. However, objective evaluation was lacking. For example, Bloom (4) deplored the tendency of projects to use "after only" or "before and after" studies with no control group, a practice that might identify ineffective programs, but could not show causal relationships between program and outcome. Theorists also gave increased attention to the conditions in which social marketing efforts were most successful and to the constraints and difficulties likely to be encountered.

Contraceptive social marketing provided early, well-documented successes. *Population Reports* (61) summarized the results of 30 contraceptive social marketing projects in 27 countries, with a lengthy bibliography. The report concluded that social marketing was successful in providing protection against unwanted pregnancies at a lower cost than most other approaches. Nevertheless, parallels between commercial and social marketing were imperfect. Rothschild (54), for example, identified problematic differences with regard to product, price, segmentation, and, especially, the construct of involvement. He suggested that the public's involvement with social causes may be bimodal (very high or very low), whereas public involvement with consumer goods is typically middle-range, thus making the promotional tools used for marketing commercial consumer goods inadequate for social tasks.

Bloom & Novelli (5) produced a litany of problems that marketers faced in the public health arena. They cited the following difficulties: obtaining consumer research and data, especially behavioral data; sorting the relative influence of determinants of behavior; classifying and narrow-targeting segments; formulating and shaping simple product concepts; pricing; choosing channels and designing appeals; pretesting methods and materials; implementing long-term positioning strategies; and ignoring those segments most vulnerable and often most negatively oriented to the message. Organizational problems included poor understanding of marketing activities; treatment of plans as archival, rather than action, documents; and "institutional amnesia."

Further problems occur because, rather than encouraging people to do something, as commercial marketers do, social marketers must often discourage behaviors that may be attractive to the audience or deeply ingrained. Solomon (62) concluded that "marketing concepts cannot be applied wholesale to social campaigns without a great deal of thought and sensitivity." A veteran marketer has said, "It's a thousand times harder to do social marketing than packaged goods marketing" (15). Social marketing finished its first decade with cautious optimism, a more realistic estimation of both its limits and its potential.

INCREASING ACCEPTANCE   By the late 1980s, social marketing had become an accepted practice, while taking some surprising new forms. However, fundamental questions still have not been answered: Does social marketing deliver what it promises? What is the impact of connecting marketing and social causes? What effect does it have at the sustainable behavior level? Is it cost-effective? Is it ethical?

Since the late 1980s, there have been more publications to guide the social marketer, including a comprehensive text by Kotler & Roberto (30). Lefebvre & Flora (37) reviewed the social marketing field from the perspective of health promotion/education. They cited the orientation to consumer needs as social marketing's most important contribution, despite such barriers as the propensity of public health programs to be "expert-driven." They concluded that although not a panacea, "health marketing has the potential of reaching the largest possible group of people at the least cost with the most effective, consumer-satisfying program," if practitioners thoroughly understand its concepts and limitations and have mastered its skills. Although there has been a broader acceptance of marketing principles in many health spheres, some remain critical of social marketing's ethical dimensions, its impact, and its capacity to deliver what it promises.

Concerns about Social Marketing

ETHICAL ISSUES   Questions about the ethics of social marketing surfaced soon after the concept was introduced. As early as 1979, Laczniak et al (32) polled more than 300 experts, such as professors of ethics, psychology, and economics and marketing practitioners, and found a wide range of ethical concerns. Some respondents feared that marketers were getting in over their heads, by acquiring social power without a full sense of the issues or their responsibility. In the words of one, "social marketing could ultimately operate as a form of thought control by the economically powerful." Marketers were, in general, more favorable toward the new discipline, but they too had their concerns. Some feared that the public would associate marketing with controversial causes and, thus, perceive them as "neopropagandists" (that is, the field of marketing would suffer from the taint of social causes). This is a surprising assertion, because the shoe is usually on the other foot in debates about the marketing of causes. Laczniak et al found general concern that social marketing would likely operate without any control and regulation, in contrast with health education, whose professional associations gave serious attention to self-imposed ethical codes.

Because advertising is a key component of marketing, the debate on the ethical aspects of advertising has some bearing on social marketing. Some feel that the negative aspects of advertising outweigh the benefits of a social marketing campaign, no matter how noble the cause. Pollay (53) reported the consensus of 50 noted humanities and social science scholars: Advertising's effect, among other things, is to trivialize real experience and engender materialism, cynicism, anxiety, disrespect for age and tradition, loss of self-esteem, and a preoccupation with sex and competition. Holbrook (20) responded that advertising is a mirror of societal norms, which reflects many wholesome values, such as family affection, generosity, patriotism, positive anticipation, and joy. These opposite points of view probably stem from different assessments of the merit of the consumer society and its capacity to provide human fulfillment.

Health educators also expressed ethical concerns about the new discipline. Some concerns related to the concept of victim-blaming and the debate about persuasion versus coercion, current in the 1970s and 1980s (11, 12, 18, 51, 57, 68). Victim-blaming occurs when individuals are held responsible for their problems, thus obscuring institutional and societal forces over which they may have little control (for example, economic status, working conditions, public policies, and laws). Marketing efforts usually address individuals and encourage individual behavior change, thus implicitly holding individuals responsible for the solutions to problems.

It can also be argued, however, that social marketing is a tool, like the telephone, which can be used for a positive end, such as fostering human interaction, or for a negative purpose, such as obscene calls. In this review, we regard social marketing as an instrument, but the ethical dimensions of social marketing clearly deserve continuing attention.

DISEMPOWERMENT   In addition to ethical concerns, social marketing has been criticized as ineffectual or even counterproductive. For instance, Werner (56) criticized social marketing's emphasis on commercial products, by claiming that it is at odds with the philosophy of community empowerment. Werner alleged that oral rehydration solution (ORS) manufacturers, both private and government, were reluctant to accept a cereal-based ORS for fear of encouraging home-based mixes. According to this view, even the selling of ORS creates dependency and detracts from the empowering knowledge of the principle of treating diarrhea.

Social marketing has also been criticized for reaching the wrong audiences. Luthra (46) pointed out that in Bangladesh, mass media channels, such as television and the press, are primarily accessible to men and the urban elite. She argues that a literacy rate of 16% among women makes instructional billboards and newspapers useless for most mothers. Furthermore, important information about contraceptive use and side effects was not made available in a form appropriate to the target audience until after sales decreased because of user dissatisfaction. Luthra concluded that social marketing is not responsive to the needs and concerns of the user, but is driven by marketing and sales signals defined by Western commercial marketing practice.

THE COMMERCIALIZATION OF HEALTH INFORMATION   In the 1980s, with the general ascendancy of supply side economics and the popular acknowledgment of the success of market mechanisms during the latter half of the decade, the bias against commercialism subsided. Commercial terms gained increasing acceptance, even in countries where the economies had long been centrally planned. Public health services became "products," people became "clients" and "consumers," and organizations with a product to distribute became "vendors." The decade saw a marked growth in the practice of social marketing for health, as well as health-related commercial marketing and cause-related marketing.

Health-related commercial marketing emerged in the late 1980s, when the Kellogg Company cited National Cancer Institute (NCI) findings in marketing its high-fiber All-Bran cereal. Kellogg "educated" the public, while increasing its market share from 36% to 42%; thus, it started a major marketing trend (16). Kellogg claimed that after the campaign, over 90% of Americans knew the fiber-cancer message and had heard it an average of 35 times. The educational aspects of the campaign were questioned by Levy & Stokes (38), however, because the benefits did not generalize to other high-fiber cereals until those companies mounted their own cancer education/marketing campaigns. Although nonprofit sources generally enjoy greater credibility than profit sources, the Kellogg-NCI combination is perceived as almost as credible as the nonprofit source alone (19). Thus, Kellogg may have raised its credibility, while NCI gained greater exposure at no cost, as a result of what Freimuth et al (16) called "seductive" collaboration.

Cause-related marketing is a similar commercial/social marketing blend. In this strategy, corporations donate a percentage of their profits to a cause, thus lending marketing expertise and support to a cause, while enhancing their images and making profits. In the early 1970s, for example, the US Committee for the United Nations International Children Emergency Fund (UNICEF) cooperated with several companies that announced in their marketing efforts their support to UNICEF, thus tying the amount of their contributions to the volume of sales of their products. Caesar (7) describes other examples, such as American Express' pledge to donate one cent to the Statue of Liberty renovation fund each time its card was used. During that period, American Express raised $1.7 million for the renovation project, while increasing the use of its cards by 30%. Studies to measure impact for the corporate sponsors, as well as for public health, are needed (16).

As the 1990s begin, our review of the literature shows that social marketing has become more pervasive in public health. Although some complain that it is often adopted piecemeal and without a system of operational procedures, it has arrived at the end of its second decade with a measure of maturity— generally considered a useful practice, but still not fully understood by many health professionals.

Examples of Social Marketing from Developing Countries

Although marketing is deeply rooted in business practice in the United States and other developed countries, the deliberate practice of marketing for public health has found its most complete expression in the less developed countries. Various social marketing activities have been undertaken for nutrition, family planning, and other public health projects in Asia since the late 1960s and early 1970s; subsequently, these activities were extended to Africa, Latin America, and the Middle East. Public health problems in the developing nations are so large and urgent that both immediate actions and innovative approaches are required. For the adoption of public health marketing practices in developing countries, it is fortuitous that the few modern mass media available are usually government owned and operated and, therefore, more obliged in principle to devote time to social development activities. The overwhelming and sometimes monopolistic power of these centralized media was evident to public health professionals. The family planning pioneers in developing countries knew that their cause was controversial and were eager to argue their case in various public fora, particularly through the media. Thus, family planning has often led the way in innovative communication strategies, including social marketing techniques.

Nine illustrative projects, chosen for their variety of subjects, approaches, and geographic representation, have been divided into three groups (see Table 1). The information is based on documents and reports provided by the institutions responsible for the projects. The descriptions are necessarily brief. Readers are encouraged to refer to the sources and institutions cited for more complete information, including statistical data.

The above-mentioned standard social marketing procedures were used in these projects, except where particular techniques are mentioned. These examples do not yet demonstrate long-term impact on behavioral change; therefore, the cost of behavioral change is not available. More evaluations and studies are needed to determine cost-effectiveness.

TANGIBLE PRODUCTS   A diarrheal disease control program in Egypt achieved impressive results. In December 1984, one year into the campaign, approximately 90% of the mothers surveyed recognized the dangers of de-

Table 1   Examples of social marketing

Program	Organizations Involved	Date
Tangible Products		
Egypt—National Control of Diarrheal Diseases Project (NCDDP)	John Snow Public Health Group	1983–1988
Dominican Republic-Contraceptive Social Marketing	Futures Group, AED, Doremus, Porter & Novelli, John Short Associates	1984–1989
Bangladesh—Contraceptive Social Marketing	Population Services International, Manoff Int.	1974–1987
Kenya—Condom Promotion	Population Services International	1972–1974
Sustained Health Practices		
Cameroon—Weaning Project	CARE, Manoff Int., Educational Development Center	1985–1989
Indonesia—Weaning Project	Manoff International	1984–1989
Malaysia—PEMADAM Dadah/Drug Prevention	Government of Malaysia	1976–present
Services Utilization		
Colombia—National Vaccination Crusade	UNICEF, WHO, PAHO	1984–1994
Philippines—Expanded Program Immunization	HealthCOM, AED	1984

hydration, compared with 32% in May 1983; 95% knew of oral rehydration therapy (ORT); and, among those who used ORT in 1984, approximately 60% mixed the solution correctly, compared with 25% in 1983 (58).

In the Dominican Republic, contraceptive social marketing implemented by Profamilia, a local family planning association, achieved its objectives: increased availability of Microgynon birth control pills, increased use among lower socioeconomic women, increased contraceptive prevalence, and increased involvement from the private sector with consequent expanded market outlets. In collaboration with a private sector orals manufacturer, Profamilia reduced the price of Microgynon by 50% and sold the oral under a new logo. In a five-year period, Profamilia generated enough sales revenue to recover all operating costs and become self-sufficient. Microgynon purchasers represented an expanded market (34% new acceptors), as well as brand switchers already in the commercial market (66%). Some 89% of the clients surveyed planned to continue using Microgynon (17, 63). Equally impressive, however, is the overall trend in the total orals market. During the five-year period, the contraceptive social marketing program contributed to a 30% increase in the total orals market, without eroding the market shares of other leading orals manufacturers.

Bangladesh is acclaimed as having one of the most successful contraceptive social marketing projects. In one decade, the program sold over 130 million condoms and over 2.2 million cycles of oral contraception. In 1984, the project served 40% of all contraceptive acceptors (many being rural) by selling low-cost products through retail and wholesale outlets. Qualitative research techniques, such as focus group discussions and in-depth interviews, were used to identify the major resistance points to using contraception. Investigators concluded that men should be the primary target audience of the media program, because they were the most resistant, ignorant, and unwilling to consider family planning. Research concerning current users confirmed that husbands were an important source of instruction. Fourteen months after the radio portion of the campaign began, the number of persons who believed that modern family planning methods are unsafe decreased and interpersonal discussions about family planning and recognition of the personal economic benefits of family planning increased. Contraceptive social marketing efforts in Bangladesh drew attention to both the private and public sectors, expanded the market, and used indigenous institutions in program planning, operation, and evaluation (33, 46, 58).

Through mass media in Kenya, social marketing emphasized the quality image of Kinga condom, reflected in product design, package, and moderate cost. Commercial shopkeepers and a mobile sales team were used as condom distribution channels and proved effective in extending accessibility to rural areas. The promotional campaign had a significant impact on contraceptive practice. Current method users among survey respondents rose from 21% to

35% in one year, whereas the control group showed little change. In addition to promoting sales, the campaign created a high level of brand awareness. After six months of marketing, 85% of male survey respondents were aware of Kinga condoms. Of those who had heard of Kinga, 80% were able to describe its purpose as a contraceptive, rather than as a venereal disease prophylactic, a function that was deliberately included in the campaign messages. Before being educated about Kinga, only 23% of survey respondents spontaneously mentioned condoms when discussing contraceptive methods. Six months into the campaign, this figure had risen to 57% (3).

SUSTAINED HEALTH PRACTICES   The Cameroon Weaning Project indicates that social marketing techniques can be successful in strengthening community-based health education in remote areas. The Cameroon Project provided a unique opportunity to employ social marketing under extremely tough conditions, because of the limited resources of the implementing agency (a private voluntary organization) and the difficult social and ecological environment. Despite the difficult circumstances under which the program was undertaken, moderate gains were demonstrated. Improved skills of CARE staff in conducting quantitative and qualitative research, applying appropriate communications skills, and disseminating simplified information improved knowledge levels and infant feeding practices among illiterate, rural mothers (21).

The Indonesia Weaning Project was designed to develop low-cost, nutritionally-sound, sustainable solutions to reduce weaning problems. In addition to radio, posters, and recipe leaflets, community leaders and health workers channeled nutrition education to mothers. Evaluation using control and case groups showed that knowledge of weaning methods, nutritionally-sound feeding practice, and child growth increased most among communities that also received face-to-face communication from health workers (47, 48), thus showing the importance of a marketing approach, rather than a media-based advertising campaign.

The Dadah/drug prevention program (PEMADAM) in Malaysia is exceptional, because it markets social policies. The comprehensive campaign combines marketing principles and other strategies, such as community and national-level involvement, in a broad approach to drug prevention education that aims to make drug abuse socially unacceptable. PEMADAM is attempting to instill societal principles through social marketing, aimed at linking an understanding of human behavior with effective social planning at a time when social issues are critical (65, 71).

SERVICE UTILIZATION   In Colombia, the drive for universal child immunization combined communication and marketing strategies, mobilization of political will and support from various sectors of society, and deployment of volunteers at a grass-roots level. Local leaders and health promoters were influential in disseminating information in the community through home visits. The strategy of bringing demand in contact with the service, which they called channeling, helped increase immunization coverage from 20% in 1979 to 60% among children under one and 80% under four in 1984 (23). The experience prompted UNICEF to institute a broad approach to its immunization programs in other parts of the world.

In the Philippines immunization project, mass media motivated mothers to bring their children to the clinic for face-to-face education. This strategy is progressing towards the goal of 85% immunization coverage by 1993. In a 1990 survey sample, computed coverage among 12–23-month-old children was 64%. Although the coverage effect has been moderate, a substantial effect in timeliness of coverage has been observed. The percentage of children who completed the entire series of vaccinations before their first birthday increased from 32.2% to 56.2% within one year. In addition, a significant improvement in client knowledge, especially concerning the logistics of vaccination, was noted. Mobilized national support has been responsible for much of the success to date (6).

In these illustrative cases, social marketing has been effective in increasing acceptance of tangible products, such as the condom and the ORS packet. To change health practices, however, social marketing needs to be part of a broader strategy that includes linkages with service delivery, skills learning, and community education. If the goal is sustained behavior change, and if the change has structural implications, social marketing per se has less impact.

Views from Practitioners

For this review, we contacted 15 practitioners for a modified Delphi inquiry. The five who responded corroborated the findings in the example projects of tangible products. Family planning projects have found social marketing particularly effective in getting their products accepted. Contraceptive social marketing programs are providing protection to over 8 million couples in the developing countries, which represents 1.5–2 million births avoided annually, or about a 2% decrement in annual world population growth (P. D. Harvey, Population Services International).

To measure impact, the quantity of each contraceptive sold is converted into couple years of protection (CYPs). A survey of 63 family planning projects, which marketed contraception and sterilization in ten developing countries, found that the cost of providing CYPs was $2–6 per year, significantly lower than other methods of delivering family planning in the countries studied (22). However, measures other than cost, such as pre- and post-surveys of population, should be used to evaluate impact, because distribution or sales of contraceptives does not always mean that the devices are effectively used (J. Rimon, Population Communication Services).

As a result of its effectiveness in marketing tangible products, some practitioners now plan to use social marketing to promote other products, such as Vitamin A supplements against xerophthalmia, antimalarial drugs, and prophylaxis and treatment for sexually transmitted diseases (P. D. Harvey).

Some practitioners raised concern over the high cost of mounting a social marketing project. If a large proportion of budgets is spent on advertising and packaging, mostly at full price, then social marketing projects are hardly sustainable (J. Rimon). In such cases, dependence upon external subsidies and technical assistance must continue.

Practitioners also expressed concerns about cost and accessibility. One prominent practitioner argued that social marketing family planning projects provide services that are not patronizing and do not undermine the dignity of recipients, because the products are purchased through an essentially neutral market system in which virtually all groups participate (P. D. Harvey). However, even subsidized products, such as the ORS packet, can come close to a day's wage in many countries. If products that must be purchased are the sole focus of a social marketing project, certain segments of the population, usually the poorest, will be excluded. Thus, numerous approaches are needed to achieve coverage, including health education, communication, training, and social marketing with differential pricing targeted for various population segments to achieve coverage (56).

Several practitioners urged stricter professional standards, such as greater rigor in segmenting audiences and tailoring messages for more impact on behavior. These standards would require an accommodation between the marketing perspective, which targets segments most likely to change, and the public health/epidemiological perspective, which is typically concerned with the poorest, highest risk, and least accessible populations (M. Rasmuson, Academy for Educational Development).

Interpersonal communication strategies are important. The Stanford Three-Community Heart Disease Study and the subsequent Five City Project reported that quality media campaigns can inform, motivate, and produce changes, but face-to-face communication is needed for skill-building, monitoring, and feedback (14, 37). Though often cited as a project that included marketing, the Three-Community Study did not consciously employ marketing strategies at the time (N. Maccoby, Stanford Center for Research in Disease Prevention).

When social marketing first appeared, enthusiastic supporters thought it might solve many public health problems. However, practitioners, while arguing for its effective use, have been cautious about its impact and aware of requisite conditions. More rigorous analysis and objective evaluation of social marketing projects would clearly help validate the effectiveness and cost-effectiveness of the practice.

STRENGTHS AND WEAKNESSES

Strengths of the Social Marketing Approach in Public Health

KNOWING THE AUDIENCE   Social marketing has had a beneficial impact on how the public health sector educates the public and persuades communities and individuals to adopt healthy practices. With its emphasis on clients, social marketing has sharpened the focus on the public. It has brought more precision to audience analysis and segmentation. In addition to demographics, psychographic data (attitudes, preferences, personality traits) and social structure data (church, worksite, family) are increasingly seen as vital in designing projects. These data provide critical information for the formulation of better targeted and more effective messages, thus leading to more appropriate message design, more effective delivery, and, above all, better reception by the public, the ultimate beneficiaries of public health measures.

SYSTEMATIC USE OF QUALITATIVE METHODS   Marketers are diligent users of focus groups and other qualitative research methods, which add insight to the quantitative information gathered by such instruments as questionnaires. Health educators have long used group discussion primarily to resolve community issues. But, their more recent use of focus groups to obtain customers' views of their campaigns and products and to pretest messages reveals the positive influence of marketing.

USE OF INCENTIVES   Social marketers make deliberate and systematic use of incentives and special promotion efforts, such as contests and competitions, which use rewards to draw clients to the market place. This method was not a regular feature of the motivational efforts of public health projects in the past. Purists might consider any offer of reward a kind of bribery, but the competition for attention in the midst of the exploding commercial clutter has made it an acceptable practice.

CLOSER MONITORING   Most public health projects pay insufficient attention to monitoring and often neglect management. Social marketers are committed to close tracking of progress, an important management principle.

STRATEGIC USE OF MASS MEDIA   Social marketers use of mass media in delivering messages to specific audiences to create awareness or foster and reinforce certain health practices contrasts sharply with the media outreach of the majority of public health projects. Marketing projects, which usually include intensive and prolonged use of broadcast media, purchase air time slots specifically aimed at targeted audiences, whereas underfunded public health projects often depend on the largess of the media for free air time. In the latter situation, it is the media program directors who, as an obligation to a good cause, decide which PSAs to air and when. When PSAs are broadcast during slack hours once or twice a month, they can hardly be expected to have the same impact as a systematic, well-targeted media campaign.

REALISTIC EXPECTATIONS   Although risk-taking is part of the commercial world, entrepreneurs do not take on impossible odds and would refuse any hopeless venture. Social marketers follow that tradition. In public health, however, officials are too often asked to undertake a $10,000/5-person job with $500 and one person. Such doomed projects erode credibility, which, in turn, hurts public health's standing in its competition with other development priorities. Social marketing cannot help but improve the chances of public health programs through more realistic estimations of the requirements for success.

ASPIRING TO HIGH STANDARDS   Just as important, social marketing, with its roots in the commercial world, often aspires to attain the best information materials and talent. This has alerted many public health professionals who have all too often been compelled to accept second rate work as a result of perennial budgetary constraints.

RECOGNITION OF PRICE   Operating from the conceptual framework of the 4 Ps, marketers accept that there is a price for any new product or behavior even in a voluntary exchange, although not necessarily in monetary terms. Public health professionals have only recently accepted that cost comes in many forms, such as inconvenience, opportunity costs, and incongruence with local culture. The notion, if it is good for you, you must want it, still lingers in the health field, but social marketers do not make such an assumption. In fact, marketers ask, "How can we make people want it?"

Weaknesses and Negative Aspects of Social Marketing in Public Health

TIME, MONEY, AND HUMAN REQUIREMENTS   Marketing practices require a heavy investment of time, money, and human resources that many public health agencies cannot afford. However well designed a project may be, without proper financing and staff, it will not succeed. A special event to generate support and promote a health practice requires careful preparation and implementation; it cannot be handled by volunteers alone.

Social marketing will continue to run into bureaucratic obstacles, such as unrealistic time frames, inadequate funding, and understaffing. Because governments are principal players in public health, especially in the developing countries, many of these bureaucratic constraints will not go away. Social marketing practitioners should develop innovative ways to overcome these obstacles and adapt themselves to the realities of development and the constraints of the bureaucratic environment. Otherwise, social marketing may face a gradual diminution of its role in public health.

MARKETING ELEMENTS MISSING   Marketing is part of a commercial enterprise with many elements, some of which are missing in the public health arena. Checking the requirements of commercial marketing against the realities of social marketing for public health programs is a good way to identify inherent problems. The commercial equation typically includes research for new products; market surveys of public interest in potential new products; manufacture of products with quality control; the dynamic price-product-need triangle and the interaction with wholesale and retail networks to get products distributed and made accessible; commissions and/or bonuses to motivate sales force; dismissal of incompetents; bankruptcies for mismanagement; dividends for share holders; and government regulatory oversight. Any one of these elements affects the others, as each serves as a check and balance for the entire enterprise. Too often, several of these elements are missing in public health initiatives.

Perhaps the four most intractable obstacles to the success of social marketing in public health are aspects of the 4 Ps (52). Public health does not have the flexibility to adjust products and services to clients' interests and preferences. Commercial companies often drop a product line when products prove unpopular. It is more difficult to discontinue a needed public health service. In social marketing, price, or the clients' assessment of the cost of the service or product, may include such factors as travel time, effort expended, physical discomfort, and the social consequences of innovative behavior, which may transgress taboos, norms, or the client's perception of his or her ability to change. For example, the cost in terms of effort and inconvenience for rural women to take their children to be immunized is the enemy of many immunization programs. Although a network of retail points at convenient locations is a sine qua non for any successful commercial marketing effort, there is a limit on the number of places at which public health products are available. Behavior change through social marketing requires the commitment to a sustained promotional effort. However, few public health projects have the resources to support prolonged promotion activities.

THE DEATH OF PSAs AND OTHER FREE SERVICES?   Social marketers' practice of buying air time may have a serious negative impact on the future of

PSAs. The health sector has depended on broadcasting services to give free air time to PSAs. In many countries, once the broadcast media have been paid to air public health spots, they are no longer willing to give free air time to health (39). The same could be true for the print media. Paying for time and space creates a serious problem for the tradition of free promotion for public health. Efforts to influence public service air time policies may be a good starting place to tackle this issue.

A BROADER APPROACH

Allied Practices

Because social marketing is not the only practice in the field of social change, it is useful to touch upon the allied practices of development communication, health education and promotion, and public relations. Although they have different starting points, and each has developed a theoretical framework for its methods of work, they all encourage people to change attitudes and behavior and facilitate the adoption of new behavior. They all tend to have an eclectic approach and have benefited variously from psychology, anthropology, and sociology. Indeed, each of these practices is quick to incorporate that which it perceives to be of value.

Development communication specialists are concerned with interpersonal, group, and mediated communication. Many of them come from a background of mass communication; others have their roots in interpersonal communication. Both groups stress the importance of the two-way dialogue, especially when working with communities, which emphasizes the critical importance of meeting people's felt needs. Development communication strategies now include education and social marketing elements.

For decades, health education has championed the principle of community involvement. Health educators are expected to put the interest of the community first in designing any project. They consider communication a skill and marketing a tool. Health educators also emphasize understanding the various determinants of health behavior. Health education students are now required to take communication and social marketing courses as part of their training. As an example of this dovetailing of disciplines, the World Health Organization's (WHO) expert committee on new approaches to health education in primary health care urged health education practitioners in 1982 to adopt a people-oriented approach. The committee also called for strengthening the communication skills of health education specialists (70).

Public relations began as a way to improve public perception for institutions and individuals. Many of its early practitioners came from journalism. Through evolution, it now encompasses media outreach, special events, in-house communication, and community education. Many universities that grant public relations degrees now offer courses in communication, advertising, journalism, and marketing. Public relations specialists not only project their institution's or client's views to the public, but also reflect the public's interest and perception in their feedback to employers and help devise policies and strategies beneficial to both their employers and the public. Both the health education specialists and public relations practitioners in the US have recently introduced an accreditation program to ensure professional and ethical standards among their ranks.

Social marketing and its allied practices all claim that their respective approaches are comprehensive. They most certainly have overlapping claims and methodologies. All of them require their practitioners to analyze audiences, design tailored messages to suit specific segments, and pretest approaches and materials. They all work with mass media, stress operations research and data collection, facilitate behavior change, practice empathy, orient themselves closely to their audiences, and recognize the principles of involvement and empowerment (40).

A Prospective Look

With the advent of the lifestyle illnesses, social marketing, which depends heavily on media, is likely to play a bigger role in public health. Lifestyle illnesses, such as cancer, heart diseases, psychosocial disorders, malnutrition and overnutrition, accidents, and sexually transmitted diseases, are, in fact, transmittable by the impact of words and images on lifestyle. Similarly, words and images are needed to combat them. With the explosion of human interaction and communication, abetted by more than 400 million annual travelers in recent years, these diseases need to be approached not as noncommunicable diseases, as most are currently classified, but as new "communicable" diseases. With its disciplined approach to mass media work, social marketing can and should play a useful role in combating these new communicable diseases (39).

Since social marketing carved out its niche in public health in the 1970s and 1980s, many health professionals and development specialists have realized that social change is a complex and challenging process. Health behavior cannot be separated from such issues as policy; economic and social circumstances; personal attitudes; political and religious allegiances; societal norms; and the entrenched interests of businesses, institutions, and certain professional groups. Increasingly, health and development specialists are advocating a broader look at these problems and tackling them in a more comprehensive way. At the international level, WHO and UNICEF, now support a broader approach to change.

WHO'S HEALTH PROMOTION   The World Health Organization recently called for action in health promotion, a broader version of health education, which includes advocacy for health supportive laws and public policies, intersectoral solidarity, alliances with various social institutions, partnership with mass media, and grass-roots education strategies to empower people for health action. Dr. Hiroshi Nakajima, Director General of WHO, has said: " . . . Health is a product of social action . . . Active community participation and supportive social policies are necessary for progress" (69). The evolving WHO concept encompasses lifestyles and other social, economic, environmental, and personal factors conducive to health.

UNICEF'S SOCIAL MOBILIZATION   In launching its Child Survival and Development initiative 1983, UNICEF has found it necessary to mobilize various societal sectors for several inexpensive interventions to save millions of lives. Social mobilization (SOCMOB), as this multisectoral effort is called, is a process that seeks to facilitate and enhance the approach to development issues that aims at "going to scale," from a micro level up to national scale.

Social mobilization enables national governments and development assistance agencies to move beyond the project phase of many development progams. It first aims to create the political will for constructive change and then to translate that will into the establishment of viable social service policies and actions to meet basic needs.

A continuum of mutually reinforcing, well-researched, carefully targeted, rigorously implemented activities is required for the mobilization process. The umbrella of SOCMOB covers advocacy, marketing, media, training, community education, and grass-roots organization activities.

Often, these activities are undertaken by various groups, without a broad strategy that considers the critical linkages between and among them. They often wind up as isolated, sometimes spectacular, efforts that fizzle out like fireworks (42). The SOCMOB approach aims at avoiding this fireworks syndrome.

Because many development objectives involve far reaching changes, SOCMOB is a promising strategy for specific health programs, as well as more global issues that affect development generally. Where needed, SOCMOB can be used to generate the critical political will that is essential for development; it also aims at the involvement of individuals at the community level in adopting positive behaviors.

There is a place for marketing in both these approaches, as they stress the need to understand people and tailor inputs to the specific requirement of the communities concerned. The elements of marketing considered most critical for promoting healthy behavior include consumer or market research, product or service quality, a distribution network, product or brand image, price and consumer affordability, accessibility, consumer satisfaction, and promotion

(H. S. Dhillon, WHO). Mass media, which have a special place in marketing, are partners, not merely channels for health messages (41).

Toward the beginning of the 1980s, Fox & Kotler (15) predicted that within the decade, marketing would be a regular feature of a growing number of nonprofit organizations. This is certainly the case, as far as the health sector is concerned. Social marketing, which helps stimulate demand and fine-tune the design and delivery of health messages and services, has a secure place in public health. The new thrusts of UNICEF and WHO, two of the key development organizations at the global level, are likely to confirm this in the years to come.

Nevertheless, social marketing cannot solve public health problems on its own. Within the ranks of marketers, there is an active push for integrated marketing communication, which includes communication and education approaches. Social marketing, too, may be moving toward the broader approach. Not long ago, frustrated social marketers complained that health was simply not part of the marketing domain. It may still be so, but marketing is fast becoming part of the health domain.

Literature Cited

1. Andreasen, A. 1981. *Power Potential Channel Strategies in Social Marketing.* Working paper #743. Urbana, Ill: Bur. Econ. Bus. Res. Univ. of Ill.
2. Bartels, R. 1974. The identity crisis in marketing. *J. Mark.* 38:73–76
3. Black, R. L., Harvey, P. D. 1976. A report on a contraceptive social marketing experiment in rural Kenya. *Stud. Fam. Plann.* 7:101–7
4. Bloom, P. N. 1980. Evaluating social marketing programs: Problems and prospects. In *Marketing in the 80's: Changes and Challenges,* ed. R. P. Bagozzi et al., pp. 460–63. Chicago: Am. Mark. Assoc.
5. Bloom, P. N., Novelli, W. D. 1981. Problems and challenges in social marketing. *J. Mark.* 45:79–88
6. Cabanero-Verzosa, C., Bernaje, M. G., De Guzman, E. M., Hernandez, J. R. S., Reodica, C. N., Taguiwalo, M. M. 1989. *Managing a Communication Program on Immunization.* Washington, DC: Acad. Educ. Dev. 45 pp.
7. Caesar, P. 1986. Cause-related marketing: The new face of corporate philanthropy. *Bus. Soc. Rev.* 59:15–19
8. Dawson, L. M. 1971. Marketing science in the age of the aquarius. *J. Mark.* 35:66–72
9. El Ansary, A. I., Kramer, O. E. 1973.

Social marketing: The family planning experience. *J. Mark.* 37:1–7
10. Deleted in proof
11. Faden, R. 1987. Ethical issues in government sponsored public health campaigns. *Health Educ. Q.* 14:27–37
12. Faden, R., Faden, A. 1980. The ethics of health education as a public health policy. In *Health Education Monographs,* ed. B. P. Mathews, 2:5–23. Oakland, Calif: Third Party
13. Feldman, L. P. 1971. Societal adaptation: A new challenge for marketing. *J. Mark.* 35:54–60
14. Flora, J. A., Maccoby, N., Farquar, J. W. 1989. Communication campaigns to prevent cardiovascular disease: The Stanford community studies. In *Public Communication Campaigns.* ed. R. E. Rice, C. K. Atkin, pp. 233–52. Newbury Park/London/New Delhi: Sage. 367 pp. 2nd ed.
15. Fox, K. F. A., Kotler, P. 1980. The marketing of social causes: The first 10 years. *J. Mark.* 44:24–33
16. Freimuth, V. S., Hammond, S. L., Stein, J. A. 1988. Health advertising: Prevention for profit. *Am. J. Public Health* 78:557–61
17. Green, E. C. 1987. Contraceptive social marketing of microgynon in the Dominican Republic—Progress of the

campaign. *Occasional Papers*. Washington, DC: Futures Group. 9 pp.
18. Green, L. W. 1987. Letter to the editor. *Health Educ. Q.* 14:3–6
19. Hammond, S. L. 1987. Health advertising: The credibility of organizational sources. *Communication Yearbook 10*. Beverly Hills, Calif: Sage
20. Holbrook, M. B. 1987. Mirror, mirror, on the wall, what's unfair in the reflections on advertising? *J. Mark.* 51:95–103
21. Hollis, C. *The Cameroon Weaning Project: A PVO's Use of Social Marketing Techniques*. Newton, Mass: Educ. Dev. Cent.
22. Huber, S. C., Harvey, P. D. 1989. Family planning programs in ten developing countries. *J. Biosoc. Sci.* 21:267–77
23. Hurtado, M. P. 1990. *Colombian Case Study: The National Child Survival Development Plan—The Use of Appropriate Technology*. Cali, Colombia: Minist. Health 10 pp.
24. Israel, R. C., Foote, D., Tognetti, J. 1987. *Operational Guidelines for Social Marketing Projects in Public Health and Nutrition*. Nutr. Educ. Ser., Issue 14. Paris: UNESCO. 68 pp.
25. Kelley, E. J. 1971. Marketing's changing social/environmental role. *J. Mark.* 35:1
26. Kotler, P. 1982. *Marketing for Nonprofit Organizations*. Englewood Cliffs, NJ: Prentice-Hall. 528 pp. 2nd ed.
27. Kotler, P. 1979. Strategies for introducing marketing into nonprofit organizations. *J. Mark.* 43:37–44
28. Kotler, P., Levy, S. J. 1971. Demarketing, yes, demarketing. *Harv. Bus. Rev.* 49:74–80
29. Kotler, P., Levy, S. J. 1969. Broadening the concept of marketing. *J. Mark.* 33:10–15
30. Kotler, P., Roberto, E. L. 1989. *Social Marketing Strategies for Changing Public Behavior*. New York: Free Press. 401 pp.
31. Kotler, P., Zaltman, G. 1971. Social marketing: An approach to planned social change. *J. Mark.* 35:3–12
32. Laczniak, G. R., Lusch, R. F., Murphy, P. E. 1979. Social marketing: Its ethical dimensions. *J. Mark.* 43:29–36
33. Laing, J. E., Walker, D. 1986. *A Reassessment of the Bangladesh USAID Social Marketing Project's Objectives and Information Needs*, pp. 36–67. Arlington, Va: Int. Sci. Technol. Inst.
34. Lavidge, R. 1970. The growing responsibilities of marketing. *J. Mark.* 34:25–28
35. Lazer, W. 1969. Marketing's changing social relationships. *J. Mark.* 33:3–9
36. Lazer, W., Kelley, E. J., eds. 1973. *Social Marketing: Perspectives and Viewpoints*. Homewood, Ill: Irwin
37. Lefebvre, C. R., Flora, J. A. 1988. Social marketing and public health intervention. *Health Educ. Q.* 15:299–315
38. Levy, A. S., Stokes, R. C. 1987. Effects of health promotion advertising campaign on sales of ready-to-eat cereals. *Public Health Rep.*
39. Ling, J. C. 1990. Communicating disease through words and images. *Dev. Commun. Rep.* 71:1–11
40. Ling, J. C. 1985. Int. Union for Health Educ. Presented at World Conf. on Health Educ., Dublin, Ireland. Cited in *HYGIE Int. J. Health Educ.* 1986. 5:22–25
41. Ling, J. C. Oct. 1984. Prescribing health communications. *Far East. Econ. Rev.* pp. 40–41
42. Ling, J. C. 1983. *Fireworks Syndrome*. Presentation at Int. Conf. on Oral Rehydration Ther., Washington, DC. Reprinted in *Dev. Commun. Rep.* 1985. 51:10
43. Lovelock, C. H., ed. 1977. *Nonbusiness Marketing Cases*, 8:378. Boston: Intercoll. Case Clearing House
44. Lovelock, C. H., Weinberg, C. B. 1977. *Cases in Public and Nonprofit Marketing*. Palo Alto, Calif: Scientific Press
45. Luck, D. J. 1969. Broadening the concept of marketing—too far. *J. Mark.* 33:53–55
46. Luthra, R. 1988. *Contraceptive Social Marketing in the Third World: A Case of Multiple Transfer*, pp. 1–24. Madison: Univ. of Wisc.
47. Manoff Group Inc. 1989. *The Indonesian Weaning Project*. Washington, DC: Manoff
48. Manoff Group Inc. 1987. *Nutrition Communication and Behavior Change Project*. Washington, DC: Manoff
49. Manoff, R. K. 1985. *Social Marketing: New Imperative for Public Health*. New York: Praeger. 293 pp.
50. Martin, N. A. 1968. The outlandish idea: How a marketing man would save India. *Mark. Commun.* 297:54–60
51. McLeroy, K. R., Gottlieb, N. H., Burdine, J. N. 1987. The business of health promotion: Ethical issues and professional responsibilities. *Health Educ. Q.* 14:91–109
52. Novelli, W. D. 1989. *Marketing Health and Social Issues: What Works?* Presented to Natl. Workshop on Project

LEAN, Sponsored by Cent. Dis. Control and Kaiser Fam. Found.

53. Pollay, R. W. 1986. The distorted mirror: Reflections on the unintended consequences of advertising. *J. Mark.* 50:18–36

54. Rothschild, M. L. 1979. Marketing communications in nonbusiness situations or why it's so hard to sell brotherhood like soap. *J. Mark.* 43:11–20

55. Rothschild, M. L. 1977. *An Incomplete Bibliography of Works Relating to Marketing for Public Sector and Nonprofit Organizations,* 9:577–771. Boston: Intercoll. Case Clearing House. 2nd ed.

56. Roundtable. 1990. The politics of the solution. *Links* pp. 9–15

57. Ryan, W. 1971. *Blaming the Victim.* New York: Random House

58. Sherris, J. D., Kavenholt, B. B., Blackburn, R. 1985. Contraceptive social marketing: Lessons from experience. *Popul. Rep.* 13:774–806

59. Sheth, J. N., Frazier, G. L. 1982. A model of strategy mix choice for planned social change. *J. Mark.* 46:15–26

60. Shruptine, F. K., Osmanski, F. A. 1975. Marketing's changing role: Expanding or contracting? *J. Mark.* 39:58–66

61. Social marketing: Does it work? 1980. *Popul. Rep.* 13:393–405

62. Solomon, D. 1989. A social marketing perspective on communication campaigns. In *Public Communication Campaigns,* ed. R. E. Rice, C. K. Atkin, pp. 87–104. Newbury Park/London/New Delhi: Sage. 367 pp. 2nd ed.

63. Stover, J. 1987. The impact of CSM prevalence in the Dominican Republic. *Occasional Papers.* 11 pp.

64. Takas, A. 1974. Societal marketing: A businessman's perspective. *J. Mark.* 38:2–7

65. Teh, W. M. B. P. 1980. *The Challenge of the Media in the 80s "Dadah Menace."* Malaysia: Minist. Inf. 14 pp.

66. Deleted in proof

67. Wiebe, G. D. 1951–1952. Merchandising commodities and citizenship on television. *Public Opin. Q.* 15:679–91

68. Wikler, D. 1987. Who should be blamed for being sick? *Health Educ. Q.* 14:11–25

69. World Health Org. 1990. *A Call for Action: Promoting Health in Developing Countries.* Summ. Rep. Work. Group Health Promot. Dev. Ctries. Geneva: WHO

70. World Health Org. 1983. New approaches to health education in primary health care. *Tech. Rep. Ser.* 690:7–43

71. Yusoff, M. 1982. *Social Marketing in Malaysia—PEMADAM's Experience.* Dep. of Commun., Natl. Univ. of Malaysia. 15 pp.

Annu. Rev. Publ. Health 1992. 13:363–83

UNNECESSARY SURGERY

Lucian L. Leape

Department of Health Policy and Management, Harvard School of Public Health, Boston, Massachusetts 02115

KEY WORDS: appropriateness, second opinions, geographic variations, consensus panels, practice guidelines

INTRODUCTION

In 1974, the Congressional Committee on Interstate and Foreign Commerce held hearings on unnecessary surgery. McCarthy et al (35) presented the most important evidence. Their findings from the first surgical second opinion program (SSOP) indicated that 17.6% of recommendations for surgery were not confirmed. The Congressional Subcommittee on Oversight and Investigations extrapolated these figures to estimate that nationwide there were 2.4 million unnecessary operations performed annually, resulting in a cost of $3.9 billion and 11,900 deaths (47).

This claim fell on the receptive ears of payers, including the Health Care Financing Administration (HCFA), who were beginning to feel the burden of accelerating increases in health care costs. Reducing costs by 15–20% was an appealing prospect, and several payers subsequently instituted mandatory SSOP. About the same time, HCFA and commercial insurance companies implemented preprocedural review programs for operations widely considered overutilized.

It is worth recalling that before 1970 public policy was concerned not with overuse, but with the problems of underuse of health services and perceived shortages of doctors and hospitals (16). But, as the full costs of Medicare became evident, cost containment entered the public agenda. Increasing cost pressures in the private sector, which resulted from technologic advances, also led private payers to search for ways to reduce health care expenditures.

363

0163-7525/92/0501-0363$02.00

Unnecessary surgery was an obvious target. Doctors have had less interest in unnecessary surgery, because they have tended to dissociate themselves from the debates concerning cost containment and because most do not recognize unnecessary surgery as a significant problem. No surgeon believes that what he or she does is unnecessary, and physicians are generally reluctant to pass judgment on their colleagues.

The 1970s witnessed a remarkable profusion of mechanisms designed to change, or at least challenge, physicians' decisions. In addition to SSOP and precertification programs, analysis of geographic variations of use of procedures was provided to physicians as "feedback" with the hope of influencing their patterns of use. "Managed care" was invented: an overt second-guessing of doctors' decisions aimed at reducing days of hospitalization and use of expensive services. The government provided subsidies for the development of health maintenance organizations (HMO) and began to encourage Medicare patients to enroll in them.

Although significant reductions have subsequently been reported in hospital stay or in the use of a particular procedure, it has been difficult to demonstrate that these programs have had the significant effect on utilization and costs that were anticipated. In fact, health care costs have continued to rise at two or more times the inflation rate. More imporantly, there is no evidence that these attempts to reduce utilization have had any effect on the quality of care. Recent reports suggest high (10–20%) rates of inappropriate use of a variety of services (3, 9, 20, 29, 37, 58, 59). Clearly, unnecessary surgery is still with us.

Surgery has been a primary focus of attention for those interested in overuse of health care services for several reasons. First, it is easy to study: Most operations are reasonably standardized, outcomes are obvious, and the delivery of the service can be reliably ascertained from discharge or payment claims data. Second, operations are costly, in terms of both surgical fees and hospitalizations. More can be saved by reducing rates of surgery than by curtailing the use of most other therapeutic or diagnostic services. Third, surgical care is generally riskier than other forms of therapy. There is a finite mortality risk associated with almost every major operation. The combination of risk and potential for dramatic cure gives surgery an aura of excitement lacking in other forms of therapy. Abuse is, therefore, more serious and more intriguing.

Finally, the current interest in unnecessary surgery also reflects recent increases in the number and types of operations performed in the United States. Many operations that are now performed frequently, such as coronary artery bypass, hip replacements, carotid endarterectomy, arthroscopy, laparoscopy, and heart and liver transplantation, were unkown just 25 years ago. Not surprisingly, some of the indications for these procedures are controversial. There has also been a substantial increase in the rates of performance of well established operations, such as cataract extraction and cesarean section, which raises questions of overuse (3). Overall, the surgery rate grew at twice the rate of the population from 1979 to 1986 (27). Unnecessary surgery is, in many ways, a "disease of medical progress," which reflects the hazards, as well as the benefits, of technological advances. A concern about its impact is timely, because the implications of unnecessary surgery are greater than ever, in terms of both the number of patients at risk and the aggregate cost.

Recently, there has been a deliberate shift in federal emphasis. Responding to imprecations from the research community, Congress established the Agency for Health Care Policy and Research (AHCPR) in 1989. This new agency within the Public Health Service supervises and funds research into clinical outcomes and the development of practice guidelines, and it has launched a major effort in both areas. In addition, HCFA has pursued the development and implementation of analysis of large clinical data bases to demonstrate patterns of use that can be fed back to physicians or used by the Peer Review Organizations (PRO) as quality measures.

Physicians have also become concerned about unnecessary surgery, as their colleagues have produced more convincing and sophisticated evidence of inappropriate use of some operations and procedures (8, 59). Professional specialty societies, individually and through the Council of Medical Specialty Societies and the American Medical Association, have started to develop practice guidelines to help physicians choose appropriate care (50).

Why does unnecessary surgery occur? Why haven't the above-mentioned programs worked? More importantly, will outcomes research, data base analysis, and practice guidelines get us where we want to go?

In this review, I first consider how best to define the term unnecessary surgery and then summarize the evidence for its presence. Next, I examine the theories regarding the occurrence of unnecessary surgery, which leads logically to a consideration of methods that have been recommended for reducing it. Finally, I consider the policy implications of these recommendations.

WHAT IS UNNECESSARY SURGERY?

The term "unnecessary surgery" has many meanings. The person who has had an operation that failed to relieve his symptoms may understandably conclude that the operation was unnecessary, even if the operation is successful in most individuals and its use is unquestioned. Others confuse unnecessary with "elective," a term used by doctors in reference to timing, not as a synonym for "optional." In contrast to an "urgent" or "emergent" operation, an elective operation is one that can be scheduled at a time of convenience, because the underlying condition does not pose an immediate threat to life or health.

The most common association of the term unnecessary surgery is with high frequency of use. Some cesarean sections are considered unnecessary when the rate of performance in a region exceeds some threshold number. One learns that there are "too many" hysterectomies performed, or that Dr. X performs unnecessary surgery because he does a higher number of a certain operation than his colleagues. Some carry this type of thinking to the extreme: Lower rates of surgery of all types must be evidence of higher quality medical care! This stands in interesting contrast to the use of vaccines, for example, for which most people associate higher use with better quality care. The difference is that vaccines are considered an unequivocal low-risk good, whereas operations carry greater risk and have been suspected of overuse.

Although it might seem simplest to consider as unnecessary any operation that is not clearly necessary, this definition creates more problems than it solves. Webster defines necessary as something that "must be by reason of the nature of things," "cannot be otherwise," or "determined and fixed and inevitable" (53). No operation qualifies, for the simple reason that no operation "must be" or is "inevitable" for any patient. A host of variables enter into the decision for surgery, of which the patient's own values are among the most important. Individuals vary in their tolerance of risk, fear of surgery, desired activity level, tolerance of pain, and fear of death. They also vary in how they value different probabilities of good and bad outcomes. Clearly, it is not possible to define what is necessary for an individual—what is necessary for me may be totally unacceptable to you.

In contrast, Webster's definition of unnecessary, "useless," is easy to use, as it can be based entirely on objective data. No operation is necessary if it is ineffective, i.e. if it does not accomplish its objective for a given clinical situation.[1] For example, if the objectives of coronary artery bypass graft (CABG) surgery are to relieve pain and prolong life, CABG is ineffective— and, therefore, unnecessary—for an asymptomatic patient with coronary artery disease that causes blockage of only one of the three coronary arteries, because studies have shown that CABG does not increase longevity in patients with single vessel disease. An unnecessary operation, then, is one that is ineffective or useless. An operation is also unnecessary if it confers no clear advantage over a less risky alternative. In both instances, the operation does not represent a net benefit to the patient. The patient will not be better off. This is the definition we will use.

---

[1]Rarely is an operation totally ineffective. Internal mammary ligation for the treatment of angina pectoris and glomectomy for asthma are examples. These operations were ultimately discredited by randomized trials. More commonly, an operation is effective for its initial use, but as experience is gained, the indications are broadened to conditions for which it is useless.

One other aspect of ineffectiveness must be considered: occult or un-recognizable unnecessary surgery. For many indications for operations, the evidence for effectiveness is clear-cut. But, there are other indications for some operations for which the evidence is absent or equivocal, and expert judgments are divided on its benefit. Some indications in this "gray zone" of effectiveness will one day be found to be inappropriate. Therefore, these operations represent occult unnecessary surgery, unrecognizable at the present state of knowledge. Operations performed for indications in this uncertain or equivocal category cannot now be fairly labeled as unnecessary, but some of them eventually will be. Other operations currently labeled as effective will be found to have only marginal benefit as more data are accumulated from outcomes studies. These, too, represent occult unnecessary surgery.

Clearly, we cannot measure what is not recognizable, so it would be highly speculative to estimate the extent of occult unnecessary surgery. However, the implication is clear that the full extent of unnecessary surgery is greater than is measured by any of the current methods. For now, we must confine our analysis to what is known, i.e. to clinical situations in which the best available evidence or informed expert judgment indicates that an operation is ineffective or useless. What do we know?

THE EVIDENCE

Evidence for unnecessary surgery comes from three types of studies: circum-stantial evidence from studies of variations of rates of use of various op-erations among different geographic regions and between different types of practices, denial rates of second opinion and precertification programs, and attempts to measure inappropriate use directly.

Geographic Variations

It is not unreasonable to assume that if an operation is being performed ten times as frequently in one area as in another, the high use must represent unnecessary surgery, although an equally logical conclusion is that the low rate represents underuse. There is probably some truth in both interpretations.

In 1969, Lewis (31) published the results of a study of variations in rates of use of six common surgical procedures by Blue Cross enrollees in 11 health planning regions in Kansas. He found that rates varied by as much as 3.8 times and attributed the higher rates to overutilization. Wennberg & Gittel-sohn subsequently found similar variations in Vermont (57) and Maine (56) and they also attributed the higher rates to overuse. Significant (as high as tenfold) variations have been noted for some operations, and regional varia-tions in use have been found throughout the US, as well as in Canada (43,

51), the United Kingdom, and Norway (36). Although most studies have compared small areas (counties or hospital-service regions), significant variations have also been observed between large areas (states or parts of states) (8).

Many studies have been performed to identify the factors that lead to geographic variations and to determine if variations do, in fact, represent unnecessary surgery. The simplest and most obvious explanation for differences in rates of surgery would be differences in the incidence of disease. Curiously, this aspect of geographic variations has not been extensively investigated, perhaps because the magnitude of the variations in use of operations far exceeds any likely differences in underlying disease rates. In addition, most studies have compared adjacent small regions, in which similar populations and environments would be expected to result in similar rates of disease. In one of the few specific attempts to correlate surgical rates with disease incidence, Roos et al (45) found no relationship between rates of respiratory infection and rates of tonsillectomy.

Geographic variations could reflect differences in supply or demand. Demographic predictors of the demand for surgical services have been extensively studied. Surgical utilization is higher in older patients, women, those with higher incomes, and noncollege graduates (4, 22, 44). However, none of these factors explains more than a small fraction of geographic variations (22, 44, 56). Physicians and their spouses have higher rates of surgical treatment (6), but these differences also have not been related to geographic variations.

The effect of supply on geographic variations in use is conflicting. Health maintenance organizations and other managed care plans reduce the use of surgical care (33), but HMO participation rates have not been linked to geographic variations. Lewis (31), Wennberg & Gittelsohn (57), and Stockwell & Vayda (46) found that the number of available hospital beds was strongly related to geographic variations, but Roos (42) found no relationship between hysterectomy rates and bed availability. The number of surgeons has been correlated with regional surgical rates (1, 5, 31, 57), again with some exceptions (45).

Variations resulting from differences in demand and supply do not necessarily represent evidence of unnecessary surgery. These variations could reflect differences in the ability of patients to access useful health care. Certainly, Bunker's (6) finding that physicians and their spouses have higher surgical rates than others supports that possibility.

Many investigators consider that the practice style of physicians is the most important determinant of regional variations. Wennberg has noted remarkable consistency from year to year in regional use rates and has referred to these patterns of high or low use as "surgical signatures." He considers these local practice styles the most important variable that explains variations (55). Individual surgeons' caseloads can have a significant effect on overall regional rates, especially in small areas where a few high-volume surgeons can markedly alter the local rate (30, 45).

Why do surgeons' practice patterns vary so much? Wennberg (54) and others claim that variations in practice style reflect the degree of uncertainty in surgical decision-making. Eddy (13) has noted that as a result of the rapid pace of biomedical advances, the degree of uncertainty about the effectiveness of many forms of therapy is greater than ever. Uncertainty leads to variations in how physicians perceive the value of a procedure and, hence, to variations in its use.

If the practice style hypothesis is correct, then geographic variations in the use of operations will be greatest when the level of uncertainty as to their value is high and least when it is low. That is what has been found. In all geographic variations studies, surgery for inguinal hernia and fractured hip show the least differences. There is little disagreement about the indications for surgical treatment for these conditions. Controversial operations, such as carotid endarterectomy and laminectomy (disc operations), have the greatest variations (8, 25, 59). It is also of interest that when physicians were informed that their individual rates were substantially above state averages they reduced their rates, which suggests that they recognized some overuse (54).

Two studies have attempted to measure the contribution of unnecessary surgery to regional variations in use rates directly. Roos et al (45) studied the relationship between tonsillectomy rates and adherence to standards for indications. Although they found high rates of inappropriate use, there was no correlation with rates of tonsillectomy. The RAND Health Services Utilization Study examined the relationship between the appropriateness of indications, as determined by an expert panel, and utilization of three procedures that showed substantial variations in use between large regions (states). For the one operation studied, carotid endarterectomy, they found a high rate of inappropriate use (32%), but no difference in the rate of inappropriate use between high and low use areas (9). Analysis of the data for one state also showed no differences in rates of inappropriate use among small areas (counties) (29).

In summary, although geographic variations in the use of surgical procedures result from a multitude of factors, the most important seems to be variations in physician perceptions of the value of the operation in question. These differences result from lack of professional consensus about the value of many procedures for many potential indications. Thus, geographic variations are primarily a measure of professional uncertainty. In the few instances in which unnecessary surgery has been directly measured, the extent is greatest for procedures about which there is little professional consensus.

Thus, large geographic variations in the use of an operation suggest that a significant fraction is unnecessary. The extent of variation is not a direct measure of the extent of unnecessary surgery, however, as inappropriate use represents only a minor share of the differences.

Variations by Method of Payment

Another type of variation in practice patterns that has been cited as evidence of inappropriate care is the difference in surgical rates between HMOs and private practice. Patients who receive care in HMOs are one-half to one-fourth as likely to be operated on as patients in the fee-for-service sector (132, 49). Overall, reductions in use of medical services in HMOs does not have a deleterious effect on outcomes (10), so it can be inferred that the difference in surgical rates is at least partly due to unnecessary surgery.

Second Surgical Opinion Programs

Although the specific purpose of SSOP is to reduce the rate of unnecessary surgery, 17 years after their introduction we still do not know whether they do. McCarthy, who introduced the first SSOP in 1974, did not claim that it identified unnecessary surgery, but carefully stated that its purpose was "to help the patient make a more informed decision" (34). Others were less restrained. The Congressional Subcommittee on Oversight and In-vestigations, which as mentioned above equated McCarthy's 17.6% nonconfirmation rate in his mandatory SSOP with unnecessary surgery and thus estimated that 2.4 million unnecessary operations were performed an-nually, later strongly recommended the use of a second opinion program in the Medicare and Medicaid programs. The Department of Health and Human Services promptly instituted a national voluntary second opinion program for Medicare, and seven states introduced mandatory second opinion programs in their Medicaid programs. Private health insurers began to offer second opin-ion programs, and by 1984, 28% had mandatory SSOP, including 60 Blue Cross/Blue Shield plans. Employers also instituted mandatory second opinion programs; by 1988, a survey of 240 major US firms found that 62% reduced coverage if a second opinion was not obtained (39).

It is clear that the major reason for instituting second opinion programs has been to control costs by reducing rates of surgery. In the absence of controlled studies, it is not possible to conclude whether nonconfirmation rates or nonoperative rates measure unnecessary surgery, but overall rates of surgery have been reduced by SSOPs—at least initially (28). At Senate hearings in 1985, the Inspector General reported that Medicaid mandatory programs in three states had reduced utilization 20–35% and saved $7.5 million (48). In their study of the Massachusetts Medicaid SSOP, Poggio et al (41) estimated a total reduction in rates of performance of the targeted operations of 24%. Almost all of this reduction was due to the "sentinel effect"—a decline in recommendations for surgery because of the physicians' knowledge that a second opinion would be obtained. The direct effect of the nonconfirmations (allowing for those who decide to have the operation anyway) only reduced the surgical rate by 2%. Few studies have addressed the effect of second opinion programs on health status, and none have assessed health status of the target population before and after the surgical decision.

Recently, enthusiasm for SSOPs has cooled as more and more programs report high confirmation rates (and, therefore, little direct savings.) Lacking plan-specific information about the sentinel effect, many payers apparently do not consider its savings to be relevant. Several insurers and large companies have given up their programs because they cost more than they save (39). Finally, HCFA, which never fully implemented the Congressional mandate for SSOPs, has recently withdrawn its proposed regulations for mandatory SSOPs for both Medicaid and Medicare, citing controversies over cost-effectiveness, concern over creating barriers to care, and its desire to decrease the number of mandated programs (39).

What does the experience with second opinion programs tell us about the extent of unnecessary surgery? Unfortunately, less than one might hope. Although many studies have been made of nonconfirmation rates and cost savings, none have directly addressed the question of whether nonconfirmation accurately identifies operations that should not be performed. In the absence of controls, it is not even possible to tell if the supposed benefits of forgone operations are, in fact, realized. The absence of outcome data even prevents evaluation of the supposed benefits to SSOP patients of nonconfirmation.

More fundamentally, the characteristics of second opinion programs make it unlikely that they either identify or diminish the rate of unnecessary surgery. Second opinion programs are a form of unstructured implicit review, i.e. the second surgeon makes a judgment based on his own knowledge and experience, not according to any explicit or agreed-upon criteria of appropriateness. In other clinical studies, unstructured implicit reviews have had low reliability and questionable validity. Second, the process does not distinguish between differences of opinion, in which evidence is scant and experienced surgeons disagree, and differences of fact, in which one of the surgeons (either one) has supporting scientific knowledge that the other is unaware of.

Finally, the use of peers (specialists of equal qualification) to provide the second opinion insures that SSOPs do not improve the quality of care, but actually make it worse (28). If each surgeon has a similar, independent, random error rate, the errors will be cumulative. For example, for controversial operations, we can reasonably assume that each surgeon is wrong in his judgment 10% of the time. Ten percent of the first surgeons's recommendations for surgery will be inappropriate. If the second opinion surgeon also has a 10% error rate that is independent of the first's, he or she will approve surgery for 90% of all of those for whom it was recommended. Thus, surgery will be approved for 90% (9/10) of those whose first recommendation was erroneous. And, it will be disapproved for 10% (9/90) of those for whom the first recommendation was appropriate, and who would benefit from surgery. Thus, inappropriate treatment will be advised for 18% of patients, instead of 10% if the second opinion had not been obtained.

For all of these reasons, it is not possible to draw any conclusions about the extent of unnecessary surgery from the experiences of second opinion programs.

Precertification Programs

Precertification programs are designed to identify potentially unnecessary operations before they are performed. Denial rates (the fraction of proposed operations for which payment is denied by the carrier) thus may be measures of unnecessary surgery, as these operations presumably would have been performed if payment had not been denied. For competitive reasons, commercial carriers do not release information about denial rates. However, information is available for public programs, particularly the results from the PRO, which performs the quality assurance function for Medicare. For certain designated operations, i.e. those that are widely considered overused, the PRO requires the surgeon to obtain approval before the patient can be admitted to the hospital or have the operation. A two-stage process of review is used. Nurses assess the appropriateness of the proposed surgery according to whether the patient meets explicit screening criteria for that procedure. If the patient does not, the case undergoes implicit review by a PRO physician. Screening criteria are developed by the PROs individually and vary widely (26). They are often oriented toward establishing the presence of disease, not whether the proposed operation is appropriate for the individual patient. Consideration may not be given to severity of disease, comorbidity, possible alternative treatments, or even outcome probabilities. Thus, the aggregate denial rate for PROs nationwide was, not surprisingly, only 2.3% in 1988 and 1.6% in 1990 (A. Webber 1988, personal communication).

Recently, several large insurance companies have instituted computerized preprocedural review programs by using a commercial product that applies highly detailed criteria that have been developed with the RAND/UCLA appropriateness methodology. Blue Cross/Blue Shield reported the results of a pilot program that used these criteria for 21 procedures in six states over a one-year period ending in July 1990. The overall rate of inappropriate proposed use was 11.2%; individual rates of inappropriateness varied from 0% for CABG to 21.5% for hysterectomy and 27.1% for tonsillectomy (27).

Direct Measurement

In 1953, Doyle (11) attempted one of the first direct measurements of unnecessary surgery. He reviewed the records of 6248 hysterectomies performed in Los Angeles and found that 39% were "unjustified." Because these were implicit judgments, his findings are open to the same criticisms leveled at second opinion programs: absence of specific criteria and lack of distinction between difference of opinion and difference of expertise. In a recent study of multiple reviews of 50 cases of cesarean section performed for fetal distress, Barrett et al (2) found that five reviewers agreed in their judgments in only 28% of cases. Nonetheless, 30% of the operations were judged inappropriate by four of five reviewers.

Because of dissatisfaction with implicit reviews, serious students of quality assessment have turned to explicit criteria that can be applied in a standardized fashion. The development and application of these methods has expanded dramatically in the past few years. Valid judgments require that explicit criteria be comprehensive, detailed, and clinically relevant, and that they clearly specify the conditions under which an operation is either appropriate or inappropriate. To develop criteria, investigators have used evidence in the literature, judgments of experts, or a combination of the two. The process may be informal and qualitative or highly structured and semiquantitative (17, 38). The source of information about the patients also varies. Although reimbursement claims data have been used by some, the level of clinical detail recorded is seldom adequate to permit judgments of appropriateness, so most investigators have relied on review of medical records.

Table 1 summarizes the findings from the literature of studies of unnecessary surgery by using explicit criteria. These findings are the most convincing evidence of unnecessary surgery, which appears to occur in 8–86% of patients, depending on the procedure studied and the criteria used. Although these figures are disturbingly high, it is important to note that they are not a fair representation of surgery in general. These operations were selected for study precisely because they were controversial, because of either substantial geographic variations in use or other evidence of overuse.

In summary, the evidence for unnecessary surgery is largely circumstantial. Geographic variations reflect uncertainty and, thus, indicate the presence of unnecessary surgery, but do not measure its extent. Second opinion program results represent only differences of opinion between two individuals, a thin reed upon which to make a judgment of inappropriate use. Criteria studies, and the results from the related use of explicit criteria for precertification

Table 1   Explicit criteria studies

Year	Operation	Number	% Unnecessary	Source	Type of criteria	Reference
1977	Tonsillectomy	3072	86	C	L	(45)
1986	Carotid endarterectomy	107	13	R	S	(39)
1988	Carotid endarterectomy	1302	32	R	S	(9)
1988	CABG	386	14	R	S	(58)
1988	Pacemaker insertion	382	20	R	G	(20)
1990	Hysterectomy	257	8	R	G	(18)
1990	CABG	320	16	R	S	(19)
		5826	56			

C = Payment claims.
R = Patient record review.
L = Criteria developed from literature review.
S = Criteria developed by structured process of literature analysis and consensus of experts.
G = Criteria developed by group of experts.

programs, do provide concrete evidence of unnecessary surgery. From these studies, it is reasonable to conclude that 10% or more of surgical procedures are unnecessary. For controversial operations, the fraction may be substantially higher.

WHY DOES UNNECESSARY SURGERY OCCUR?

Why do surgeons perform unnecessary surgery? It is difficult to believe that many do so deliberately, out of greed or malice. A judgment that a physician is performing unnecessary surgery implies that the operation is known to be inappropriate for a given condition. But, no one knowingly performs a useless operation. Therefore, the surgeon either does not know that it is inappropriate or does not accept the evidence.

Unfortunately, it is often not clear what is "known" in medicine. Contrary to popular assumptions, most accepted medical therapy is not based on scientific evidence of effectiveness. Acceptable therapy, therefore, includes both those treatments for which there is good evidence of effectiveness and those for which the evidence is scant, but the weight of professional opinion is favorable. Further, science is what scientists say it is, so even the acceptability of scientific data relies on the belief that the conclusions are valid. In the absence of a consensus, whether based on evidence or expert opinion, a judgment regarding the necessity of a given treatment is impossible.

Several considerations determine whether a consensus will develop and whether an individual physician will know and accept the consensus judgment on the appropriate use of any treatment: the methods by which scientific knowledge is developed, the manner by which it is disseminated, and a host of social and psychological factors.

Knowledge Development

The development of information about the usefulness of a new technology takes place in stages, starting with the demonstration that a procedure works. The inventor typically provides evidence from a clinical trial that shows that the procedure is effective for treating a certain condition. Ideally, this demonstration of potential value should lead to a randomized clinical trial, but in practice most operations are not evaluated systematically early in their dissemination. More typically, the innovator and others next explore the range of applications for the new therapy and discover and report on complications and problems associated with its use. If the apparent benefits are substantial and the risks are not excessive, widespread use may rapidly follow. Identification of conditions for which the new technology is not useful occurs slowly over time as experience accumulates. Like other negative findings (7), inappropriate use is often not reported. Rarely, and almost always much later, a new treatment may be the subject of a randomized clinical trial.

Knowledge Dissemination

The primary sources of scientific information that the physician turns to are reports of clinical research in medical journals. This research, usually carried out at an academic medical center, establishes the efficacy of a procedure, i.e. how it works under controlled experimental conditions, not the effectiveness, i.e. how the procedure works in practice. In addition, clinical research is usually directed at defining whether an operation works, not at identifying the circumstances under which it may not be of value.

Journal articles have other limitations. Because of their academic origins, the studies may reflect environments in which personnel and equipment resources are more extensive than in community practice. There is a referral bias, in that patients referred to academic medical centers are not a cross-section of those in the community. As a consequence, results from population-based studies of outcomes are almost invariably inferior to those reported in journal articles from academic centers. Journal reports are also biased toward favorable outcomes. Rarely are poor results reported. The volume of journal articles is virtually overwhelming. It is impossible for any physician to read regularly all of the journal articles that contain information relevant to his or her practice. For all of these reasons, journal articles alone are not an adequate basis for determining when an operation is indicated.

Another problem with journal articles is that clinicians can rarely use them to make decisions for a specific patient, because the information is fragmented, unconnected, and difficult to evaluate. A variety of treatment options are presented without adequate information needed to evaluate and compare them. This is both a quantitative problem—the volume of information is staggering—and a qualitative one: how to sort out useful information from a plethora of irrelevancy. It is clearly impossible for individual physicians to evaluate all forms of therapy for all of the conditions that they are called upon to treat (13).

Development of Clinical Consensus

Because of the voluminous, fragmentary, and disconnected nature of medical scientific information, physicians turn to various authorities—experts—for assistance in forming their conclusions about the value of a treatment or procedure. They obtain expert advice through textbooks, medical meetings, continuing education courses, and informal contacts.

Textbooks and continuing education courses provide comprehensive overviews and perspectives on the state of practice in the use of operations. Emphasis is usually placed on the rationale for use of operation and the details of diagnosis and management. Rarely is much attention given to explicit consideration of contraindications, the conditions under which an operation is not indicated. Medical meetings provide physicians with multiple opportunities to learn from their colleagues. Presentations, like journal articles and textbooks, tend to concentrate on outcomes and problems for broad general groupings of patients, e.g. "Limb salvage in 600 patients undergoing femoral-popliteal bypass." However, meetings provide physicians with an opportunity to question the experts. Discussions with colleagues help physicians shape their own perception of the value and use of a procedure.

Physician Use of New Information

Because the fragmented and biased nature of available information makes it difficult for the average surgeon to keep up, some unnecessary surgery undoubtedly results from ignorance. But, sometimes the information is received and rejected. Like others, physicians resist change and they have learned not to believe everything they hear from the experts. Most physicians can readily recall examples of brilliant ideas that were eventually discredited. If new information is contrary to personal experience or an expert opinion seems ill-founded, the wise clinician adopts a wait and see attitude. This may be true even when there is an expert consensus on an issue. In a study of the adoption of recommendations of the National Institutes of Health Consensus Conferences, Kanouse et al (24) found that the availability of new information concerning the value of a procedure or treatment was insufficient to bring about changes in practice patterns.

Psychosocial Factors

Individual personality and character traits are important determinants of practice style. Age, experience, personality, and specialty influence how physicians use tests (15). Family practitioners and internists approach patient care differently than surgeons, who may be less risk averse. Training and tradition play an important role: Doctors tend to continue doing something the way they always have if it seems successful. Motivation, which is a complex interplay of self-image, personal standards, and preferences for certain types of practice style or patients, is also a key factor (14, 55). Much has been made of economic motivation in recent years, but it is unlikely that many surgeons recommend useless operations solely because of greed. It seems probable, however, that in questionable cases, they are more likely to recommend a service they provide. As we have seen, there is evidence that doctors in fee-for-service practice recommend more operations than doctors in prepaid plans (32, 49).

Practice patterns may be influenced more by social factors than by personal ones (21). Studies of the adoption of new technologies have shown that acceptance of a new treatment occurs as a result of a consensus of peers, and that endorsement by a local opinion leader is usually required before general use will occur (21). Community physicians tend to distrust the scientific literature, as much of it is inaccessible or irrelevant. Consequently, they rely more heavily on word of mouth and the evaluations of colleagues. Local norms, which may vary considerably from region to region, are developed (the "surgical signatures" of Wennberg). Interestingly, although there has been scientific interest in the factors that lead to adoption of new technologies, few investigators have studied the process by which ineffective treatments are abandoned. Unless abuses are egregious and the evidence is unequivocal, leaders seldom speak out against an outdated procedure. In the absence of social pressure, physicians are often slow to change.

The net effect of our system of generation, dissemination, and incorporation of medical scientific information is to leave practicing physicians without clear guidance as to effective treatment in many situations. There is often little or no consensus, or if there is a consensus among experts, the community physician may not be aware of it.

Lack of Consensus

Lack of consensus has a profound effect on the nature of medical practice. Lack of consensus leads different groups of doctors to different conclusions about the value of an operation, the major cause of geographic variations. Lack of consensus leads to differences of second opinions from the first. And, uncertainty stemming from lack of consensus leads surgeons to recommend operations for patients who desire them but who will not benefit.

In summary, although many factors play a role in the occurrence of unnecessary surgery, the root cause is the inadequate production, evaluation, dissemination, and use of information. If the limits of effectiveness of an operation were established for all of its uses, and if that information was widely accepted and widely disseminated, the opportunities for misuse would be greatly diminished.

WHAT CAN BE DONE ABOUT UNNECESSARY SURGERY?

It is evident that utilization review, second surgical opinion programs and geographic variation analysis with feedback are blunt instruments for improving quality. Each takes advantage of the pervasive uncertainty in medical practice to intimidate or exert peer pressure on physicians to conform. Although these programs may decrease the volume of services that are provided, they do so unselectively. As we have seen, there is no evidence that any of these programs specifically reduces inappropriate care, and, in the case of SSOP, it possibly increases. Without a focus, these programs are unlikely to lead to identifiable improvements in quality.

To decrease unnecessary surgery, it is first necessary to define it. Physicians need better information on effectiveness and better dissemination and use of that information. Finally, attention must be given to developing more effective ways to get doctors to accept and use new information. Outcomes research attempts to improve the information base, whereas practice guidelines make it more accessible to physicians.

Outcomes Research

The randomized clinical trial is widely accepted as the gold standard for measuring effectiveness, but the costs and logistic problems of conducting these trials limit their applicability. In recent years, the effectiveness of a treatment has increasingly been evaluated by sophisticated analyses of patient outcomes. As noted, the AHCPR has launched a major effort—the Medical Treatment Effectiveness Program—to evaluate the outcomes of treatment of several important diseases, such as cataract, myocardial infarction, and back pain.

Although the importance of studying outcomes is unassailable, expectations regarding the usefulness of this information may be exaggerated. Meaningful information from outcomes studies requires evaluation of numerous health factors in addition to the presence of disease. Controlling for these variables can be difficult and expensive; thus, effectiveness studies of all variants of patient and disease are not possible. Consequently, it is unlikely that outcomes studies can ever provide information on more than a minor fraction of the thousands of diseases and treatments.

This is not to say that outcomes studies should not be carried out. On the contrary, they offer the most practical hope of obtaining valuable information that will both validate treatments that work and lead to elimination of those that do not. But for maximum efficiency, outcomes studies should be focused on specific treatments for which the information will be of greatest value, i.e. on those that are performed in large numbers, show wide geographic variations, and are controversial. Despite its limitations, outcomes research is the best current hope for improvement in knowledge generation.

Practice Guidelines

The other challenge, getting physicians to accept and use effectiveness information, may be more difficult. The current movement to develop practice guidelines is an attempt to accomplish this mission. The objective of practice guidelines is to make effectiveness information accessible and acceptable to doctors by providing authoritative statements regarding the appropriateness of a procedure for all of its possible indications. These statements are based on available evidence and expert opinion. As we have seen, even when there is good scientific data, guidelines are needed to translate that information into a useable form. If well done, guidelines provide practicing physicians with a better informed, more objective, and, therefore, wiser evaluation than they can readily obtain from the literature and personal experience. The development of comprehensive practice guidelines is an urgent first priority for anyone who wishes to decrease the rate of unnecesssary surgery. Fortunately, the urgency of that need has risen to national attention within the past several years and has been accepted both within the medical profession and by the government.

Practice guideline development is the second major responsibility of the AHCPR. Recently, at the agency's behest, a committee of the Institute of Medicine issued a set of attributes and principles for the guideline development process (23). The report stressed the importance of credibility and accountability and the need for the link between guidelines and scientific evidence to be explicit. It strongly recommended that the guideline development process "include participation by representatives of key affected groups and disciplines" to insure that all relevant evidence is located, that practical problems are identified, and that affected groups will cooperate in implementation (23).

Professional specialty societies have also begun to develop comprehensive and highly specific practice guidelines (50). Early experience suggests that these guidelines will be used and will make a difference. For example, following the 1987 universal adoption by Massachusetts anesthetists of the American Society of Anesthesiologists' "Standards for Basic Intra-Operative Monitoring," the number of deaths from hypoxia decreased to zero in the following year, and for the first time no lawsuits were filed for hypoxic damage (40).

Ultimately, the validity of practice guidelines will depend on the advances in scientific knowledge provided by randomized clinical trials and outcomes studies. The commitment of Congress to support outcomes studies is, therefore, encouraging. These efforts are complementary. Outcomes data provide evidence to be used in guideline development, while the guideline process helps focus outcomes research by identifying common clinical conditions for which effectiveness information is lacking.

POLICY IMPLICATIONS

As Eddy (12) has described, medical practice is in the middle of a profound transition. Once it was assumed that physician's decisions were, by definition, correct; however, evidence now indicates that many are not, and mechanisms have been established to second-guess physician judgments. Eddy points out, however, that much of medical care is effective, doctors are not practicing fraud, and the problems are no one's fault. Physicians make errors because they must make decisions every day on the basis of inadequate information. And, they must deal not only with vagaries of scientific knowledge, but also with variations in patient preferences and expectations, changing systems of reimbursement, threats of malpractice, and peer pressure.

The pace of technologic progress is now such that it has become impossible for researchers to provide the information on effectiveness of new treatments as rapidly as they are developed. Further, our methods of information dissemination are not adequate to make even that which is known accessible to the physician. As a result, it is not surprising that evidence from a variety of sources suggests a substantial amount of surgery is unnecessary. The solutions to these problems will not come quickly or easily, but the movement to practice guidelines should ultimately lead to more rational and more acceptable medical decision-making.

Credibility of practice guidelines requires that the judgments be made by respected clinical experts, leaders in their fields. But, that may not be enough. Surgeons, in particular, are unlikely to accept these recommendations without professional endorsement. Surgical leaders must accept the process and support the results. The AHCPR has been slow to enlist the support or participation of organized medicine—either the American Medical Association or the relevant specialty societies. Also, the academic establishment's position is unclear. Some health services researchers are very interested in various aspects of guideline development, but they have had limited input into the federal process. Without either professional or academic support, it is hard to believe that federal guidelines will be accepted. A related question is whether the government will require physicians to follow the federally developed guidelines. Such a requirement would result in the de facto nullification of one of the highest functions of a profession: control of its standards. It seems improbable that either organized medicine or individual doctors will readily accept such an outcome. If the legitimacy of federal guidelines is challenged, as it almost certainly will be, it is not likely that either Congress or the courts will support the right of the federal government to practice medicine. To be viable, therefore, practice guidelines must be supported by either the academic establishment or organized medicine, preferably both.

The use of practice guidelines will result in significant changes in the way doctors practice medicine. For the first time, the identification and significant reduction of inappropriate care and unnecessary surgery will be possible. Whether this potential will be realized will be determined within the next few years by the interplay of government policies and professional reactions. If means to cooperate cannot be found, reductions in unnecessary surgery may be long in coming.

Literature Cited

1. Am. Coll. Surg. and Am. Surg. Assoc. 1975. *Surgery in the United States: A Summary Report of the Study on Surgical Services for the United States.* Chicago: Am. Coll. Surg./Am. Surg. Assoc.
2. Barrett, J. F. R., Jarvis, G. J., Macdonald, H. N., Buchan, P. C., Tyrrell, S. N., et al. 1990. Inconsistencies in clinical decisions in obstetrics. *Lancet* 336:549–51
3. Barron, J. Apr. 16, 1989. Unnecessasry surgery. NY Times Mag.
4. Bombardier, C., Fuchs, V. R., Lillard, L. A., Warner, K. E. 1977. Socioeconomic factors affecting the utilization of surgical operations. *N. Engl. J. Med.* 297:699–705
5. Bunker, J. P. 1970. Surgical manpower. A comparison of operations and surgeons in the United States and in England and Wales. *N. Engl. J. Med.* 282:135–44
6. Bunker, J. P., Brown, B. W. 1974. The physician-patient as an informed consumer of surgical services. *N. Engl. J. Med.* 290:1051–55
7. Chalmers, T. C. 1987. Meta-analysis in clinical medicine. *Trans. Am. Clin. Climatol. Assoc.* 99:144–50
8. Chassin, M. R., Brook, R. H., Park, R. E., Keesey, J., Fink, A., et al. 1986. Variations in the use of medical and surgical services by the Medicare population. *N. Engl. J. Med.* 314:285–90
9. Chassin, M. R., Kosecoff, J., Park, R. E., Winslow, C. M., Kahn, K. L. 1987. Does inappropriate use explain geographic variations in the use of health care services? *J. Am. Med. Assoc.* 258:2533–37
10. Dorsey, J. L. 1983. Use of diagnostic resources in health maintenance organizations and fee-for-service practice settings. *Arch. Int. Med.* 143:1863–65
11. Doyle, J. C. 1953. Unnecessary hysterectomies. *J. Am. Med. Assoc.* 151:360–65
12. Eddy, D. M. 1990. The challenge. *J. Am. Med. Assoc.* 263:287
13. Eddy, D. M. 1984. Variations in physician practice: the role of uncertainty. *Health Aff.* 3:74–89
14. Eisenberg, J. M. 1985. Physician utilization: The state of research about physicians' practice patterns. *Med. Care* 23:461–83
15. Eisenberg, J. M., Nicklin, D. 1981. Use of diagnostic services by physicians in community practice. *Med. Care* 19:297
16. Evans, R. G., Barer, M. L., Hertzman, C. 1991. The 20-year experiment: Accounting for, explaining, and evaluating health care cost containment in Canada and the United States. *Annu. Rev. Public Health* 12:481–518
17. Fink, A., Kosecoff, J., Chassin, M., Brook, R. H. 1984. Consensus methods: characteristics and guidelines for use. *Am. J. Public Health* 74:979–83

18. Gambone, J. C., Reiter, R. C., Lench, J. B. 1990. Quality assurance indicators and short-term outcome of hysterectomy. *Obstet. Gynecol.* 76:841–45
19. Gray, D., Hampton, J. R., Bernstein, S. J., Kosecoff, J., Brook, R. H. 1990. Audit of coronary angiography and bypass surgery. *Lancet* 335:1317–20
20. Greenspan, A. M., Kay, H. R., Berger, B. C., Greenberg, R. M., Greenspan, A. J., et al. 1988. Incidence of unwarranted implantation of permanent cardiac pacemakers in a large medical population. *N. Engl. J. Med.* 318:158–63
21. Greer, A. L. 1988. The state of the art versus the state of the science. *Int. J. Tech. Assess. Health Care* 4:5–25
22. Hulka, B. S., Wheat, J. R. 1985. Patterns of utilization: The patient perspective. *Med. Care* 23:438–60
23. Inst. Med. 1990. Clinical practice guidelines: directions for a new program. Washington, DC: Nat. Acad. Press
24. Kanouse, D. E., Winkler, J. D., Berry, S. H., Brook, R. H. 1987. *Physician Awareness of the NIH Consensus Development Program.* R-2980 3060 Santa Monica: RAND
25. Keller, R. B., Soule, D. N., Wennberg, J. E., Hanley, D. F. 1990. Dealing with geographic variations in the use of hospitals. *J. Bone Joint Surg.* 72-A:1286–93
26. Kellie, S. E., Kelly, J. T. 1991. Medicare Peer Review Organization preprocedure review criteria. *J. Am. Med. Assoc.* 265:1265–70
27. Kramon, G. Feb. 24, 1991. Medical second-guessing—in advance. *NY Times*
28. Leape, L. L. 1989. Unnecessary surgery. A Pew Memorial trust policy synthesis: 7. HSR: Health Serv. Res. 24 (3):351–407
29. Leape, L. L., Park, R. E., Solomon, D. H., Chassin, M. R., Kosecoff, J., Brook, R. H. 1990. Does inappropriate use explain small area variations in the use of health care services? *J. Am. Med. Assoc.* 263:669–72
30. Leape, L. L., Park, R. E., Solomon, D. H., Chassin, M. R., Kosecoff, J., Brook, R. H. 1989. Relation between surgeons' practice volumes and geographic variation in the rate of carotid endarterectomy. *N. Engl. J. Med.* 321:653–57
31. Lewis, C. E. 1969. Variations in the incidence of surgery. *N. Engl. J. Med.* 281:880–84
32. LoGerfo, J. P., Efird, R. A., Diehr, P. K., Richardson, W. C. 1979. Rates of surgical care in prepaid group practices and the independent setting. *Med. Care* 17:1–10
33. Manning, W. G., Leibowitz, A., Goldberg, G. A., Rogers, W. H., Newhouse, J. P. 1984. A controlled trial of the effect of a prepaid group practice on use of services. *N. Engl. J. Med.* 310:1505–10
34. McCarthy, E. G., Finkel, M. L. 1978. Second opinion elective surgery programs: Outcome status over time. *Med. Care* 16:984–94
35. McCarthy, E. G., Widmer, G. W. 1974. Effects of screening by consultants on recommended elective procedures. *N. Engl. J. Med.* 291:1331–35
36. McPherson, K., Wennberg, J. E., Hovind, D. B., Clifford, P. 1982. Small-area variations in the use of common surgical procedures: An international comparison of New England, England, and Norway. *N. Engl. J. Med.* 307:1310–14
37. Merrick, N. J., Brook, R. H., Fink, A., Solomon, D. H. 1986. Use of carotid endarterectomy in five California Veterans Administration medical centers. *J. Am. Med. Assoc.* 256:2531–35
38. Park, R. E., Fink, A., Brook, R. H., Chassin, M. R., Kahn, K. L. et al. 1986. Physician ratings of appropriate indications for six medical and surgical procedures. *Am. J. Public Health* 76:766–72
39. Peebles, R. J. 1991. Second opinions and cost-effectiveness: the questions continue. *Am. Coll. Surg. Bull.* 76:18–25
40. Pierce, E. C. 1990. The development of anesthesia guidelines and standards. *QRB* 16:61–64
41. Poggio, E., Goldberg, H. B., Kronick, R., Schmitz, R., Van Harrison, R., Ertel, P. 1985. *Second Surgical Opinion Programs: An Analysis of Public Policy Options.* Natl. Tech. Inf. Serv.
42. Roos, N. P. 1984. Hysterectomy: Variations in rates across small areas and across physicians' practices. *Am. J. Public Health* 74:327–34
43. Roos, N. P., Roos, L. L. 1982. Surgical rate variations: Do they reflect the health or socioeconomic characteristics of the population? *Med. Care* 20:945–58
44. Roos, N. P., Roos, L. L. 1981. High and low surgical rates: Risk factors for area residents *Am. J. Public Health* 71:591–600
45. Roos, N. P., Roos, L. L., Henteleff, P. D. 1977. Elective surgical rates—do high rates mean lower standards? *N. Engl. J. Med.* 297:360–65
46. Stockwell, H., Vayda, E. 1979. Vari-

ations in surgery in Ontario. *Med. Care* 17:390–96

47. US Congr. House Subcomm. Oversight Invest. 1976. *Cost and Quality of Health Care: Unnecesssry Surgery.* Washington, DC: GPO

48. US Congr. Senate Comm. Aging. 1985. *Unnecessary Surgery: Double Jeopardy for Older Americans.* Washington, DC: GPO

49. US Dep. Health Educ. Welf. 1971. *The Federal Employees Health Benefits Program—Enrollment and Utilization of Health Services, 1961–1968.* Washington, DC: GPO

50. US Gen. Account. Off. 1991. *Practice Guidelines: The Experience of Medical Specialty Societies.* Publ. GAO/PEMD-91-11. Washington, DC: GAO

51. Vayda, E., Barnsley, J. M., Mindell, W. R., Cardillo, B. 1984. Five-year study of surgical rates in Ontario's counties. *Can. Med. Assoc. J.* 131:111–15

52. Deleted in proof

53. *Webster's 3rd New International Dictionary.* 1976. Springfield: Merriam

54. Wennberg, J. E. 1984. Dealing with medical practice variations: a proposal for action. *Health Aff.* 3:6–31

55. Wennberg, J. E., Gittelsohn, A. 1982. Variations in medical care among small areas. *Sci. Am.* 246:120–34

56. Wennberg, J. E., Gittelsohn, A. 1975. Health care delivery in Main I: Patterns of use of common surgical procedures. *J. Main. Med. Assoc.* 66:123–49

57. Wennberg, J., Gittelsohn, A. 1973. Small area variations in health care delivery. *Science* 142:1102–8

58. Winslow, C. M., Kosecoff, J. B., Chassin, M., Kanouse, D. E., Brook, R. H. 1988. The appropriateness of performing coronary artery bypass surgery. *J. Am. Med. Assoc.* 260:505–9

59. Winslow, C. M., Solomon, D. H., Chassin, M. R., Kosecoff, J., Merrick, N. J. et al. 1988. The appropriateness of carotid endarterectomy. *N. Engl. J. Med.* 31:721–27

Annu. Rev. Publ. Health. 1992. 13:385–98

CAUSES OF LOW PRESCHOOL IMMUNIZATION COVERAGE IN THE UNITED STATES[1]

Felicity T. Cutts, Walter A. Orenstein, and Roger H. Bernier

Immunization Division, Centers for Disease Control, Atlanta, Georgia 30333

KEY WORDS: immunization programs, health seeking behavior, health services, immunization compliance

BACKGROUND

In 1978, the United States established the objective of completing the basic immunization series of at least 90% of children by age two years by the year 1990. Although state school immunization laws have led to the immunization of over 95% of school enterers (32), the situation among preschoolers is less encouraging. Recent outbreak investigations in many inner city areas have estimated that only 40–60% of children have completed the series by age two years (12, 13, 55). This low coverage among preschoolers is reflected in the recent resurgence of measles (7, 11, 57). In 1990, the number of reported measles cases (provisional total 27, 672) was the highest since 1977 (55, 201 cases reported), compared with a nadir of 1497 cases in 1983. Approximately one half of reported cases in 1990 were among preschool children; among vaccine-eligible preschoolers aged 16–59 months, 79% were unvaccinated (10a).

There is no mechanism similar to school immunization laws to achieve universal immunization of preschoolers. State day care immunization laws only affect licensed centers, which care for an estimated 20% of children

---

[1]The US Government has the right to retain a nonexclusive royalty-free license in and to any copyright covering this paper.

under age 6 years who have working parents (70). There is, therefore, a need to design appropriate interventions to increase coverage among preschoolers.

Determinants of receipt of immunization are complex and interwoven. In this paper, we review published studies of determinants of receipt of immunization in the US. We classify factors relating to receipt of immunization in two broad categories: consumer demand for services and the supply of services. Although there is great interplay between the different factors, we use this classification to help identify potential interventions to increase preschool immunization coverage.

CONSUMER DEMAND FOR IMMUNIZATION SERVICES

Factors affecting consumer demand for immunization include beliefs about health care and illness and socioeconomic characteristics of the individual and of the social group with which the individual interacts.

Health Beliefs

Many theoretical models that share common dimensions have been developed to explain utilization of such preventive health services as immunization (17). One of the frameworks most commonly used to understand and predict health-promoting behavior is the "health belief" model, which was formally developed by Rosenstock and colleagues (63). This model has four components: "perceived susceptibility," which refers to the subjective perception of risk of vulnerability to a health threat; "perceived severity," which consists of one's perception of the seriousness of the health threat; "perceived benefits," which consists of the belief that the health-promoting behavior will be effective; and "perceived barriers," which refers to the assessment of the negative consequences associated with the behavior, such as cost, inconvenience, negative perceptions of health services, and side effects.

Early descriptive studies, which used the health belief framework, were conducted on the acceptance of the Salk polio vaccine (14, 27, 50). More recently, analytic studies have been conducted on the receipt of influenza or swine flu vaccine by adults (1, 18, 38, 66). Janz & Becker (35) reviewed studies of health-promoting behavior, clinic utilization, and behavior during illness. Perceived barriers had the most frequently reported impact on behavior (93%), followed by perceived susceptibility (86%), benefits (74%), and severity (50%).

Health beliefs motivate the individual to act, but the appropriate behavior may not occur unless a cue to action is present. Such cues can be internal (e.g. symptoms) or external (e.g. mass media messages, advice from friends or the medical profession) (2). Persons who seek vaccination are likely to discuss vaccination with friends, peer groups, or physicians or to consider that most of their friends have been vaccinated (14, 18, 20, 27, 28, 50). Persons of higher socioeconomic status are more likely to have a wide circle of friends and to seek advice outside the family (14).

More recently, the health belief framework has been further extended to include the individual's assessment of his or her ability to carry out the health-promoting behavior successfully ("self-efficacy"). This "protection-motivation" theory includes many of the components of the health belief model, with the addition of the role of self-efficacy (60). Self-efficacy influences not only the initiation of the health-promoting behavior, but also a person's persistence in the face of obstacles.

In summary, motivation to undertake a health-promoting action is increased when the individual feels vulnerable to a severe threat to health, perceives that the action is effective and that he/she can confidently carry out the action, and when perceived costs and barriers associated with the action are small. Positive motivation is most likely to lead to effective action in the presence of a "cue." Sociodemographic characteristics may act through any of these components to affect the likelihood of a health-promoting act.

Socioeconomic Status

Economic and demographic measures of socioeconomic status, particularly parental education, income, family size, and race, have consistently been shown to influence receipt of immunization (4, 14, 18, 26, 27, 29, 43, 44, 46, 48, 50, 52, 58, 62). A national telephone survey of access to health care, conducted in 1986 by the Robert Wood Johnson Foundation, found that children who were uninsured, poor, or nonwhite were less likely to have seen a physician in the past year, and uninsured children under age 5 were less likely to have up-to-date immunizations. According to parental history, 19% of uninsured children, 6% of children with private insurance, and 1% of children on Medicaid were not up-to-date (74).

Many persons at or near the poverty line lack health insurance. In 1986, approximately 16% of children under age 13 were covered by public health insurance (usually Medicaid), and 18% were uninsured. Medicaid availability varies between states, which may impose limitations on eligibility for services, the frequency and number of services provided, and physician reimbursement (47, 64). Fees are often well below those paid by the private sector; thus, physicians are discouraged from participating in Medicaid (77). Medicaid's complex administrative procedures also obstruct use (5, 68, 77). In 1986, Medicaid covered less than half of eligible children (64). Pediatrician participation in Medicaid is lowest in large metropolitan areas, in which the risk of early acquisition of vaccine-preventable diseases is highest (77). Medicaid children, like uninsured children, receive more of their care in hospital outpatient departments, emergency rooms, and public clinics, than in physician's offices.

Provision of health insurance increases service utilization, but does not guarantee high immunization rates (21, 41, 65, 74). Dutton (21) and Rundall & Wheeler (65) showed that perceived service barriers, negative attitudes of consumers towards the type of health services available to the poor, and lower belief in susceptibility to illness were greater influences on the receipt of immunization by lower socioeconomic groups than the direct effect of payment for services.

In the United Kingdom, despite the availability of free medical care for all, use of preventive care services varies greatly between deprived and endowed communities (45). In a recent study, Peckham et al (58) mailed questionnaires to 1793 health professionals and 3394 parents, in seven districts with "high" and eight districts with "low" coverage for measles and pertussis vaccines. They developed scores for practice organization, physician knowledge, and parental attitudes and combined these with indicators of socioeconomic status in multivariate analyses.

In the practice organization score, a point was assigned when all members of the practice team, and not only the physician, could obtain consent for vaccination, give injections, and conduct patient recall. In the physician knowledge score, a point was assigned for correct knowledge of contraindications to each vaccine. In the parental attitude score, a point was assigned for each positive attitude expressed towards severity and infectivity of target diseases, efficacy, and safety of vaccines.

Family and parental factors associated with low immunization uptake were low social class, large family size, presence of a chronically ill child in the family, and low parental attitude score. Of these, parental attitude score had the greatest influence. Only 30% of children whose parents had the lowest attitude score had received measles vaccine, and coverage increased to 90% among children whose parents had the highest score. Practice factors reducing immunization uptake were low practice organization score (measles vaccine coverage was 72% in practices scoring zero, and 90% in practices scoring high), and low physicians knowledge score (measles vaccine uptake was 77% among children who visited the lowest scoring physicians, and 90% among children who visited the highest scoring physicians).

Each group of variables was interrelated. The practice organization score was positively correlated with both the physician knowledge and the parental attitude scores. Practice organization scores were lower in socially deprived areas. Low socioeconomic groups were thus served by practices that were less well organized and staffed by less knowledgeable practitioners. This reinforced the parents' negative attitudes towards the health services and led to incomplete immunization.

SUPPLY OF IMMUNIZATION SERVICES

Published and unpublished reports document the failure of the health system to provide easily available and acceptable immunization services to persons in the lower socioeconomic groups. The system adversely affects immunization rates by creating barriers that restrict access and policies that impede attendance, thus missing opportunities to vaccinate persons who do attend and failing to use education and follow-up to keep children in the system.

Barriers to Utilization of Immunization Services

In May 1990, 57 immunization projects that receive federal grant funds, including projects in all 50 states, the District of Colombia, and some large cities and counties, were surveyed by the Centers for Disease Control. Fifty-four project managers responded (Table 1). Half stated that children were not receiving vaccines in one or more localities because of barriers, particularly insufficient clinic staff (70%), insufficient clinic hours (56%), and inaccessible clinic locations (15%). These barriers arose because of inadequate local resources for vaccine delivery.

In addition, clinic policies, which tend to impede attendance, have been observed in areas affected by preschool measles outbreaks since 1986. Such policies include visits by appointment only; waits of several weeks for appointments; vaccination on only certain days of the week; limits on the number of clients registered per day; long waiting times; residency restrictions (not accepting out-of-county residents); the need for physician referral; comprehensive physical examinations before vaccination; vaccinations administered only by physicians; charges for vaccine administration, either flat-rate or sliding scale; and the need to sign a statement of inability to pay a private physician (56).

Table 1 Barriers to immunization identified by 27 of 54 immunization program managers[a,b]

Potential barrier	n	%
Insufficient staff	19	70
Insufficient clinic hours	15	56
Inadequate clinic location	4	15
Appointment-only systems	25	93
Prior physical examinations required	15	56
Physician referral needed	11	41
Immunizations given only in well-baby clinics	10	37
Financial screening/vaccine fees	6	22

[a] 27 program mangers did not identify any barriers to immunization in their immunization projects.
[b] From Ref. 56.

Missed Immunization Opportunities

Missed opportunities may occur when a child attends immunization services, but does not receive all the vaccines for which he or she is eligible (nonsimultaneous vaccination), or when a child who is eligible for vaccination attends other health care services (e.g. acute care visits), but is not immunized. They may occur because of failure to screen a child's immunization eligibility, failure to provide vaccination at the same locale as curative services, or inappropriate policies on contraindications to vaccination.

Table 2 summarizes studies on missed immunization opportunities in the US. Record audits at emergency rooms (40), public clinics (24), and pediatric inpatient facilities (69) showed that up to 75.5% of children who attended did not receive all the vaccines for which they were eligible. A Utah study (39) indicated that illness of the child was a major reason for failure to immunize. In 1973, health department audits in Tennessee indicated that 10–24% of children had a missed immunization opportunity, most often because of delay

Table 2   Studies on missed immunization opportunities in the US

Year	Site	Number of records audited	Percent of children vaccinated	Type of missed opportunity	Percent with ≥ 1 missed opportunity	Ref. number
1973	Health department	294	78.6	Non-sim[c]+ curative	10.5	30
	Health department	133	42.1	Non-sim+ curative	24	
1986	Health department	. . .[a]	41.0	Non-sim	21	31
1987	Health department	2360	42.0	Non-sim	19	36
1986	Community	31	*[b]	Non-sim+ curative	42	33
1986	Pediatric inpatients	102	64.0	Curative	19	69
1989	Emergency room	278	. . .	Curative	76	40
1989	Public clinic	253	67.0	Non-sim+ curative	30	24

[a] . . . no information
[b] *only unvaccinated children studied
[c] non-simultaneous vaccination

of measles vaccination for tuberculin testing (30). In Gainesville, Georgia in 1986 (31) and in Virginia in 1987 (36), health department audits showed that 21% of 21–23-month-olds and 19% of 24-month-olds, respectively, had a missed opportunity for simultaneous vaccination.

Simplifying clinic procedures to reduce missed opportunities has dramatically increased adult immunization rates. A standing order, which gave nurses the responsibility to identify and vaccinate patients at a general medical clinic, increased influenza immunization rates from 28% before the intervention to 81% during the intervention (42). Immunization rates in control clinics, in which a specific physician's order was required, remained at 29%.

Missed opportunities have also been reduced by systems that prompt providers to screen the vaccination status of all clinic attendees. In a busy internal medicine clinic, reminder questionnaires were attached to patient's charts during the influenza season (25). Immunization rates for influenza and pneumococcal vaccines rose from 2.9% and 5.5% of eligible patients pre-intervention to 75% and 67%, respectively, during the intervention. In an infant primary care clinic, for children with appointments, clerks attached an immunization information label to the clinic note to be used by the physician (6). Receipt of third dose diphtheria-tetanus-pertussis/oral polio vaccine (DTP/OPV) by age 190 days increased significantly, from 25% preintervention to 33% postintervention, even though approximately 50% of infants in the intervention period had unscheduled visits without appointments and thus did not have the label placed on the clinic note.

The feasibility and acceptability of immunizing children at curative services has also been shown (72, 73). In a 1966–1967 study in a pediatric emergency room in Los Angeles County, a health aide or public health nurse completed a record of the immunizations required. The physician signed the record if there were no contraindications, and the nurse then vaccinated the child and gave a written return appointment. Follow-up was conducted seven days after a broken appointment, first by postcard, then by a second postcard, telephone, or telegram. Fifty-two percent of children kept their scheduled appointment. An additional 27% returned after the reminders (73).

Potential immunization opportunities exist outside the health sector at other public assistance programs. Parents of children with measles were interviewed in Milwaukee, Chicago, Dallas, and Los Angeles in 1989–1990 (34). Of 397 vaccine eligible measles cases, 40–91% were enrolled in one or more social programs. Children under one year of age were more likely to be enrolled in the Women, Infants, and Children (WIC) program; those one year or older were more likely to receive Aid for Dependent Children (AFDC).

Most children have contacts with the health system. The National Medical Care Utilization and Expenditure survey showed that even among the poor, over 87% of children had at least one contact with a health care provider in the previous year (9). These contacts are opportunities to immunize children and to keep the children in the system, by educating and motivating parents to return and by conducting active follow-up.

Patient Education

Although many studies have shown that physicians' advice influences parents (1, 14, 18, 27), we have not found published intervention studies of the effect of clinic-based education. One paper has evaluated the effect of health education in the hospital setting, one through the mass media, and one in the school setting.

A 1986 study in St. Louis compared three hospital-based educational interventions with a control group. Postpartum mothers were randomly assigned to receive an "immunization packet" (containing an immunization record for the child and a booklet on the importance of immunizations), the packet plus a video presentation, or both of these plus a phone call reminder when the child was two months of age. There was no significant difference between groups in the percentage that received first dose DTP/OPV (average 94.5%) or three doses of DTP and two of oral polio (average 69%) (16).

Peterson (59) reported no increase in vaccination activities after a 1975–1977 mass media campaign to promote routine immunization in Missouri. However, during an outbreak, vaccination activities increased when mass publicity was combined with the provision of extra clinics.

School-based health education was evaluated in Denver before the school laws (71). Parents of 2028 children received a colorful pamphlet and newsletters about immunization. Students and parent-teacher organizations participated in immunization-oriented projects. Three months after the education campaign, only ten of 569 immunization-deficient children had been immunized. This contrasted to schools that sent reminders to parents and provided immunization on site, where 66% of 653 immunization-deficient children were immunized in the same period.

Although none of these studies showed an impact of the educational program on immunization rates, the educational interventions were not designed after an assessment of the specific informational needs or of the most appropriate communication methods for those populations, and mass media techniques have developed considerably since 1976. It is, therefore, difficult to draw conclusions about the potential effectiveness of health education activities.

Follow-up Systems

Active follow-up of children can be conducted by general reminders, which provide information on the importance of immunization, or specific reminders, which inform parents of their own child's needs and where immunizations can be obtained. They may be distributed to all parents (universal) or only to "high risk" families, and can be sent before a scheduled appointment ("tickler systems") or after a child has defaulted ("recall"). The increase in percentage of the target group receiving immunization after follow-up has varied greatly: 0–28% for general, universal reminders (3, 10, 16, 46); 5–16% for general, high-risk reminders (15, 76); and 13–33% for specific reminders (51, 75; K. Tollestrup and B. B. Hubbard 1989, unpublished data, Washington State Department of Health and Social Services). All studies of specific reminders showed significant increases in attendance. There was no consistent difference in response rates to mailed or telephone reminders. Most studies reported difficulty in locating families: Approximately one third of families were untraceable because of inaccurate addresses, lack of telephones, or migration from the area.

The cost of follow-up varied greatly. In the early 1980s, Yokley & Glenwick (75) found that a specific letter combined with a lottery ticket incentive was more effective in the short term than a specific letter alone or combined with increased clinic hours, and all were more effective than a general mailout. However, by three months postintervention, the specific letter alone was the most cost-effective intervention, at an estimated cost of $2.27 per additional child immunized, compared with $6.91 for the specific letter plus lottery ticket, $6.28 for the specific letter and increased clinic hours, and $3.64 for the general mailout.

The most effective reminder contains specific information about the child's own vaccine requirements and reinforces health beliefs about susceptibility to disease. Mailed reminders appear equally effective as telephone reminders.

DISCUSSION

Studies on the receipt of immunization have used different methods and conceptual approaches. Few studies have examined the role of health beliefs, socioeconomic factors, and service delivery factors in equal depth. Furthermore, many studies had potential methodological problems (49). Sampling bias and variation in determinants of receipt of vaccination across cultures sometimes limited the generalizability of findings (1, 4, 44). Many studies relied on self-reporting of vaccinations received, which may have led to misclassification of vaccination status (1, 4, 14, 18, 27, 38, 39, 50, 64).

The interpretation of data on health beliefs is complex. In retrospective studies, it is difficult to attribute cause and effect to statistical relationships. Even with prospective studies, prior experience may shape consumer attitudes, and attitudes may not remain constant over time (8, 37). Major controversies, such as the Cutter incident, in which 260 paralytic poliomyelitis cases were caused by the use of lots of Cutter polio vaccine that contained active virus (53), and the 1976 swine flu episode, during which cases of Guillain-Barre syndrome followed a mass campaign of swine flu vaccination (67), may have influenced attitudes towards vaccine safety in studies conducted shortly afterwards. Findings from adult immunization studies may not be applicable to the preschool population.

Despite potential methodological problems, studies have given consistent results. Most children begin the immunization series; coverage of first dose DTP was over 90% in many studies (9, 16, 29, 39, 44). The major problem is failure to complete the immunization schedule on time. Lower socioeconomic groups are least likely to be immunized on time. Improved financial access to health care increases utilization, but does not eliminate socioeconomic differentials, because of other barriers associated with the health services available to the poor and near-poor and the negative attitudes towards health services that these barriers create. Favorable health benefits affect intention to obtain vaccination, but may be neither sufficient nor necessary conditions for vaccination (50).

The causes of low immunization coverage among preschoolers are multifactorial, and studies to date have not demonstrated which factors are the most important. However, the characteristics of persons who are least motivated to obtain timely vaccinations for their children are known, as are the characteristics of the health services that deter these families from seeking vaccination. Although we are not able to say which single factor is the most important in predicting receipt of immunizations, we have identified potentially correctable causes of low immunization coverage among preschoolers.

This review has identified five priority areas for improvement of service provision within the existing health care system. First, barriers to immunization must be removed by increasing clinic staff and clinic hours of operation. Second, clinic policies should allow vaccination on demand and minimize bureaucratic obstacles. Third, existing contacts with families must be used to immunize, through simultaneous administration of vaccines and screening of eligibility and vaccination at curative services. Fourth, active follow-up, with specific, rather than general, reminders, should be conducted. Fifth, other potential contacts with the high-risk population should be exploited. Immunization should be linked to such services as WIC, AFDC, or housing programs. Where resources permit, immunization should be provided on site. At a minimum, the child's immunization status should be assessed and the parent should be referred for immunization.

Concurrently with action to improve the provision of immunization services, operational research should be conducted to clarify issues relating to consumer demand. The influence of clinic organization and health workers' knowledge and attitudes on consumer behavior in the US should be studied and appropriate interventions should be developed. In depth studies of different methods of health education should be conducted. Such methods include a home-based immunization record, which is designed to educate the mother about the immunization schedule and remind her of appointments (as in developing countries), and clinic-based education by persons who have authority that is recognized by parents. Positive incentives, such as the lottery tickets used by Yokley & Glenwick (75), may be helpful in the short term to raise coverage quickly during an outbreak, for example. Their long-term cost-effectiveness requires careful evaluation. Links with influential community groups should be explored, and the applicability to the US of community mobilization techniques used in developing countries should be evaluated.

To implement these recommendations, resources must be invested in the public sector. Increases in federal assistance to the immunization program in the 1980s have only compensated for the exponential increase in vaccine costs and have not always been matched by increased state resources. Federal funding for such programs as the Maternal and Child Health Services block grant and the Community Health Centers program decreased in real terms by 11–43% between 1978 and 1986, and only a minority of those in need are reached (70). Recent changes in the Medicaid program have the potential to increase coverage of pregnant women and infants (54). However, unless reimbursement fees are increased and administrative procedures are streamlined, pediatrician participation in Medicaid will probably continue to fall (77). In the long term, there is a need to work towards a universal, equitable health care system (19, 22, 54, 61).

The World Health Organization has emphasized the need for political will to achieve universal childhood immunization (23). Though it is tempting for health care providers to attribute low immunization uptake to consumer apathy, much evidence points to correctable deficiencies of the health care system. The nation's preschool immunization objectives will only be reached if society has the commitment to respond to needs.

Literature Cited

1. Aho, W. R. 1979. Participation of senior citizens in the swine flu inoculation program: An analysis of health belief model variables in preventive health behavior. *J. Gerontol.* 34:201–8
2. Becker, M. H., Haefner, D. P., Kasl, S. V., Kirscht, J. P., Maiman, L. A., Rosenstock, I. M. 1977. Selected psychosocial models and correlates of individual health-related behaviors. *Med. Care* 15 (Suppl.):27–46
3. Beets, C. 1988. Effectiveness of hospital-based follow-up. See Ref. 11a, pp. 161–62
4. Belcher, J. C. 1958. Acceptance of the Salk polio vaccine. *Rural Soc.* 23:158–70

5. Bergner, L., Yerby, A. S. 1968. Low income and barriers to use of health services. *N. Engl. J. Med.* 278:541–46
6. Brink, S. 1989. Provider reminders. Changing information format to increase infant immunizations. *Med. Care* 27:648–53
7. Brunell, P. A. 1990. Measles one more time. *Pediatrics* 86:474–78
8. Buchner, D. M., Carter, W. B., Inui, T. S. 1985. The relationship of attitude changes to compliance with influenza immunization, a prospective study. *Med. Care* 23:771–78
9. Butler, J. A., Winter, W. D., Singer, J. D., Wenger, M. 1985. Medical care use and expenditure among children and

youth in the United States: analysis of a national probability sample. *Pediatrics* 76:495–507

10. Byrne, E. B., Schaffner, W., Dini, E. F., Case, G. E. 1970. Infant immunization surveillance: cost vs. effect. A prospective, controlled evaluation of a large-scale program in Rhode Island. *J. Am. Med. Assoc.* 212:770–73

10a. Cent. Dis. Control. 1991. Measles—United States, 1990. *Morbid. Mortal. Wkly. Rep.* 40:369–72

11. Cent. Dis. Control. 1990. Measles-United States, 1989 and first 20 weeks 1990. *Morbid. Mortal. Wkly. Rep.* 39:353–63

11a. Cent. Dis. Control. 1988. *Proc. 22nd Immun. Conf.*, San Antonio, Texas, June 20–24. Atlanta: Cent. Dis. Control

12. Cent. Dis. Control. 1987. Measles-Dade County, Florida. *Morbid. Mortal. Wkly. Rep.* 36:45–48

13. Cent. Dis. Control. 1986. Measles-New Jersey. *Morbid. Mortal. Wkly. Rep.* 35:213–15

13a. Cent. Dis. Control. 1978. Measles—United States, 1977–78. *Morbid. Mortal. Wkly. Rep.* 27:235–37

14. Clausen, J. A., Seidenfeld, M. A., Deasy, L. C. 1954. Parent attitudes towards participation of their children in polio vaccine trials. *Am. J. Public Health* 44:1526–36

15. Crankshaw, R. L. 1988. Identification and follow-up of high risk children in Utah. See Ref. 11a, pp. 157–58

16. Crowe, J. D. 1988. Evaluation of selected educational interventions. See Ref. 11a, pp. 133–42

17. Cummings, K. M., Becker, M. H., Maile, M. C. 1980. Bringing the models together: An empirical approach to combining variables used to explain health actions. *J. Behav. Med.* 3:123–45

18. Cummings, K. M., Jette, A. M., Brock, B. M., Haefner, D. P. 1979. Psychosocial determinants of immunization behavior in a swine influenza compaign. *Med. Care* 17:639–49

19. Davies, N. E., Felder, L. H. 1990. Applying brakes to the runaway American health care system. *J. Am. Med. Assoc.* 263:73–76

20. Deasy, L. C. 1956. Socioeconomic status and participation in the poliomyelitis vaccine trials. *Am. Sociol. Rev.* 21:185–91

21. Dutton, D. B. 1978. Explaining the low use of health services by the poor: Cost, attitudes, or delivery systems. *Am. Sociol. Rev.* 43:348–68

22. Enthoven, A., Kronick, R. 1989. A consumer-choice health plan for the 1990s.

Universal health insurance in a system designed to promote quality and economy. *N. Engl. J. Med.* 320:29–37, 94–100

23. Expand. Program. Immun. 1987. Global Advisory Group. Acceleration of EPI progress. *Wkly. Epidemiol. Rec.* 62:5–9

24. Farizo, K. M., Stehr-Green, P. A., Markowitz, L. E., Frederick, P. 1990. Missed opportunities for measles vaccination in a public pediatric clinic, Los Angeles. *Epidemic Intell. Serv. Conf.*, April 23–37, (Abstr.). Atlanta: Cent. Dis. Control

25. Gelfman, D. M., Witherspoon, J. M., Buchsbaum, D. G., Centor, R. M. 1986. Short-term results of an immunization compliance program. *Va. Med. Mon.* 113:532–34

26. Gergen, P. J., Ezzati, T., Russell, H. 1988. DTP immunization status and tetanus antitoxin titers of Mexican American children ages six months through eleven years. *Am. J. Public Health* 78:1446–50

27. Glasser, M. A. 1958. A study of the public's acceptance of the Salk vaccine program. *Am. J. Public Health* 48:141–46

28. Gray, R. M., Kesler, J. P., Moody, P. M. 1966. The effects of social class and friend's expectations on oral polio vaccination participation. *Am. J. Public Health* 56:2028–32

29. Guthrie, N. 1963. Immunization status of 2-year old infants in Memphis and Shelby County, Tennessee. *Public Health Rep.* 78:443–47

30. Guyer, B., Barid, S. J., Hutcheson, R. H., Strain, R. S. 1976. Failure to vaccinate children against measles during the second year of life. *Public Health Rep.* 91:133–37

31. Hanes, A. 1988. Immunization status of reviews, efforts, and results in Georgia. See Ref. 11a, pp. 159–60

32. Hinman, A. R., Jordan, W. S. 1983. Progress toward achieving the 1990 immunization objectives. *Public Health Rep.* 98:436–43

33. Hutchins, S. S., Escolan, J., Markowitz, L. E., Hawkins, C., Kimbler, A., et al. 1989. Measles outbreak among unvaccinated preschool children: Opportunities missed by health care providers to administer measles vaccine. *Pediatrics* 83:369–74

34. Hutchins, S., Gindler, J., Laliberte, K., et al. 1990. Access of preschool-aged children to health care services and federal assistance programs. *Proc. 24th Natl. Immun. Conf.*, Orlando, Fla. May 21–25. Atlanta: Cent. Dis. Control

35. Janz, N. K., Becker, M. H. 1984. The health belief model: a decade later. *Health Educ. Q.* 11:1–47

36. Jones, J. E., White, K. E., Campbell, R. N., Farrell, J. B. 1988. Simultaneous childhood vaccine administration: A strategy to improve primary vaccine series completion. See Ref. 11a, pp. 145–48

37. Kviz, F. J., Dawkins, C. E., Ervin, N. E. 1985. Mothers' health beliefs and use of well-baby services among a high-risk population. *Res. Nurs. Health* 8:381–87

38. Larson, E. B., Olsen, E., Cole, W., Shortell, S. 1979. The relationship of health beliefs and a postcard reminder to influenza vaccination. *J. Fam. Pract.* 8:1207–11

39. Lewis, T., Osborn, L. M., Lewis, K., Brockert, J., Jacobsen, J., Cherry, J. D. Influence of parental knowledge and opinions on 12-month diphtheria, tetanus and pertussis vaccination rates. *Am. J. Dis. Child.* 142:283–86

40. Lindegren, M. L., Atkinson, W. L., Farizo, K. M., Stehr-Green, P. 1990. Vaccination in pediatric emergency rooms during a measles outbreak, Chicago. *Epidemic Intell. Serv. Conf.*, April 23–27. Atlanta: Cent. Dis. Control. (Abstr.)

41. Lurie, N., Manning, W. G., Peterson, C., Goldberg, G. A., Phelps, C. A., Lillard, L. 1987. Preventive care: Do we practice what we preach? *Am. J. Public Health* 77:801–4

42. Margolis, K. L., Lofgren, R. P., Korn, J. E. 1988. Organizational strategies to improve influenza vaccine delivery. A standing order in a general medicine clinic. *Arch. Intern. Med.* 148:2205–7

43. Markland, R. E., Durand, D. E. 1976. An investigation of sociopsychological factors affecting infant immunization. *Am. J. Public Health* 66:168–70

44. Marks, J. S., Halpin, T. J., Irvin, J. J., Johnson, D. A., Keller, J. R. 1979. Risk factors associated with failure to receive vaccinations. *Pediatrics* 64:304–9

45. Marsh, G. N., Channing, D. M. 1987. Comparison in use of health services between a deprived and an endowed community. *Arch. Dis. Child.* 62:392–96

46. Martin, D. A., Fleming, S. J., Fleming, T. G., Scott, D. C. 1969. An evaluation of immunization status of white children in a Kentucky county. *Public Health Rep.* 84:605–10

47. Mayster, V., Waitzkin, H., Hubbell, F. A., Rucker, L. 1990. Local advocacy for the medically indigent. *J. Am. Med. Assoc.* 263:262–68

48. McCormick, M. C., Shapiro, S., Star-field, B. H. 1981. The association of patient-held records and completion of immunizations. *Clin. Pediatr.* 20:270–74

49. McKinlay, J. B. 1972. Some approaches and problems in the study of the use of services—an overview. *J. Health Soc. Behav.* 13:115–22

50. Merrill, M. H., Hollister, A. C., Gibbens, S. F., Haynes, A. W. 1958. Attitudes of Californians towards poliomyelitis vaccination. *Am. J. Public Health* 48:146–52

51. Minear, R. E., Guyer, B. 1979. Assessing immunization services at a neighborhood health center. *Pediatrics* 63:416–19

52. Morris, L. 1964. Further analysis of national participation in the inactivated poliomyelitis vaccination program, 1955–61. *Public Health Rep.* 79:469–81

53. Nathanson, N., Langmuir, A. D. 1963. The Cutter incident: Poliomyelitis following formaldehyde-inactivated poliovirus vaccination in the United States during the spring of 1955. II. Relationship of poliomyelitis to Cutter vaccine. *Am. J. Hyg.* 78:29–60

54. Oberg, C. N. 1990. Medically uninsured children in the United States: a challenge to public policy. *Pediatrics* 85:824–33

55. Orenstein, W. A., Allman, K. C., Eddins, D., Snyder, M., Seastrom, G. 1988. Preschool immunization-1988. See Ref. 11a, pp. 121–28

56. Orenstein, W. A., Atkinson, W., Mason, D., Bernier, R. H. 1990. Barriers to vaccinating preschool children. *J. Hlth. Care for the Poor and Underserved* 1:315–30.

57. Orenstein, W. A., Markowitz, K. E., Hersh, B. S., Preblud, S. R., Hinman, A. R. 1989. The elusiveness of measles elimination: ten years and still counting. *Proc. 23rd Natl. Immun. Conf.*, San Diego, Calif., June, pp. 67–73. Atlanta: Cent. Dis. Control

58. Peckham, C., Senturia, Y., Ades, A. 1989. *National Immunisation Study: Factors Influencing Immunisation Uptake in Childhood.* London: Dep. Paediatr. Epidemiol., Inst. Child Health

59. Peterson, L. 1987. Prevention and community compliance to immunization schedules. In *Prevention and Health: Directions for Policy and Practice*, ed. A. H. Katz, J. A. Hermalin, R. E. Hess, pp. 79–95. New York: Hawarth

60. Prentice-Dunn, S., Rogers, R. W. 1986. Protection motivation theory and preventive health: beyond the health belief model. *Health Educ. Res.* 1:153–61

61. Relman, A. S. 1989. Universal health insurance: Its time has come. *N. Engl. J. Med.* 320:117–18

62. Riddiough, M. A., Willems, J. S., Sanders, C. R., Kemp, K. 1981. Factors affecting the use of vaccines: considerations for immunization program planners. *Public Health Rep.* 96:528–35

63. Rosenstock, I. M., Strecher, V. J., Becker, M. H. 1988. Social learning theory and the health belief model. *Health Educ. Q.* 15:175–83

64. Rowland, D., Lyons, B., Edwards, J. 1988. Medicaid: Health care for the poor in the Reagan era. *Annu. Rev. Public Health* 9:427–50

65. Rundall, T. G., Wheeler, J. R. C. 1979. The effect of income on use of preventive care: An evaluation of alternative explanations. *J. Health Soc. Behav.* 20:397–406

66. Rundall, T. G., Wheeler, J. R. C., 1979. Factors associated with utilization of the swine flu vaccination program among senior citizens in Tompkins County. *Med. Care* 17:191–200

67. Schonberger, L. B., Bregman, D. J., Sullivan-Bolyai, J. Z., Keenlyside, R. A., Ziegler, D. W., et al. 1979. Guillain-Barre syndrome following vaccination in the national influenza immunization program, United States, 1976–77. *Am. J. Epidemiol.* 110:105–23

68. Schreier, H. A. 1974. On the failure to eradicate measles. *N. Engl. J. Med.* 290:803–4

69. Tifft, C. J., Lederman, H. M. 1988. Immunization status of hospitalized preschool-age children. The need for hospital-based immunization programs. *Am. J. Dis. Child.* 142:719–20

70. US Congr. Off. Technol. Assess. 1988. Well child care. In *Healthy Children. Investing in the Future,* chap. 6, pp. 119–44, Washington DC: GPO

71. Vernon, T. M., Conner, J. S., Shaw, B. S., Lampe, J. M., Doster, M. E. 1976. An evaluation of three techniques for improving immunization levels in elementary schools. *Am. J. Public Health* 66:457–60

72. Walterspiel, J. N., Dishuck, J. F. 1989. Updating immunization status at discharge (letter). *Am. J. Dis. Child.* 143:879–80

73. Wingert, W. A., Larsen, W., Lenoski, E. F., Friedman, D. B. 1969. Immunization for children: Motivating families to complete a series. *Calif. Med.* 110:207–12

74. Wood, D. L., Hayward, R. A., Corey, C. R., Freeman, H. E., Shapiro, M. F. 1990. Access to medical care for children and adolescents in the United States. *Pediatrics* 85:666–73

75. Yokley, J. M., Glenwick, D. S. 1984. Increasing the immunization of preschool children, an evaluation of applied community interventions. *J. Appl. Behav. Anal.* 17:313–25

76. Young, S. A., Halpin, T. J., Johnson, D. A., Irvin, J. J., Marks, S. S. 1980. Effectiveness of a mailed reminder on the immunization levels of infants at high risk of failure to complete immunizations. *Am. J. Public Health* 70:422–24

77. Yudkowsky, B. K., Cartland, J. D. C., Flint, S. S. 1990. Pediatrician participation in Medicaid: 1978 to 1989. *Pediatrics* 85:567–77

Annu. Rev. Publ. Health 1992. 13:399–410

ACCESS AND COST IMPLICATIONS OF STATE LIMITATIONS ON MEDICAID REIMBURSEMENT FOR PHARMACEUTICALS

Stuart O. Schweitzer and S. Renee Shiota

University of California School of Public Health, Los Angeles, California 90024

KEY WORDS: cost containment, drug expenditures, Medicaid restrictions, Medicaid reductions, drug formulary

INTRODUCTION

Pharmaceuticals contribute a small share of total health care expenditures, but have nonetheless generated a large share of public sector regulatory attention. In 1986, drugs and medical sundries constituted only 6.5% of total health expenditures, which represents a decline from a 13.6% proportion in 1950 and 1960, a 10.7% share in 1970, and 7.6% share in 1980 (10). Even in terms of annual changes, expenditures for pharmaceuticals are modest when compared with those for all other categories, although growth rate for pharmaceuticals has exceeded the consumer price index since 1975. As overall health expenditures rise, however, and states attempt to constrain ever-rising costs of their Medicaid programs, any major expenditure category must be considered for reductions. As a result, pharmaceuticals appear an attractive target to cost-containment mechanisms. This paper examines one approach to the attempted reduction in Medicaid program costs—the imposition of restrictions on access to pharmaceuticals reimbursed through Medicaid programs.

0163-7525/92/0501-0399$02.00

BACKGROUND

In January 1966, the United States Social Security Act, Title XIX was enacted, thus creating the Medicaid program. Federal matching funds were provided to states for the provision of basic medical care to low income populations. Medicaid, along with the Medicare program, emerged as the largest public assistance system in the US. Because Medicaid programs are entirely administered by the separate states, Medicaid eligibility requirements are among the most complex of any public assistance programs. States may also elect to provide optional services.

Under certain federal conditions, states that provide optional services may impose limitations on service delivery by utilizing cost-sharing requirements and other stringent restrictions. One optional service, prescription drug coverage, is offered as a benefit by almost all state Medicaid programs, except those in Alaska and Wyoming (8). However, significant variation in these states' prescription drug programs exists. For example, imposition of copayments, limitation in the number of prescriptions per recipient, and reimbursement restrictions of varying degrees of severity are common among states that provide this service.

Medicaid programs have been faced with shrinking financial resources, while also facing increases in program expenditures caused by health care inflation. Currently, Medicaid accounts for approximately one third of state and local government health care expenditures, and often represents the largest program in a state's budget (9). The political climate regarding rising health care costs has provided Congress, as well as state legislatures, with the impetus to restrict government spending on all health programs. In 1981, Congress passed the Omnibus Budget Reconciliation Act, which effectively cut federal support for Medicaid and conferred to states greater flexibility and responsibility for developing cost-containment policies.

Medicaid Drug Formularies

Responding to this intense economic pressure, states have implemented cost-containment measures to control, for example, prescription drug costs. Many states have implemented drug formularies, which are statewide lists of basic drugs, as criteria for Medicaid reimbursement to reduce drug and overall Medicaid costs. Thus, restrictions on the use of certain drug products or entire therapeutic categories are often adopted.

Drug formularies are categorized as either open or restricted. Restricted, or closed, drug formularies are characterized by a state's policy not to pay for prescription drugs unless they are specifically listed. Open drug formularies provide prescribing guidelines that generally pay for all prescribed drugs, regardless of their inclusion on a drug list. States with open formularies, which provide some guidance in drug reimbursement, as well as states with no formal drug reimbursement policy, are referred to as open formulary states.

It is difficult to compare Medicaid formularies across states accurately, because of differences in important related administrative policies. For example, some states with a restrictive drug formulary may provide other mechanisms, such as prior authorization protocol, to enable Medicaid patients to have access to nonformulary drugs.

Prior authorization is an example of treatment authorization requests required by Medicaid for additional treatment or, in this case, prescription drugs that are not specified as reimbursable by the program. Prior authorization for prescription drugs requires that a physician or pharmacist document the need of a Medicaid patient for an unreimburseable drug product. This request is then submitted, usually by telephone or mail, to a Medicaid field office for approval or denial. If the majority of prior authorization requests are approved, a restrictive formulary with prior authorization may actually provide more availability of drugs to beneficiaries than would a less restrictive formulary with no exemption process. California, for example, is a state that has a restrictive formulary, but also administers a formal prior authorization program, the treatment authorization request (TAR).

Another characteristic of a drug formulary is the concept of positive versus negative formulary lists. A positive formulary is a list of drugs that are fully reimbursable by the payor of services. This type of formulary usually lists drugs of choice based upon scientific and clinical evidence. Choices are usually determined with strong medical and pharmaceutical input on the basis of cost, efficacy, and safety. In contrast, a negative formulary is a list of drugs or therapeutic categories that are not reimbursable by the payor of services. For example, drugs that treat anorexia or weight gain, fertility, hair growth, smoking cessation, and coughs and colds are often included on negative formularies.

Literature Review on Medicaid Drug Formularies

Research regarding Medicaid drug formularies has centered around the issue of restrictive versus open formularies. Significant controversy has been elicited, as restrictive formulary proponents commend fiscal restraints, while opponents criticize drug formularies as an obstacle to the efficient practice of high quality medicine. Additionally, wide variation of conclusions in the literature concerning the effect of restrictive formularies makes interpretation difficult, especially because most studies (including 1, 4, 6, 7) are funded at least in part by the pharmaceutical industry.

Although many studies of the effects of restricted drug access exist, their results are not generalizable, because of differences in the state Medicaid programs analyzed. Among the current research studies, two types of analyses have been employed: single state studies and multistate studies.

Single state studies are the most common among Medicaid formulary evaluations. However, because these analyses are limited to the experience in a single state, they tend to reflect the idiosyncracies of formulary restrictions in the state, e.g. the prior authorization process or TAR in California. In addition, single state studies, as a result of comparing expenditures before and after a formulary policy change, inadvertently attribute any differences to that change without critically examining other policy or environmental changes that might concur with the state specific formulary policy. Therefore, conclusions are often difficult to validate as true causal effects. Finally, pre-post single state studies monitor only short-term effects of formulary restrictions, which does not consider long-term consequences of new physician prescribing or treatment patterns.

Factors that are often controlled in multistate studies, but lack in single state studies, include program size, composition, and reimbursement trends. These variables are important, because Medicaid program costs are a function of program size, therefore subject to changes in the number of eligibles. However, even per-eligible costs vary with the severity and duration of economic cycles. Additionally, the composition of those persons on Medicaid varies, which is particularly evident in California and New York, two very populous states facing the AIDS epidemic. Also, state reductions in Medicaid reimbursement levels affect Medicaid access, as the number of participating Medicaid providers changes according to reimbursement levels.

In the following literature review, we only discuss published studies. Thus, seven studies are examined, of which two (4, 7) are published by the National Pharmaceutical Council. Additionally, we separate formulary studies on the basis of Medicaid cost results and Medicaid drug access. We first present Medicaid cost studies, which are further classified into multistate and single state studies.

In 1972, Hammel (3) conducted an early multistate study, which examined open and restrictive formularies. His evaluation examined Medicaid expenditures of nine Western states and ten Southern states, by using data provided by the Department of Health, Education, and Welfare. The 19 states were categorized as either open or restrictive, and Medicaid expenditures were compared between those classifications. Hammel concluded that in both the West and South, restrictive formulary policies resulted in higher state per capita Medicaid expenditures than did open formularies. This study is weak, however, because it is old and insufficient in controlling differences in eligibility requirements and variations in benefits among the different West and South Medicaid programs.

The multistate study by Smith & Simmons (7) utilized a combined time series cross-sectional methodology to examine the effects of formulary limitations in Medicaid drug programs from 1973 to 1980. A multivariate analysis was developed that included independent variables specific to formulary restrictions: drug price, utilization limitations, and other Medicaid policies. Medicaid drug expenditures per eligible and recipient, as well as a participation rate ratio of recipients to eligibles were used as the dependent variables.

Smith & Simmons did not find strong results in their model. Independent variables were highly intercorrelated, thus giving imprecise parameter estimates. Additionally, the multivariate analysis results were mixed regarding formulary restrictions. In some cases, formulary restrictions appeared to reduce Medicaid expenditures on drugs; in most cases, however, formulary restrictions were associated with an increase in Medicaid expenditures. This conclusion was not statistically convincing, because of the high multicollinearity between the independent variables.

A more recent multistate expenditure study, by Schweitzer et al (6), investigated the relationship between formulary restrictiveness and Medicaid expenditures. The authors tested the hypothesis that restrictive drug access lowers total expenditures. They used cross-section regression analysis to determine the financial impact of restrictive drug formularies by analyzing drug expenditures as a function of formulary policy and other variables. Seven states—California, Illinois, Kentucky, Mississippi, New York, South Carolina, and Washington—were analyzed.

Schweitzer et al found that restrictive formularies did not appear to reduce Medicaid drug expenditures. But, in contrast to the findings of the earlier, more limited studies, the authors observed that total Medicaid expenditures were reduced in restrictive formulary states. The authors reasoned that the restrictive formularies may not directly cause this reduction in expenditures, but may merely represent a proxy for general Medicaid restrictive cost-containment programs.

Schweitzer et al's contrasting results of reduced total Medicaid expenditure may be attributed to a more thorough control of external variables. Schweitzer's regression model controlled to a greater extent such factors as medical practice patterns, health status, demography, and prevailing illness patterns among each state's total population, not just the Medicaid population. Thus, he better accounted for interstate differences in patterns of medical care, health care costs trends, demographic differences, and variations in morbidity across states. Additionally, Schweitzer et al examined a longer period (ten years), thus monitoring longer term effects than other multistate studies that utilized shorter time series.

Although Schweitzer et al's research is plausible and adequately controls for numerous variables, the study fails to link the association between restrictive drug access and lower overall Medicaid expenditures to a causality. Schweitzer addresses this issue in his conclusion by stating, "The associations do not appear to be simple or obvious." Schweitzer's study also differs from the other multistate studies, in that substitution effects are not considered.

Several unpublished studies of specific drug restrictions determined that if close substitutes for a drug are not on the formulary, the total cost of treatment for an episode of illness can increase dramatically. One must weigh the higher cost of a new drug against the cost of other health services, such as physician office visits and hospital admissions, which often act as substitutes and are orders of magnitude more expensive. The net effect depends on many factors, such as the extent of potential unnecessary use of the more expensive drug and the likelihood that nonuse will lead to the other increased services. For some exclusions, it is certainly possible that the net costs may rise. Whether this is a broadly observed phenomenon depends on the characteristics of a formulary.

Although single state studies are less generalizable than multistate studies, their relative abundance provides interesting state specific information. Meyer et al (5) evaluated Tennessee's Medicaid drug program qualitatively. They described Tennessee's attempt to adapt features of an unrestricted drug formulary and drug utilization review. The authors supported Tennessee's efforts and anticipated that the program would benefit the citizens of the state. However, because this study lacked adequate quantitative validation, the conclusions should be viewed with skepticism.

In 1980, Hefner (4) conducted a study that compared two states, to control for the effects of general trends by Medicaid recipients' use of services. Hefner compared Texas, which has an open formulary, with Louisiana which has a closed formulary. Louisiana instituted a negative formulary in July 1976, which excluded anorexics, cough and cold remedies, minor tranquilizers, multiple-ingredient anti-anemia preparations, certain gastrointestinal drugs, certain vitamins, enzymes, and other miscellaneous products. Louisiana Medicaid officials estimated that the restrictive formulary would decrease drug expenditures by 15.68% and save $5.6 million.

Hefner's method involved two approaches: a longitudinal study of the Medicaid program utilization patterns before and after the 1976 Louisiana restrictions and integration of the frequency of disease patterns associated with provider encounters into the longitudinal results. Hefner utilized an 18-month study period, which was divided into three six-month periods: a six-month preperiod or control period, a six-month adjustment period, and a six-month comparison period. Hefner also matched samples of eligibles for the control and comparison study periods by population characteristics, such as aid category, sex, age, race, and residence. Additionally, Hefner examined specific units of service that represented the largest cost items in the Medicaid program.

Hefner's study found that cost increases associated with increased utilization for other medical services were 3.5 times the savings from a restrictive drug formulary. Although this study's method to control for general trends was an improvement over an earlier Hefner unpublished single state study, he failed to distinguish the effect of other nonpolicy influences on Medicaid program costs. Also, the implementation of Louisiana's negative formulary policy was not viewed as substantial enough to warrant such large increases in hospitalizations in a relatively short period of study.

In 1989, Dranove (1) evaluated the cost-effectiveness of formulary restrictions in Illinois. In 1984, Illinois's Department of Public Aid eased restrictions on anti-infective drug products for Medicaid reimbursement. Dranove studied this new policy effect on both the use of physicians' services and the cost of treating bacterial infections. Dranove constructed a sample of Medicaid ambulatory patients with bacterial infections in 1983 and 1984. By using regression analysis, Dranove concluded that the number of physician visits per patient decreased after the addition of new anti-infective drug products. However, he also concluded that this physician utilization decrease did not offset higher drug costs of the new policy. Although Dranove's method for assessing the impact of new policy is interesting, a strong link between relaxing formulary restrictions and increased utilization of other services lacks controls for other influences. Additionally, Dranove did not include an evaluation of the formulary change on inpatient hospital costs that could have strengthened his finding of increased utilization of other services.

Because Dranove's study lacks statistically significant results and excludes the impact of formulary changes on inpatient hospital costs, his conclusions on decreased physician visit utilization with the addition of new anti-infective drug products is not convincing. Dranove's results indicate that no association exists between easing formulary restrictions and physician utilization and cost.

Although there is evidence, albeit tentative and statistically weak, that Medicaid expenditures may actually rise in response to formulary restrictions, the overall view is indeterminant. Numerous narrowly focused studies derive an opposite association between restrictive Medicaid formularies and expenditures, whereas the more thorough, multistate Schweitzer study finds an association, but cannot attribute causality. In conclusion, there is not a strong case that formularies either raise or reduce Medicaid expenditures.

NEW RESEARCH AND FUTURE DEVELOPMENT

Drug formularies have become an increasingly popular cost-minimization strategy. Supporting this trend is the fact that in 1988, only four of 48 Medicaid programs had completely "open" formularies, which reimbursed for all Food and Drug Administration (FDA) approved drug products (8). In the remaining Medicaid programs, approval of a new drug product by the FDA does not guarantee Medicaid recipients access to new drugs. Products must be approved by Medicaid programs before reimbursement is secured.

In the case of California's Medicaid drug formulary, the formulary is updated by an ongoing process of adding newer drug products and deleting older, inferior drug products. The Department of Health Services uses five criteria: cost, essential need, safety, efficacy, and misuse potential. Each state's formulary drug determinations vary depending on the state's policy. In general, the criteria seem to be based on cost and availability of substitutes; however, substitutes are often not very close.

In the area of social policy and Medicaid drug formularies, Schweitzer et al (6) and Grabowski (2) examined Medicaid beneficiaries' access to new drug products. The Schweitzer et al study investigated the "social drug lag" between the time a drug is approved for marketing by the FDA and the time it is available to a state's indigent population through the Medicaid program.

In this study, Schweitzer established a drug lag index for comparing states and analyzing time trends. In particular, the drug lag index measured the fraction of time that a new drug is available to a state's Medicaid beneficiaries during the first two years of market life from FDA approval.

Schweitzer found that from 1970 to 1980, the FDA approved 120 new drug products for marketing. But, the approval of these new drug products adopted by formulary states ranged from 19% to 73%. Of the seven states in the study, Illinois, Washington, South Carolina, Mississippi, and New York had relatively short average lengths of time for approval. In the other two states, California and Kentucky, the average lengths of time for approval were relatively long.

The range in the approval lag was very large. For those drugs that were eventually approved, Kentucky, averaged more than five years for approval, whereas Washington averaged a little more than one year. Additionally, Schweitzer et al discovered that the drug approval lag trend decreased over the period of study for all states combined.

Grabowski's study also examined the effects of drug formularies on the availability of new drugs to Medicaid beneficiaries. The study analyzed the impact of drug formulary time delays on the marketing exclusivity periods and related factors that influence drug innovation incentives. Grabowski's research showed three categories of drugs to be the least available: psychotherapeutics, anti-infectives, and antifertility products. Grabowski also found that a typical new drug product was available to Medicaid patients only two of the first five years of market life. Thus, the study showed that Medicaid patients in restrictive formulary states had significantly restricted access to new drug products. Furthermore, restrictions were not limited to duplicate drug products, but included drugs that exhibited strong, non-Medicaid market performance, as well as high FDA therapeutic importance.

As demonstrated by Schweitzer's and Grabowski's research, wide variation exists in the restrictiveness of state formularies. In some cases, the delay between the first marketing of a new drug product and its availability to Medicaid beneficiaries lasts only months; in other states, the lag is frequently several years. And, in many states, products are never approved for Medicaid reimbursement.

A recent unpublished study by Grabowski and colleagues (1991, The Medicaid Drug Lag: Adoption of New Drugs by State Medicaid Formulas, Duke University), which was funded by Glaxo Pharmaceutical, investigated indigent patients' access to new drugs in various states with Medicaid formularies. This study was an extension of the two previous analyses of the Medicaid approval process by Schweitzer et al and Grabowski. In this paper, however, a larger sample of states with Medicaid formularies was examined for a longer time period, 1970–1985. Time trends were presented for this extended period and for the more recent period of 1979–1985. As in Grabowski's earlier study, therapeutic categories and market sales were also investigated. The experiences of nine states with Medicaid formularies (California, Illinois, Kentucky, Mississippi, Missouri, New York, South Carolina, Tennessee and Washington) were examined in more detail.

The study found that Medicaid patients continue to face significant restrictions regarding new outpatient drugs. Although a positive trend toward increasing availability was observed during the 1970s, this was not the case in 1979–1985. In this period, the typical new drug compound experienced lags of 20 months in securing a position onto these formularies and were available less than 40% of the time during the first four years of market life. Furthermore, certain categories of drugs, such as anti-infectives and psychopharmacologics, were particularly restricted by Medicaid formularies. New drugs of commercial and therapeutic importance in these and other therapeutic categories also experienced significant restrictions on availability. In addition, greater drug availability was observed for drug products with higher market sales.

The experience with respect to Medicaid formularies varied dramatically across the nine states. As noted previously, California had the most restrictive formulary of these states, as only about one third of the FDA approved new drugs gained acceptance onto the Medicaid formulary. These acceptances had a lag of roughly four years from the date of first marketing approval. By contrast, New York, which had a closed Medicaid formulary only since 1977, exhibited an acceptance rate of over 80%, with an average time delay of only eight months.

After constructing a picture of California's and New York's Medicaid drug adoption process from interviews and literature, the difference between restrictive and liberal policies appears less distinct. Although, California's Medi-Cal formulary does not offer as many new drug products during the first four years of market life as New York, California's prior authorization program enables some access to nonformulary drug products. However, it is not clear whether California's 70% approval of prior authorization requests significantly improves Medicaid beneficiaries access to new drug products or merely creates further obstacles to an already restrictive drug formulary.

New Legislation

Congress's concern over the cost and accessibility of pharmaceuticals to Medicaid programs led to sweeping legislative reform in 1990. This legislation, the Prudent Purchasing Act of 1990 [Public Law (PL) 101-508] contains several parts. Beginning January 1, 1991, federal Medicaid funds may be withheld from states for prescription drugs if the drug manufacturer of a Medicaid reimbursed drug product does not enter into an agreement to provide specified quarterly rebates to states. In response to this mandate, the federal government has offered to assist states with start-up administrative costs by providing 75 cents, rather than the usual 50 cents, of each dollar spent on the program in fiscal 1991.

In addition to the rebate requirement, the federal legislation specifies a list of drugs that a state may exclude from coverage, such as drugs that treat anorexia or weight gain, fertility, smoking cessation, and coughs and colds. The Health and Human Services Secretary is required to update the list periodically to add or delete drugs determined to be clinically abusive or inappropriately utilized.

The federal rebates are applied to single source and multiple source drugs. There are two possible rebates for single source drugs: the greater of 12.5% of the average manufacturer price (AMP) or the difference between the AMP and "best price," which the manufacturer sells to any other customer. However, this legislation exempts from best price contract sales to the Department of Veterans Affairs. Rebates for multiple source drugs, better known as generics and over-the-counter drugs, are 10% of the AMP for 1991–1993 and 11% thereafter. To facilitate the best price agreement, manufacturers, wholesalers, and direct sellers of drugs must provide pricing information, which is termed confidential. If this legislative requirement is not fulfilled, violators are subject to fines of up to $100,000.

States receive manufacturer rebates by submitting, no later than 60 days after the end of each calendar quarter, information on the total number of dosage units of each covered outpatient drug dispensed under the Medicaid discount plan during the quarter. States collect dosage information from pharmacies that submit Medicaid drug reimbursement claims to the state. Under these operating procedures, pharmacies are not directly affected, because reimbursement rates remain unchanged between the state and pharmacies. After submitting the rebate claims to the manufacturers, the state receives the appropriate rebate from the manufacturer. Thus, the states benefit from the rebates, while maintaining business as usual with the pharmacies.

A prior authorization mechanism is required through which states grant specific permission for use of a nonformulary drug before reimbursement is permitted under the new legislation. States that currently have a prior approval program are required to respond to a drug request within 24 hours, with the assurance that a patient have access to a 72-hour emergency supply.

Drugs newly approved by the FDA are not eligible for prior authorization until after six months of availability and, in the case of FDA 1-A (major therapeutic innovations) classified drugs, prior authorization requirements are clearly restricted.

The federal legislation has also addressed issues of generic substitution, pharmacy reimbursement, and, most interesting, utilization review issues along with education. Under this new legislation, prospective and retrospective drug review is required. Prospective drug review specifies screening for potential problems caused by drug interactions, contraindications, allergies, dosage forms, and misuse factors. Retrospective drug review focuses on analyzing claims data and other records for fraud, overutilization, and inappropriate use by physicians, pharmacists, and patients. Acquired information from these two utilization programs will assist the states in required outreach to educate physicians with the goal of improving prescribing and dispensing practices.

It is interesting to examine policy changes in California, which has had the most restrictive formula in the country (2, 8; Grabowski et al 1991, unpublished). In July 1990, new California legislation mandated a drug discount program to be implemented immediately by California's Medi-Cal pharmaceutical program. Close behind California's drug discount legislation, Congress passed a similar drug discounting policy applicable to all Medicaid drug formulary programs.

California's legislation differs from the federal best price criterion, because it does not specify a target percent discount, but rather allows for flexibility in negotiations. The California legislation states that best price means the negotiated price, or the manufacturer's lowest price available to any class of trade organization or entity. In addition, California does not exempt the Department of Veterans Affairs from the contracted best price as specified in the federal legislation.

The anticipated benefits of the new legislation are not only to decrease Medicaid program costs, but to provide the possibility of increased Medicaid beneficiaries' access to new drug products. After preliminary evaluation of California's drug discount legislation, it appears that the original Medi-Cal drug formulary list has significantly expanded in a shorter period of time than previously witnessed. Additionally, the prior authorization program has benefited from an increase in state funds to improve service response time to providers. This improvement is difficult to evaluate so soon after phase-in of this legislation, but is viewed as a positive step in alleviating the burden of the prior authorization process to providers.

Although decreased program costs will produce a windfall for state Medicaid programs, analysts predict that pharmaceutical prices may increase for other payors. Specifically, a shift in prices may adversely affect private pay patients, including Medicare beneficiaries who do not qualify for Medicaid, if pharmaceutical companies attempt to recover lost revenue through price discrimination. However, this scenario may not be realistic if pharmaceutical companies are pricing correctly in the market. Thus, the issue of drug pricing may come under closer scrutiny. Additionally, pharmaceutical companies may face unintended risks of Medicaid discounting, as other public and private customers may increase pressure for similar discounts.

With legislation so new, it is impossible to evaluate the impact of PL 101-508 on either Medicaid drug program costs or prescribing and dispensing patterns. Also, there is little information on whether this new legislation will reduce the wide variation across states in Medicaid program access to new drug products.

In summary, the literature review of restrictive Medicaid formularies and its effects on Medicaid expenditures is inconclusive. Although many studies conclude that Medicaid expenditures may actually increase in reaction to formulary restrictions, this evidence is tentative and statistically weak. However, the conclusion that restrictive formularies delay access of new drug products to Medicaid beneficiaries is supported in the literature. Also, this delayed access varies dramatically across restrictive Medicaid formulary states, which seems to reflect an individual state's administration of their formulary. Future issues regarding Medicaid formularies points to new cost-containment developments, such as the new Medicaid discount legislation. As a result of the pressure on federal and state governments to control high health care costs, more cost-containment measures, such as this legislation, will be forthcoming. Understanding the impact of these changes on cost and access is important for future health policy legislation and program implementors.

Literature Cited

1. Dranove, D. 1989. Medicaid drug formulary restrictions. *J. Law Econ.* 32: 143–62
2. Grabowski, H. 1988. Medicaid patients' access to new drugs. *Health Aff.* Winter:102–14
3. Hammel, R. W. 1972. Insights into public assistance medical care expenditures. *J. Am. Med. Assoc.* 219:13:1740–44
4. Hefner, D. L. 1980. *Cost-Effectiveness of a Restrictive Drug Formulary: Louisiana vs. Texas*, pp. 1–14. Washington, DC: Nat. Pharm. Counc.
5. Meyer, M. C., Bates, H., Swift, R. G. 1974. The role of state formularies. *J. Am. Pharm. Assoc.* NS14:12:663–66
6. Schweitzer, S. O., Salehi, H., Boling, N. 1985. The social drug lag: An examination of pharmaceutical approval delays in Medicaid formularies. *Soc. Sci. Med.* 21:10:1077–82
7. Smith, M. C., Simmons, S. 1982. A study of the effects of formulary limitations in Medicaid drug programs. *Proc. Natl. Pharm. Counc.*, pp. 117–41. Washington, DC: Natl. Pharm. Counc.
8. Soumerai, S. B., Ross-Degnan, D. 1990. Experience of state drug benefit programs. *Health Aff.* Fall:36–54
9. Systemetrics/McGraw-Hill. 1990. *Pharmaceutical and Health Care Expenditures in Medi-Cal 1984–1989: Final Report*, pp. 1–25. Santa Barbara, Calif: Systemetrics/McGraw-Hill
10. US Dep. Health Hum. Serv. 1988. *Program Statistics: Medicare and Medicaid Data Book*, p. 72. Washington, DC: Health Care Finance. Adm.

Symposium on Selected Clinical Syndromes
Associated with Aging

Introduction, Gilbert S. Omenn, Symposium Editor

The aging of society in the developed countries is the dominant demographic phenomenon of our time. The number of persons aged 65 and over in the United States has grown from 3.1 million in 1900 (4% of the population) to over 30 million today (12%). Projections indicate that there will be 35 million in the year 2000, 39 million in 2010, 52 million in 2020, and 66 million (22% of the population) in 2030 as the post-World War II baby-boom population ages. The percentage growth in the over-85 population is even faster. Thus, there is understandable concern among health economists, bugeteers, and planners—and among physicians, as well—that the high utilization of medical care by an aging population will reinforce the runaway health care inflation of recent years.

This section of the *Annual Review of Public Health* reflects a strongly held view of our Editorial Committee and a growing perception nationally that prevention has a major place in the care of older women and men. We have chosen several major clinical problems of older people—acute confusional states, cognitive impairment, physical inactivity, falls, and nonfall injuries—to explore the multifactorial causes and the evidence for effective preventive measures. The authors provide authoritative reviews of the issues and evidence.

Research on health promotion and disease prevention in older men and women was long neglected. In retrospect, it is striking that the major cardiovascular prevention trials reported in the 1970s and 1980s enrolled only middle-aged men—in MRFIT, men aged 35–57 and in the Coronary Primary Prevention Trial of the Lipid Research Centers, men aged 35–59. Since the establishment of the National Institute on Aging, the National Institutes of Health has been rectifying this deficiency.

Throughout the Public Health Service, attention to older people in health promotion/disease prevention programs has been growing. The 1989 *Guide to Clinical Preventive Services* included a specific schedule of screening, counseling, and immunization services recommended for older adults. The highest priority is to improve functional status and quality of life, rather than just extending life. The 1979 report of the Surgeon General, *Healthy People,* and *Health Objectives for the Nation 1990* the following year set as the primary goal for older adults 25% reduction in the number of days of restricted activity. In *Healthy People 2000,* the first overarching goal is to "increase the span of healthy life for Americans." The 1980 figures were 73.7 years for life expectancy at birth, of which 11.7 years were dysfunctional, on average.

There is ample time for effective health promotion actions to take effect in older people; for example, women and men who reach age 65 can expect to live into their eighties. But, there is no assurance that the same risk factors have the same relative importance in older people as in middle-age. Specific research is required. What is known for several key risk factors and preventive interventions is well-summarized in the February 1992 *Clinics in Geriatric Medicine,* which was designed to be complementary to this Symposium. As with younger age groups, however, the biggest challenge is to entice those who most need to participate—sedentary, smoking, low-income, socially isolated, sensory-impaired, multiply medicated, or depressed individuals. As always, those of us in public health and preventive medicine must emphasize ways to reach the whole population and especially those most at risk.

Preventive actions, in both clinical and community arenas, seem to face far more scrutiny of their likely costs than do diagnostic tests and treatments. Total costs of population-based health promotion programs can become rather substantial if screening tests, confirmatory tests, and counseling are provided to large numbers of people to prevent relatively few adverse events per year. The benefit-to-risk ratio drops further when future benefits are discounted against present costs, if high-risk individuals are disproportionately missed, if identified individuals fail to follow through with recommended behavior changes or medicines, or if the target population is heterogeneous for conditions screened and for appropriateness of interventions.

As I have noted in the Summer 1990 issue of *Health Affairs* devoted to prevention, generalized analyses of health promotion and disease prevention programs can be misleading. It is essential to specify the target populations by age, sex, racial and ethnic group, underlying incidence of predisposing preventable risk factors, portion of the risk attributable to each of those factors and their combinations, willingness to participate, and compliance with recommendations.

The classic differentiation among primary, secondary, and tertiary prevention efforts is useful, too. Primary prevention aims to avert the initiation of the disease process; secondary, to detect early signs of disease before the person is clinically affected; and tertiary, to prevent serious and often costly complications of already-diagnosed disease. Some of these considerations make the benefit/cost ratio of efficacious preventive services potentially more favorable among older men and women than in their middle-aged counterparts.

Primary prevention may seem less useful in older adults if it must precede the onset of the disease process by many years. However, smoking cessation seems to reduce coronary mortality promptly and with similar magnitude in older and middle-aged individuals; the aggregate benefit per 1000 persons is much higher in older adults because the mortality rate is so much higher. Because incidence, morbidity, and mortality rates of the common cancers rise sharply with age, any secondary prevention program that works in older adults should generate more lives saved per 1000 people screened.

Two major efforts are under way to assess cost-effectiveness of various preventive interventions for Medicare-eligible elderly persons. The first is a series of literature reviews and analyses by the Congressional Office of Technology Assessment. The second is a set of demonstrations in North Carolina, southern California, Baltimore, Pittsburgh, and Seattle to assess the costs, potential cost savings, and changes in health-related quality of life after introduction of experimental packages of preventive services.

It is ridiculous to expect health promotion and disease prevention to accomplish grand-scale cost containment in the health care sector in the face of continuing escalation of expenditures for diagnosis, treatment, and long-term care. However, it is reasonable to expect well-selected health promotion and disease prevention initiatives to achieve improvement in health status, maintenance of functional independence, and moderation of increases in health care expenditures.

Annu. Rev. Health. 1992. 13:415–430

ACUTE CONFUSIONAL STATES IN OLDER ADULTS AND THE ROLE OF POLYPHARMACY

Ronald B. Stewart

Department of Pharmacy Practice, College of Pharmacy, University of Florida, Gainesville, Florida 32610

William E. Hale

Florida Geriatric Research Program, Dunedin, Florida 34698

KEY WORDS: adverse drug reactions, geriatrics, drug-induced disease, cognitive dysfunction, delirium

INTRODUCTION

Cognitive impairment in the elderly represents a major public health problem as the proportion of elderly persons in the population increases. Epidemiologic data show that 1.4% of persons aged 65–74 years have a dementing illness; this figure rises to 20.8% for persons over age 85–89 years (45, 91).

Acute confusional state (ACS), or delirium, which is a form of dementia, differs from Alzheimer's disease by its speed of onset. Also, the delirium patient may fluctuate between full alertness and coma, and the condition is usually reversible (21). Lipowski (56) has defined delirium as "a transient organic mental syndrome of acute onset, characterized by global impairment of cognitive functions, a reduced level of consciousness, attentional abnormalities, increased or decreased psychomotor activity, and a disordered sleep-wake cycle." Acute confusion is a common occurrence among institutionalized elderly persons (72, 92).

Confusional states presumedly reflect disturbances in cerebral metabolism.

415

0163-7525/92/0501-0415$02.00

In elderly persons, confusional states can be caused by many physical or psychological alterations, including cerebrovascular accidents, seizures, infections, hypoxia, myocardial infarction, depression, and drugs (55, 57).

Acute confusional state is a clinical entity that includes specific *Diagnostic and Statistical Manual of Mental Disorders III* criteria for the diagnosis (21). In this review, we expand the definition of delirium to all forms of cognitive impairment that result from multiple drug therapy, which is an important etiologic factor of cognitive impairment in the elderly (67).

Larson and associates (52) found drug-induced dementia to be a cause of cognitive impairment in 11.6% of patients with suspected dementia. Furthermore, the relative odds of drug-induced dementia increased from 1.0 in patients taking 0–1 drug to 9.3 in those taking 4–5 drugs, which suggests that polypharmacy is an important risk factor of cognitive impairment in the older person.

We can define polypharmacy as the use of more than one drug to treat symptoms or disease. There are many examples of beneficial drug combinations (15). Antimicrobial combinations have been used to broaden the spectrum of antimicrobial coverage and decrease toxicity by use of lower drug concentrations (13). Similarly, levodopa has been combined with carbidopa to increase the concentration of levodopa in the brain (9).

The term polypharmacy has also been used to describe the situation in which drugs, usually in large numbers, are used to manage multiple symptoms and diseases in an individual patient. We use this definition in our discussion. Polypharmacy is a particularly common problem among older persons (12, 81). In this review, we describe the problems of ACS that result from specific drugs, examine the evidence that points to confusional states with polypharmacy, and outline methods that can be employed to prevent the occurrence of the problem.

EPIDEMIOLOGY

Although ACS in the geriatric patient is recognized as a common problem by health care providers, epidemiologic data on the incidence of this syndrome, particularly in ambulatory elderly, are lacking. Most information concerning the frequency of this condition has been obtained from studies of institutionalized elderly persons (92). Incidence estimates vary greatly because of different diagnostic criteria and methods employed by investigators and because of the different settings in which patients were studied (58).

Studies of ACS among hospital admissions have found that 10–40% of elderly patients were acutely confused on admission. Estimates depend on the type of institution (psychiatric hospital, general medical ward, or geriatric unit) to which patients were admitted (58). Estimates of acute confusional disorder in elderly patients admitted to general medical wards have usually been much lower. According to Hodkinson (40), about one fourth of geriatric patients in a multicenter study of 21 geriatric departments were acutely confused on admission. Bergmann & Eartham (7) found that 15% of geriatric patients admitted to a general medical ward suffered from ACS. Seymour et al (75) found that 16% of patients over age 70 who were admitted as emergencies to a general medical unit were acutely confused.

In about 25–35% of geriatric patients with normal cognitive states on admission, ACS develops during the first month of their hospital stay (40). The elderly are at much greater risk of ACS than younger age groups. In one prospective study, 29.5% of patients over age 70 exhibited confusion within six weeks of their admission to general medical wards, compared with 3.6% of those under age 70 (27). Warshaw et al (89) found confusion and advanced age to be significantly correlated: 61% of female patients over age 84 were moderately to severely disoriented. Unfortunately, no information could be found on the incidence of ACS in the ambulatory elderly population. One would expect that most elderly persons in the ambulatory setting would be immediately brought to the attention of a physician if this condition developed and would be hospitalized.

DRUG-RELATED ACUTE CONFUSIONAL STATES

Numerous causes of ACS in the elderly have been identified. Most authorities believe that the condition results from multifactorial etiologies, rather than a single cause. The combination of these factors alters cerebral function and produces the syndrome (54). Because most clinical conditions thought to be associated with ACS, including cardiovascular, neurologic, and psychologic conditions, are commonly treated with drug therapy, it is difficult to separate the contribution of drugs to ACS.

Larson et al (53) studied 200 consecutive patients over age 60 with suspected dementia and found 69.5% had dementia of the Alzheimer type. Drug toxicity was the most common treatable form of the suspected dementia and was present in ten (5.0%) of the patients.

For physicians to attribute ACS to a drug or combination of drugs, they must have an index of suspicion that the drug could be responsible. Morrison & Katz (67) have concluded that mechanisms do not currently exist to evaluate appropriately the potential for specific drugs to cause cognitive deterioration.

POLYPHARMACY AND THE ELDERLY

Older adults in the US represent about 12% of the population, yet they consume 31% of all prescription medications and use a disproportionate share of nonprescription drugs (3, 24). Studies of drug use in patients who attended a general medical clinic associated with a teaching hospital revealed that the average number of medications used per person was 3.2, and the number increased to 5.0 for patients over age 65 (81). Cross-sectional studies of elderly populations (conducted in 1982–1985) have shown that the elderly use an averge of 1.7 to 2.7 prescribed medications in addition to one nonprescribed drug, and the number of drugs used increases with increasing age (36, 38). In 1977, patients in the US received 4.3 new and refill prescriptions, but that number rose to 10.7 for patients over age 65 (47).

Many clinicians and researchers have questioned the wisdom and rationale of polypharmacy in the elderly (5, 49, 51, 61, 70). The use of multiple concurrent medications may predispose the older person to iatrogenic illness, including adverse drug reactions, drug-drug interactions, and decreased medication compliance (41) (Figure 1). Although most experts discourage the use of multiple medications to treat symptoms and disease in the elderly, investigations have shown that the number of medications used by ambulatory elderly persons has increased from 1978–1979 to 1987–1988 (83). Furthermore, numerous factors will increase the likelihood of polypharmacy in the elderly in the future (80). New advances in diagnostic techniques will increase the number of detectable diseases in the elderly, and physicians may feel impelled to treat those conditions. New drugs will become available through traditional pharmacologic research and new biotechnological breakthroughs. Considering the prevalence of potentially treatable disease in the elderly, polypharmacy will become the rule, not the exception.

COGNITIVE IMPAIRMENT RESULTING FROM MONOTHERAPY

Ample evidence is available to show that certain drugs can impair cognitive function in specific situations (93). By using scientific methods, researchers have shown that anticholinergic agents and psychotropic drugs cause cognitive impairment (67). For many other classes of drugs, including antihypertensives, nonsteroidal anti-inflammatory drugs, and corticosteroids, documentation of cognitive impairment is less convincing (67). The majority of evidence relating cognitive impairment or ACS to drugs has been derived from individual case reports (67).

Anticholinergic agents have repeatedly been demonstrated to alter memory of normal volunteers (14). By using a double-blind crossover study, Sunderland and colleagues (84) have shown that patients with Alzheimer's disease are more sensitive to cognitive impairment from scopolamine than normal, age-matched controls. The effect of low-dose intramuscular scopolamine on cognitive function in elderly medical inpatients has been investigated by Miller and associates (66). Patients were randomly assigned to receive in-

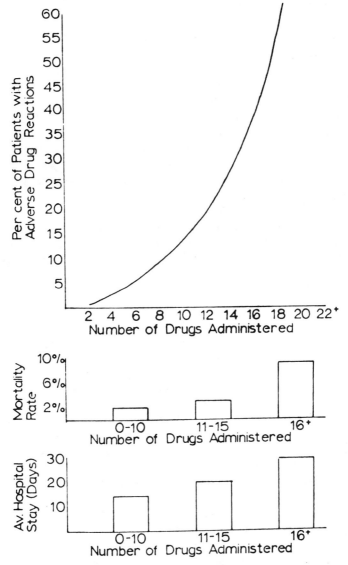

Figure 1 The relationship of rate of adverse drug reactions to number of drugs administered, mortality rate, and duration of hospitalization. (Reprinted with permission from Ref. 76.)

tramuscularly 0.005 mg/Kg of either scopolamine or placebo two hours before surgery. Scopolamine produced mild cognitive impairment, which was observed on a Delirium Symptom Checklist and the Rey Auditory-Verbal Learning instruments.

Trihexyphenidyl causes memory impairment in normal elderly volunteers. In one study, volunteers received a four-day course of treatment with either trihexyphenidyl 4 mg bid or amantadine 100 mg bid. Subjects who received trihexyphenidyl complained of confusion and exhibited memory impairment on objective memory tests, but no memory impairment was noted when amantadine was administered (64).

Because most tricyclic antidepressants have anticholinergic properties, their effect on cognitive state has been investigated (62). Cole and associates (19) reported that confusion or agitation developed in about 5% of elderly depressed patients receiving amitriptyline or imipramine. Amitriptyline significantly impaired cognitive performance in a placebo controlled study of elderly depressed outpatients with pretreatment evidence of mild cognitive impairment (11). Not all investigators have noted clinically significant confusion that resulted from the use of anticholinergics in the elderly. Seifert and colleagues (74) studied the use of drugs with anticholinergic effects in 29 confused and 54 nonconfused elderly nursing home patients. No patient received higher than the equivalent recommended daily dose of atropine, when calculated in terms of relative anticholinergic potency. No statistically significant correlation was found between confusion and the amount of anticholinergic administered. The authors noted that medication with significant anticholinergic effects were often prescribed for patients who already had confusion and cognitive impairment.

Cognitive impairment resulting from benzodiazepine administration has been extensively investigated by using well designed methodology. Impaired learning of verbal and visual information was demonstrated in both anxious and normal nonelderly volunteers (26, 73). Bond & Lader (10) have shown that the cognitive impairment associated with long-acting benzodiazepines persists for an extended period of time.

The effect of chronic administration of benzodiazepines on cognitive function in the elderly has received less study. Larson et al (52) found that in 35 of 308 patients with suspected dementia, the condition resulted from chronic drug use. Dementia was attributed to the chronic administration of a single benzodiazepine in 13 patients in this group. However, the authors also found that the risk of dementia increased with the number of concurrent drugs administered. Other investigators have failed to find cognitive impairment with chronic benzodiazepine administration. Viukari and associates (88) performed a randomized, double-blind crossover study of the effects of 1 mg flunitrazepam and 5 mg nitrazepam on cognitive tests in hospitalized elderly psychiatric patients. They found little effect on performance.

High blood pressure is a common disease in elderly persons, occurring in about 40% of the population over age 65. High blood pressure is a risk factor for cognitive impairment, primarily as a result of multi-infarct dementia, but antihypertensive drugs have also been implicated as a cause of cognitive dysfunction (1). In this case report, five patients complained of such symptoms as decreased memory, inability to perform calculations, and reading impairment. Solomon and colleagues (77) conducted a controlled study to demonstrate cognitive impairment in patients treated with methyldopa and propranolol. Croog and associates (33) also provided evidence that methyldopa could cause decreased visual-motor performance and lead to decreased quality of life.

Hypotension, particularly the iatrogenic–induced syndrome, frequently has been cited as a cause of ACS in the elderly (28). Aggressive reduction of blood pressure in the elderly may cause decreased perfusion to the central nervous system and precipitate adverse effects on cognitive and behavioral function. Goldstein and colleagues (28) evaluated this phenomenon by performing a battery of psychometric tests on hypertensive patients over age 60. A group of patients were tested after successful blood pressure reduction with antihypertensive drugs and then compared with a placebo-treated control group. There was no difference in cognitive function, motor skills, memory, or affect between the two groups. Neither blood pressure reduction nor medication impaired cognitive function in this elderly population.

Digoxin is one of the most frequently used medications by persons over age 65 (36, 38). Closson (16) and Grubb (34) have shown that digoxin intoxication can cause psychiatric side effects, including delirium and dementia. Tucker & Ng (85) demonstrated a significant correlation between plasma digoxin concentration and performance on the Buschke selective reminding test and the facial recognition test. There have been numerous case reports of cognitive impairment to many other drug classes, including nonsteroidal anti-inflammatory agents, meperidine, corticosteroids, and H-2 receptor antagonists (18, 22, 23, 29, 87).

The studies cited above demonstrate that anticholinergic drugs, as well as several other drug groups, can produce cognitive impairment. Most effects of drug-induced cognitive impairment have been minor and only detectable with sensitive testing instruments. Several investigators have been unable to demonstrate gross cognitive impairment when using such screening tests as the Mini-Mental State Examination (4, 25, 82).

Administration of drugs in most of the above-mentioned studies did not produce an actual acute confusional state. Other factors, including disease, nutrition, psychological stressors, and drug interactions probably play an important role in the acute confusional state of elderly persons.

COGNITIVE IMPAIRMENT RESULTING FROM POLYPHARMACY

In the cases described above, acute cognitive impairment was usually attributed to a single drug. Because the elderly usually administer several drugs concurrently, cognitive impairment could result from the combined effect of drugs.

Very few reports of ACS caused by polypharmacy are published in national refereed journals. Several examples of ACS resulting from polypharmacy have appeared in practice-oriented journals. Bressler (12) described a 75-year-old man who was drug-free until atrial fibrillation developed. The patient then received digoxin, warfarin, hydrochlorothiazide, and diazepam. Two weeks later, he was rehospitalized with complaints of visual disturbance, diffuse headache, lethargy, fatigue, impaired memory, and daytime somnolence. On admission to the hospital, he had elevated concentrations of serum digoxin (2.8 ng/ml) and diazepam (2.4 mcg/ml; normal is 0.5–1.0 mcg/ml) and the prothrombin time was 28 seconds (normal 10–14). His lethargy, somnolence, and memory deficit were attributed to diazepam overdose, even though the medications were prescribed at usual adult doses. This case illustrates the pharmacokinetic and pharmacodynamic changes that place older persons at risk of adverse drug reactions.

Gordon & Preiksaitis (30) described three elderly patients who suffered from acute confusion as a result of multiple medications. One patient, an 80-year-old man, was brought to the geriatric care center for evaluation of a seven-month history of increasing confusion. His prescribed medications included carbidopa/levodopa (25/100 mg tid), enteric coated aspirin (650 mg bid), diltiazem (60 mg qid), allopurinol (300 mg daily), hydrochlorothiazide/amiloride (every other day), digoxin (0.125 mg daily), nitropaste (qid), ranitidine (150 mg at bedtime), and diazepam (5 mg bid, as needed). Diazepam, hydrochlorothiazide/amiloride, and allopurinol were discontinued, and dosage reduction was accomplished for aspirin, diltiazem, and digoxin. Within two weeks, there was a marked improvement in mental and physical functioning. The authors concluded that the patient suffered from polypharmacy with psychoactive and nonpsychoactive drugs.

Other authors have described similar situations of multiple drug therapy that caused acute agitation and confusional states in older persons (65, 69, 71). These authors have called for a more cautious approach to multiple drug use in the elderly.

We have studied factors that correlate with cognitive decline in 1264 elderly participants who attended a health screening program (82). Mini-Mental State Examination scores were used to identify risk factors for cognitive decline. Age, self-reported memory loss, and the presence of multiple disease states were the most important predictors of cognitive decline. The total number of drugs used was not an important predictor of cognitive function. Only one drug, dipyridamole, was associated with decreased scores on the Mini-Mental State Examination.

Magaziner and colleagues (60) studied medication use and functional decline in 609 women, aged 65 or older, in 20 contiguous census tracts of Baltimore, Maryland. After controlling for age, education, physical health, number of chronic conditions, and baseline functional status, prescription medication use was associated with a decline in ability to perform physical activities of daily living and an increase in symptoms of depression over a one-year period; however, no change was noted in cognitive functioning. The average number of medications reported was 3.45, and 10% of the women reported the use of five or more prescription medications.

POLYPHARMACY AS A CAUSE OF ACS: BARRIERS OF ATTRIBUTION AND CAUSALITY

Numerous factors have contributed to our lack of knowledge concerning the role of polypharmacy in producing ACS in the elderly. The most important factors are our present paradigm of adverse drug reaction reporting, lack of drug testing for cognitive impairment, and the nature of ACS. Current models for identifying and reporting drug-induced illness have discouraged reports of ACS caused by combination drug therapy. Most information on drug-induced disease has been derived from spontaneous reporting via the Food and Drug Administration's (FDA) voluntary reporting program and from published literature reports in the letters and brief communication sections of medical and pharmaceutical journals (43). Many investigators have proposed models to assist clinicians in detecting adverse drug reactions and assessing causality or attribution to a drug or drugs (8, 42, 43, 46, 50, 68). These models and the FDA reporting system (1639 reporting form) focus on the identification of a specific drug, or sometimes a drug interaction, as the causative agent that produces an adverse effect. To be identified as the etiologic agent, a drug should usually be known to cause the reaction and its administration should be temporally related to the adverse event. Ideally, the reaction should resolve on discontinuance of the drug (dechallenge) and recur when the drug is administered (rechallenge) to the patient (43, 50).

In the setting of an acute confusional state caused by the combination of ten different drugs, those criteria will not be fulfilled. An index of suspicion will probably not be raised to multiple drugs in combination as a cause of ACS. In most instances, physicians will not discontinue (dechallenge) all drugs, and if the patients' confusional state improved after dechallenge, a rechallenge would rarely be attempted. Most journal editors would lack interest in articles that describe ACS when the causative agent cannot be more clearly delineated (43, 44). As a result, there is a paucity of published reports describing ACS caused by polypharmacy. Another factor contributing to our lack of knowledge in this area is that little research had been conducted to evaluate the effect of drug therapy on cognitive impairment in the elderly. For many years, geriatric specialists have called for the FDA to establish requirements for drug testing in the elderly (79), as the pharmacokinetics and pharmacodynamics of many drugs differ in older pesons because of alterations in elimination and distribution.

Because multiple drug therapy is commonplace, new drugs should be tested to determine their propensity to interact with drugs commonly prescribed for older persons. Unfortunately, the FDA took nearly a decade to establish guidelines for drug testing in the elderly (79, 86). The new regulations should lead to safer, more effective drug therapy, but the guidelines still do not provide for evaluation of drug-induced cognitive impairment. Existing mechanisms do not ensure an appropriate evaluation of the potential for specific drugs, let alone drug combinations, to cause cognitive deterioration.

The nature of ACS makes it very difficult to assess drug-induced causes, especially to combination drug therapy. The clinical setting of an elderly patient with ACS is likely to be quite unstable. A patient who has eight to ten drugs prescribed by a physician probably has several acute or chronic illnesses that could each be a cause of ACS. The patient is probably anxious and concerned about issues of hospitalization, institutionalization, separation from spouse or family members, and death. Therefore, the patient likely has a drug or drug combination, a medical condition, and a psychologic state that could precipitate ACS. In this setting, nutrition and hydration usually are compromised as well. An ambulatory patient in this difficult state is also less able to follow medication administration instructions correctly, and medication errors may further complicate the situation.

When an ACS is recognized, several factors typically change rapidly. A patient with ACS quickly gains the attention of physicians and is admitted to a hospital. Fluid and electrolyte balance are assessed, and treatment is immediately started. Numerous drugs in the patient's regimen may be discontinued, while new drugs may be administered; health care workers ensure that drugs and dosages are administered correctly. The patient immediately receives increased attention, which may provide comfort and allay anxiety. Nutritional status probably improves, and better care is provided for the patient's acute and chronic illnesses. In 24–72 hours, the patient's ACS may improve or completely resolve. One then must determine whether the patient's improvement resulted from increased attention, changes in hydration and electrolyte balance, drug therapy, nutrition, or a combination of these factors. The settings of ACS clearly make attribution of drugs a difficult task.

POLYPHARMACY: AN UNCONTROLLED EXPERIMENT

It is impossible to predict the outcome of combining eight to ten different medications in an elderly patient. A scientist working in the laboratory would never add ten different chemicals at random to a test tube without first preparing for possible explosive consequences. Yet, ten, and sometimes more, medications are often given almost randomly to elderly persons without a clear understanding of possible untoward consequences. The ease of rationalizing expected therapeutic benefit from prescribing multiple drugs contrasts with our ability to predict deleterious side effects (59).

The interaction of two drugs administered to a patient has been a major area of interest for many scientists for nearly two decades (37). Even with carefully controlled experiments, it has been difficult to identify interacting properties when two drugs are given together. We are not aware of any attempts to conduct a scientifically designed study to determine the pharmacologic effects of combining five to ten drugs in the same patient. Loewe (59) attempted to apply scientific principles to the study of interactions between drugs more than two decades ago. However, he was never able to devise a satisfactory method for the simultaneous study of the effect of more than two drugs in combination. Therefore, one might consider it an uncontrolled experiment each time multiple drugs are prescribed for an older person.

The multiple pharmacologic effects possessed by a drug make it difficult to predict results of combination therapy. Few drugs have precise and narrow ranges of action. Thiazide diuretics, for example, produce many different effects, including decreased body water, sodium, chloride, and potassium and increased serum glucose, calcium, uric acid, cholesterol, and triglycerides (90). Any drug that has effects similar or opposite to these actions may interact with thiazide diuretics, thus producing additive or antagonistic effects. The difficulty of accurately predicting the effects of combining ten drugs can be appreciated.

There is ample evidence to demonstrate the hazards of multiple drug therapy. Smith et al (76) found an adverse reaction rate of 40% in patients given 16–20 drugs, compared with a rate of 7% in those given 6–10 drugs. May et al (63) studied the effects of multiple drug administration on adverse drug reactions in 10,518 patients who were hospitalized on a general medical service. They found a higher risk of adverse drug reactions for patients who received multiple drugs and speculated that the increased risk may result from drug interactions. Generally, the incidence of adverse drug reactions increases with the number of drugs administered (6, 17, 20, 31, 35, 39, 42, 48, 78).

It seems logical that if one drug is beneficial in treating one disease, then several drugs could benefit an elderly person with multiple diseases. Unfortunately, we have not reached the level of sophistication in pharmacology and therapeutics to test the above hypothesis. Until methods are developed to examine pharmacologic effects of multiple drug therapy, physicians caring for older persons must be continually vigilant for ACS from polypharmacy.

FUTURE STRATEGIES TO PREVENT POLYPHARMACY IN THE ELDERLY

The problems identified above clearly indicate that numerous factors contribute to polypharmacy in older persons. Currently, we do not know whether multiple drug therapy in the elderly is optimal or if it has a beneficial or detrimental effect on the quality of life. Therefore, this issue requires a concerted effort on the part of political leaders, educational institutions, governmental agencies, and the pharmaceutical industry to develop future strategies to deal with the concerns of polypharmacy.

Educational Strategies

A major effort is needed to develop educational programs about geriatric drug therapy for health professionals and consumers. Although the greying of the population has been predicted for many years, educational programs have not been implemented to accommodate these changes. Most physicians and other health care practitioners caring for the elderly have not had the benefit of geriatric education. Education planners, political leaders, government agencies, and private foundations should join forces to develop geriatric education programs that include rational use of medication in the curriculum of all health care providers.

A broad system of continuing education for current practitioners is needed to upgrade their knowledge base on drug therapy. Simultaneously, educational programs should be provided to elderly consumers concerning the risks and benefits of drug therapy and the techniques they can employ to make drug therapy safer, more effective, and less costly.

Drug Utilization Review

Sophisticated computer software will be needed to monitor therapy of the elderly prospectively and screen patients' therapy for inappropriate drug combinations. Computers could alert the pharmacists and prescribing physicians of multiple drug therapy in time to take corrective action.

The Medicare Catastrophic Care Act of 1988 included a provision that would have required participating pharmacies to maintain pharmacy records for all drugs dispensed and to offer to counsel patients on appropriate use of a dispensed drug and on potential interactions between drugs (32). Participating pharmacies also had to agree to use the electronic point-of-sale claim processing system through a computer terminal in the pharmacy. Although the legislation has been repealed, similar legislation has been enacted for Medicaid (2).

In our opinion, computerized records of prescriptions received by patients would be an important step to prevent problems of polypharmacy in the elderly.

Research

Research efforts must be intensified to document the problems of multiple drug therapy and ACS in the elderly. Many physicians can relate personal experiences in which ACS developed in an elderly person as a result of polypharmacy, yet there is a paucity of these reports in the medical and pharmacy literature. Health professionals should be encouraged to report these instances and document the public health importance of the problem.

Research is also needed to determine factors that predispose older persons to the problem of ACS and to identify the drug or drug combinations most likely to cause the problem.

SUMMARY

Cognitive impairment resulting from drug therapy in older persons has been well documented for numerous classes of drugs. Unfortunately, the problem of ACS caused by polypharmacy is rarely reported in the medical literature, although we believe that it occurs frequently. Health professionals need more education concerning the risks of drug therapy in older persons and methods of reducing the use of multiple drug therapy. Finally, more research is needed to identify patient and drug factors that lead to drug-induced ACS and cognitive decline in the elderly.

Literature Cited

1. Adler, S. 1974. Methyldopa-induced decrease in mental activity. *J. Am. Med. Assoc.* 230:1428–29

2. Am. Soc. Hosp. Pharm. Gov. Aff. Div. 1990. Summary of 1990 Medicaid drug rebate legislation. *Am. J. Hosp. Pharm.* 48:114–17

3. Baum, C. Kennedy, D. L., Forbes, M. B., Jones, J. K. 1984. Drug use in the United States in 1981. *J. Am. Med. Assoc.* 251:1293–97

4. Bedry, R., Dartigues, J. F., Gagnon, M. 1990. The role of benzodiazepine consumption on cognitive functioning in elderly French community residents. *J. Clin. Res. Pharmacoepidemiol. Abstr.* 4:135

5. Beers, M. H., Ouslander, J. G. 1989. Risk factors in geriatric drug prescribing: a practical guide to avoiding problems. *Drugs.* 37:105–12

6. Bennett, B. S., Lipman, A. G. 1977. Comparative study of prospective surveillance and voluntary reporting in determining the incidence of adverse drug reactions. *Am. J. Hosp. Pharm.* 34:931–36

7. Bergmann, K. Eastham, E. J. 1974. Psychogeriatric ascertainment and assessment for treatment in an acute medical ward setting. *Age Aging* 3:174–88

8. Berry, L. L., Segal, R., Sherrin, T. P., Fudge, K. A. 1988. Sensitivity and specificity of three methods of detecting adverse drug reactions. *Am. J. Hosp. Pharm.* 45:1534–39

9. Bianchine, J. R., Shaw, G. M. 1976. Clinical pharmacokinetics of levodopa in Parkinson's disease. *Clin. Pharmacokinet.* 1:313–38

10. Bond, A., Lader, M. 1981. After effects of sleeping drugs. In *Psychopharmacology of Sleep,* ed. D. Wheatley, pp. 177–97. New York: Raven

11. Branconnier, R. J., Cole, J. O., Ghazvinian, S., Rosenthal, S. 1982. Treating the depressed elderly patient: The comparative behavioral pharmacology of mianserin and amitriptyline. *Advances Biochem. Psychopharmacol.* 32:195–212

12. Bressler, R. 1987. Multiple Drug Use in an Elderly Man. *Hosp. Pract.* 111:127

13. Bushby, S. R. M., Hitchings, G. H. 1968. Trimethoprim, a sulfonamide potentiator. *Br. J. Pharmacol. Chemother.* 33:72–90

14. Caine, E. D. Weingartner, H. Ludlow, C. L., Cudahy, E. A., Whery, S. 1981. Qualitative analysis of scopolamine-induced amnesia. *Psychopharmacology* 74:74–80

15. Caranasos, G. J., Stewart, R. B. 1985. Clinically desirable drug interactions. *Annu. Rev. Pharmacol. Toxicol.* 25:67–95

16. Closson, R. G. 1983. Visual hallucinations as the earliest symptoms of digoxin intoxication. *Arch. Neurol.* 40:386

17. Cluff, L. E., Thornton, G., Seidl, L. 1965. Epidemiological study of adverse drug reactions. *Trans. Assoc. Am. Physicians* 78:255–68

18. Cohen, S. A. 1988. Delirious woman with disabling headaches. *Hosp. Pract.* 20:45–52

19. Cole, J. O., Branconnier, R., Saloman, M., Dessain, E. 1983. Tricyclic use in the cognitively impaired elderly. *J. Clin. Psychol.* 44:14–19

20. Colt, H. G., Shapiro, A. P. 1989. Drug-induced illness as a cause for admission to a community hospital. *J. Am. Geriatr. Soc.* 37:323–26

21. *Diagnostic and Statistical Manual of Mental Disorders.* Revised, 1987. Washington, DC: Am. Psychiatr. Assoc. 3rd ed.

22. Eisendrath, S. J., Goldman, B., Douglas, J., Dimatteo, L, VanDyke, G. 1987. Meperidine-induced delirium. *Am. J. Psychol.* 144:1062–65

23. Eisendrath, S. J., Ostroff, J. W. 1990. Ranitidine-associated delirium. *Psychosomatics* 31:98–100

24. Fincham, J. E., 1986. Over-the-counter drug use and misuse by the ambulatory elderly: a review of the literature. *J. Geriatr. Drug Ther.* 1:3–21

25. Folstein, M. F., Folstein, S. E., McHugh, P. R. 1975. Mini-mental state. *J. Psychiatr. Res.* 12:189–98

26. Ghoneim, M. M., Hinrichs, J. V., Mewaldt, S. P. 1984. Dose-response analysis of the behavioral effects of diazepam. I. Learning and memory. *Psychopharmacology* 82:291–95

27. Gillick, M. R., Serrell, N. A., Gillick, L. S. 1982. Adverse consequences of hospitalization in the elderly. *Soc. Sci. Med.* 16:1033–38

28. Goldstein, G., Materson, B. J., Cushman, W. C., Reda, D. J., Freis, E. D., et al. 1990. Treatment of hypertension in the elderly: II. Cognitive and behavioral function. *Hypertension* 15:361–69

29. Goodwin, J. S., Regan, M. 1982. Cognitive dysfunction associated with naproxen and ibuprofen in the elderly. *Arthr. Rheum.* 25:1013–15

30. Gordon, M., Preiksaitis, H. G. 1988. Drugs and the aging brain. *Geriatrics* 43:69–78

31. Gray, T. K., Adams, L. L., Fallon, H. J. 1973. Short-term intense surveillance of adverse drug reactions. *J. Clin. Pharmacol.* 13:61–67

32. Greenberg, R. B. 1988. Catastrophic coverage act of 1988. *Am. J. Hosp. Pharm.* 45:2518–25

33. Croog, S. H., Levine, S., Testa, M. A., Brown, B., Bulpitt, C. J., et al. 1986. The effects of antihypertensive therapy on the quality of life. *N. Engl. J. Med.* 314:1657–64

34. Grubb, B. P. 1987. Digitalis delirium in an elderly woman. *Digitalis Toxic.* 18:329–30

35. Grymonpre, R. E. Mitenko, P. A., Sitar, D. S., Aoki, F. Y., Montgomery, P. R. 1988. Drug-associated hospital admissions in older medical patients. *J. Am. Geriatr. Soc.* 36:1092–98

36. Hale, W. E., May, F. E., Marks, R. G., Stewart, R. B. 1987. Drug use in an ambulatory elderly population: a five year update. *Drug Intell. Clin. Pharm.* 21:530–35

37. Hansten, P. D., Horn, J. R., eds. 1989. *Drug Interactions.* Philadelphia: Lea & Febiger. 6th ed.

38. Helling, D. K., Lemke, J. H., Semla, T. P., Wallace, R. B., Lipson, D. P., Cornoni-Huntley, J., 1987. Medication use characteristics in the elderly: the Iowa 65+ Rural Health Study. *J. Am. Geriatr. Soc.* 35:4–12

39. Hoddinott, B. C., Gowdey, L. W., Coulter, W. K., Parker, J. M. 1967. Drug reactions and errors in administration on a medical ward. *Can. Med. Assoc. J.* 97:1001–6

40. Hodkinson, H. H. 1973. Mental impairment in the elderly. *J. R. Coll. Physicians London* 7:305–15

41. Hurwitz, N., Wade, O. L. 1969. Intensive hospital monitoring of adverse drug reactions to drugs. *Br. Med. J.* i:531–36

42. Hutchinson, T. A., Leventhal, J. M., Kramer, M. S., Karch, F. E., Lipman, A. G., Feinstein, A. R. 1979. An algorithm for the operational assessment of adverse drug reactions. II. Demonstration of reproducibility and validity. *J. Am. Med. Assoc.* 242:633–38

43. Jones, J. K. 1982. Criteria for journal reports of suspected adverse drug reactions. *Clin. Pharm.* 1:554–55

44. Jones, J. K. 1985. Adverse drug reaction considerations in geriatric drug research. *Drug Inf. J.* 19:459–68

45. Jorm, A. F., Korten, A. E., Henderson, A. S. 1987. The prevalence of dementia: A quantitative integration of the literature. *ACTA Psychiatr. Scand.* 76:465–79

46. Karch, F. E., Lasagna, L. 1977. Toward the operational identification of adverse drug reactions. *Clin. Pharmacol. Ther.* 21:247–54

47. Kasper, J. A., 1982. *Prescribed Medicines: Use, Expenditures and Source of Payment* (data preview 9, Natl. Health Care Expend. Study) Washington, DC: US Dep. Health Human Serv. Publ. No. (PHS) 82:3320

48. Kellaway, G. S. M., McCrae, E. 1973. Intensive monitoring of adverse drug effects in patients discharged from acute medical wards. *N. Z. Med. J.* 78:525–28

49. Kovar, M. 1977. Health of the elderly and use of health services. *Public Health Rep.* 92:9–19

50. Kramer, M. S., Leventhal, J. M., Hutchinson, T. A., Feinstein, A. R. 1979. An algorithm for the operational assessment of adverse drug reactions. I. Background, description and instructions for use. *J. Am. Med. Assoc.* 242:623–32

51. Kroenke, L. T. C. K., Pinholt, E. M. 1990. Reducing Polypharmacy in the Elderly: A Controlled Trial of Physicians Feedback. *J. Am. Geriatr. Soc.* 38:31–36

52. Larson, E. B., Kukull, W. A., Buchner, D., Reifler, B. V. 1987. Adverse drug reactions associated with global cognitive impairment in elderly persons. *Ann. Intern. Med.* 107:169–73

53. Larson, E. B., Reifler, B. V., Sumi, S. M., Canfield, C. G., Chinn, N. M. 1985. Diagnostic evaluation of 200 elderly outpatients with suspected dementia. *J. Gerontol.* 40:536–543

54. Levkoff, S. E., Besdine, R. W., Wetle, T. 1986. Acute confusional states (delirium) in the hospitalized elderly. *Annu. Rev. Gerontol. Geriatr.*, ed. C. Eisdorfer, 6:1–26. New York: Springer

55. Lipowski, Z. J. 1984. Acute confusional states (delirium). In M. L. Albert (Ed) *Clinical nerurology of aging*. (pp. 279–297). New York: Oxford University Press

56. Lipowski, Z. J. 1990. *Delirium: Acute Confusional States*, pp. 38. London: Oxford Univ. Press

57. Lipowski, Z. J. 1990. See Ref. 56, pp. 109

58. Lipowski, Z. J. 1990. See Ref. 56, pp. 47

59. Loewe, S. 1953. The problem of synergism and antagonism of combined drugs. *Arzneim. Forsch.* 3:285–90

60. Magaziner, J., Cadigan, D. A., Fedder, D. O., Hebel, J. R. 1989. Medication use and functional decline among community-dwelling older women. *J. Aging Health.* 1:470–85

61. Martin, D. C., Morycz, R. K., McDowell, J., Snustad, D., Karpf, M. 1985. Community-based geriatric assessment. *J. Am. Geriatr. Soc.*, 33:602–6

62. Mattila, M. J., Saarialho-Kere, U., Mattila, M. E. 1988. Effects of sertraline and amitriptyline on performance of healthy subjects over 50 years of age. *J. Clin. Psychol.* 49(Suppl. 8):52–58

63. May, F. E., Stewart, R. B., Cluff, L. E. 1977. Drug interactions and multiple drug administration. *Clin. Pharmacol. Ther.* 22:322–28

64. McEvoy, J. P., McCue, M., Spring, B., Mohs, R. C., Lavori, P. W., Farr, R. M. 1987. Effects of amantidine and trihexyphenidyl on memory in elderly volunteers. *Am. J. Psychol.* 144:573–77

65. Miller, F., Menninger, J., Whitcup, S. M. 1986. Lithium-neuroleptic neurotoxicity in the elderly bipolar patient. *J. Clin. Psychopharmacol.* 6:176–78

66. Miller, P. S., Richardson, S., Jyu, C. A., Lemay, J. S., Hiscock, M. 1988. Association of low serum anticholinergic levels and cognitive impairment in elderly presurgical patients, *Am. J. Psychiatr.* 145:342–45

67. Morrison, R. L., Katz, I. R. 1989. Drug-related cognitive impairment: Current progress and recurrent problems. In *Annu. Rev. Gerontol. Geriatr.* 9:232–79. New York: Springer

68. Naranjo, C. A., Busto, V., Sellers, E. M., Sandor, P., Ruiz, I. 1981. A method for estimating the probability of adverse drug reactions, *Clin. Pharmacol. Ther.* 30:239–45

69. O'Neil, C. K., Poirier, T. I. 1990. Confusion in the elderly patient. *US Pharm.* Aug:74–80

70. Ouslander, J. G. 1981. Drug therapy in the elderly. *Ann. Int. Med.* 95:711–22

71. Preskorn, S. H., Berber, J. H., Faul, J. C., Hirschfeld, R. M. A. 1990. Serious adverse effects of combining fluoxetine and tricyclic antidepressants. *Am. J. Psychiatr.* 147:532

72. Rep. R. Coll. Physicians, Coll. Comm. Geriatr.: Organic mental impairment in

the elderly. 1981. *J. R. Coll. Physicians London* 15:141–67

73. Scharf, M. B., Khosla, N., Lysaght, R., Brocker, N., Moran, J. 1983. Anterograde amnesia with oral lorazepam. *J. Clin. Psychol.* 44:362–64

74. Seifert, R., Jamieson, J., Gardner, R. 1983. Use of anticholinergics in the nursing home: An empirical study and review. *Drug Intell. Clin. Pharm.* 17:470–73

75. Seymour, D. G., Henschke, P. J., Cape, R. D. T., Campbell, A. F. 1980. Acute confusional states and dementia in the elderly: The role of dehydration, volume depletion, physical illness and age. *Age Ageing* 9:137–46

76. Smith, J. W., Seidl, L. G., Cluff, L. E. 1966. Studies on the epidemiology of adverse drug reactions. V. Clinical factors influencing susceptibility. *Ann. Intern. Med.* 65:629–40

77. Solomon, S., Hotchkiss, E., Saravay, S., Bayer, C., Ramsey, P., Blum, R. 1983. Impairment of memory function by antihypertensive medication. *Arch. Gen. Psychol.* 40:1109–12

78. Steel, K., Gertman, P. M., Crescenzi, C. 1981. Iatrogenic illness on a general medical service at a university hospital. *N. Engl. J. Med.* 304:638–42

79. Stewart, R. B. 1985. Clinical research in the elderly, An assessment of needs. *Clin. Res. Pract. Drug Regul. Aff.* 3:477–500

80. Stewart, R. B. 1990. Polypharmacy in the Elderly: A Fait Accompli? *Drug Intell. Clin. Pharm.* 24:321–23

81. Stewart, R. B., Cluff, L. E. 1971. Studies on the epidemiology of adverse drug reactions. VI: Utilization and interactions of prescription and nonprescription drugs in outpatients. *Hopkins Med. J.* 129:319–31

82. Stewart, R. B., Moore, M. T., May, F. E., Marks, R. G., Hale, W. E. 1991. Correlates of cognitive dysfunction in an ambulatory elderly population. *Gerontology* 37:272–80

83. Stewart, R. B., Moore, M. T., May, F. E., Marks, R. G., Hale, W. E. 1991. Changing patterns of therapeutic agents

in the elderly: A ten-year overview. *Age Ageing* 20:182–88

84. Sunderland, T., Tariot, P. N., Cohen, R. M., Weingartner, H. Mueller, E. A. III, Murphy, D. L. 1987. Anticholinergic sensitivity in patients with dementia of the Alzheimer's type and age-matched controls. *Arch. Gen. Psychol.* 44:418–26

85. Tucker, A. R., Ng, K. T. 1983. Digoxin-related impairment of learning and memory in cardiac patients. *Psychopharmacology* 81:86–88

86. US Dept. Health Human Serv. 1989. *Guidelines for the Study of Drugs Likely to Be Used in the Elderly.* Washington, DC: Public Health Serv., Food Drug Admin.

87. Varney, N. R., Alexander, B., MacIndoe, J. H. 1984. Reversible steroid dementia in patients without steroid psychosis. *Am. J. Psychiatr.* 141:369–72

88. Viukari, M., Jaatinen, P., Kylmamaa, T. 1983. Flunitrazepam, nitrazepam and psychomotor skills in psychogeriatric patients. *Curr. Ther. Res.* 33:828–34

89. Warshaw, G. A., Moore, J. T., Friedman, S. W., Currie, C. T., Kennie, D. C., et al 1982. Functional disability in the hospitalized elderly. *J. Am. Med. Assoc.* 248:847–50

90. Weiner, I. M. 1990. Diuretics and other agents employed in the mobilization of edema fluid. In *Goodman and Gilman's The Pharmacological Basis of Therapeutics,* ed. A. Gilman, T. Rall, A Nies, P. Taylor, pp. 718–21. New York: Pergamon. 8th ed.

91. White, L. R., Cartwright, W. S., Coronoi-Huntley, J., Brock, D. W. 1986. Geriatric epidemiology. In *Annu. Rev. Gerontol. Geriatr.,* ed. C. Eisdorfer, 6:215. New York: Springer

92. Williams, M. A., Campbell, E. B., Raynor, W. J., Musholt, M. A., Mlynarczyk, S. M., Crane, L. F. 1985. Predictors of acute confusional states in hospitalized elderly patients. *Res. Nurs. Health* 8:31–40

93. Wood, K. A., Harris, M. J., Morreale, A. 1988. Drug-induced psychosis and depression in the elderly. *Psychiatr. Clin. North Am.* 11:167–93

Annu. Rev. Publ. Health. 13:431-49

COGNITIVE IMPAIRMENT:
Dementia and Alzheimer's Disease

Eric B. Larson, Walter A. Kukull, and Robert L. Katzman

Departments of Medicine, Epidemiology, and Health Services, University of Washington, Seattle, Washington 98195; Department of Neurology, University of California, San Diego, California 92093

KEY WORDS: aging, epidemiology

INTRODUCTION

Of all the age-related syndromes, perhaps none is more strongly associated with aging than dementia. Dementia is defined as a syndrome of global loss of cognitive function, especially memory, sufficient to impair social or occupational function. Before the mid-1970s, dementia was considered a natural, indeed normal, consequence of aging. Alzheimer's disease (AD) was primarily considered a cause of presenile dementia, whereas so-called "senile dementia" (age 65+) was largely ignored by both the public and medical practitioners. Now we know that AD affects adults of all ages, but only rarely those under age 60. The prevalence increases dramatically for each age group over age 65, and AD is the most common condition to cause disability in "old old" persons over age 85. Concomitant with the aging of most advanced societies, the past decade has seen increasing awareness that dementia is a problem of immense importance to public health (1).

THE SYNDROME OF DEMENTIA

As a clinical term, dementia describes a syndrome of generalized mental deterioration that causes functional impairment (2). The most widely accepted formal definition of dementia is from the third edition of *Diagnostic & Statistical Manual of the American Psychiatric Association* (DSM-III) (3):

431

0163-7525/92/0501-0431$02.00

Dementia consists of impairment in short- and long-term memory, along with disturbances of other cognitive functions (e.g. abstract thinking, judgment, language, recognition) and/or personality change. The disturbance must be sufficient to interfere significantly with work, usual social activities, or relationships with others. Dementia is explicitly distinguished from an acute or short-lived episode of delirium and from focal loss of function, like isolated language problems (aphasia) or circumscribed memory loss (amnesia).

As individuals age beyond 65, decline is more variable. Furthermore, although environment and educational achievement clearly affect cognitive function at all ages, these effects are probably more important in older age groups. Because most dementing illnesses begin insidiously, the distinction between so-called "normal" age-related functional decline and early or mild dementia can be difficult until more information is known about the rate of decline and associated functional problems (2, 4, 5, 7). One key distinguishing feature is that age-related decline does not usually cause significant impairment of function (7). These persons are able to compensate and function independently. Also, the pace of decline due to dementing illness is greater (6), based on serial, layperson observations of general function and repeated neuropsychological measures of cognitive function (8, 9), usually after one year or at most two years of observation.

Underdetection or underrecognition of dementia by 20% or more has been demonstrated repeatedly in community-based studies and in hospital settings (10). The extent varies in different settings and depends on where one places the boundary between normal and abnormal age-related decline and the willingness of providers to examine mental function.

The dysfunction of dementia makes persons vulnerable in many ways (1). Demented persons are at risk of socioeconomic victimization and abuse. If they are isolated, they frequently suffer because of an inability to handle personal business and household affairs. They are at high risk of personal injuries from falls and accidents and can injure others if they operate complex machines, like automobiles. Finally, there are clear "medical" risks of dementia (11). Patients may not be able to take medication reliably or safely (12). They often cannot report problems to family or caregivers; as a result, medical problems are not detected until they are relatively far advanced (7). There are many causes of dementia; some causes, which can be effectively and easily treated, may lead to irreversible damage if not cared for promptly (11, 13). For these reasons, we conclude that underrecognition of dementia, especially in older persons, is a potentially serious problem.

CAUSES OF DEMENTIA

Like other common syndromes in medicine, dementia may be caused by many illnesses, which may present singly or in various combinations. It is a serious mistake to equate dementia with AD, even though in most countries it is probably the most common cause of dementia (1, 15). The distribution of illnesses that cause dementia has been the subject of much clinical research in recent years (13, 14). We know that in the US and Canada, AD is the most common cause (15). However, the distribution of Alzheimer's and other causes, especially multiinfarct dementia, the second most common cause, varies depending on the nature of the underlying population (13, 14). In predominantly Caucasian, middle-class, community-based populations, AD may be the cause of dementia in up to 90% or more cases (16). By contrast, in populations with larger numbers of blacks, especially with a high prevalence of untreated high blood pressure or diabetes, the proportion of multiinfarct dementia will be relatively greater, although AD is usually still more common (13, 14).

The Canadian Consensus Conference on Assessment of Dementia evaluated the overall prevalence of conditions that cause dementia (17). After AD and multiinfarct dementia, conditions judged to have moderate prevalence were Parkinson's disease, alcohol abuse, drug toxicity, and depression (though not an isolated cause of dementia). A long list of other causes includes chronic degenerative diseases of the nervous system (Pick's disease, Huntington disease, progressive supranuclear palsy), postanoxic or posttraumatic brain damage, brain tumor, normal pressure hydrocephalus, certain metabolic disorders (hypo- or hyperthyroidism, hyponatremia, hypercalcemia, hypoglycemia, renal failure, B12 deficiency, and other nutritional deficiencies), certain central nervous system infections [human immunodeficiency virus (HIV), neurosyphilis, and Creutzfeld-Jakob disease], neurotoxins (aluminum, mercury, and aromatic hydrocarbons), and the remote effects of carcinoma on the central nervous system (2, 17).

Some causes of dementia are more likely to contribute to the severity of dementia and patient dysfunction than they are to be the sole cause of dementia. Drug toxicity is a good example (12). Hearing loss, depression, and acute or subacute infections, like urinary tract infection, do not themselves cause dementia, but can make dementia worse and are called "sources of excess disability" (18, 19).

The heterogeneity of dementias is important for clinicians, investigators, and policy makers. Clinicians need to perform careful evaluations of patients to determine the causes and plan appropriate treatment and follow-up (11).

Research involving patients with AD can only begin after a careful diagnostic evaluation, which consists of a general history, physical, neurological, and neuropsychological evaluation, and laboratory investigation, to look for other causes of dementia. At present, there is no specific diagnostic test for Alzheimer's (20); the clinical diagnosis is probabilistic, with optimal sensitivity and specificity about 85–90% (21, 22).

For health planning, AD has a median survival of eight to ten years after onset (range 1–20 years) (23). Survival of multiinfarct dementia patients is usually shorter, although also highly variable and likely to be improved by control of risk factors for strokes and use of antiplatelet drugs, like aspirin or ticlopidine.

POPULATION AND AGE-SPECIFIC DISEASE RATES

Prevalence of Alzheimer's Disease and Dementia

There are two current approaches to estimate the prevalence of dementia and AD. The first is characterized by population sampling, a screening examination, diagnosis of the screen positives, and usually examination of a sample of the screen negatives to estimate the false-negative rate of the screening battery. The second approach identifies cases from well-documented medical records.

In European countries, the prevalence of dementia was 1–6% in persons aged 65 years or more, either based on National Health Service reports for primary identification of cases, or by using a screening instrument for cognitive impairment followed by a physician's examination to define the case (24–31).

From a sample of 6634 community-dwelling persons aged 55 or greater in Shanghai, China, Zhang et al (32) screened 5055 for cognitive impairment by using the Mini-Mental State Examination (33). Different cutoff scores were used depending on level of education. Screening was empirically estimated to have a sensitivity of 85% and a specificity of 93%. All screen positives, plus a 5% random sample of screen negatives, were subjected to a differential diagnosis of dementia. The prevalence of dementia was 4.6% among those persons aged 65 and older and 24.3% among those aged 85 and older; rates similar to those derived in the European studies are cited above (24–31). Approximately 65% of demented persons were classified as having AD. Female sex and low educational level were strongly related to dementia.

Pfeffer et al (34) used a similar design to estimate the prevalence of dementia in a retirement community. Persons scoring in the abnormal range on screening, plus a 14% sample of those who scored in the normal range, were referred for diagnosis. The screening battery included the Mini-Mental State Exam (33), a structured interview for demographics and past medical history, and an assessment of depression. Persons continuing to the next phase were examined by a neurologist, whose findings were reviewed blindly by another neurologist, followed by a consensus conference. Dementia of Alzheimer's type occurred in 15.3% of the community surveyed, including 35.8% of the 80+ age group. By excluding cases classified as questionable, the estimate decreased to 6.2% of those 65+ and 15.8% of those over age 80. Of course, the retirement community may have been enriched with cognitively impaired persons.

A widely cited study (16), which used the survey/screening approach, began with a census of persons over age 65 in East Boston, of whom 3623 (81%) received the initial memory testing. The sample receiving the full diagnostic examination for dementia included 52% (196) of 378 with poor memory, 9% (101) of 1108 with intermediate memory, and 8% (170) of 2137 with good memory. Sampling after screening, rather than before, was an innovation from the design used by Pfeffer et al (34). Standardized criteria (35, 36) were applied to the dementia diagnosis, but determining whether the observed intellectual deficit was "sufficient to interfere with social and occupational functioning" (a DSM-III criterion) was difficult in their survey, because the expected social and occupational functioning was closely tied to the social role expectations. Instead of measuring dysfunction, the investigators imputed from the examination and test scores the size of a deficit that would be expected to affect function. An accompanying editorial (37) noted that this procedure may overestimate prevalence by labeling persons ill who appear to fulfill their roles adequately.

The prevalence of AD in East Boston (16) was 10.3% in persons aged 65+, compared with 6.2% (or 15.3%) of the US retirement community (34), and 3.1% in Shanghai (32). For the over-85 age group in East Boston, the prevalence of AD was estimated to be 47%. Evans (15) estimates that 7.5–14.3 million persons in the US will have AD by the year 2050, of whom 4.7–10.5 million would be aged 85 of more, based on East Boston rates.

The three studies cited above went into the community to find cases. Kokmen et al (38) used the database of the Mayo Clinic and affiliated hospitals to determine the prevalence of dementia and AD in Rochester, Minnesota, by using a list of 26 diagnoses that possibly lead to dementia. Records of all persons alive on prevalence day (January 1, 1975) were searched for the existence of any of the diagnoses between 1959 and 1982, which then led to a detailed medical record review and evaluation of the person's dementia status according to established criteria (35, 36). For persons aged at least 65 years, the age and sex adjusted prevalence of dementia was approximately 3.5%; the prevalence of AD was 2.4% (12.6% for the 85+ age group). These rates are similar to those reported for Shanghai (32). The stability of the population-base in Rochester and the depth of the medical database available for computerized search make this type of study possible. However, dementia could go unrecognized either because one of the potential diagnoses was not used in the medical record, or because sufficient information was not available on review to make a diagnosis based on the criteria. We conclude that the results in Rochester and East Boston probably constitute lower and upper bounds for US estimates of prevalence of dementia and AD. In all studies, prevalence rates increase dramatically with age.

Incidence

The incidence of "medium and severe age psychosis" and organic brain syndrome per 100 person-years for the population over age 60 in Lundby, Sweden, during 25 years of observation (1947–1972) was calculated to be 1.6 for 1947–1957 and 1.1 for 1957–1972 (39). (For consistency, rates are reported here in person-years, even though some were originally estimated as cumulative incidence per annual population.) Incidence increased sharply with age: 5.8 and 3.3 per 100 person-years for the two time periods for the 80–89 age group (39).

Treves et al (40) conducted a study with the Israeli national neurologic disease register and a review of medical records of potential cases. For the data when "the first change in mental function consistent with a diagnosis of dementia" was noticed, the incidence of presenile dementia of the Alzheimer's type (ages 40–60) was found to be 0.002 per 100 person-years (2.4 per 100,000 population). Rates of disease appeared to increase with age in the same manner as dementia rates among older age groups. Thus, the authors inferred that presenile and "senile" disease may be part of the same continuum, rather than two separate diseases (40).

A longitudinal follow-up study (41) from the Bronx, New York, involved 434 nondemented persons aged 75 to 85, who were followed over a five-year period as part of a volunteer cohort. All subjects received a standardized examination at entry into the study and were evaluated annually with a cognitive test battery. If the test battery indicated abnormal decline, subjects were referred for a detailed dementia work-up. The cohort was 90% white, 64.5% female, and 70% Jewish. During the study, new cases of dementia were diagnosed, which led to an incidence rate of 3.5 per 100 person years, a result similar to the Lundby study (39). The incidence rate for Alzheimer's was 2.0 per 100 person years. Interestingly, higher scores (fewer errors) on the initial mental status test were associated with lower risk of subsequent (new) AD.

Studies utilizing the Mayo Clinic database and the population of Rochester, Olmsted County, Minnesota, involved cases with onset in 1960–1964 (42) and for three consecutive five-year periods ending in 1974 (43). Based on 178 dementia cases, the age-specific rates for AD increased from 0.1 per 100 person-years in the 60–69 age group to 0.5 in the 70–79 age group and to 1.4 per 100 person-years in the over 80 age group; these results are close to those for the 75–85-year-old cohort in the Bronx. The second study (43) confirmed the pattern of age-specific rates and concluded that the incidence of AD did not change during the 15-year time period. The 20-year follow-up through medical records allowed time for the diagnosis of AD to be substantiated, a feature unavailable to conventional cohort studies. Schoenberg (44) cautions that even the Rochester rates may be underestimates, because persons still may have not reached medical care or may have been unrecognized by providers. [However, these studies (41–43) serve as a benchmark for the incidence of AD in the US.]

EPIDEMIOLOGY OF ALZHEIMER'S DISEASE

Analytic epidemiologic studies have tested a wide variety of conditions and exposures for association with the onset of AD (see 44–47). In addition, a consortium of original investigators has analyzed pooled data from the major epidemiologic case control studies to arrive at potentially more stable estimates of risk, especially for those studies in which the numbers of subjects were small or the power low (48). Here, we summarize findings and describe how possible sources of bias might affect the strength of association with putative risk factors.

Family History

Estimates of increased risk to family members of AD patients are the most consistent of any factor investigated, except age (46). The estimates range from 1.0 (49) to 7.7 (50), with a crude mean of about 4.0 among seven case control studies (49–55).

One possibility for bias lies in the ascertainment of cases and controls and how the family members were diagnosed as AD. Because nondifferential misclassification of exposure (in this case family history) should reduce the risk estimate toward the null, any elevated (or decreased) observed risk is likely to be an underestimate of the true risk. If the misclassification is differential, rather than nondifferential, then the resulting risk estimate could be biased in either direction (56). The degree to which cases are self-selected to attend a referral-level specialty clinic for the diagnosis of AD arguably may be related to the family's previous experience with the disease. If the disease has occurred in other relatives, the patient or patient's caregiver may be more likely to recognize the onset of the disease and seek help. Because referral or specialty centers are the most commonly used source of cases for research studies, the occurrence of AD in relatives of cases that enter studies could be spuriously high. Another possible source of bias, which has not been studied, is a recall bias: Case informants may be more likely to recall dementia in other relatives than control informants. This is plausible, as informants' close association with the case may increase their awareness of dementia symptoms in more distant relatives, whereas control informants may be more likely to consider mild to moderate symptoms of dementia in other relatives just normal aging.

The definition of "family history" varies across studies; most often it is, appropriately, the occurrence of the AD in at least one other first-degree relative (parent, sibling, or child). Some studies loosely include any other family member who either has or had AD. Obtaining an accurate diagnosis of the affected relative based on the report of an informant relative is a significant problem (57); autopsy findings or medical records should be sought, but are often unavailable. Further problems arise from failure to consider the size of the family, the age of living family members, the age at death and cause of death of deceased family members, the age at onset of AD, or an estimate of the age-specific incidence of the disease (58, 59). Hughes (1991, in preparation) has developed a "familial risk" score for each family, which utilizes the items mentioned above. The classification of cases as familial or sporadic, therefore, becomes a stochastic process, by which some individuals have high probability of being true familial cases and others have a high probability of being true sporadic (nonfamilial) cases. The remainder, which is likely to be a substantial proportion, would have some intermediate probability attached to them and would necessarily remain unclassified.

Genetic linkage studies seek large pedigrees with many affected members to search for genetic markers. A family-history-positive pedigree that included a proband and one other relative would be of little value for genetic linkage studies. Large pedigrees with multiple affecteds are quite rare, and genetic heterogeneity appears to exist (63, 64). The relative importance of genetics in the etiology of AD is still a key question, but it is unlikely that crude measurements, such as "family history," identify homogeneous disease subgroups that could provide new information about genetic or environmental risk factors.

Head Trauma

Prior head trauma as a potential risk factor for AD has been evaluated in many of the current case-control studies (42–52, 55, 65–69). The rationale for the possible association of head injury and AD is based on the occurrence of dementia pugilistica (DP), the punch-drunk syndrome seen in boxers, in which continuous insult ultimately leads to neuron loss. Until recently, the pathological findings of DP and AD were thought to be distinct; the former exhibited an excess of neurofibrillary tangles and no amyloid plaques, the latter exhibited both plaques and tangles. Roberts et al (70) immunocytochemically demonstrated diffuse deposits of β-amyloid that were not evident previously with conventional staining methods. Thus, at least based on this molecular marker, DP and AD may share common pathogenetic mechanisms that lead to tangle and plaque formation.

Most studies have found that head trauma (with recovery) before the onset of AD occurs more frequently in AD cases than in controls. Point estimates of the odds ratio, which average about 2.9, vary from 0.6 (66) to 6.0 (49); however, the 95% confidence intervals for the odds ratios exclude 1.0 in only three of nine case control studies (50, 65, 67). History of head injury is usually obtained from surrogate respondents, who may be more likely to recall previous head injury as they seek explanations for the onset of AD.

Chandra et al (68) utilized the medical record system of the Mayo Clinic to identify all persons with head injuries and loss of consciousness who came to medical attention in a cohort of incident AD cases and matched control subjects. Of the 274 pairs, nine were discordant for head injury with loss of consciousness: five in which the case was injured, and four in which the control was injured. Because of the relative rarity of head injuries among the controls, the power to detect a true difference was diminished, even though the overall sample size was large. The authors concluded that, because their study found no difference and had no recall bias, head trauma with loss of consciousness was unlikely to be related to the onset of AD. They did not assess whether minor head injuries differed between cases and controls; this aspect may have been the basis of the findings of previous studies. Katzman et al (41) followed a cohort of 434 persons aged 75–85 for five years to determine the incidence of dementia and AD. No difference in the occurrence of prior head trauma was found for those who became cases. Recall bias was also minimized in this study, as head trauma data were collected before the clinical onset of disease.

The following are key questions that surround the evaluation of head trauma as a risk factor for AD:

1. What dose, in terms of frequency or severity, increases the risk of AD?
2. What proportion of AD is associated with head trauma? Is the AD associated with head trauma a specific subtype?
3. What is the optimum time at-risk between head injury and onset of AD?
4. Will seeking to prevent head injury have a measurable impact on public health by reducing the incidence of AD?
5. Is there a valid biologic marker for exposure to head injury?

If head trauma is a risk factor for AD, answers to these questions could lead to intervention strategies aimed at the prevention of head injury and, thus, AD.

Aluminum Exposure

Aluminum compounds have been found in the neurofibrillary tangles and the cores of plaques that occur in the brains of AD patients (71). Jacobs et al (72), however, found no difference in the levels of aluminum in AD and control brains. Aluminum is neurotoxic and has been implicated as a possible cause of encephalopathies related to dialysis (71, 73, 74), which have different clinical and pathologic characteristics from AD. But, aluminum is also very common, and daily intake, primarily from foodstuffs, may exceed 20 mg.

Attempts to monitor tissue concentrations of aluminum in serum, blood, hair, and urine have shown that these concentrations were not associated with dietary intake or age, nor were they stable over time (75).

Martyn et al (76) recently reported an increased risk of AD for persons who reside in water districts in which the aluminum content was 0.11 mg/l or greater, compared with 0.01 mg/l, associated with an estimated relative risk 1.5 (95% confidence interval 1.1–2.2). Alzheimer's cases included in the study were only those aged less than 70 years who had attended a cranial computed tomography clinic. No dose-response trend was evident.

A recent case-control study (77) of AD reported an association between aluminum-containing antiperspirants and onset of AD with an odds ratio of 1.6 (1.0, 2.4). A dose-response trend was observed for frequency of use. Paradoxically, the odds ratio for use of aluminum-containing antacids was 0.7 (0.3, 2.0), which possibly reflects differences in bioavailability of aluminum administered in different forms.

Among 1353 Canadian gold and uranium miners (78) who inhaled aluminum powder (McIntyre powder) before entering the mine, as prophylaxis against silicotic lung disease, neuropsychological testing classified significantly more exposed miners than nonexposed as having cognitive impairment, with relative risk of 2.6. The proportion of impaired miners rose with the years of exposure (78), but there was no greater occurrence of neurological problems or AD.

To carry the study of aluminum in the etiology of AD beyond the stage of controversy and conjecture, the biochemistry of aluminum and the identification of the particular forms specific to pathogenesis of AD must be described in detail. If AD and aluminum are linked, prevention will require methods for determining exposure and its temporal relation to the onset of disease.

Viruses

Infectious particles, e.g. prions, can cause spongiform encephalopathies, such as Creutzfeld-Jakob disease, scrapie, Kuru, and Gerstmann-Strausslar syndrome (79–81). Manuelidis et al (82) attempted to transmit AD to hamsters injected with buffy coat from AD patients. Their results were inconclusive; the affected hamsters developed spongiform changes and not AD pathology, which raises the possibility of contamination with spongiform agents.

Postmortem AD brain tissue has been tested for herpes viral DNA, with negative results (83, 84). Comparison of patients with AD, Down syndrome, and other causes of dementia with age-matched normal control subjects for cross-reactive antibodies to HIV type 1, caprine arthritis encephalitis virus, and equine infectious anemia virus revealed no cross reactive antibodies in cerebrospinal fluid or serum (85). Renvoize et al (86) found no difference in titer for Adenovirus, Chlamydia Group B, Coxiella burnettii, Cytomegalovirus, Herpes simplex virus, Influenza A, Influenza B, Measles, and Mycoplasma pneumoniae in 33 clinical AD patients and 28 psychiatric patients (86).

If AD is an infectious process, it is more likely to result from an unconventional virus or infectious protein than from more common viruses (80, 81, 86). However, detection techniques used to date (86) may not be sufficiently sensitive, and/or the tissues tested may not reflect the genesis of the disease.

Other Factors

Equivocal or unsubstantiated increased risk estimates have been found for maternal age, Down syndrome in relatives, thyroid disease, smoking, and sedentary lifestyle (44–47). Kokmen et al (87) have recently reported no increased risk for therapeutic radiation. Many other possible factors have been evaluated in the reported case-control studies without significant result.

Because molecular genetics has been proceeding rapidly in the study of AD (61–64), and because genetic heterogeneity is likely, the possibility of interactions between genotype and external risk factors must be considered in future epidemiologic studies. Ottman (88) recently outlined five generic ways in which the effects of risk factors and genotypes could combine.

BIOLOGY OF ALZHEIMER'S DISEASE

The biology of AD has been dominated for almost a century by the remarkable morphological changes, which were described in 1907 by Alois Alzheimer, in the brain of a patient who died at age 55 with a progressive dementia that involved memory, language, and behavioral changes (89): atrophy of the brain, especially involving the neocortex; the presence of abnormally staining neurons, the neurofibrillary tangles; and the presence of numerous neuritic plaques, focal collections of degenerating nerve terminals that surround a core of an abnormal fibrillar protein, β-amyloid (90, 91). The accelerating pace of AD research during the past several years has led to a series of remarkable findings, including quantitative analysis of the cellular changes, clinical-pathological correlations, and initial identification of the molecular aspects of these abnormal structures. These advances have made it possible to begin forming a clearer picture of AD as a chronic disorder in terms of the changes in the brain that characterize it.

One fundamental question is now being answered: "What causes dementia in Alzheimer's disease?" Cognitive impairment, measured by mental status testing, is caused by the loss of synapses (and neurons), particularly in frontal and parietal association neocortex. Important losses of nerve cells and synapses occur in other regions of the brain, such as the hippocampus, which is especially involved in new learning, and the amygdala, hypothalamus, and olfactory cortex, which are involved in emotional and behavioral changes. There is also major involvement of the basal forebrain cholinergic nuclei, the locus coeruleus noradrenergic nuclei, and dorsal raphe serotonergic nuclei. These are all systems that project primarily to neocortex and hippocampus, thus contributing their terminals as the presynaptic component to neocortical and hippocampal synapses.

Loss of synapses has been shown electron microscopically (92) and histologically (93, 94). Masliah et al (94) used antisynaptophysin, an antibody to one of the proteins that coat synaptic vesicles, to determine the density of synapses in association neocortex. The density of synapses measured with this antibody correlated extraordinarily well ($r > 0.7$) with measures of cognitive functions (95), including the Mini-Mental State Exam, the Information Memory Concentration test, and the Mattis Dementia Rating Scale, which were carried out during the year before death (95). These highly significant correlations were obtained on a cohort of AD patients that did not include cognitively normal subjects. By using a stepwise linear regression, approximately 90% of the variance in cognition during the last year of life could be accounted for by a model that primarily used the midfrontal and inferior parietal synaptic densities.

If the dementia is due to loss of synapses in neocortex, the next question is, "What causes this loss?" What is the sequence of events that leads to the abnormal changes in nerve cell bodies (neurofibrillary tangles), the development of neuritic plaques with their β-amyloid core, and the loss of synapses? Although the answer is unknown, the earliest stages in the pathogenetic sequence, as well as some aspects of later stages, are beginning to be understood.

One major hypothesis of pathogenesis concerns the role of the β-amyloid. This protein fragment has been sequenced (96), and the gene for the amyloid precursor protein (APP) has been mapped to chromosome 21 (97). The gene itself has now been sequenced (98); it codes for an interesting series of isoforms of APP, which differ by the presence or absence of a serine protease inhibitor insert. Amyloid precursor protein is a molecule produced normally by cells, including neurons, and is probably required for cell viability. The abnormal breakdown product, β-amyloid, accumulates in the core of the neuritic plaque, and a fragment of this polypeptide may itself be neurotoxic (99). The regulatory region for the APP gene contains primarily GC signals; thus, APP probably is a normally produced protein with a "housekeeping function." The region also contains two regulatory sites that could respond to injury, ischemia, and other insults—that is, a heat shock regulatory region and a C-fos regulatory region (100).

One hypothesis that has strong circumstantial support is that the first step in the development of AD, in at least some persons, is the laying down of small focal collections of the β-amyloid protein and its precursor protein (APP) in "diffuse plaques." Diffuse plaques precede neuritic plaques and neurofibrillary tangles by some years in at least the form of AD that develops in individuals with Down syndrome (101, 102). In Down syndrome, there is a triplication of chromosome 21, which results in three gene doses, not the two doses normally present on two chromosomes. The gene for APP is on chromosome 21 and is close to the beginning of that section of the chromosome involved in the production of Down syndrome. One could, therefore, assume that in Down syndrome, unusually large amounts of APP are formed, some of which are then broken down to the β-amyloid. Diffuse plaques are found as early as age 10 in brains studied at autopsy, whereas the full-fledged Alzheimer changes typically do not occur until age 30–40. Thus, a 10–25-year lag period may exist between the first production of the diffuse plaques and the development of further changes.

A second condition in which an abnormality of the APP gene produces amyloid disease occurs in a particular genetic form of familial AD. These particular kindreds have a mutation on the APP gene at a DNA nucleotide adjacent to the beginning of the sequence (near the carboxy terminal) for the β-amyloid peptide itself (63). This mutation probably makes the breakdown or degradation of APP into this peptide more likely to occur, thus leading to development of an early onset form of AD with symptoms often manifested during the fifth decade of life. Schellenberg et al (64) have provided evidence that this particular mutation is rare.

If head injury is a risk factor for AD (45–51), it could act, in part, by leading to the release of β-amyloid, with the production of diffuse plaques and eventual later onset of Alzheimer's. In this regard, the production of diffuse plaques might be analogous to various initiation events that precede malignancies. In the development of cancer, initial events often require some further carcinogenic event to set off the malignant process. For example, the first event in the pathogenesis of cervical cancer is infection by particular types of papilloma virus. But, a second carcinogenic event is required before the cells become malignant. Is this also true of AD? Does the production of the diffuse amyloid plaques simply act as an initiating factor, which then requires some second event to set off the full disorder?

During the symptomatic phase of AD, neuritic plaques and neurofibrillary tangles are formed, and nerve cells, particularly large neurons, and synapses are lost. The process of cell death in AD is not understood, but each neurofibrillary tangle is now known to be a degenerating neuronal body that contains thousands of abnormal fibrils, which are most commonly present in pairs of long, very thin fibers wound around each other in a helical fashion, the so-called paired helical filaments (103). These fibrils consist, at least in part, of accumulation of an abnormally phosphorylated form of a group of proteins, the Tau proteins. Tau proteins are normally expressed in nerve cell bodies during early development and are present in abundance only on axons during normal adult life; but, they accumulate in the cell body of neurons affected by the Alzheimer process. The "Alz-50" antibody, which has been used to identify Alzheimer brains immunochemically, reacts with a specific phosphorylated Tau epitope. Thus, the intracellular fibrous proteins in the nerve cells in the Alzheimer brain become abnormally phosphorylated. In addition to Tau and ubiquitin, otherwise normal neurofilaments present in these neurons become abnormally phosphorylated. There are alterations in several of the kinases, enzymes that control phosphorylation. Specifically, α-2 protein kinase C is markedly reduced (104). Casein kinase is elevated in cells associated with neurofibrillary tangles, but is generally reduced in the AD brain (105).

If these changes are essential to the development of the Alzheimer process, they suggest possibilities by which the disease might be modified or prevented pharmacologically. The laying down or abnormal degradation of APP into β-amyloid and the intracellular events, including the abnormal phosphorylation, that occur in later stages is of interest to several laboratories, including biotechnology and drug firms. Neurotrophic factors may be helpful. The cholinergic system in rat brains is controlled by a particular neurotrophic nerve growth factor (NGF). Administration of NGF to rats not only protects the cholinergic projection system from the basal nucleus of the forebrain to the cortex following experimental injury, but also improves the maze learning performance of impaired elderly rats. Whether a similar effect would occur in primates and humans is of intense interest.

The basal forebrain cholinergic projection system to neocortical association areas and hippocampus has received special attention, since its markers were found to be decreased by 70–90% (90, 91). The loss of choline acetyltransferase, a marker of cholinergic neurons, correlates well with degree of dementia, although not to the degree that loss of synapses does. The early finding of this cholinergic deficit led to numerous attempts to treat the disease by using cholinomimetic drugs that act directly upon the system or drugs that inhibit the breakdown of the remaining acetylcholine that is formed in the Alzheimer brain. One of the latter drugs, tetrahydroaminoacridine, whose chemical name is now tacrine, has received widespread publicity from a recent large national trial; tacrine does seem to produce mild cognitive improvement that lasts several months in a subset of Alzheimer patients (106). Although not yet well studied in humans, we suspect that an agent like NGF, which also acts primarily on this cholinergic system, may ultimately be more useful as therapy than cholinomimetic agents; at present, however, there is no convincing evidence that existing treatments modify the course of AD.

SUMMARY

The importance of dementia, a syndrome of global cognitive impairment, has gained widespread recognition in the past two decades. The most common cause, Alzheimer's disease, may be the single greatest source of dysfunction among persons over age 85. The disease, distinct from normal aging, is progressive, has a highly variable course, and can have tremendous impact on families. Duration of symptoms averages eight to ten years from onset, four to five years from diagnosis. Diagnosis is often delayed, because of the insidious nature of the illness.

Prevalence and incidence rates may vary severalfold between different studies. One consistent finding is the dramatic increase with age; prevalence rates are 25–48% for persons over age 85. The two most consistent risk factors for AD are age and positive family history. Another likely risk factor is head trauma. Alzheimer's disease is almost certainly due to heterogeneous causes.

Biologic understanding of AD is primarily based on study of distinctive pathologic changes in the brain. Increasingly well-characterized pathologic changes precede the clinical manifestation of disease. Ultimately, the pathologic cause of AD is loss of neurons and neuronal connections in the brain, especially in the frontal and parietal association neocortex. Many systems are involved, but the most affected system is the cholinergic system, followed by the noradrenergic and serotonergic neurotransmitter systems.

Drug treatment and other intervention strategies to prevent or delay progression of the disease have been limited, primarily because so little is known about the cause or risk factors for the disease. Current palliative treatments are attempts to minimize the morbidity of abnormal behaviors and medical complications associated with dementia. Ideally, treatment would either involve replacement therapy or drugs, which prevent or delay the pathologic changes that occur in AD. Two of the more promising experimental therapeutic attempts involve interruption of the pathogenetic events involving β-amyloid and its precursor proteins and administration of NGF. Public health attempts at risk factor reduction are clearly premature.

The next decade or two will likely witness improved understanding of the pathogenesis of Alzheimer's disease. Epidemiologic study will contribute to our knowledge of pathogenesis and may reveal heretofore unrecognized and, hopefully, modifiable risk factors. Social and clinical strategies to deal with a disease of such immense importance also needs development and evaluation. The public's interest in this disease is intense, and it looks to the scientific community for progress in understanding and managing this often tragic illness.

Literature Cited

1. US Congr., Off. Technol. Assess. 1987. *Losing a Million Minds: Confronting the Tragedy of Alzheimer's Disease and Other Dementias*. OTA-BA-323. Washington, DC: GPO
2. Larson, E. B., Lo, B., Williams, M. E. 1986. Evaluation and care of elderly patients with dementia. *J. Gen. Intern. Med.* 1:116–26
3. *Diagnostic and Statistical Manual of Mental Disorders*, pp. 103–7. 1987. Washington, DC: Am. Psychiatr. Assoc. 3rd ed.
4. Adams, R. A., Victor, M. 1977. *Principles of Neurology*, pp. 396–405. New York: McGraw-Hill
5. Schock, N. W. 1962. The physiology of aging. *Sci. Am.* 206:100–18
6. Wang, H. S. 1985. Dementia in old age. In *Dementia*, ed. C. E. Wells. Philadelphia: Davis
7. Larson, E. B., Featherstone, H. J., Reifler, B. V., Canfield, C. G., Chinn, N. W. 1985. Medical aspects of care of elderly patients with cognitive impairment. *Dev. Neuropsychiatry* 2:145–71
8. Krenz, C., Larson, E. B., Buchner, D. M., Canfield, C. G. 1988. Characterizing patient dysfunction in Alzheimer's type dementia. *Med. Care* 26:453–61
9. van Belle, G., Uhlmann, R. F., Hughes, J. P., Larson, E. B. 1990. Reliability of estimates of changes in mental status test performance. *J. Clin. Epidemiol.* 43:589–95
10. Roca, R. P., Klein, L. E., Kirby, J. M. 1984. Recognition of dementia among medical inpatients. *Arch. Intern. Med.* 144:73–75
11. Larson, E. B., Reifler, B. V., Featherstone, H. J., English, D. R. 1984. Dementia in elderly outpatients: A prospective study. *Ann. Intern. Med.* 100:417–23
12. Larson, E. B., Kukull, W. A., Buchner, D. M., Reifler, B. V. 1987. Adverse drug reactions associated with global cognitive impairment in elderly persons. *Ann. Intern. Med.* 107:169–73
13. Clarfield, A. M. 1988. The reversible dementias: Do they reverse? *Ann. Intern. Med.* 109:476
14. Barry, P. B., Moskowitz, M. A. 1988. The diagnosis of reversible dementia in the elderly: A critical review. *Arch. Intern. Med.* 148:1914
15. Evans, D. A. 1990. Estimated prevalence of Alzheimer's disease in the United States. *Milbank Fund. Q.* 68:267–289

16. Evans, D. A., Funkenstein, H. H., Albert, M. S., Silers, P. A., Cook, N. R., et al. 1989. Prevalence of Alzheimer's disease in a community population of older persons: Higher than previously reported. *J. Am. Med. Assoc.* 262:2251–56
17. Can. Consens. Conf. Assess. Dementia. 1991. Toronto: Can. Print. Off.
18. Larson, E. B., Buchner, D. M., Uhlmann, R. F., Reifler, B. V. 1986. Caring for elderly patients with dementia. *Arch. Intern. Med.* 146:1909–10
19. Reifler, B. V., Larson, E. B. 1988. Excess disability in demented elderly outpatients. *J. Am. Geriatr. Soc.* 36:82–83
20. Hughes, J. P., van Belle, G., Kukull, W. A., Larson, E. B., Teri, L. 1989. On the uses of registries for Alzheimer's disease. *Alzheimer's Dis. Relat. Disord. J.* 3(4):205–17
21. Kukull, W. A., Larson, E. B., Reifler, B. V., Lampe, T. H., Yerby, M. S., Hughes, J. S. 1990. The validity of three clinical diagnostic criteria for Alzheimer's disease. *Neurology* 40:1364–69
22. McCormick, W. C., Larson, E. B. 1990. Pragmatism and probabilities in dementia. *Hosp. Pract.* Dec:93–104
23. Walsh, J. S., Welch, H. G., Larson, E. B. 1990. Survival of outpatients with Alzheimer-type dementia. *Ann. Intern. Med.* 113(6):429–34
24. Akesson, H. O. 1969. A population study of senile and arteriosclerotic psychoses. *Hum. Hered.* 19:546–66
25. Broe, G. A., Akhtar, A. J., Andrews, G. R., Caerd, F. I., Gilmore, A. J. J., et al. 1976. Neurological disorders in the elderly at home. *J. Neurol. Neurosurg. Psychiatry* 39:362–66
26. Kay, D. W. K., Beamesh, P., Roth, M. 1964. Old age mental disorders in Newcastle upon Tyne. Part I: a study of prevalence. *Br. J. Psychiatry* 110:146–58
27. Kay, D. W. K., Bergman, K., Foster, E. M., McKechnie, A. A., Roth, M. 1970. Mental illness and hospital usage in the elderly: a random sample followed-up. *Compr. Psychiatry* 11:26–35
28. Molsa, P. K., Marttila, R., Rinne, U. K. 1982. Epidemiology of dementia in a Finnish population. *Acta Neurol. Scand.* 65:541–52
29. Sulkava, R., Wikstrom, J., Aromaa, A., Raitasalo, R., Lehtinen, V. et al. 1985. Prevalence of severe dementia in Finland. *Neurology* 35:1025–29

30. Primrose, E. J. R. 1962. *Psychological Illness, a Community Study*. Springfield: Thomas

31. Essen-Moller, E. 1956. Individual traits and morbidity in a Swedish rural population. *Acta Psychiatr. Scand.* (Suppl. 100)

32. Zhang, M., Katzman, R., Salmon, D., Jin, H., Cai, G. et al. 1990. The prevalence of dementia and Alzheimer's disease in Shanghai, China: the impact of age, gender, and education. *Ann. Neurol.* 27:428–37

33. Folstein, M. F., Folstein, S. E., McHugh, P. R. 1975. Mini-Mental State: a practical method of grading the cognitive state of patients for the clinicians. *J. Psychiatr. Res.* 12:189–98

34. Pfeffer, R. I., Afifi, A. A., Chance, J. M. 1987. Prevalence of Alzheimer's disease in a retirement community. *Am. J. Epidemiol.* 125:420–36

35. McKhann, G., Drachman, D., Folstein, M., Katzman, R., Price, D., et al. 1984. Clinical diagnosis of Alzheimer's disease: report of the NINCDS-ADRDA work group under the auspices of the Department of Health and Human Services task force on Alzheimer's disease. *Neurology* 34:939–44

36. Am. Psychiatr. Assoc. 1980. *Diagnostic and Statistical Manual of Mental Disorders*. Washington, DC: Am. Psychiatr. Assoc.

37. Larson, E. B. 1989. Alzheimer's disease in the community (editorial). *J. Am. Med. Assoc.* 262:2591–92

38. Kokmen, E., Beard, M., Offord, K. P., Kurland, L. T. 1989. Prevalence of medically diagnosed dementia in a defined United States population: Rochester Minnesota, January 1, 1975. *Neurology* 39:773–76

39. Hagnell, O., Lanke, J., Rorsman, B., Ojesjo, L. 1981. Does the incidence of age psychosis decrease? A prospective longitudinal study of a complete population investigated during the 25-year period 1947–1972: the Lundby study. *Neuropsychobiology* 7:201–11

40. Treves, T., Korczyn, A. D., Zilber, N., Kahana, E., Leibowitz, Y., et al. 1986. Presenile dementia in Israel. *Arch. Neurol.* 43:26–29

41. Katzman, R., Aronson, M., Fuld, P., Kawas, C., Brown, T., et al. 1989. Development of dementing illnesses in an 80-year-old volunteer cohort. *Ann. Neurol.* 25:317–24

42. Schoenberg, B. S., Kokmen, E., Okazaki, H. 1987. Alzheimer's disease and other dementing illnesses in a defined United States population: incidence rates and clinical features. *Ann. Neurol.* 22:724–29

43. Kokmen, E., Chandra, V., Schoenberg, B. S. 1988. Trends in the incidence of dementing illness in Rochester, Minnesota in three quinquennial periods 1960–1974. *Neurology* 38:975–80

44. Henderson, A. S. 1986. The epidemiology of Alzheimer's disease. *Br. Med. Bull.* 42:3–10

45. Rocca, W. A., Amaducci, L. A., Schoenberg, B. S. 1986. The epidemiology of clinically diagnosed Alzheimer's disease. *Ann. Neurol.* 19:415–24

46. Rocca, W. A., Amaducci, L. A. 1991. Epidemiology of Alzheimer's disease. In *Neuroepidemiology*, ed. D. W. Anderson, pp. 55–96. Boca Raton, Fla: CRC

47. Schoenberg, B. S. 1986. Epidemiology of Alzheimer's disease and other dementing illnesses. *J. Chron. Dis.* 39:1095–1104

48. van Duijin, C. M., Stidnen, T., Hofman, A. for the EURODEM risk factors group. 1991. Risk factors for Alzheimer's disease: Overview of the EU-RODEM collaborative reanalysis of case-control studies. *Int. J. Epidemiol.* 2(Suppl. 2):S4–12

49. Chandra, V., Philipose, V., Bell, P. A., Lazaroff, A., Schoenberg, B. S. 1987. Case-control study of late onset "probable Alzheimer's disease." *Neurology* 37:1295–1300

50. Heyman, A., Wilkinson, W. E., Stafford, J. A., Helms, M. J., Sigmon, A. H., et al. 1984. Alzheimer's disease: a study of epidemiological aspects. *Ann. Neurol.* 15:335–41

51. Amaducci, L. A., Fratiglioni, L., Rocca, W. A., Fieschi, C., Livrea, P., et al. 1986. Risk factors for clinically diagnosed Alzheimer's disease: a case-control study of an Italian population. *Neurology* 36:922–31

52. Shalat, S. L., Seltzer, B., Pidcock, C., Baker, E. L. Jr. 1987. Risk factors for Alzheimer's disease: a case-control study. *Neurology* 37:1630–33

53. Graves, A. B., White, E., Koepsell, T. D., Reifler, B. V., van Belle, G., et al. 1990. A case-control study of Alzheimer's disease. *Ann. Neurol.* 28:766–74

54. Hofman, A., Schulte, W., Tanja, T. A., van Duijin, C. M., Haaxma, R., et al. 1989. History of dementia and Parkinson's disease in 1st-degree relatives of patients with Alzheimer's disease. *Neurology* 39:1589–92

55. Broe, G. A., Henderson, A. S., Creasy, H., McCusker, E., Korten, A. E., et al. 1990. A case-control study of Alzheim-

er's disease in Australia. *Neurology* 40:1698–1707

56. Kleinbaum, D. G., Kupper, L. L., Morgenstein, H. 1982. *Epidemiologic Research Principles and Quantitative Methods*. Belmont, Calif: Lifetime Learning

57. Kukull, W. A., Larson, E. B. 1989. Distinguishing Alzheimer's disease from other dementias: questionnaire responses of close relatives and autopsy results. *J. Am. Geriatr. Soc.* 37:521–27

58. Cupples, L. A., Terrin, N. C., Myers, R. H., D'Agostino, R. B. 1989. Using survival methods to estimate age-at-onset distributions for genetic diseases with an application to Huntington's disease. *Genet. Epidemiol.* 6:361–71

59. Farrer, L. A., Myers, R. H., Cupples, L. A., St. George-Hyslop, P. H., Bird, T. D., et al. 1990. Transmission and age-at-onset patterns in familial Alzheimer's disease, evidence for heterogeneity. *Neurology* 40:395–403

60. Deleted in proof

61. St. George-Hyslop, P. H., Tanzi, R. E., Polinsky, R. J., Haines, J. L., Nee, L., et al. 1987. The genetic defect causing familial Alzheimer's disease maps to Chromosome 21. *Science* 235:885–89

62. Schellenberg, G. D., Bird, T. D., Wijsman, E. M., Moore, D. K., Boehnke, M., et al. 1988. Absence of linkage of Chromosome 21 q 21 markers to familial Alzheimer's disease. *Science* 241:1507–10

63. Goate, A., Chartier-Harlin, M., Mullen, J., Brown, F., Crawford, L., et al. 1991. Segregation of a missense mutation in the amyloid precursor protein gene with familial Alzheimer's disease. *Nature* 349:704–6

64. Schellenberg, G. D., Anderson, L., O'Dahl, S., Wijsman, E. M., Sadovnick, A. D., et al. 1991. APP 717, APP 693 and PRIP gene mutations are rare in Alzheimer's disease. *Am. J. Hum. Genet.* 49:511–17

65. Mortimer, J. A., French, L. R., Hutton, J. T., Schuman, L. M. 1985. Head injury as a risk factor for Alzheimer's disease. *Neurology* 35:264–67

66. Sulkava, R., Erkinjuntti, T., Palo, J. 1985. Head injuries in Alzheimer's disease and vascular dementia. *Neurology* 35:1804

67. Graves, A. B., White, E., Koepsell, T. D., Reifler, B. V., van Belle, G., et al. 1990. The association between head trauma and Alzheimer's disease. *Am. J. Epidemiol.* 131:491–501

68. Chandra, V., Kokmen, E., Schoenberg, B. S., Beard, C. M. 1989. Head trauma

with loss of consciousness as a risk factor for Alzheimer's disease. *Neurology* 39:1576–78

69. Gedye, A., Beattie, B. L., Tuokko, H., Horton, A., Kosarek, E. 1989. Severe head injury hastens the onset of Alzheimer's disease. *J. Am. Geriatr. Soc.* 37:970–73

70. Roberts, G. W., Allsop, D., Bruton, C. 1990. The occult aftermath of boxing. *J. Neurol. Neurosurg. Psychiatry* 53:373–78

71. McLachlan, D. R., Lukiw, W. J., Kruck, T. P. 1989. New evidence for an active role of aluminum in Alzheimer's disease. *Can. J. Neurol. Sci.* 16 (Suppl. 4):490–97

72. Jacobs, R. W., Duong, T., Jones, R. E., Trapp, G. A., Scheibel, A. B. 1989. A re-examination of aluminum in Alzheimer's disease: analyses by energy-dispersive x-ray microprobe and flameless atomic absorption spectrophotometry. *Can. J. Neurol. Sci.* 16 (Suppl. 4):498–503

73. Roskams, A. J., Connor, J. R. 1990. Aluminum access to the brain: a role for transferrin and its receptor. *Proc. Natl. Acad. Sci. USA* 87:9024–27

74. Hewitt, C. D., Savory, J., Wills, M. R. 1990. Aspects of aluminum toxicity. *Clin. Lab. Med.* 10:403–22

75. Naylor, G. J., Sheperd, B., Treliving, L., McHarg, A., Smith, A., et al. 1990. Tissue concentration stability over time, relationship to age, and dietary intake. *Biol. Psychiatry* 27:884–90

76. Martyn, C. N., Barker, D. J., Osmond, C., Harris, E. C., Edwardson, J. A., et al. 1989. Geographical relation between Alzheimer's disease and aluminum in drinking water. *Lancet* 1(8629):59–62

77. Graves, A. B., White, E., Koepsell, T. D., Reifler, B. V., van Belle, G., et al. 1990. The association between aluminum-containing products and Alzheimer's disease. *J. Clin. Epidemiol.* 43:35–44

78. Rifat, S. L., Eastwood, M. R., McLachlan, D. R., Corey, P. N. 1990. Effect of exposure of miners to aluminum powder. *Lancet* 336:1162–65

79. Prusiner, S. B. 1987. Prions and neurodegenerative diseases. *N. Engl. J. Med.* 317:1571–81

80. Masters, C. L., Beyreuther, K. 1987. Neuronal origin of cerebral amyloidogenic proteins: their role in Alzheimer's disease and unconventional virus diseases of the nervous system. *Ciba Found. Symp.* 126:49–64

81. Masters, C. L., Beyreuther, K. 1988. Neuropathology of unconventional virus

infections: molecular pathology of spongeform change and amyloid plaque deposition. *Ciba Found. Symp.* 135:24–36

82. Manuelidis, E. E., deFigueiredo, J. M., Kim, J. H., Fritch, W. W., Manuelidis, L. 1988. Transmission studies from blood of Alzheimer's disease patients and healthy relatives. *Proc. Natl. Acad. Sci. USA* 85:4898–91

83. Deatly, A. M., Haase, A. T., Fewster, P. H., Lewis, E., Ball, M. J. 1990. Human herpes virus infections and Alzheimer's disease. *Neuropathol. Appl. Neurobiol.* 16:213–223

84. Walker, D. G., O'Kusky, J. R., McGeer, P. L. 1989. In situ hybridization analysis for herpes simplex virus nucleic acids in Alzheimer's disease. *Alzheimer Dis. Assoc. Disord.* 3:123–31

85. Friedland, R. P., May, C., Dahlberg, J. 1990. The viral hypothesis of Alzheimer's disease absence of antibodies to lentiviruses. *Arch. Neurol.* 47:177–78

86. Renvoize, E. B., Awad, I. O., Hambling, M. H. 1987. A sero-epidemiological study of conventional infectious agents in Alzheimer's disease. *Age Aging* 16:311–14

87. Kokmen, E., Beard, C. M., Bergstrath, E., Anderson, J. A., Earle, J. D. 1990. Alzheimer's disease and prior therapeutic radiation exposure: a case-control study. *Neurology* 40:1376–79

88. Ottman, R. 1990. An epidemiologic approach to gene-environment interaction. *Genet. Epidemiol.* 7:177–85

89. Alzheimer, A. 1907. Uber eine eigenartige Erkrankung der Hirnrinde. *Alg. Z. Psychiatrie* 64:164–68

90. Katzman, R. 1986. Alzheimer's disease. *N. Engl. J. Med.* 314:964–73

91. Katzman, R., Saitoh, T. 1991. Advances in Alzheimer's disease. *FASEB J.* 5:278–86

92. DeKosky, S. T., Scheff, S. W. 1990. Synapse loss in frontal cortex biopsies in Alzheimer's disease: Correlation with cognitive severity. *Ann. Neurol.* 27:457–64

93. Hamos, J. E., DeGennaro, L. J., Drachman, D. A. 1989. Synaptic loss in Alzheimer's disease. *Neurology* 39:355–61

94. Masliah, E., Terry, R. D., DeTeresa, R., Hansen, L. A. 1989. Immunohistochemical quantification of the synapse related protein synaptophysin in Alzheimer disease. *Neurosci. Lett.* 103:234–38

95. Terry, R. D., Masliah, E., Salmon, D.,

Butters, N., DeTeresa, R., et al. 1991. Physical basis of cognitive alterations in Alzheimer disease: Synapse loss is the major correlate of cognitive impairment. *Ann. Neurol.* In press

96. Glenner, C. G., Wong, C. W. 1984. Alzheimer's disease: Initial report of the purification and characterization of a novel cerebrovascular amyloid protein. *Biochem. Biophys. Res. Commun.* 120: 885–90

97. Goldgaber, D., Lerman, M. I., McBride, O. W., Saffiotti, U., Gajdusek, D. C. 1987. Characterization and chromosomal localization of a cDNA encoding brain amyloid of Alzheimer's disease. *Science* 235:877–80

98. Kang, J., Lemaire, H. G., Unterbeck, A., Salbaum, M. J., Masters, C. L., et al. 1987. The precursor of Alzheimer's disease amyloid A4 protein resembles a cell-surface receptor. *Nature* 325:733–36

99. Yankner, B. A., Dawes, L. R., Fisher, S., Villa-Komaroff, L., OsterGranite, M. L., Neve, R. L. 1989. Neurotoxicity of a fragment of the amyloid precursor associated with Alzheimer's disease. *Science* 245:417

100. Salbaum, J. M., Weidemann, A., Lemaire, H. L., Masters, C. L., Beyreuther, K. 1988. The promoter of Alzheimer's disease amyloid A4 precursor gene. *EMBO J.* 7:2807–13

101. Giaccone, G., Tagliavini, F., Linoli, G., Bouras, D., Frigeri, O. L., et al. 1989. Down patients: Extracellular preamyloid deposits precede neuritic degeneration and senile plaques. *Neurosci. Lett.* 97:232–38

102. Rumble, B., Retallack, R., Hilbich, C., Simms, G., Multhaup, G. B. 1989. Amyloid A4 protein and its precursor in Down's syndrome and Alzheimer's disease. *N. Engl. J. Med.* 320:1446–52

103. Kosik, K. S. 1989. The molecular and cellular pathology of Alzheimer neurofibrillary lesions. *J. Gerontol.* 44:B55–58

104. Masliah, E., Cole, G., Shimohama, S., Hansen, L., DeTeresa, R., et al. 1990. Differential involvement of protein kinase C isozymes in Alzheimer's disease. *J. Neurosci.* 10:2113–24

105. Iimoto, D. S., Masliah, E., DeTeresa, R., Terry, R. D., Saitoh, T. 1990. Aberrant casein kinase II in Alzheimer's disease. *Brain Res.* 507:273–80

106. Eagger, S. A., Levy, R., Sahakian, B. J. 1991. Tacrine in Alzheimer's disease. *Lancet* 337:989–92

Annu. Rev. Publ. Health. 1992. 13:451–68

EFFECTS OF PHYSICAL ACTIVITY ON HEALTH STATUS IN OLDER ADULTS I: Observational Studies[1]

Edward H. Wagner[1] and Andrea Z. LaCroix[2]

Center for Health Studies, Group Health Cooperative of Puget Sound, Seattle, Washington 98101; Departments of [1]Health Services and [2]Epidemiology, University of Washington, Seattle, Washington 98195

David M. Buchner[3] and Eric B. Larson

Departments of Health Services and Medicine, University of Washington, Seattle, Washington; [3]Northwest Health Services Research and Development Field Program, Seattle VA Medical Center, Seattle, Washington

All authors associated with Center for Health Promotion in Older Adults, School of Public Health, University of Washington, which is supported by grant R48/CCR002181-05 from the Centers for Disease Control.

KEY WORDS: exercise, disability

All parts of the body which have a function, if used in moderation and exercised in labors to which each is accustomed, become thereby well-developed and age slowly; but if unused and left idle, they become liable to disease, defective in growth and age quickly.

Hippocrates

INTRODUCTION

The prevention of disability and the preservation of independence have become the clinical and policy priorities for the health care of older adults

451

(84). Aging is characterized by a diffuse loss of physiologic capacity and reserve and reduced ability to adapt to challenges. Almost without exception, both cross-sectional and cohort studies demonstrate declines in average physiologic performance or capacity with advancing age. There had been a tendency to assume that such functional declines were genetically programmed and, as a result, inevitable. However, in reviewing the various declines in function with age found by the Baltimore Longitudinal Study of Aging, Shock (77) noted that "the effects of age are highly individual, and chronological age alone is a poor index of physiologic function."

Investigators have noticed that many older subjects evidenced minimal or no decline. Rowe & Kahn (72) suggested that this preservation of function represents "successful aging" and that the steep mean declines in function assumed to be "normal" or "usual" may not be inevitable consequences of growing older. The challenge inherent in this revised view of aging is to identify the extrinsic determinants of decline (36, 72) and intervene upon those that are mutable.

In this paper, we examine the observational evidence concerning the effects on physical health of one potentially deleterious and mutable extrinsic factor—inactivity. Our primary focus is on the evidence linking inactivity to disability and frailty or reduced physiologic reserve. We also discuss the closely related literature concerning the association in older adults between inactivity and depression, fractures, coronary heart disease, and mortality.

A companion paper (15) considers the experimental evidence that increasing activity reduces or eliminates functional decline. The experimental data to date are limited by short follow-up intervals, highly selected participants, and interventions largely aimed at increasing vigorous activities. The observational evidence reviewed in this paper, therefore, furnishes complementary information about the health effects of the full distribution of physical activities in broader segments of the population over longer time periods.

The methodologic limitations of observational studies of activity and health have been well described (52). Observational studies are limited by the well-known difficulties of validly measuring physical activity (53) and the selective forces that lead individuals to adopt various patterns of activity. In this review, we pay close attention to the method of measuring activity in key studies. Because healthier individuals are more likely to remain active, we give greater emphasis to longitudinal studies that can control for differences in baseline health status.

Inactivity and Disability

Figure 1 depicts the various interrelated pathways by which inactivity can produce or accelerate the onset of disability and death. The model is derived from several sources (17, 21, 34, 86). Although inactivity increases the risk of disabling health events, such as myocardial infarction, its major impacts on functional status are probably more protracted and subtle. We propose that inactivity accelerates the rates of decline of major physiologic adaptive systems (deconditioning), which eventually reach the point at which the individual's ability to prevent or recover from acute stresses is impaired. The aging individual's ability to cope with such stresses and preserve subsequent function depends upon the maintenance of adequate physiologic reserves, particularly neurologic control, mechanical performance, and energy metabolism (4, 17), and is also assisted by such modifying factors as positive affect.

The Disuse Hypothesis

Bassey (5) and Bortz (11) noted the similarities between the structural and functional declines associated with aging and the effects of enforced inactivity, such as bed rest or space flight. They also noted the ability of activating interventions, like exercise programs, to slow the rate of decline. Bortz defined a "disuse syndrome" (10), characterized by loss of cardiovascular reserve, obesity, "musculoskeletal fragility," and depression, and argued forcefully for the potential of exercise to prevent or reverse the syndrome.

Acute inactivity and deconditioning account for some of the steep declines in function seen in hospitalized older patients (37, 38). Whether slowly progressive deconditioning due to habitual inactivity contributes to reductions in function and reserve is one focus of this review. We hypothesize that the deconditioning effects of inactivity account for a substantial proportion of the negative slope in functional capacity with increasing age and that programs to increase activity can reverse some of these effects. Although most of the evidence available pertains to physical activity, inactivity in other aspects of life—intellectual, social, interpersonal—might also have adverse health consequences.

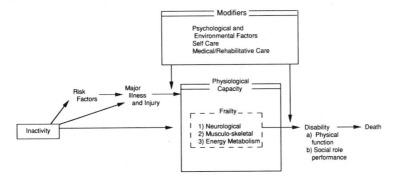

Figure 1 The relationship of inactivity to disease, disability, and death: a conceptual model.

What Do We Mean by Physical Activity?

Physical activity is purposeful body movement, whereas exercise refers to deliberate efforts to increase activity beyond that needed to perform social roles. Investigators have tended to consider activities in terms of their usual energy expenditure (calories/unit time) and impact on cardiovascular fitness as measured by aerobic capacity. This limited view may obscure other dimensions of physical activity that are important to the health of older adults. Besides the duration and intensity of energy expenditure, activities also vary in such dimensions as the parts of the body affected, the nature and strength of the forces acting on those body parts, the degree of central nervous system processing required for the activity, and the quantity of endorphins released. These additional dimensions may be critical to producing specific health effects. For example, activities with similar energy expenditures, but different degrees of stress on bones (e.g. swimming and jogging), may have very different effects on bone density (79). Characterizing activities based on their impact on other physiologic capacities, such as bone density, muscle strength, or balance, is a fruitful research direction. In the meantime, estimation of time spent doing various specific activities would seem to preserve the most information (26).

Activity Patterns in Older Adults

The proportion of older persons who are inactive varies with the definition of physical activity or exercise used and the population studied. In a well-to-do retirement community, only 10% reported no exercise at all (56). However, 43% of a national sample of individuals 65 years and older were categorized as sedentary (20), and 61% of respondents to the Behavioral Risk Factor Surveys who were 55 years and older (89) and 53% of a random sample of older (age 65+) residents of Nottinghamshire, England, reported no leisure physical activity (26). Evidence from repeated Canadian surveys suggests that physical activity among seniors has increased over time (19).

Self-reported physical activity declines with increasing age. Most of the decline in physical activity with age involves more strenuous activities (56, 58). Only about 10% of older adults report such activities as running or swimming, which are vigorous enough and performed with sufficient regularity to meet the Public Health Service's national objectives (20, 56, 84). Substantial proportions of all surveyed senior populations report involvement in less vigorous activities, such as gardening and walking, as exercise. In fact, these two activities account for much of their total leisure energy expenditure when activities are aggregated (15, 26, 56, 58). The vigor of gardening and walking is likely to be highly variable, which adds to the difficulties of validly assessing activity levels in older individuals. Gardening and walking are reported as exercise far less frequently by younger adults. One potential explanation for this age difference in what might be considered as "exercise" is the observation that older adults rate the exertion needed to achieve a given heart rate elevation more highly than younger counterparts (78).

What accounts for the reduction in activity, particularly vigorous activities, with increasing age? Mobily (57) identified two sets of barriers to exercise in the elderly: environmental or normative messages to slow down and personal frustrations associated with illness or the perceived difficulty of engaging in strenuous exercise. A common perception is that social norms urge older people to relax, yet most surveys indicate that older people associate well-being and life satisfaction with higher levels of activity (12). However, one of the few empiric studies of attitudes about exercise showed that older respondents viewed participation in more vigorous activities as less appropriate for older persons (61). Attitudes about participation in physical activity may be changing, particularly among more affluent and educated seniors (56), but data are sparse.

The Effects of Illness on Activity

The higher rates of ill health among older adults account for some of their decline in activity. Ill health appears to be a major reason for drop-outs from exercise programs (47). Discomfort may be an important reason; one survey found that declines in physical activity among seniors were strongly correlated with increased symptoms (30).

A second reason may be that older persons are more cautious than their younger counterparts (12) and more likely to reduce activities after acute health events for fear of a recurrence or other injury. Fear of falling has now been recognized as a threat to health that is, perhaps, more consequential than falling itself (55). Fallers and near-fallers experience declines in health and increases in health care utilization out of proportion to the extent of the injuries incurred (46, 85). We suspect similar scenarios with other health problems, although this important issue needs further research.

Well-meaning efforts by medical providers, family, and friends to protect older persons from possible harm related to activity probably contribute to activity limitation (12, 51, 88). This tendency to protect the elderly may become even more intense in the face of medically diagnosed illnesses, like coronary heart disease, diabetes, or arthritis, or visible reductions in the steadiness of gait or balance. As activities become more and more restricted, physiologic deficits due to deconditioning may become more visible, and the process escalates. The health care system may further contribute to the view of activity as dangerous through unsubstantiated "community standards," such as those requiring that older adults protect their arthritic joints from the stress of exercise (31) or engage in treadmill testing before embarking on a moderate exercise regimen (75).

We conclude that the impacts of illness or injury on activity go beyond their pathophysiologic effects to include fear of harm from activity and, perhaps, well-intentioned discouragement of activity by medical providers and others.

PHYSICAL ACTIVITY AND HEALTH

The observational evidence linking activity and health in older adults comes from two principal study strategies: comparisons of athletes with nonathletes and comparisons within more representative populations that exhibit a range of activity levels. The former strategy predominates in studies that examine the relationship between activity and physiologic indicators, whereas the latter comprises most studies that link activity level to disease or functional status. A comparison of athletes with nonathletes is, of course, treacherous, because of the relationships between long-term favorable physiologic, lifestyle, and health characteristics and sustaining athletic activities.

Physiologic Capacity or Reserve

The maintenance of optimal functional status requires adequate physiologic capacity and reserve. Badley et al (4) suggested that three areas have the greatest relevance for subsequent function: neurologic control, mechanical performance, and energy metabolism.

NEUROLOGICAL CONTROL   Maintenance of function requires the performance of complex tasks, which in turn require well-functioning central and peripheral nervous systems. Tests of neurologic function are strongly associated with current functional status (45, 90), future institutionalization (90), and risk of falls (60, 83). The relationship between impaired cognitive function, a crucial element in neurologic control, and disability is also clear. Does regular physical activity preserve neurologic control in the aging individual?

Several cross-sectional studies have compared reaction and movement times in response to various stimuli among individuals of differing ages and levels of regular exercise (22, 23, 69, 81). Mostly, these studies suggest that older exercisers perform better than older sedentary individuals and, in some studies, as well as much younger individuals. Similarly, some studies have found that physically active seniors have better cognitive function than inactive ones (1, 22, 23). The effects of exercise programs on cognition have been less positive, but the programs have been of short duration, and statistical power has been limited by small samples (15).

Spirduso (81) speculated that the effects of activity on psychomotor speed might be mediated by either enhancements of cerebral circulation or trophic influences on synaptic or neurocellular function. Rogers et al (70) recently supported the first hypothesis. They examined cerebral blood flow and cognitive function in three cohorts of older volunteers (mean age, 65 years): a group continuing to work, active retirees as measured by an activity inventory, and inactive retirees. The first two groups engaged in similar amounts of activity at baseline and maintained their baseline cerebral blood flow levels over the four-year follow-up period, whereas the inactive retirees experienced a significant decline in cerebral blood flow. Although cognitive function was measured only at the end of follow-up, it too was significantly lower in the inactive cohort. The second hypothesis, trophic effects, has received support from promising efforts to preserve cognition by increasing intellectual activity (74).

MECHANICAL PERFORMANCE

Muscle strength   Reduced muscle strength, particularly in the lower extremities, is associated with reductions in functional status and increased risk of falling (16). Muscle loss may also account for a substantial proportion of the age-related decline in aerobic capacity (33). The relationship between physical activity and muscle strength in older adults is controversial; some studies relate inactivity to age-related decline (2, 3, 24), and others fail to support such a relationship (42). This may not be surprising, as prevalent activities in older adults, like gardening and walking, may not include sufficient resistance exercise to improve strength. Bassey et al (6) did find that the calf strength of seniors correlated significantly with measures of walking speed, walking quantity (as measured by an accelerometer), and self-reported leisure activity. Although suggestive, the impact of less vigorous activities, such as walking and gardening, on lower extremity muscle strength remains uncertain. This would appear to be a critical question, given the increasing recognition of lower extremity weakness as a risk factor for falls (16).

Bone density   Both inactivity and aging are associated with losses in bone mineral density, a major risk factor for fractures of the hip, vertebrae, and wrist. Bone loss begins in early adulthood, accelerates around the menopause, and returns to a stable rate of decline for the remainder of the life span (68). Rather dramatic losses of bone mass follow enforced bed rest (48). This loss may not be recouped if an older, bed-confined patient does not return to full activities. The role of less extreme forms of inactivity on bone density has been the subject of considerable speculation and some research.

Athletes, particularly runners, tend to have higher bone density than nonathletes, particularly in bones most affected by their sport. For example, Lane et al (50) compared bone density in 14 runners and matched controls over age 50. Bone density in the first lumbar vertebra was 40% higher in runners than in controls. However, there is very little observational evidence as to the effects of less vigorous activities, like walking, on bone density.

Two epidemiologic studies have examined the relationship between activity and fractures in older adults. Cooper et al (25) compared recent activity levels and muscle strength in a community-based group of hip fracture patients with matched controls from the same community. They found that activity during the six weeks before the fracture, measured by an inventory of weight-bearing activities like standing and walking, was associated with reduced risk of hip fracture. Because fractures occur in sicker patients, recent activity may have been reduced by an illness that predisposed to fall and fracture. Sorock et al (80) assessed the relationship between activity and self-reported fracture over the next year in a retirement community by asking about involvement in nine different exercise activities. Among those participants reporting regular walking, the risk of fracture was less than for those who were sedentary. However, walking may reduce fractures by preventing falls, rather than by strengthening bones. Further studies of the effects of less vigorous activities on bone density are sorely needed.

ENERGY METABOLISM   Studies of aerobic capacity, or the ability to perform work by using oxygen in response to maximal stress (VO_2max), have generated much speculation and research about age-related functional decline and the role of activity in that decline. Because aerobic capacity quantitates the ability to work, it should be closely related to functional status, and some evidence indicates that it is. For example, reduced VO_2max limits the speed of walking or stair climbing (28, 41).

Several studies of older athletes suggest that those remaining active in their sports experience a slower decline of VO_2max than their more sedentary counterparts (76). However former athletes who have given up their sport decline at the usual rate. Buchner & Wagner (18) reviewed six longitudinal studies (27, 28, 39, 40, 44, 65) that compared changes in VO_2max over time in active and sedentary older adults. In every study, the rate of decline was lower in the active cohort, who declined at annual rates of 0.24–0.78 ml/kg/min, than in the sedentary control individuals, who declined at rates of 0.30–1.62 ml/kg/min annually. The active subgroups in most of these studies participated in intense exercise, again leaving unsettled the impact of less strenuous activity.

Modifiers: Depression

Depression has powerful adverse effects on physical health and functional status (87). Inactivity is associated with negative affect and depressive symptoms, but the direction of the relationship has been uncertain, because activity reduction is a well-recognized manifestation of depression. Two recent population-based cohort studies provide stronger evidence that inactivity can precede depressive symptoms (18, 32). Farmer et al (32) used data from the National Health and Nutrition Examination Survey to examine the association between reported physical activity in 1975 and depressive symptoms on resurvey in 1982–1984. Women who reported little or no recreational activity at baseline had significantly more depressive symptoms than more active women. Among members of the Alameda Population Laboratory cohort (18), those with low leisure activity levels at baseline were significantly more likely to report depressive symptoms nine years later, and those whose exercise levels declined over the nine-year interval had more depressive symptoms a decade later.

Coronary Heart Disease

Physical activity may affect the risk of coronary heart disease (CHD) through its direct effects on cardiac function (e.g. by increasing cardiac output, stroke volume) and through its indirect effects on levels of coronary risk factors (e.g. lipids, blood pressure, glucose metabolism, body composition) (52). Several recent reviews evaluated the strength of the epidemiologic evidence that relates physical activity levels to the occurrence of coronary outcomes mostly in middle-aged men (8, 62, 66). Berlin (9) found overall relative risks for the association of moderate or sedentary compared with high levels of nonoccupational physical activity to be 1.5 for CHD incidence (95% confidence interval, 1.4–1.7) and 1.6 for CHD death (95% confidence interval, 1.1–2.4). These studies provide very little information on the effects of physical activity on CHD risk in older men and virtually no information on older women.

One exception is the Honolulu Heart Program cohort, which included men aged 65 and older (29). Physical activity was measured with an index created by multiplying the estimated oxygen consumption associated with basal, sedentary, slight, moderate, or heavy activities by the number of hours spent doing each activity during a usual day. Relative risks for the incidence of CHD during 12 years of follow-up, which compared men in the lowest tertile (inactive) with those in the highest tertile of physical activity (active), were 1.5 for men aged 45–64 (95% confidence interval, 1.1–1.9) and 2.3 for men aged 65 and older (95% confidence interval, 1.0–5.3). In older, retired men, for whom the physical activity index would reflect leisure-time activity exclusively, the relative risk among inactive men was 3.4.

The effects of exercise on CHD may be explained, at least in part, by its impacts on lipids. Epidemiologic studies have consistently shown that physical activity improves lipid profiles in older adults (67, 73, 91). In general, those who exercise regularly at moderate intensity levels or higher have higher high density lipoprotein (HDL) cholesterol levels and lower low density lipoprotein cholesterol and triglyceride levels. One study (67) found that in women, the highest HDL cholesterol levels were seen in light to moderate intensity exercisers.

Other Chronic Diseases

In another analysis of initially healthy Honolulu men from the Heart Program cohort, the physical activity index was associated with remaining free of more than eight major chronic conditions during a 12-year follow-up period after adjustment for age (7). Additional adjustment for body mass index, blood pressure, and other risk factors diminished the association between physical activity index and remaining healthy, which suggests that the association between physical activity and major chronic diseases may be mediated by favorable levels of other risk factors.

Disability

The investigation of the effect of activity on functional outcomes is relatively new; initial studies have been conducted within the context of ongoing prospective studies of older adults. Four studies have directly examined the association between baseline physical activity and subsequent function. Three have shown compelling associations between physical activity and maintaining function (13, 49, 59), whereas the fourth found no effect of baseline activity status (64).

Branch (13) found that men and women aged 65 and older, who reported having slowed down their physical activities, were twice as likely to have functional disabilities five years later. Mor et al (59) used data from the Longitudinal Supplement on Aging, a national probability sample of older adults, to investigate factors associated with functional decline in persons aged 70–74. Two indicators of physical activity were available: engaging in a regular routine of physical exercise and walking a mile or more without resting. Among men and women who were functionally intact at baseline, inactivity was associated with a 50% greater risk of losing function during a two-year follow-up period. A regular routine of physical exercise was the more predictive item for men, whereas the frequency of walking a mile or more was the more predictive item for women.

In three communities of the National Institute on Aging Established Populations for Epidemiologic Studies of the Elderly, 6981 older men and women with intact mobility at baseline (i.e. able to climb stairs and walk a half mile without help) were followed annually for four years to determine factors associated with maintaining mobility (49). The frequency of three types of physical activity was examined: walking, gardening, and doing vigorous exercise. For each of the three activities, age-adjusted rates of maintaining mobility were highest in those who engaged in the activity three or more times per week and lowest in those who rarely or never engaged in the activity. None of the activities was clearly superior to the others in maximizing the rates of maintaining mobility. Based on a composite index of physical activity, which summed the frequency of all three activities, men and women with high activity levels were 40% less likely to lose mobility during the four years of follow-up than those with low activity levels.

Conversely, analysis of the Framingham data showed no association between an activity index based on hours spent in sedentary, slight, moderate, and heavy activity and a cumulative disability index assessed 21 years later (64). The lengthy interval between activity measurement and assessment of outcome raises the question as to whether the baseline measure of activity indexed a consistent pattern over the follow-up interval. Sustained activity appears to be necessary for health benefits (62).

Mortality

Several studies have examined the association between activity and mortality in older adults. Table 1 summarizes the results of eight recent prospective studies. Of the eight studies, four focused on simple dichotomies by comparing some regular physical activity with sedentary lifestyle (35, 43, 71) or slowed down activities with not slowed down (14). Inactivity was associated with a 30–40% increased risk of death in two of the studies (43, 71), and a threefold increased risk of death in the third (35). A fourth study of Swedish men born in 1913 found a twofold increased risk of death during 15 years of follow-up among those who rated their physical fitness level as bad or very bad on a seven-point scale, compared with men who reported excellent physical fitness levels (82). These studies provide no information as to the type, amount, or intensity of activity associated with the protective effect.

In contrast, a study of Harvard alumni measured physical activity in terms of energy expenditure based on number of blocks walked, stairs climbed, and time spent in sports play (63). Men aged 60–84 who expended more than 2000 kilocalories per week, compared with those who expended less than 500, were only half as likely to die during 12–16 years of follow-up. Similarly, physical fitness, as measured by total treadmill time, was strongly associated with mortality during a 4–15-year follow-up in initially healthy men and women aged 60 and older (9). In this study, the association between physical fitness and mortality was stronger in older adults (>60 years) than in the younger age groups (20–59 years). Social activity, as measured by such leisure time activities as going to movies, dancing, sightseeing, and picnicking, was not associated with risk of death in an eight-year study recently reported (54).

This evidence suggests that regular physical activity reduces the risk of death in persons aged 60 and older. Paffenbarger & Hyde (62) emphasize that physical activity must be a current practice to be beneficial; exercise in mid-life that is discontinued in late life is of no benefit, whereas exercise initiated in late-life, even after a sedentary middle-age, may result in substantial gains in life expectancy. Too few studies have focused on the relation-

Table 1 Prospective studies of activity and mortality in older adults

Reference	Study population	Years of follow-up	Measure of physical activity	Variables adjusted	Rate ratio (95% confidence interval)	Comments
Branch & Jette (13)	766 women and 467 men aged 66–98 years from the Massachussets Health Care Panel Study	5	Slowed down activity pace vs. not slowed down	Age, self-assessed health, income	Crude: Women 1.32 (0.81–1.83) Men 2.28 (1.26–3.30) Multivariate: Women 0.79 (0.47–1.31) Men 1.12 (0.64–1.96)	
Paffenbarger et al (63)	Harvard alumni aged 60–74 at entry (a subset of the total 16,936 men aged 35–74)	12–16	Energy expenditure (kcal per week) based on blocks walked, stairs climbed, and sports play	None	Age group 60–69: ≥2000 kcal vs. <500 0.53 500–1999 kcal vs. <500 0.63 Age group 70–84: ≥2000 kcal vs. <500 0.51 500–1999 kcal vs. <500 0.72	
Kaplan et al (43)	Men and women aged 60–94 years in Alameda County, California; 890 aged 65–70 564 aged ≥ 70	17	Inactive vs. regular physical activity	Age, self-assessed health status, smoking, relative weight, alcohol consumption, hours of sleep, eating breakfast, snacking	Age group 60–69: 1.38 (1.09–1.75) Age group 70+: 1.37 (1.09–1.72)	
Blair et al (19)	Men and women aged 60 and older in Dallas, Texas (a	4–15	Total treadmill time in seconds	None	Age group ≥60: Men Fitness quintile 5 vs. 1 8.3	Increase in death rates across quintiles of physical

	subset of the total 13,344 men and women aged ≥20)				4 vs. 1 4.5 3 vs. 1 2.0 2 vs. 1 1.6 Women Fitness quintile 5 vs. 1 4.9 4 vs. 1 1.9 3 vs. 1 1.9 2 vs. 1 1.2	fitness 1 = highest, 5 = lowest) was greatest in older men and women.
Rotevatn et al (71)	2631 men aged 65–74 residing in Norway	11	Amount of daily physical activity classified as "little or none" vs. "much or moderate"	None	1.29[a]	
Grand et al (35)	645 men and women aged ≥60 residing in rural areas of Southwest France	4	Physical exercise (yes vs. no)	Age	0.32 (0.20–0.49)	
Lee & Markides (54)	508 men and women aged ≥60 residing in San Antonio, Texas	8	10 item scale of social activities (distance traveled from home, frequency of movies, dances, visiting zoos or museums, sports events, hunting or fishing, parades or fiestas, games, sight-seeing, picnicking)	Age, sex, ethnicity, years of school, and self-related health	0.97[b]	Activity level was significantly related to mortality in unadjusted survival models but not after adjustment for age
Svardsudd & Tibblin (82)	787 men aged 60 residing in Gothenburg, Sweden	15	Self-rated physical fitness classified on a 7-point scale ranging from "excellent" (=1) to "very bad" (=7)	None	Physical fitness scores 5–7 vs. 1 1.90[a]	

[a] p <0.05—not statistically significant.
[b] not statistically significant.

ship between social activity and mortality in older adults to draw firm conclusions.

CONCLUSIONS

Older adults reduce their activity levels as they age, and larger proportions are sedentary. Planning feasible interventions requires a far better understanding of the determinants of this behavior pattern than currently exists. We must determine the extent to which well-meaning advice by formal and informal caregivers leads to activity reductions following falls, near-falls, other accidents, or illnesses.

Whatever the reason for its occurrence, strong and consistent evidence indicates that chronic inactivity has important adverse health consequences. The studies also provide encouraging evidence that even modestly increased physical activity levels in older adults may have major public health benefits. Increased activity in older adults appears to result in diminished age-related declines in physiologic reserve, fewer depressive symptoms, reduced risk of CHD, fewer osteoporotic fractures, higher rates of maintaining function and avoiding functional loss, and lower mortality.

The method of measuring physical activity varies widely across studies, as does the level of activity at which health benefits begin. Future research must answer crucial questions about the type, intensity, and duration of activity required to achieve various health effects. Whether increasing physical activity levels in previously sedentary older adults will achieve the same health benefits as naturally selected activity patterns is a crucial and testable hypothesis for experimental studies. Existing studies are discussed in the companion article (15).

ACKNOWLEDGMENTS

The authors are very grateful for Ms. Rita Weikal's invaluable efforts in preparing the manuscript and bibliography.

Literature Cited

1. Abourzek, T. 1988. The effects of regular aerobic exercise on short-term memory efficiency in the older adult. In *Aging and Motor Behavior,* ed. A. C. Ostrow, pp. 105–13. Indianapolis: Benchmark
2. Aniansson, A., Grimby, G., Rundgren, A. 1980. Isometric and isokinetic quadriceps muscle strength in 70-year-old men and women. *Scand. J. Rehabil. Med.* 12:161–68
3. Aoyagi, Y., Katsuta, S. 1990. Relationship between the starting age of training and physical fitness in old age. *Sport Sci.* 15(1):65–71
4. Badley, E. M., Lee, J., Wood, P. H. N. 1987. Impairment, disability, and the ICIDG model II: The nature of the underlying condition and patterns of impairment. *Int. Rehabil. Med.* 8(3):118–24
5. Bassey, E. J. 1978. Age, inactivity and some physiological responses to exercise. *Gerontology* 24:66–77

6. Bassey, E. J., Bendall, M. J., Pearson, M. 1988. Muscle strength in the triceps surae and objectively measured customary walking activity in men and women over 65 years of age. *Clin. Sci.* 74:85–89

7. Benfante, R., Reed, D., Brody, J. 1985. Biological and social predictors of health in an aging cohort. *J. Chron. Dis.* 38(5):385–95

8. Berlin, J. A., Colditz, G. A. 1990. The meta-analysis of physical activity in the prevention of coronary heart disease. *Am. J. Epidemiol.* 132(4):612–28

9. Blair, S. N., Kohl, H. W. III., Paffenbarger, R. S. Jr., Clark, D. G., Cooper, K. H., et al. 1989. Physical fitness and all-cause mortality: A prospective study of healthy men and women. *J. Am. Med. Assoc.* 262: (17):2395–2401

10. Bortz, W. M. II. 1984. The Disuse Syndrome. *West. J. Med.* 141(5):691–94

11. Bortz, W. M. II. 1982. Disuse and aging. *J. Am. Med. Assoc.* 248(10):1203–8

12. Botwinick, J. 1984. *Aging and Behavior.* New York: Springer. 437 pp. 3rd ed.

13. Branch, L. G. 1985. Health practices and incident disability among the elderly. *Am. J. Public Health* 75(12):1436–39

14. Branch, L. G., Jette, A. M. 1984. Personal health practices and mortality among the elderly. *Am. J. Public Health* 74(10):1126–29

15. Buchner, D. M., Beresford, S. A., Larson, E. B., LaCroix, A. Z., Wagner, E. H. 1992. Effects of exercise on functional status in older adults: Interventional studies. *Annu. Rev. Public Health.* 13:469–88

16. Buchner, D. M., deLateur, B. J. 1991. The importance of skeletal muscle strength to physical function in older adults. *Ann. Behav. Med.* 13(3):91–98

17. Buchner, D. M., Wagner, E. H. 1991. Can frail health be prevented? *Clin. Geriatr. Med.* 8(1): In press

18. Camacho, T. C., Roberts, R. E., Lazarus, N. B., Kaplan, G. A., Cohen, R. D. 1991. Physical activity and depression: Evidence from the Alameda County Study. *Am. J. Epidemiol.* 134(2):220–31

19. Can. Fit. Surv. 1982. *Fitness and Aging.* Ottawa: Gov. Can., Fit. Amat. Sport.

20. Caspersen, C. J., Christenson, G. M., Pollard, R. A. 1986. Status of the 1990 physical fitness and exercise objectives—evidence from NHIS 1985. *Public Health Rep.* 101(6):587–92

21. Chamie, M. 1990. The status and use of the international classification of impairments, disabilities and handicaps (ICIDH). *World Health Stat. Q.* 43 (4):273–80

22. Clarkson-Smith, L., Hartley, A. A. 1990. Structural equation models of relationships between exercise and cognitive abilities. *Psychol. Aging* 5:437–46

23. Clarkson-Smith, L., Hartley, A. A. 1989. Relationships between physical exercise and cognitive abilities in older adults. *Psychol. Aging* 4:183–89

24. Clement, F. J. 1974. Longitudinal and cross-sectional assessments of age changes in physical strength as related to sex, social class, and mental ability. *J. Gerontol.* 29:423–29

25. Cooper, C., Barker, D. J. P., Wickham, C. 1988. Physical activity, muscle strength, and calcium intake in fracture of the proximal femur in Britain. *Br. Med. J.* 297:1443–46

26. Dallosso, H. M., Morgan, K., Bassey, E. J., Ebrahim, S. B. J., Fentem, P. H., et al. 1988. Levels of customary physical activity among the old and the very old living at home. *J. Epidemiol. Community Health* 42:121–27

27. Dehn, M., Bruce, R. 1972. Longitudinal variations in maximal oxygen intake with age and activity. *J. Appl. Physiol.* 33(6):805–7

28. Dill, D. B., Robinson, S., Ross, J. C. 1967. A longitudinal study of 16 champion runners. *J. Sports Med.* 7:4–27

29. Donahue, R. P., Abbott, R. D., Reed, D. M., Yano, K. 1988. Physical activity and coronary heart disease in middle-aged and elderly men: The Honolulu heart program. *Am. J. Public Health* 78(6):683–85

30. Ebrahim, S., Dallosso, H., Morgan, K., Bassey, J., Fentem, P., et al. 1988. Causes of ill health among a random sample of old and very old people: possibilities for prevention. *J. R. Coll. Physicians London* 22(2):105–7

31. Ekdahl, C., Andersson, S. I., Moritz, U., Svensson, B. 1990. Dynamic versus static training in patients with rheumatoid arthritis. *Scand. J. Rheumatol.* 19:17–26

32. Farmer, M. E., Locke, B. Z., Moscicki, E. K., Dannenberg, A. L., Larson, D. B., et al. 1988. Physical activity and depressive symptoms: The NHANES I epidemiologic follow-up study. *Am. J. Epidemiol.* 128:1340–51

33. Fleg, J. L., Lakatta, E. G. 1988. Role of muscle loss in the age-associated reduction in $V_{O_{2}max}$. *J. Appl. Physiol.* 65:1147–51

34. Fried, L., Herdman, S. J., Kuhn, K. E., Rubin, G., Turano, K. 1991. Preclinical disability: Hypotheses about the bottom of the iceberg. *J. Aging Health* 3(2):285–300

35. Grand, A., Grosclaude, P., Bocquet, H., Pous, J., Albarede, J. L. 1990. Disability, psychosocial factors and mortality among the elderly in a rural French population. *J. Clin. Epidemiol.* 43(8):773–82

36. Grimley Evans, J. 1984. Prevention of age-associated loss of autonomy: Epidemiological approaches. *J. Chron. Dis.* 37(5):353–63

37. Hirsh, C. H., Sommers, L., Losen, A., Mullen, L., Hutner Winograd, C. 1990. The natural history of functional morbidity in hospitalized older patients. *J. Am. Geriatr. Soc.* 38:1296–1303

38. Hoenig, H. M., Rubenstein, L. Z. 1991. Hospital-associated deconditioning and dysfunction. *J. Am. Geriatr. Soc.* 39:220–22

39. Hollman, W. 1966. Diminution of cardiopulmonary capacity in the course of life and its prevention by participation in sports. *Proc. Int. Congr. Sports Sci., Tokyo,* pp. 91. Jpn. Union Sports Sci.

40. Irving, J. B., Kusumi, F., Bruce, R. A. 1980. Longitudinal variations in maximal oxygen consumption in healthy men. *Clin. Cardiol.* 3(2):134–36

41. Jette, M., Sidney, K., Blumchen, G. 1990. Metabolic equivalents (METS) in exercise testing, exercise prescription, and evaluation of functional capacity. *Clin. Cardiol.* 13(8):555–65

42. Kallman, D. A., Plato, C. C., Tobin, J. D. 1990. The role of muscle loss in the age-related decline of grip strength: Cross-sectional and longitudinal perspectives. *J. Gerontol.* 45(3):M82–88

43. Kaplan, G. A., Seeman, T. E., Cohen, R. D., Knudsen, L. P., Guralnik, J. 1987. Mortality among the elderly in the Alameda County study: Behavioral and demographic risk factors. *Am. J. Public Health* 77(3):307–12

44. Kasch, F. W., Boyer, J. L., Van Camp, S. P., Verity, L. S. 1990. The effect of physical activity on aerobic power in older men (a longitudinal study). *Phys. Sportsmed.* 18:73–83

45. Kaye, K., Grigsby, J., Robbins, L. J., Korzun, B. 1990. Prediction of independent functioning and behavior problems in geriatric patients. *J. Am. Geriatr. Soc.* 38:1304–10

46. Keil, D. P., O'Sullivan, P., Teno, J. M., Mor, V. 1991. Health care utilization and functional status in the aged following a fall. *Med. Care* 29(3):221–28

47. Kriska, A. M., Bayles, C., Cauley, J. A., Laporte, R. E., Sandler, R. B., et al. 1986. A randomized exercise trial in older women: Increased activity over two years and the factors associated with compliance. *Med. Sci. Sports Exerc.* 18:557–62

48. Krolner, B., Toft, B. 1983. Vertebral bone loss: An unheeded side effect of therapeutic bed rest. *Clin. Sci.* 64:537–40

49. LaCroix, A. Z., Guralnik, J. M., Berkman, L. F., Wallace, R. B., Evans, D. A. 1990. *Maintaining mobility in late life: The role of smoking, alcohol consumption, and physical activity.* Presented at 118th, Annu. Meet. Am. Public Health Assoc., New York

50. Lane, N. E., Bloch, D. A., Jones, H. H., Marshall, W. H., Wood, P. D., et al. 1986. Long distance running, bone density, and osteoarthritis. *J. Am. Med. Assoc.* 255(9):1147–51

51. Lampman, R. M., Savage, P. J. 1988. Exercise and Aging: A review of benefits and a plan for action. In *The Endocrinology of Aging,* ed. J. R. Sowers, J. V. Felicetta, pp. 307–35. New York: Raven

52. Laporte, R. E., Adams, L. L., Savage, D. D., Brenes, G., Dearwater, S., et al. 1984. The spectrum of physical activity, cardiovascular disease and health: An epidemiologic perspective. *Am. J. Epidemiol.* 120(40):507–15

53. Laporte, R. E., Montoye, H. J., Caspersen, C. 1985. Assessment of physical activity in epidemiologic research: Problems and prospects. *Public Health Rep.* 100(2): 131–47

54. Lee, D. J., Markides, K. S. 1990. Activity and mortality among aged persons over an eight-year period. *J. Gerontol.* 45(1):S39–42

55. Maki, B. E., Holliday, P. J., Topper, A. K. 1991. Fear of falling and postural performance in the elderly. *J. Gerontol.* 46(4):M123–31

56. McPhillips, J. B., Pellettera, K. M., Barrett-Connor, E., Wingard, D. L., Criqui, M. H. 1989. Exercise patterns in a population of older adults. *Am. J. Prev. Med.* 5(2):65–72

57. Mobily, K. E. Motivational aspects of exercise for the elderly: Barriers and solutions. *Phys. Occup. Ther. Geriatr.* 1(4):43–54

58. Montoye, H. J. 1975. *Physical Activity and Health: An epidemiology study of an entire community.* Englewood Cliffs, NJ: Prentice Hall

59. Mor, V., Murphy, J., Masterson-Allen, S., Willey, C., Razmpour, A., et al. 1989. Risk of functional decline among well elders. *J. Clin. Epidemiol.* 42(9):895–904

60. Nevitt, M. C., Cummings, S. R., Black, D. 1989. Risk factors for recurrent non-syncopal falls: A prospective study. *J. Am. Med. Assoc.* 261:2663–68

61. Ostrow, A. C., Dzewaltowski, D. A. 1986. Older adults' perceptions of physical activity participation based on age-role and sex-role appropriateness. *Res. Q. Exerc. Sport* 57(2):167–69

62. Paffenbarger, R. S. Jr., Hyde, R. T. 1984. Exercise in the prevention of coronary heart disease. *Prev. Med.* 13:3–22

63. Paffenbarger, R. S. Jr., Hyde, R. T., Wing, A. L. 1986. Physical activity, all-cause mortality, and longevity of college alumni. *N. Engl. J. Med.* 314(10):605–13

64. Pinsky, J. L., Leaverton, P. E., Stokes, J., III. 1987. Predictors of good function: The Framingham Study. *J. Chron. Dis.* (Suppl.) 40:159S-67S

65. Plowman, S. A., Drinkwater, B. L., Horvath, S. M. 1979. Age and aerobic power in women: A longitudinal study. *J. Gerontol.* 34:512–20

66. Powell, K. E., Thompson, P. D., Caspersen, C. J., Kendrick, J. S. 1987. Physical activity and the incidence of coronary heart disease. *Annu. Rev. Public Health* 8:253–87

67. Reaven, P. D., McPhillips, J. B., Barrett-Connor, E. L., Criqui, M. H. 1990. Leisure time exercise and lipid and lipoprotein levels in an older population. *J. Am. Geriatr. Soc.* 38:847–54

68. Riggs, B. L., Jowsey, J., Kelly, P. J., Hoffman, D. L., Arnaud, C. D. 1976. Effects of oral therapy with calcium and vitamin D in primary osteoporosis. *J. Clin. Endocrinol. Metab.* 42:1139–44

69. Rili, R., Busch, S. 1986. Motor performance of women as a function of age and physical activity level. *J. Gerontol.* 41(5):645–49

70. Rogers, R. L., Meyer, J. S., Mortel, K. F. 1990. After reaching retirement age physical activity sustains cerebral perfusion and cognition. *J. Am. Geriatr. Soc.* 38:123–28

71. Rotevatn, S., Akslen, L. A., Bjelke, E. 1989. Lifestyle and mortality among Norwegian men. *Prev. Med.* 18:433–43

72. Rowe, J. W., Kahn, R. L. 1987. Human aging: Usual and successful. *Science* 237:143–49

73. Sallis, J. F., Haskell, W. L., Fortmann, S. P., Wood, P. D., Vranizan, K. M.

1986. Moderate-intensity physical activity and cardiovascular risk factors: The Stanford Five-City Project. *Prev. Med.* 15:561–68

74. Schaie, K., Willis, S. L. 1986. Can decline in adult intellectual functioning be reversed? *Dev. Psychol.* 22(2):223–32

75. Shepard, R. J. 1990. The scientific basis of exercise prescribing for the very old. *J. Am. Geriatr. Soc.* 38(1):62–70

76. Shepard, R. J. 1987. *Physical Activity and Aging.* Rockville, Md: Aspen. 354 pp. 2nd ed.

77. Shock, N. W. 1984. Energy metabolism, caloric intake, and physical activity of the aging. In *Normal Human Aging: The Baltimore Longitudinal Study of Aging*, pp. 372–83 (Append.). US Dep. Health Hum. Serv., NIH Publ. No. 84-2450

78. Sidney, K. H., Shephard, R. J. 1977. Perception of exertion in the elderly, effects of aging, mode of exercise and physical training. *Percept. Mot. Skills* 44:999–1010

79. Sinaki, M. 1989. Exercise and osteoporosis. *Arch. Phys. Med. Rehabil.* 70:220–29

80. Sorock, G. S., Bush, T. L., Golden, A. L., Fried, L. P., Breuer, B., et al. 1988. Physical activity and fracture risk in a free-living elderly cohort. *J. Gerontol.* 43(5):M134–39

81. Spirduso, W. W. 1980. Physical fitness, aging, and psychomotor speed: A review. *J. Gerontol.* 35(6):850–65

82. Svardsudd, K., Tibblin, G. 1990. Is quality of life affecting survival? *Scand. J. Prim. Health Care Suppl.* 1:55–60

83. Tinetti, M. E., Speechley, M. 1989. Prevention of falls among the elderly. *N. Engl. J. Med.* 320:1055–59

84. US Off. Assist. Secr. Health and Surg. Gen. 1979. *Healthy People: The Surgeon General's Report on Health Promotion and Disease Prevention*, Washington, DC: GPO [DHEW Publ. No. (PHS) 87-1232]

85. Vellas, B., Cayla, F., Bocquet, H., de Pemille, F., Albarede, J. L. 1987. Prospective study of restriction of activity in old people after falls. *Age Ageing* 16:189–93

86. Verbrugge, L. M., Lepkowski, J. M., Imanaka, Y. 1989. Comorbidity and its impact on disability. *Milbank Mem. Fund Q.* 67(3–4):450–84

87. Wells, K. B., Stewart. A., Hays, R. D., Burnham, A., Rogers, W., et al. 1989. The functioning and well-being of depressed patients. *J. Am. Med. Assoc.* 262:914–19

88. Wenger, N. K. 1981. Rehabilitation of

the elderly cardiac patient. *Cardiovasc. Clin.* 12:221–30

89. White, C. C., Powell, K. E., Hogelin, G. C., Gentry, E. M., Forman, M. R. 1987. The behavioral risk factor surveys: IV. The descriptive epidemiology of exercise. *Am. J. Prev. Med.* 3(6):304–10

90. Williams, M. E., Hornberger, J. C. 1984. A quantitative method of identifying older persons at risk for increasing long-term care services. *J. Chron. Dis.* 37:705–11

91. Yano, K., Reed, D. M., Curb, J. D., Hankin, J. H., Albers, J. J. 1986. Biological and dietary correlates of plasma lipids and lipoproteins among elderly Japanese men in Hawaii. *Arteriosclerosis* 6(4):422–33

Annu. Rev. Publ. Health 1992. 13:469–88

EFFECTS OF PHYSICAL ACTIVITY ON HEALTH STATUS IN OLDER ADULTS II: Intervention Studies[1]

David M. Buchner

Departments of Health Services and Medicine, University of Washington, Seattle, Washington; Northwest Health Services Research and Development Field Program, Seattle VA Medical Center, Seattle, Washington 98195

Shirley A. A. Beresford[1] and Eric B. Larson[2]

Departments of [1]Epidemiology and [2]Medicine and Health Services, University of Washington, Seattle, Washington 98195

Andrea Z. LaCroix[3] and Edward H. Wagner[4]

Center for Health Studies, Group Health Cooperative of Puget Sound, Seattle, Washington; Departments of [3]Epidemiology and [4]Health Services, University of Washington, Seattle, Washington 98195

All authors associated with Center for Health Promotion in Older Adults, School of Public Health, University of Washington

KEY WORDS: exercise, aged, bone density, frail elderly

INTRODUCTION

Older adults often say "staying active" is important to healthy aging. Physical activity is usually emphasized, but intellectual and social activities are also important. A growing body of scientific evidence addresses this subject. In the preceding article, we critically reviewed the epidemiologic evidence that activity patterns are associated with health (96). Here, we discuss the experimental evidence that interventions that "activate" older adults promote their health and maintain or improve physical and mental functioning during normal daily activities.

The distinction between physiologic and functional status effects of exercise is critical to this review. The International Classification of Impairments, Disabilities, and Handicaps definitions of impairments and disabilities embody this distinction. An impairment is a "loss or abnormality of psychological, physiological, or anatomical structure or function" (26). A disability is a "restriction or lack . . . of ability to perform an activity in the manner or within the range considered normal for a human being" (26). A great deal is known about the therapeutic role of exercise on physiologic impairments in such diseases as ischemic heart disease, hypertension, noninsulin dependent diabetes mellitus, chronic obstructive pulmonary disease, obesity, and depression. We do not discuss these areas in any detail, as they are covered by other review articles and in Bouchard et al's (18) recent text book. Much less is known about exercise and "functional status."

We begin by considering the physiologic measures of physical fitness, evidence that exercise can improve fitness in older adults, and theoretical reasons why exercise should improve functional status in older adults. We review experimental evidence that addresses whether exercise improves functional status in older adults and focus on balance, gait, and physical health status; cognitive status; and rate of bone loss.

EXERCISE AND PHYSICAL FITNESS

There are five common measures of physical fitness (86): muscle strength and endurance, flexibility, body composition, anaerobic capacity (abilities), and aerobic capacity (abilities). Exercise affects these measures of fitness in healthy, younger adults. Because age-related decline in strength and aerobic capacity is hypothesized to be important to disability, we focus on these measures. Joint flexibility, body composition, and anaerobic capacity also show age-related changes, but have received little attention as to their role in the pathogenesis of frail health.

Aerobic Capacity

DEFINITION AND MEASUREMENT   Aerobic capacity can be defined as the ability of the body to produce energy by using oxygen. It is a principal measure of the ability of the body to do sustained work (86). It is usually assessed as maximal aerobic power, or VO_2 max, and measured as (maximal) milliliters of oxygen consumed per kilogram of body weight per minute (ml/kg/min), or as metabolic equivalents (METS) (1 MET = the rate of oxygen consumption at rest, about 3.5 ml/kg/min) (56).

AGE-RELATED DECLINE   Much attention has been paid in gerontology to the decline in aerobic capacity with age (13, 20, 37, 57, 83). Between the ages of 30 and 80, about 50% of aerobic capacity is lost. Even so, variation in aerobic capacity is large enough that the range in older adults overlaps that of younger adults (55, 62, 72). Absolute rates of decline are higher in sedentary adults than active adults (23, 37, 57). A recent study estimated that exercising adults lose 0.25 ml/kg/min in aerobic capacity each year, which is one-third the yearly loss rate of 0.71/ml/kg/min for nonexercisers (57).

EFFECTS OF EXERCISE   Many studies report that aerobic exercise improves aerobic capacity in older adults (1, 4, 9, 10, 14, 17, 21, 33, 35, 39, 41, 48, 53, 61, 69, 70, 73, 79, 81, 84, 91, 93). Improvement with 3–12 months of exercise is modest and ranges from 5% to 20%.

Skeletal Muscle Strength

DEFINITION AND MEASUREMENT   Strength can be defined as the maximum force exerted by a muscle (38). Strength is not just a property of muscle, but depends upon neurological function (44). Strength can be measured as the maximum weight lifted (isotonic strength), as the maximum force exerted against a fixed object (isometric strength), or as the peak torque produced at a given speed of muscular contraction (isokinetic strength).

AGE-RELATED DECLINE   Age-related decline in strength is well documented. Typical cross-sectional data suggest a 30–40% loss of back, leg, and arm strength between ages 30 and 80 (50). Longitudinal studies suggest that the rate of decline is curvilinear and underestimated by cross-sectional data (32). For example, longitudinal studies show a 60% loss in grip strength between ages 30 and 80 (32). Other longitudinal studies report that healthy older adults lose 10–25% of their quadriceps strength in seven years (6, 8).

EFFECTS OF EXERCISE   There are fewer studies of the effects of strengthening exercise in older adults than of aerobic exercise (2, 4, 5, 7, 27, 28, 33, 45, 46, 49, 58, 60, 67, 70, 71). Most studies are small, nonrandomized trials of a few months of resistance training, although a randomized controlled trial was recently reported (28). Almost all studies report that resistance training increases the strength of older adults (46, 91). Earlier studies of low and moderate intensity resistance training reported modest increases (10–25%) in strength with exercise (7, 60, 67, 71). More recent studies in healthy adults (28, 49) and frail adults (46, 47) showed that more vigorous exercise produces far greater gains in strength (100–200% in a three-month training program). Because elderly adults are often relatively weak, expressing improvement in terms of percent gain obscures the fact that absolute gains in strength are modest.

Although resistance exercise can increase strength in older adults, the mechanism underlying the gain is debated. An early article argued that although older adults increased strength with exercise, their muscles did not hypertrophy (67); rather, neural factors (learning effects) could account for the increased strength. Later studies showed that resistance exercise can cause muscular hypertrophy (46, 49), yet neural effects may still be important. The cross-sectional area of a muscle and its strength are highly correlated in younger adults (63) and probably in older adults, as well (75). However, short-term training programs typically increase strength far more than muscle cross-sectional area (63). This finding also appears true in older adults, as studies report that 10–20% increases in muscle area are accompanied by 100–200% increases in strength (46, 49). Thus, the excess strength, not accounted for by hypertrophy, may be due to various neural factors (68).

THEORETICAL RELATIONSHIP BETWEEN FITNESS AND FUNCTIONAL STATUS

The pathogenesis of disability is complex. Part I of this series describes a model of disability. We describe below in more detail the theoretical relationship between fitness and functional status and the rationale for why exercise should improve functional status.

Physical Functional Status

The usual mechanism involved to explain why exercise should improve functional status focuses on aerobic capacity (20, 82, 97). The energy needed to do a given task can be estimated by measuring oxygen consumption during steady-state performance of the task. For example, walking on a level grade at 5 km/h requires 3.2 METS (56). Loss of aerobic capacity with inactivity or illness eventually causes aerobic capacity to fall below the level required for daily tasks. Because exercise can increase aerobic capacity, it should improve functional status when aerobic capacity is below the threshold needed for daily activities.

There is a roughly parallel explanation focusing on strength (22, 97). The amount of strength needed to perform a task can be estimated from biomechanical studies. To stand up, for example, the typical person requires about 120 Newton-meters of knee torque to transfer his body weight from a chair to his lower extremities (59). Suppose strength falls below the level required for standing up. Increasing maximal strength should improve function, because of an elegant logarithmic mathematical relationship between peak strength and endurance at submaximal tasks (38, 85). Suppose maximal strength for about one second is 20 kg. If, after an exercise program, maximum strength improves to 40 kg, the person should be able to lift the 20 kg weight for 60 seconds. That is, increasing strength should improve performance on sub-maximal tasks of daily life.

Note that both explanations involve a threshold effect. Levels of fitness below the threshold are associated with impaired ability to do the activity. If fitness exceeds the threshold, the activity can be performed. Figure 1 illustrates this relationship.

Cognitive Functional Status

The argument that exercise that improves cognitive status depends mainly upon epidemiologic evidence that older adults who exercise perform better on neuropsychological tests. Our preceding article comments on this evidence. The physiologic mechanism underlying the association is unclear. Exercise could improve cognition by improving either blood flow to the brain (78) or oxygen metabolism in the brain (41).

INTERVENTION STUDIES

Exercise Effects on Gait, Balance, and Physical Function

Several intervention studies address the effect of exercise on gait and balance in older adults (Table 1). Seven studies of gait and balance reported some statistically significant improvements attributable to exercise (11, 34, 45, 46, 54, 76, 95). Another positive study is not included in Table 1 because it did

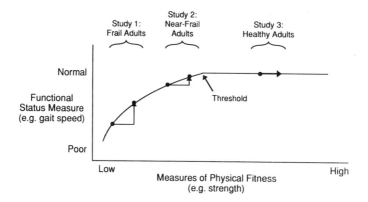

Figure 1   Theoretical relationship between physical fitness and functional status. The curvilinear relationship shows a threshold effect: above the threshold level of fitness, functional status is normal; below it, function is impaired. A curvilinear relationship implies that the benefit from exercise depends upon the target group. Three hypothetical exercise studies are shown. Each study produces the same absolute improvement in fitness. In the frail adults of Study 1, exercise produces a large improvement in functional status. In the healthy adults of Study 3, no benefit is seen. Study 2 shows intermediate benefits.

Table 1 Studies of the effect of exercise on gait and balance in older adults[a]

Study	Sample	RCT[b]	N per Group[c]	Outcome Measure[d]	%[e] Improvement	Effect Size[f]	Improved Fitness?[g]
Fiatarone et al (46)	Long-term care facility	No	9[h]	Tandem gait speed	48*	0.81	Yes
				Gait speed	ns[i]	—	
Barry et al (11)	Community	No	~7	Heel stand EO	51*	0.69	Yes
				Heel stand EC	35*	0.32	
				One foot stand	15*	0.19	
				Agility walk	0	0.0	
Hopkins et al (54)	Sedentary, community	Yes	~26	One foot stand	13*	0.42	Yes
				Agility walk	11*	0.55	
				Arm agility	4*	0.23	
Brown & Holloszy (19)	Community	No	~20	One foot stand EO	31	0.59	Yes
				One foot stand EC	24	0.25	
				Gait Speed	3	0.16	
Rikli & Edwards (76)	Sedentary, community	No	~17	One foot stand	32*	0.66	Yes
Era (45)[j]	Community	Yes	~14	Force plate measures:			Yes
				Lateral sway EO	~18*	—	
				Lateral sway EO (tandem)	~0	—	
				Lateral EC	~20	—	
				AP Sway EO	~18*	—	
				AP Sway EO (tandem)	~26	—	
				AP Sway EC	~24	—	

Vanfraechen (95)	Sedentary	No	10	One foot stand	104*	5.9	?
Crilly et al (34)	Healthy, sedentary, community	Yes	~24	Gait speed[k]	?	no data	?
				Force plate measures[l]:			
				Lateral sway EO	7	0.13	
				Lateral EC	10	0.20	
				AP Sway EO	4	0.10	
				AP Sway EC	-4	-0.07	
Gutman et al (52)	Community	No	~14	Balance beam	11	—	?
Clark et al (31)	Institutionalized mental patients	No	~8	Toe stand	-28	—	?
				One foot stand	-6	—	
				Balance beam	-45	—	

[a] Studies by Roberts (77) and Bassett et al (12) are omitted from the table because raw data were not reported.
[b] RCT = randomized controlled trial.
[c] N per group = the average group size in the analysis.
[d] EO = eyes open; EC = eyes closed; AP = Antero-posterior.
[e]* Results were reported as statistically significant.
[f] Effect size is a standardized measure of an intervention effect, typically used in meta-analysis. Effect size = net improvement on an outcome variable due to the intervention, divided by the standard deviation of the outcome variable. If effect size is missing, either mean and/or variance data were not reported.
[g] Did exercise improve measures of physical fitness?
[h] N = 5 in the analysis of tandem gait speed.
[i] Raw data on gait speed not reported, but results described as nonsignificant.
[j] Results reported only for strength training intervention. Group means estimated from graphs, as numeric data were not reported. Statistical analysis did not compare improvement over time between experimental and control group, but tested if improvement in the experimental group was significant.
[k] Raw data on gait speed not reported, but results described as significant.
[l] Sway was measured as the root mean square of the amplitude of sway.

not report detailed data (77). Three studies reported no significant effects of exercise on gait and balance (19, 31, 52). Another study, not included in Table 1 because it did not report detailed data, was also negative (12).

Several factors may account for the variation in findings among the studies in Table 1. If there is a curvilinear relationship between fitness and functional status (Figure 1), exercise should not improve gait and balance in adults whose fitness levels exceed a certain threshold. Variation in fitness levels among study samples could explain differences in results. Possibly, the negative studies had an inadequate exercise stimulus. A counter argument is that exercise may not need to improve fitness to improve function.

Limited statistical power may explain differences in results and is reason to regard the results in Table 1 as encouraging. In studies in which effect sizes could be calculated, exercise produced an effect size of 0.15 or greater for 76% (13/17) of the outcomes studied.

The studies in Table 1 provide only preliminary evidence that exercise improves gait and balance in older adults. The lack of randomized trials is important: Subjects may show learning effects on clinical gait and balance measures (51). Most studies lacked blinded outcome measures and had small, nonrepresentative study groups. As studies lacked follow-up, it is uncertain whether exercise can produce sustained effects on gait and balance. Ongoing research, such as the Frailty and Injuries: Cooperative Studies of Intervention Techniques (FICSIT) initiative funded by the National Institute on Aging, should help clarify the situation. For example, the University of Washington FICSIT study, along with additional research funded by the Centers for Disease Control, compares the effects of six different types of exercise in a single-blinded, randomized controlled trial involving over 180 subjects.

We did not find exercise studies restricted to older adults that carefully measured functional status outcomes other than gait and balance. Exercise studies in arthritis patients have measured functional status, although most have enrolled both young and old adults. Because of the pain and joint limitations of arthritis, the public health importance of exercise is enhanced if exercise is safe and effective in arthritis patients.

Three studies of exercise in rheumatoid arthritis and osteoarthritis patients included follow-up outcome measures (Table 2). All reported improvement in functional status because of exercise. Improvements in function persisted at follow-up three months (42), eight months (47), and nine months (64) after discharge from supervised exercise classes. Studies typically reported 10–25% improvements in outcomes at follow-up compared with baseline. Notably, exercise did not make arthritic pain worse. Two studies reported that exercise relieved pain symptoms.

The studies in Table 2 provide relatively strong evidence that exercise improves functional status in arthritis patients. Studies had long-term follow-

Table 2 Selected studies of the effect of exercise on functional status in arthritis patients

Study	Age (Years)	Type of Arthritis[a]	RCT[b]	N per group[c]	Protocol	Months of Exercise	Months of Follow-up	Effects of Exercise
Minor et al (64)	21–83	OA & RA	Yes	~32[d]	Endurance training	3	9	Faster gait speed; improvement in physical activity, anxiety, and depression scales of AIMS[e]; no change in pain
Ekdahl et al (42)	23–64	RA	Yes	~30	General exercise	1.5	3	Faster gait speed; less pain; less morning stiffness
Fisher et al (47)	Mean = 68	OA	No	11	Strength training	4	8	Faster gait speed; improvement in dependence, difficulty, and pain subscales of Jette Functional Status Index

[a] OA = osteoarthritis; RA = rheumatoid arthritis.
[b] RCT = randomized controlled trial.
[c] N per group = average group size in the analysis.
[d] The analysis combined two aerobic exercise groups.
[e] AIMS = Arthritis Impact Measurement Scales.

up, and one study was single-blinded (47). Study samples were somewhat different in age and arthritis symptoms, which suggests that results may be generalizable to broad population groups. Arthritis patients are not physically fit and have reduced aerobic capacity (65) and muscular strength (47, 54). By limiting the sample to arthritis patients, studies focused on a target group capable of showing considerable improvement in functional status in a short period.

Exercise Effects on Cognition

Several experimental studies address the obvious chicken and egg issue: Does exercise make people smarter, or do smarter people simply exercise more? The first five studies in Table 3 (11, 40, 41, 74, 92) reported some significant improvement. The next five studies (17, 43, 61, 66, 70) were more rigorous and reported no improvement. There are several possible explanations for the mixed results. As noted above, it may be important to target not just sedentary adults, but specifically physically unfit adults. The exercise protocols varied in type, duration, and intensity. Samples varied from community adults to institutionalized mental patients.

A common interpretation of the negative studies is that short-term exercise is not sufficient (61, 70). Adults must exercise for long periods of time to show cognitive benefits. This interpretation is supported by the last study in Table 3 of a three-year exercise program (76). The study was not a randomized trial, but the investigators reported a modest, though significant, effect of exercise on reaction time.

Another interpretation is that existing studies lack statistical power and cannot reliably detect an effect of exercise on neuropsychological tests. Statistically significant improvement in test performance because of exercise ranged in magnitude from 3% to 35% (next to last column, Table 3). But studies reported nonsignificant trends of the same magnitude (last column, Table 3). No one has argued that exercise should have large effects on cognitive function as measured by neuropsychological tests. It seems more likely that exercise effects are modest.

In summary, the existing literature is insufficient to prove or exclude the possibility of a modest effect of exercise on cognition. An upward shift of the population mean IQ by a few points would represent an important, if not remarkable, effect of exercise. Large, long-term, well-designed, well-targeted exercise studies are needed that have the statistical power to detect modest effects of exercise on cognition.

Exercise Effects on Osteoporosis

The increased risk of osteoporosis with inactivity, particularly bed rest, has long been recognized. Later, exercise per se was identified as a protective factor that decreases fracture risk (25). Many reviews of this subject exist, including a recent review of both animal and human evidence (80) and a critical review by Block (16).

Given the large amount of interest in this subject, there are surprisingly few randomized trials. Table 4 shows nine studies in postmenopausal women that had at least one year of follow-up, only two of which are randomized controlled trials (15, 29). Six studies (29, 30, 36, 87–90) reported a positive effect of exercise on bone mass. Two studies (3, 24) were reported as negative, but had small sample sizes and little statistical power. The only large randomized trial was reported as negative (15); its walking intervention was of modest intensity, which may partly explain this result.

An interesting aspect of the studies is that bone mineral density was often measured at the radius. Changes in radial bone density would be interpreted as generalized effects of exercise, as exercise programs did not usually focus on the wrist. One study reported that strength training with aerobic exercise may increase bone density more than just aerobic exercise alone (29).

It is widely believed that exercise promotes bone strength in postmenopausal women. Part I of this series shows that research findings from observational studies support this conclusion, yet there is a lack of evidence from randomized trials. Randomized trials are needed particularly to rule out the possibility that past exercise is responsible for the apparent benefit of exercise in later years. Investigators must systematically study how type and intensity of exercise affect bone strength. Eventually, studies will need to test whether exercise reduces fracture rates.

SUMMARY

This review has focused on a specific part of the relationship of exercise to health. The overall evidence supporting the health benefits of exercise is substantial and has been critically reviewed recently (18, 94). Thus, the United States Preventive Services Task Force recommends that all adults exercise regularly (94). The conclusions summarized below regarding older adults do not affect this basic recommendation.

There is solid evidence that exercise can improve measures of fitness in older adults, particularly strength and aerobic capacity. These exercise effects occur in chronically ill adults, as well as in healthy adults. Because physical fitness is a determinant of functional status, it is logical to ask whether exercise can prevent or improve impairments in functional status in older adults.

The evidence that exercise improves functional status is promising, but inconclusive. Problems with existing studies include a lack of randomized controlled trials, a lack of evidence that effects of exercise can be sustained

Table 3 Controlled trials of the effect of exercise of neuropsychological tests in older adults

Author	Age (Years)	Sample	RCT[a]	N per group[b]	Exercise Program	Duration (months)	Significance[c]	Range of Improvement[d]	
								Significant	Not significant
Barry et al (11)	55–79	Community	No	~ 7	Aerobic	3	3/19	6–7%	−23–46%
Powell (74)	59–89	Institutionalized (mental patients)	Yes	~11	Light general	3	2/3	26% & 35%	6%
Stamford et al (92)	mean = 72	Institutionalized (mental patients)	Yes	~ 9	Aerobic	3	2/4	no raw data	no raw data
Diesfeldt & Diesfeldt-Groenendijk (40)	mean = 82	Institutionalized (mental patients)	No	20	Light general	1	2/4	20% & 26%	25% & 38%
Dustman et al (41)	55–70	Community	Yes[e]	~15	Aerobic	4	7/9	3–14%	−4–10%

Study	Age range	Setting	RCT[a]	N per group[b]	Exercise type	No. of tests[c]	Ratio[c]	Net improvement[d]	Range
Molloy et al (66)	73–90	Nursing home	Yes	~22	Light general	3	1/8	18%	−5–19%
Blumenthal et al (17)	60–83	Community	Yes	~34	Aerobic	4	0/17	—	−16–23%, 158%
Madden et al (61)	60–83	Community	Yes	~26	Aerobic	4	0/30	—	All reaction time measures
Emery & Gatz (43)	61–86	Community	Yes	~15	Aerobic	3	0/4	—	1–9%
Panton et al (70)	70–79	Community	Yes	~15	Aerobic/strength training	6	0/4	—	−3–3%
Rikli & Edwards 1991 (76)	57–85	Community	No[e]	~17	General	36	2/2	6% and 13%	—

[a] RCT = randomized controlled trial.

[b] N per group = average group size in the analysis.

[c] A ratio of the number of neuropsychological tests that improved significantly with exercise, to the total number of tests. Subscales were considered a separate test if results were analyzed separately.

[d] The net improvement in neuropsychological tests was calculated from raw scores. Results are classified as to whether the improvement was statistically significant. For example, in the study by Barry et al (11), the net improvement on three tests was statistically significant and ranged from 6% to 7%. The net improvement on 16 tests was not significant, and ranged from −23% to 46%.

[e] Study was not described as randomized by author; subjects were alternately assigned to exercise versus control groups.

Table 4 Studies of the effect of exercise on bone mineral density in older women[a,b]

Authors	Sample	Age	RCT[c]	Adjusted for estrogens	Length of follow-up	Outcome assessed	Main findings
Smith & Reddan (88)	40	69–95	No	No mention	3 yrs	BMC at distal radius (SPA)	Group with light to moderate physical activity (30 min/day 3 days/wk) sig. better than controls (P = .02)
Aloia et al (3)	18	Post-menp. Mean 53	No	No mention	1 yr	TBCa via NAA BMC of radius (SPA)	Change in calcium balance sig. better in group with physical fitness exercises (60 min/day 3 days/wk). No change in BMC
Smith et al (89)	80	69–95 Mean 82	No	No mention	3 yrs	BMC of radius (SPA)	Group with exercise program (around a chair) 30 min/day 3 days/wk sig. better than controls
Chow et al (29)	68	50–62	Yes	Not on estrogens throughout the study	14 mths	CaBI via NAA of trunk and pelvis	Both aerobic exercise group (40 mins/day 3 days/wk) and the aerobic plus strengthening group (55 min/day 3 days/wk) sig. better than controls

Chow et al (30)	38	Post-menp. Mean 65	No	No mention	1 yr	CaBI via NAA of trunk and pelvis	Hospital group had sig. more compliance with exercising (60 min/day 3 days/wk of aerobic plus strengthening) and sig. better CaBI than home group
Cavanaugh & Cann (24)	18	49–64	No	Those using HRT in last 5 years excluded	1 yr	TMD of spine via CT	Group assigned to walking (40 min/day 3 days/wk) was not sig. different from controls
Dalsky et al (36)	35	55–70	No	No, but measured	22 mths	BMC of lumbar spine (DPA)	Long-term weight-bearing exercise group (50 min/day 3 days/wk) sig. better than controls
Smith et al (90) and Smith et al (87)	212	35–65	No	Those on HRT excluded	3 yrs and 4 yrs	BMC of distal radius, ulna, and humerus (SPA)	Group with physical activity class (45 min/day 3 days/wk) sig. better at radius & ulna. At 4 years, sig. difference in humerus for postmenopausal
Black Sandler et al (15)	255	Post-menp. Mean 57	Yes	Those on HRT excluded	3 yrs	BTD and CS area of radial bone (CT)	Walking group (3 miles/day 2 days/wk) not sig. different from controls, except in those with high grip strength

[a] Only studies with at least one year of follow-up are included.

[b] wk = week, min = minutes, mod. = moderate, sig. = significantly, mths = months, BMC = bone mineral content, SPA = single photon absorptiometry, post-menp. = post menopausal, TBCa = total body calcium, NAA = neutron activation analysis, HRT = hormone replacement therapy, BDT = bone tissue density, CS = cross sectional, CABI = calcium bone index, TMD = trabecular mineral density, CT = computerized tomography, DPA = dual photon absorptiometry.

[c] RCT = randomized controlled trial.

over long periods of time, inadequate statistical power, and failure to target physically unfit individuals.

Existing studies suggest that exercise may produce improvements in gait and balance. Arthritis patients may experience long-term functional status benefits from exercise, including improved mobility and decreased pain symptoms. Nonrandomized trials suggest exercise promotes bone mineral density and thereby decreases fracture risk. Recent studies have generally concluded that short-term exercise does not improve cognitive function. Yet the limited statistical power of these studies does not preclude what may be a modest, but functionally meaningful, effect of exercise on cognition.

Future research, beyond correcting methodologic deficiencies in existing studies, should systematically study how functional status effects of exercise vary with the type, intensity, and duration of exercise. It should address issues in recruiting functionally impaired older adults into exercise studies, issues in promoting long-term adherence to exercise, and whether the currently low rate of exercise-related injuries in supervised classes can be sustained in more cost-effective interventions that require less supervision.

ACKNOWLEDGMENTS

The authors would like to thank Michelle Bugge for her assistance in preparing this manuscript. Background research for this manuscript was supported in part by grants R48/CCR002181, RO1/AG06456, and U01/AG09095, and by the Health Services Research and Development Field Program of the Seattle VA Medical Center. The opinions expressed in the manuscript are those of the authors.

Literature Cited

1. Adams, G. M., de Vries, H. A. 1973. Physiological effects of exercise training regimen upon women aged 52 to 79. *J. Gerontol.* 28:50–55
2. Agre, J. C., Pierce, L. E., Raab, D. M., McAdams, M., Smith, E. L. 1988. Light resistance and stretching exercise in elderly women: effect upon strength. *Arch. Phys. Med. Rehabil.* 69:273–76
3. Aloia, J. F., Cohn, S. H., Ostuni, J. A., Cane, R., Ellis, K., 1978. Prevention of involutional bone loss by exercise. *Ann. Intern. Med.* 89:356–58
4. Aniansson, A., Grimby, G., Rundgren, A., Svanborg, A., Olander, J. 1980. Physical training in old men. *Age Ageing* 9:186–87
5. Aniansson, A., Gustafsson, E. 1981. Physical training in elderly men with special reference to quadriceps muscle strength and morphology. *Clin. Physiol.* 1:87–98

6. Aniansson, A., Hedberg, M., Henning, G. B., Grimby, G. 1986. Muscle morphology, enzymatic activity, and muscle strength in elderly men: a follow-up study. *Muscle Nerve* 9:585–91
7. Aniansson, A., Ljungberg, P., Rundgren, A., Wetterqvist, H. 1984. Effect of a training programme for pensioners on condition and muscular strength. *Arch. Gerontol. Geriatr.* 3:229–41
8. Aniansson, A., Sperling, L., Rundgren, A., Lehnberg, E. 1983. Muscle function in 75-year-old men and women: a longitudinal study. *Scand. J. Rehabil. Med.* (Suppl.) 9:92–103
9. Badenhop, D. T., Cleary, P. A., Schaal, S. F., Fox, E. L., Bartels, R. L. 1983. Physiological adjustments to higher- or lower-intensity exercise in elders. *Med. Sci. Sports Exerc.* 15:496–502
10. Barry, A. J., Daly, J. W., Pruett, E. D. R., Steinmetz, J. R., Page, H. F., et al.

1966. The effects of physical conditioning on older individuals: I. Work capacity, circulatory-respiratory function and work electrocardiogram. *J. Gerontol.* 21:182–91

11. Barry, A. J., Steinmetz, J. R., Page, H. F., Rodahl, K. 1966. The effects of physical conditioning on older individuals. II. Motor performance and cognitive function. *J. Gerontol.* 21:192–99

12. Bassett, C., McClamrock, E., Schmelzer, M. 1982. A 10-week exercise program for senior citizens. *Geriatr. Nurs.* 3:103–5

13. Bassey, E. J. 1978. Age, inactivity, and some physiological responses to exercise. *Gerontology* 24:66–77

14. Belman, M. J., Gaesser, G. A. 1991. Exercise training below and above the lactate threshold in the elderly. *Med. Sci. Sports Exerc.* 23:562–68

15. Black Sandler, R., Cauley, J. A., Hom, D. L., Sashin, D., Kriska, A. M. 1987. The effects of walking on the cross-sectional dimensions of the radius in postmenopausal women. *Calcific. Tissue Int.* 41:65–69

16. Block, J. E., Smith, R., Friedlander, A., Genant, H. K. 1989. Preventing osteoporosis with exercise: A review with emphasis on methodology. *Med. Hypoth.* 30:9–19

17. Blumenthal, J. A., Emery, C. F., Madden, D. J., George, L. K., Coleman, R. E., et al. 1989. Cardiovascular and behavioral effects of aerobic exercise training in healthy older men and women. *J. Gerontol.* 44:M147–57

18. Bouchard, C., Shephard, R. J., Stephens, T., Sutton, J. R., McPherson, B. D., eds. 1990. *Exercise, Fitness, and Health.* Champaign, Ill: Human Kinetics

19. Brown, M., Holloszy, J. O. 1991. Effects of a low intensity exercise program on selected physical performance characteristics of 60- to 71-year olds. *Aging* 3:129–39

20. Bruce, R. A. 1984. Exercise, functional aerobic capacity, and aging—another viewpoint. *Med. Sci. Sports Exerc.* 16:8–13

21. Buccola, V. A., Stone, W. J. 1975. Effects of jogging and cycling programs on physiological and personality variables in aged men. *Res. Q.* 46:134–39

22. Buchner, D. M., de Lateur, B. J. 1991. The importance of skeletal muscle strength to physical function in older adults. *Behav. Med. Ann.* 13:In press

23. Buchner, D. M., Wagner, E. H. 1991. Can frail health be prevented? *Clin. Geriatr. Med.* In press

24. Cavanaugh, D. J., Cann, C. E. 1988. Brisk walkng does not stop bone loss in postmenopausal women, *Bone* 9:201–4

25. Chalmers, J., Ho, K. C. 1970. Geographical variations in senile osteoporosis. *J. Bone Joint Surg.* 52:667–75

26. Chamie, M. 1990. The status and use of the International Classification of Impairments, Disabilities and Handicaps (ICIDH). *World Health Stat. Q.* 43:273–80

27. Chapman, E. A., de Vries, H. A., Swezey, R. 1972. Joint stiffness: effects of exercise on young and old men. *J. Gerontol.* 27:218–21

28. Charette, S. L., McEvoy, L., Pyka, G., Snow-Harter, C., Guido, G., et al. 1991. Muscle hypertrophy response to resistance training in older women. *J. Appl. Physiol.* 70:1912–16

29. Chow, R., Harrison, J. E., Notarius, C. 1987. Effect of two randomized exercise programmes on bone mass of healthy postmenopausal women. *Br. Med. J.* 295:1441–44

30. Chow, R. K., Harrison, J. E., Sturtridge, W., Josse, R., Murray, T. M., et al. 1987. The effect of exercise on bone mass of osteoporotic patients on flouride treatment. *Clin. Invest. Med.* 10:59–63

31. Clark, B. A., Wade, M. G., Massey, B. H., Van Dyke, R. 1975. Response of institutionalized geriatric mental patients to a twelve-week program of regular physical activity. *J. Gerontol.* 30:565–73

32. Clement, F. J. 1974. Longitudinal and cross-sectional assessments of age changes in physical strength as relate to sex, social class, and mental ability. *J. Gerontol.* 29:423–29

33. Cress, M. E., Thomas, D. P., Johnson, J., Kasch, F. W., Cassens, R. G., et al. 1991. Effect of training on VO2max, thigh strength, and muscle morphology in septuagenarian women. *Med. Sci. Sports Exerc.* 23:752–58

34. Crilly, R. G., Willems, D. A., Trenholm, K. J., Hayes, K. C., Delaquerriere-Richardson, L. F. O. 1989. Effect of exercise on postural sway in the elderly. *Gerontology* 35:137–43

35. Cunningham, D. A., Rechnitzer, P. A., Howard, J. H., Donner, A. P. 1987. Exercise training of men at retirement: a clinical trial. *J. Gerontol.* 45:17–23

36. Dalsky, G. P., Stocke, K. S., Ehsani, A. A., Slatopolsky, E., Lee, W. C. et al. 1988. Weight-bearing exercise training and lumbar bone mineral content in postmenopausal women. *Ann. Intern. Med.* 108:824–28

37. Dehn, M. M., Bruce, R. A. 1972. Lon-

gitudinal variations in maximal oxygen intake with age and activity. *J. Appl. Physiol.* 33:805–7

38. de Lateur, B. J., Lehmann, J. F. 1986. Strengthening exercise. In *Principles of Physical Medicine and Rehabilitation in the Musculoskeletal Diseases,* ed. J. C. Leek, J. F. Lehmann, 3:25–61. Orlando, Fla: Grune & Stratton

39. deVries, H. A. 1970. Physiological effects of an exercise training regimen upon men aged 52–88. *J. Gerontol.* 25:325–36

40. Diesfeldt, H. F. A., Diesfeldt-Groenendijk, H. 1977. Improving cognitive performance in psychogeriatric patients: the influence of physical exercise. *Age Ageing* 6:58–64

41. Dustman, R. E., Ruhling, R. O., Russell, E. M., Shearer, D. E., Bonekat, H. W., et al. 1984. Aerobic exercise training and improved neuropsychological function of older individuals. *Neurobiol. Aging* 5:35–42

42. Ekdahl, C., Andersson, S. I., Moritz, U., Svensson, B. 1990. Dynamic versus static training in patients with rheumatoid arthritis. *Scand. J. Rheumatol.* 19:17–26

43. Emery, C. F., Gatz, M. 1990. Psychological and cognitive effects of an exercise program for community-residing older adults. *Gerontologist* 30:184–88

44. Enoka, R. M. 1988. Muscle strength and its development. *Sports Med.* 6:146–69

45. Era, P. 1988. Posture control in the elderly. *Int. J. Technol. Aging* 1:166–79

46. Fiatarone, M. A., Marks, E. C., Ryan, N. D., Meredith, C. N., Lipsitz, L. A., Evans, W. J. 1990. High-intensity strength training in nonagenarians. *J. Am. Med. Assoc.* 263:3029–34

47. Fisher, N. M., Pedergast, D. R., Gresham, G. E., Calkins, E. 1991. Muscle rehabilitation: its effect on muscular and functional performance of patients with knee osteoarthritis. *Arch. Phys. Med. Rehabil.* 72:367–74

48. Foster, V. L., Hume, G. J. E., Byrnes, W. C., Dickinson, A. L., Chatfield, S. J. 1989. Endurance training for elderly women: moderate vs. low intensity. *J. Gerontol.* 44:M184–78

49. Frontera, W. R., Meredith, C. N., O'Reilly, K. P., Knuttgen, H. G., Evans, W. J. 1988. Strength conditioning in older men: skeletal muscle hypertrophy and improved function. *J. Appl. Physiol.* 64:1038–44

50. Grimby, G., Saltin, B. 1983. Minireview: the ageing muscle. *Clin. Physiol.* 3:209–18

51. Guralnik, J. M., Branch, L. G., Cummings, S. R., Curb, J. D. 1989. Physical performance measures in aging research. *J. Gerontol.* 44:M141–46

52. Gutman, G. M., Herbert, C. P., Brown, S. R. 1977. Feldenkrais versus conventional exercises for elderly. *J. Gerontol.* 32:562–72

53. Haber, P., Honiger, B., Klicpera, M., Niederberger, M. 1984. Effects in elderly people 67–76 years of age of three-month endurance training on a bicycle ergometer. *Eur. Heart J.* (Suppl.) 5:37–39

54. Hopkins, D. R., Murrah, B., Hoeger, W. W. K., Rhodes, R. C. 1990. Effect of low-impact aerobic dance on the functional fitness of elderly women. *Gerontologist* 30:189–92

55. Irving, J. B., Kusumi, F., Bruce, R. A. 1980. Longitudinal variations in maximal oxygen consumption in healthy men. *Clin. Cardiol.* 3:134–36

56. Jette, M., Sidney, K., Blumchen, G. 1990. Metabolic equivalents (METS) in exercise testing, exercise prescription, and evaluation of functional capacity. *Clin. Cardiol.* 13:555–65

57. Kasch, F. W., Boyer J. L., Van Camp, S. P., Verity, L. S., Wallace, J. P. 1990. The effect of physical activity and inactivity on aerobic power in older men (a longitudinal study). *Phys. Sportsmed.* 18:73–83

58. Kauffman, T. L. 1985. Strength training effect in young and aged women. *Arch. Phys. Med. Rehabil.* 66:223–26

59. Kelley, D. L., Dainis, A., Wood, G. K. 1976. Mechanics and muscular dynamics of rising from a seated position. In *Biomechanics V-B. V.1B,* ed. P. V. Komi, pp. 127–34. Baltimore: University Park

60. Liemohn, W. P. 1975. Strength and aging: an exploratory study. *Int. J. Aging Hum. Dev.* 6:347–57

61. Madden, D. J., Blumenthal, J. A., Allen, P. A., Emergy, C. F. 1989. Improving aerobic capacity in healthy older adults does not necessarily lead to improved cognitive performance. *Psychol. Aging* 4:307–20

62. Mahler, D. A., Cunningham, L. N., Curfman, G. D. 1986. Aging and exercise performance. *Clin. Geriatr. Med.* 2:433–52

63. Maughan, R. J. 1984. Relationship between muscle strength and muscle cross-sectional area. *Sports Med.* 1:263–69

64. Minor, M. A., Hewett, J. E., Webel, R. R., Anderson, S. K., Kay, D. R. 1989. Efficacy of physical conditioning exercise in patients with rheumatoid arthri-

tis and osteoarthritis. *Arthritis Rheum.* 32:1396–1405

65. Minor, M. A., Hewett, J. E., Webel, R. R., Dreisinger, T. E., Kay, D. R. 1988. Exercise tolerance and disease related measures in patients with rheumatoid arthritis and osteoarthritis. *J. Rheumatol.* 15:905–11

66. Molloy, D. W., Richardson, L. D., Crilly, R. G. 1988. The effects of a three-month exercise programme on neuropsychological function in elderly institutionalized women: a randomized controlled trial. *Age Ageing* 17:303–10

67. Moritani, T., deVries, H. A. 1980. Potential for gross muscle hypertrophy in older men. *J. Gerontol.* 35:672–82

68. Moritani, T., deVries, H. A. 1979. Neural factors versus hypertrophy in the time course of muscle strength gain. *Am. J. Phys. Med.* 58:115–30

69. Niinimaa, V., Shephard, R. J. 1978. Training and oxygen conductance in the elderly. I. the respiratory system. *J. Gerontol.* 33:354–61

70. Panton, L. B., Graves, J. E., Pollock, M. L., Hagberg, J. M., Chen, W. 1990. Effect of aerobic and resistance training on fractionated reaction time and speed of movement. *J. Gerontol.* 45:M26–31

71. Perkins, L. C., Kaiser, H. L. 1961. Results of short-term isotonic and isometric exercise programs in persons over sixty. *Phys. Ther. Rev.* 41:633–35

72. Plowman, S. A., Drinkwater, B. L., Horvath, S. M. 1979. Age and aerobic power in women: a longitudinal study. *J. Gerontol.* 34:512–20

73. Posner, J. D., Gorman, K. M., Gitlin, L. N., Sands, L. P., Kleban, M., et al. 1990. Effects of exercise training in the elderly on the occurrence and time to onset of cardiovascular diagnoses. *J. Am. Geriatr. Soc.* 38:205–10

74. Powell, R. R. 1974. Psychological effects of exercise therapy upon institutionalized geriatric mental patients. *J. Gerontol.* 29:157–61

75. Reed, R. L., Pearlmutter, L., Yochum, K., Meredith, K. E., Mooradian, A. D. 1991. The relationship between muscle mass and muscle strength in the elderly. *J. Am. Geriatr. Soc.* 39:555–61

76. Rikli, R. E., Edwards, D. J. 1991. Effects of a three-year exercise program on motor function and cognitive processing speed in older women. *Res. Q. Exerc. Sport* 62:61–67

77. Roberts, B. L. 1985. Walking improves balance, reduces falls. *Am. J. Nurs.* 85:1397

78. Rogers, R. L., Meyer, J. S., Mortel, K. F. 1990. After reaching retirement age physical activity sustains cerebral perfusion and cognition. *J. Am. Geriatr. Soc.* 38:123–28

79. Sagiv, M., Fisher, N., Yaniv, A., Rudoy, J. 1989. Effect of running versus isometric training programs on healthy elderly at rest. *Gerontology* 35:72–77

80. Schoutens, A., Laurent, E., Poortmans, J. R. 1989. Effects of inactivity and exercise on bone. *Sport Med.* 7:71–81

81. Seals, D. R., Hagberg, J. M., Hurley, B. F., Ehsani, A. A., Holloszy, J. O. 1984. Endurance training in older men and women. I. Cardiovascular responses to exercise. *J. Appl. Physiol.* 57:1024–29

82. Shephard, R. J. 1990. The scientific basis of exercise prescribing for the very old. *J. Am. Geriatr. Soc.* 38:62–70

83. Shephard, R. J., Sidney, K. H. 1978. Exercise and aging. *Exerc. Sport Sci. Rev.* 6:1–57

84. Sidney, K. H., Shephard, R. J. 1978. Frequency and intensity of exercise training for elderly subjects. *Med. Sci. Sports* 10:125–31

85. Simonson, E. 1971. Recovery and fatigue. In *Physiology of Work Capacity and Fatigue,* ed. E. Simonson, 18:440–58. Springfield, Ill: Thomas

86. Skinner, J. S., Baldini, F. D., Gardner, A. W. 1990. Assessment of fitness. See Ref. 18, pp. 109–19

87. Smith, E. L., Gilligan, C., McAdam, M., Ensign, C. P., Smith, P. E. 1989. Deterring bone loss by exercise intervention in premenopausal women and postmenopausal women. *Calcif. Tissue Int.* 44:312–21

88. Smith, E. L., Reddan, W. 1976. Physical activity—a modality for bone accretion in the aged. *Am. J. Roentgenol.* 126:1297

89. Smith, E. L., Reddan, W., Smith, P. E. 1981. Physical activity and calcium modalities for bone mineral increase in aged women. *Med. Sci. Sports Exerc.* 13:60–64

90. Smith, E. L., Smith, P. E., Ensign, C. J., Shea, M. M. 1984. Bone involution decrease in exercising middle-aged women. *Calcif. Tissue Int.* 36:S129–38

91. Stamford, B. A. 1973. Effects of chronic institutionalization on physical working capacity and trainability of geriatric men. *J. Gerontol.* 28:441–46

92. Stamford, B. A., Hambacher, W., Fallica, A. 1974. Effects of daily physical exercise on the psychiatric state of institutionalized geriatric mental patients. *Res. Q.* 45:35–41

93. Suominen, H., Heikkinen, E., Liesen, H., Michel, D., Hollman, W. 1977.

Effects of 8 weeks endurance training on skeletal muscle metabolism in 56–70 yr. old sedentary men. *Eur. J. Appl. Phys.* 37:173–80

94. US Prev. Serv. Task Force: Exerc. Counsel. 1989. In *Guide to Clinical Preventive Services.* 49:297–303. Baltimore: Williams & Wilkins

95. Vanfraechem, J., Vanfraechem, R. 1977. Studies of the effect of a short training period on aged subjects. *J. Sports Med.* 17:373–80

96. Wagner, E. H., LaCroix, A. Z., Buchner, D. M., Larson, E. B. Activity and Health I: Effects of habitual activity in older adults. *Annu. Rev. Public Health* 13:451–68

97. Young, A. 1986. Exercise physiology in geriatric practice. *Acta. Med. Scand.* (Suppl.) 711:227–32

Annu. Rev. Publ. Health 1992. 13:489–508

FALLS AMONG OLDER PERSONS:
A Public Health Perspective[1]

Richard W. Sattin

Division of Injury Control, National Center for Environmental Health and Injury Control, Centers for Disease Control, Public Health Service, US Department of Health and Human Services, Atlanta, Georgia 30333

KEY WORDS: epidemiology, injury, prevention, risk factors, surveillance

INTRODUCTION

Among persons aged 65 years or older, falls are the leading cause of death from injury (66, 79). Major morbidity from falls includes more than 230,000 hip fractures per year among persons in this age group (National Center for Health Statistics 1987, unpublished data). The cost of falls among older persons is enormous, because of the high death toll, numerous disabling conditions, and extensive hospital stays; nearly $10 billion of the $158 billion lifetime economic cost of injury to our nation can be attributed to falls among older persons (79). Moreover, falls pose a particular problem for public health professionals in the development of both surveillance systems and prevention strategies.

To understand the concepts of fall prevention, one must also understand the concepts of injury control. In this article, I discuss from a public health perspective the concept of injury as a disease, the extent of the problem of falls among older persons, current concepts on the etiology of falls, the need for better surveillance, and how understanding these needs and concepts could lead us to develop a systematic approach to fall prevention.

---

[1]The US Government has the right to retain a nonexclusive royalty-free license in and to any copyright covering this paper.

INJURY AS A DISEASE

By most measures, injury ranks as one of the most serious public health problems in the United States today (15). Although the human and financial costs of injury in our society are very high, support for injury control has lagged far behind support for other public health problems (14, 79). Injuries occur at such great numbers that, until recently, they have been tacitly accepted as a normal occurrence of living in a modern society. Fortunately, in the 1985 report, *Injury in America,* the Committee on Trauma Research of the National Research Council and the Institute of Medicine proposed a national plan for injury control that focused on a public health approach to reducing injuries (14). Committee members understood that, like other diseases, injuries could be viewed as a problem in medical ecology—that is, as a relationship between a person (the host), an agent, and the environment. Unlike these other diseases, however, the underlying agent of injury is not a microbe or carcinogen. Instead, the agent is energy, most often in the form of mechanical force (37).

Injury should be considered a disease that has a short latency period. It results from the acute, rapid exposure to energy (mechanical, thermal, chemical, electrical, or radiation) or from the absence of specific body needs, such as oxygen or heat (5). The dose of energy received, the dose's distribution, duration, and rapidity, and the human's response to the transfer of the energy can determine whether an injury occurs or is prevented (14). For example, a large mechanical energy load quickly transmitted during a fall involving an older person may damage cells, tissues, and other structures, thus resulting in a fracture. If the same energy load could be transmitted at a slower velocity or dissipated over a much larger area, different responses could be mobilized, thus resulting in the prevention of injury during the fall.

EPIDEMIOLOGY OF FALLS

Definitions and Classification Schemes

The Kellogg International Work Group, from whose work most fall definitions are derived, defined a fall as "an event which results in a person coming to rest inadvertently on the ground or other lower level and other than as a consequence of the following: sustaining a violent blow; loss of consciousness; sudden onset of paralysis, as in a stroke; or an epileptic seizure" (45). Unfortunately, that and most of the derived definitions of a fall are clinically or research oriented; require extensive interviewing; are unwieldy to use in a public health setting; are subjective and, thus, allow differences in interpretation for each study setting; and are likely to miss a substantial number of falls, if the data are acquired through record review and abstracting.

Developing a definition useful to public health officials is difficult, because a fall is not a disease. Rather, a fall is often a syndrome, which represents symptoms and signs of disordered function in a disordered environment. For example, a fall might be a direct result of underlying cardiovascular or musculoskeletal disease. Depending on the amount of energy transferred, a fall itself might lead to a disease (e.g. hip fracture, traumatic brain injury) or, more often, might never attract medical or public health attention.

Various state and community public health programs have demonstrated that effective intervention strategies can be implemented by using available data on the external causes of injury, as defined by the *International Classification of Diseases, Ninth Revision, Clinical Modification* (ICD-9-CM) (33, 64). ICD-9-CM contains a standard coding system that describes diseases and the anatomical nature of injuries (N-codes). A supplemental volume, titled External Causes of Injuries (E-codes), describes the circumstances and location of the injury and is extremely useful for public health practitioners to quantify the problem of falls in their communities.

Falls can be coded according to the external causes of the injury (codes, E880–E888); however, a further definition is needed for those falls that result in nonfatal injury. The terms "fall injuries" and "fall-related injuries" are widely used, but are ambiguous, as they are often used to describe the type of anatomical injury (e.g. hip fracture, brain injury), multiple types of anatomical injuries during the same fall, or multiple fall events with at least one injury. To reduce this ambiguity, I suggest using the terms "fall injury event," which is the occurrence of a fall that resulted in at least one anatomical injury, and "fall injury," which is the type of anatomical injury sustained during the fall (such as hip fracture, skull fracture, superficial injury) (89). For those fall injury events that result in more than one anatomical injury, some researchers have developed hierarchies of fall injuries, whereby the most severe injury receives the top priority status for reporting (29, 89).

The multifaceted, multifactorial nature of falls has prompted attempts to classify falls by etiology, that is, to link specific risk factors or biologic measurements to specific types of fall (6, 9, 41, 47, 62, 67, 68, 93, 105). These classifications, however, are based on interviews with case patients or abstracts of their medical records about the circumstances of falls. Therefore, they are subject to recall and interviewer bias and have led to a lack of consistency in the literature on the association of risk factors and falls (87). Some examples of these classification schemes include unexplained falls versus falls with a self-evident etiology (e.g. syncope, seizure, stroke); and falls due to host (intrinsic) factors versus falls due to environmental (extrinsic) factors. Although these schemes might be useful in a clinical setting, they are less useful in a public health setting, because data of this extent are not readily available.

Incidence

In 1988, 9060 fatal falls (codes, E880–E888) occurred among persons aged 65 years or older (National Center for Health Statistics 1988, unpublished data). Nearly 60% of fatal falls occur in the home or in a residential institution (90). Although falls are the leading cause of death due to injury among older persons, this effect is mainly caused by its impact among those 85 or older (Table 1). More than one half of injury-related deaths of women and one third of men aged 85 or older are due to falls. The rate of deaths due to falls rises rapidly with increasing age for all race-sex groups aged 75 or older (Figure 1). White men aged 85 or older have the highest death rates associated with falls.

Pulmonary embolism is strongly associated with deaths due to falls and occurs in nearly 13% of such deaths (60). This association increases with increasing age and is much greater among those persons with fractures of the lower limbs, including femoral neck. Among those deaths from falls with no fracture listed, the prevalence of pulmonary embolism is 2.4%.

Falls can also lead to significant morbidity in older individuals. About 7% of persons over age 75 visit hospital emergency rooms for a fall injury event each year (29). Falls account for nearly 70% of all emergency room visits to treat injuries in this age group (29). In a recent study in South Miami Beach, Florida, investigators found that the rate of nonfatal fall injury events increased steadily by each five-year age group for those aged 65 or older, reaching a high of 138 per 1000 for men and 159 per 1000 for women aged 85

Table 1 Number of deaths due to injuries for persons aged 65 years or older, by cause, sex, and age group, United States, 1988[a]

| | Sex and age (years) | | | |
| | Men | | Women | |
Cause[b]	65–84	85+	65–84	85+
Falls	2,459	1,410	2,444	2,747
Motor vehicles	3,583	495	2,718	363
Drowning	315	39	119	43
Fires/Burns	707	168	566	164
Poisonings	322	53	290	132
Homicide	694	59	498	79
Suicide	4,672	498	1,086	107
Other	3,401	954	2,494	1,374
Total	16,153	3,676	10,215	5,009

[a] Source: National Center for Health Statistics, Detailed Mortality Tapes.
[b] According to the ICD-9-CM.

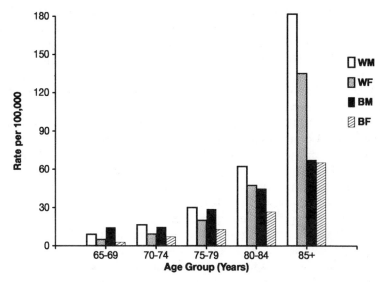

Figure 1   Rates of deaths due to falls, by age and race-sex groups, in the United States, 1988.

years or more (Figure 2). Of those fall injury events identified through the acute care setting, more than 40% resulted in hospital admissions, with an average length of stay of 11.6 days overall (89).

One specific injury type, hip fracture, increases exponentially by age in older persons, from 28 per 10,000 persons aged 65–74 to 251 per 10,000

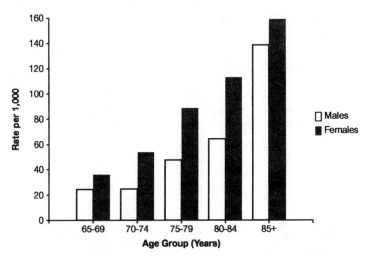

Figure 2   Rates of fall injury events, by age and sex. Study to Assess Falls Among the Elderly, Miami Beach, Florida, 1985–1987.

persons aged 85 or older (82). For persons aged 65 or older, the rate of hip fracture among white women is about twice that of white men, and white persons have about twice the rate of hip fracture as persons of all other races (4, 24, 82). More hip fractures occur in winter than summer, but this seasonal variation occurs regardless of latitude (42). Data from the National Hospital Discharge Survey, National Center for Health Statistics, indicate that in 1987, 233,432 hip fractures occurred among persons aged 65 or older. Of these, 13,138 (5.6%) resulted in death during hospitalization. If 90% of these hip fracture-related deaths were caused by falls, we could estimate that about 11,824 deaths due to falls resulted from only one type of injury. Mortality data from 1987 reveal that 8602 persons aged 65 or older died because of a fall. These and other data suggest that we have a major problem of undercounting deaths caused by falls (28).

Most falls among the elderly population result in minor or no physical injury; only a small percentage of falls cause severe injury, such as a fracture (67, 99). An estimated 25–35% of older persons fall each year (67, 98), and a higher annual incidence is reported among older persons who live in residential institutions (87). An estimated 3–6% of falls result in a fracture for persons living in the community and in nursing homes; 1% or less results in hip fractures (35, 67, 87, 99). Public health practitioners who focus prevention programs on elderly health should also consider systematically monitoring community- or nursing home-dwelling older persons for fall injury events.

Risk Factors Related to the Host

Several host factors may alter the risk of falls and fall injury events. Listed below are some of the factors that might help us identify high-risk individuals and develop screening techniques or prevention efforts (Table 2).

AGE AND SEX   In most studies of both community and institutionalized populations, researchers find that the risk of falling and being injured in-

Table 2 Potential risk factors for falls among the elderly that may help public health practitioners target intervention programs

Host	Agent	Environment
Age and sex	Mechanical energy	Lighting
Osteoporosis	Impact position	Stairs
Chronic diseases	Impact location	Rugs and flooring
Gait and balance		Bathtubs
Vision		Shelving
Mental status		Footwear
Medication use		Streets and walkways
Alcohol use		

creases with age in both sexes and is greater in females than males at most ages (9, 29, 73, 89). For example, older persons tend to have poorer responses to injury events than younger persons (5). With aging, physiologic changes occur in articular cartilage, bone, ligaments, and musculature (95). These changes can lead to osteoporosis, arthritis, decreased muscle strength and mass, decreased joint flexibility, decreased collagen elasticity and strength, and general discomfort and pain. Individuals with these changes might respond more slowly during difficult or emergency situations or develop early and excessive fatigue, which might lead to an injury (14). In addition, the most effective energy absorber in the human body, the active musculature, depends mostly on muscle strength, which decreases with age (95). During an injury event, therefore, these changes in the musculoskeletal system can lead to a decreased ability to withstand the effects of mechanical energy. Much of this variation in fall risk, however, may be due to the biologic and functional variability within age groups, rather than to simple age-dependent variations (74). If exercise and general muscle conditioning for older persons prove effective, public health practitioners could include these programs with others targeted to older persons.

Women and men may have different outcomes from a fall for several reasons. For example, osteoporosis may play a substantial role in hip and other limb fractures for women (19, 50, 59, 61). On the other hand, women might fall differently than men and absorb mechanical energy at different parts of the body (hip) than men (head) (89).

OSTEOPOROSIS   Among older persons, osteoporosis decreases bone resistance to mechanical energy, which increases the risk of compression fractures from a given force (14) and predisposes to fractures of the hip, vertebrae, distal forearm, and pelvis, especially in older, white women (19, 50, 59, 61). Considerable controversy exists over the relative importance of osteoporosis in the etiology of hip fracture. Some investigators have argued that older persons with hip fractures are no more osteoporotic than noninjured persons of similar ages (17, 18). By using biomechanics research, Lotz & Hayes (53) have shown that about one twentieth of the energy that is needed to break a hip may be available during a typical fall from standing position. On the other hand, other researchers state that data on osteoporosis and hip fracture have been misinterpreted and that the measurement of osteoporosis through bone densitometry may be used to predict the propensity for fracture and, therefore, be useful as a screening tool (43, 85). They also note that the use of estrogen replacement therapy (ERT) in peri- and postmenopausal women retards the development of osteoporosis and reduces the risk of hip fractures in older women (1, 23, 46, 104).

The use of densitometry as a basic screening tool to identify persons at high risk of hip fracture, however, is premature for several reasons. First, few, if any, longitudinal studies have observed the rate of hip fractures among women with baseline bone mass determinations at menopause (30). Without these data, determining the impact of risk factor modifications is problematic (7, 18). Second, most studies that have demonstrated a reduction in hip fracture risk among women who have ever used estrogen have not included women older than age 74, the age group at highest risk for hip fracture (1, 46, 104). One recent Swedish cohort study demonstrated a reduction in the rate of trochanteric hip fractures among women who had taken estrogen for up to five years before age 60; no effect has yet been seen for older women (63). Third, ERT's increase in the risk of endometrial and other cancers and its side effects may outweigh the risk of hip fractures for women considering the use of ERT (18). If clinical trials confirm the protective effect of ERT among women at risk of heart disease (32a), then screening for osteoporosis may play a limited role in a woman's decision to use ERT (18). Finally, for the public health practitioner, body mass index (weight in kilograms divided by height in meters squared) appears to be highly correlated with bone mass, as determined by densitometry (M. Nevitt 1991, personal communication).

The determination of the mechanism of falls and injuries and ways to alter other risk factors will likely have a greater impact on hip fracture than the use of ERT by older women (61).

CHRONIC DISEASES   Cerebrovascular, cardiovascular, and neurologic disorders may increase the number of falls among older persons (44, 51, 52, 88). In a recent population-based study (89), the most common concurrent medical diagnoses associated with a fall injury event were syncope (16%), conduction disorder/dysrhythmias (15%), chronic ischemic heart disease (9.3%), anemia (8.7%), diabetes (8.3%), and hypertensive disease (8.2%). The prevention and amelioration of these chronic ailments through chronic disease prevention activities could lead to a substantial decrease in the future number of falls and fall injury events among older persons.

Some investigators suggest that the risk of falling increases with the number of these conditions present, especially those that impair sensory, cognitive, neurologic, or musculoskeletal functioning (98, 100). Although these conditions do contribute to the occurrence of a fall, either through their physiologic effect or through a joint effect with environmental hazards, each chronic disorder probably does not contribute the same amount of risk to falling.

GAIT AND BALANCE   Gait and balance abnormalities have been repeatedly implicated in falls among older persons (41, 67, 80, 99, 100). These abnormalities may be related to changes in age, disease, or medication use or to dysfunction of the nervous, skeletal, circulatory, or respiratory systems (87). Clinically, the older person with a history of falls often has a stiff, uncoordinated gait and poor control over posture and body position (22, 87). An increasing number of clinical and laboratory measurement tools are available for assessing the complex neuromuscular functions of gait, balance, and postural control. Unfortunately, we do not yet have a way to use these clinical and laboratory measurements to develop easily administered screening procedures for public health practitioners. In addition, we do not know if physical retraining through exercise, muscle strengthening, or some other mechanism will help decrease fall injury events among older persons (see Buchner et al, this volume). The ability to influence corrective and protective response through training and education should also be investigated. An understanding of how specific gait and balance problems transform environmental features into "fall hazards" would help us focus our environmental intervention efforts.

VISION   Impaired visual acuity and depth perception have been associated with an increased risk of falling and fracturing a hip (25, 67, 100). Visual acuity might be very important in maintaining postural control among persons with neuromuscular disorders (3, 13, 25, 49, 70). Visual acuity, depth perception, contrast sensitivity, peripheral vision, visual perception, dark adaptation, and glare tolerance are all involved in the detection and avoidance of environmental hazards and can become affected by age-related vision changes, cataracts, macular degeneration, and glaucoma (98). Early detection and treatment of common conditions, such as glaucoma and cataracts, should improve visual function and might reduce falls (2). Recent study findings, however, implicate topical eye medications as increasing the risk of falling among a selected group of elderly glaucoma patients (32). Whether this effect is real or a manifestation of other chronic conditions or disease-drug interactions needs further investigation.

MENTAL STATUS   Impaired mental status and depression are associated with an increased risk of a fall injury event (6, 9, 67, 73, 99, 105). This association may be related to the increased exposure to hazardous situations, because of confusion, impaired judgment, distraction, agitation, and lack of awareness. Associated gait and balance deficits and psychomotor depression may also increase the chance of falling. Antidepressant and sedative medication used for these conditions contribute to the increased risk of falls and fall injury events (78). Simple screening tests, such as the Mini-Mental Test (31), are available to determine the person's degree of cognitive impairment. We do not yet know, however, which interventions can reduce the incidence of fall injury events in this high-risk group of older persons, while maintaining their highest level of cognitive functioning. Also, because high rates of suicide occur among older white men (58), clinicians must use caution in changing the patterns of antidepressant medication use to reduce the incidence of fall injury events.

MEDICATION USE   Ray et al (78) analyzed Michigan Medicaid data in a large and well-designed study and found a significantly increased risk of hip fracture in older persons currently taking long half-life psychotropic medications. They estimated that about 14% of these hip fractures were attributable to current use of psychotropic medications. These medications (including the widely used benzodiazepines, barbiturates, phenothiazines, and tricyclic antidepressants) may act by decreasing alertness, affecting judgment, compromising neuromuscular function, or causing dizziness and syncope. MacDonald & MacDonald (56) found a substantial excess of barbiturate use among hip fracture patients who sustained the injury at night, compared with those whose fractures occurred during the day. Studies of falling suggest that recent use of any psychotropic medication may be associated with an increased risk of falling (105). Tinetti et al (99) noted an increased risk of falling among persons who use some psychotropic medications, but the prevalence of psychotropic medication use among nonfallers was low—only one of 228 nonfallers were users—compared with prevalence reported in other surveys (67, 78).

In several studies, however, investigators have failed to find a relationship between psychotropic drug use and falling or fracturing a hip (34, 67, 71). One major reason for this discrepancy in the findings is the possible effect of an underlying condition, such as dementia, or the effect of drug-disease interactions, such as psychotropics and dementia. For example, in recent analytic studies (78, 99) that included cognitively impaired persons, researchers found an increased risk of falling or fall injury events associated with drug use, whereas the findings of studies that specifically excluded persons with cognitive impairment revealed no increase in risk (34, 67).

Falls related to multiple drug use may be an important problem (55, 98). For example, Buchner & Larson (8) found that patients with Alzheimer's disease increased their risk of falling with the increased number of drugs taken. Physicians, pharmacists, and public health practitioners need to help older persons eliminate outdated medications better and monitor medication use more closely to prevent drug-drug interactions that can cause falls.

Diuretics or antihypertensives might contribute to falling through fatigue, volume depletion, decreased mental alertness, or postural hypotension (98). Some researchers, however, have shown that use of thiazide diuretics might actually decrease the risk of a hip fracture, by decreasing urinary calcium excretion (27, 47b, 77). Because of the relatively high incidence of metabolic and other side effects associated with thiazide diuretics, these drugs are being replaced by other antihypertensives. Nevertheless, further work is warranted to investigate the preventive aspects of thiazides.

In summary, the balance of evidence suggests that psychotropic drugs play a role in the risk of falling among older persons. Effective reduction in physician prescribing practices for long half-life benzodiazepines has been accomplished through educational efforts (76). Also, New York state has recently limited excess prescribing of benzodiazepines through regulation and, thus, has decreased their use by low-income older persons by 25% (57); however, the prescribing of less acceptable medications increased (103b). Further work on drug-disease interactions and dose-specific effects, however, is needed to define more accurately who among the users of psychotropic and other medications are at highest risk of injury (36). This work is critical to designing appropriate intervention efforts.

ALCOHOL USE   Alcohol use is frequently a factor in injury. Alcohol acts as a depressant on the central nervous system and may increase the risk of falling and fall injury events by adversely affecting gait, balance, and cognition (72). Alcohol use has been frequently associated with falls in persons younger than age 65 (26, 39, 40), but most studies have not shown an association for older persons (34, 67, 73, 99). One study presents only nonanalytic evidence of an association between alcohol use and the risk of falling among older persons (103). This lack of evidence might reflect differential survival, because heavy alcohol use is strongly associated with premature mortality from a variety of causes (75). Although alcohol use is not associated with an increased risk of falls or fall injury events among older persons, the chronic use of alcohol interferes with tissue regeneration and immunologic function. An older person who drinks can, therefore, have a more severe outcome than a nondrinker who experiences the same injury event (14). In addition, the chronic use of alcohol can lead to various chronic medical conditions that predispose a person to sustain a fall or fall injury event.

Risk Factors Related to the Agent

Although we know much about the host and the environment, we know very little about the mechanism or transference of energy during a fall (14). Mechanical energy is the most common agent of injury due to falls among older persons (Table 2). Speed, violence, and concentration are key elements in transforming mechanical energy into an impact injury, which occurs by deforming tissue beyond its failure limits (102). Mechanisms that affect the risk of impact injury are the resistance of the body through inertial forces, the elastic capacity of the tissues, and the viscous tolerance of the body organs (14). Inertial forces from excessive acceleration of the skeleton lead to the tearing of an organ. An example is brain injury that results from the sudden acceleration of the skull during impact with the ground, with the loosely attached brain lagging behind. Because of its elastic capacity, the body can absorb a tremendous amount of mechanical energy and protect organs through resistance to impact. This resistance of the human body has been demonstrated by persons who have survived falls from extreme heights (14). Older persons, however, tend to have decreased elasticity of tissues and organs, which can lead to fractures of the hip, ribs, and skull. Finally, viscous tolerance, the ability of organs to withstand rapidly applied strain forces, can be exceeded during high-speed impact, thus leading to contusion and possible rupture of an organ. For example, the heart may sustain damage when the sternum is rapidly and excessively moved during a motor vehicle crash. The same compression, occurring slowly, would not necessarily damage the heart, because the organ can tolerate gradual compression.

Biomechanics is the discipline in which researchers investigate and explain the physical and physiologic responses to impact that result in injury (102). Better understanding can lead to protective devices for persons involved in potential injury events. We have yet to realize the tremendous, untapped potential in applying biomechanics to the control of injuries, other than those related to motor vehicles. Nevertheless, the biomechanics of falls and hip fractures have received growing attention over the last several years. One recent finding suggests that the position at impact, the location of impact, and the absorption of energy may be more important than the strength of the bone in determining the risk of hip fracture among older persons (53).

Risk Factors Related to the Environment

The environment has been implicated in one third to one half of all falls or fall injury events (54, 87, 92, 103). As early as 1950, Castle (10) implicated lighting and stair structure as causes of falls (Table 2). In 1955, Droller (21) implicated loose rugs and defective floors, and others (54, 83, 92) have implicated light switch hazards, thresholds, extension cords, slippery surfaces, and other household products. Architectural design of stairways and homes and visual patterns on flooring can cause missteps and increase the risk of falling (3, 13, 49, 70). Recommended solutions have included use of slip-resistant stripping in bathtubs, proper placement of shelving, removal of throw rugs, redesign of stairs, improvements in shoe design, and improvements in lighting (48, 81). These recommendations make intuitive sense, but nearly all of the studies on which these recommendations are based were descriptive, that is, they did not include valid comparison groups (81). Many of these studies have also specifically asked respondents what caused their falls, thus leading directly to interviewer and recall bias. Although environmental hazards probably contribute to falls and fall injury events in older persons, we do not know the extent of this contribution, how multiple potential hazards interact, and how this effect is modified by host and agent factors.

A particular problem in previous studies has been the instruments used to assess the environment. Most of those instruments have actually been empirically developed checklists that are based on the experience or area of interest of the investigator (12, 86, 96, 97, 101). They have also been unstandardized, have lacked definitions, and have not been evaluated to determine if they are measuring what we think they are measuring (validity) or if they are measuring it in a consistent manner (reliability) (81). The researchers using these instruments have also assumed that each hazard contributes equally to the hazard potential of the home, but no studies have confirmed this approach (actually, none have even addressed this issue).

Most of these instruments have also tended to lack specifity. For example, most current instruments do not determine which areas of a home an older person ever uses or the amount of time spent there (81). Thus, these instruments would categorize a room as hazardous, even if the hazard were present in an area in which the older person spends little or no time. Even if the room contained hazards, an older person might fall in a nonhazardous area, or the hazard might not be related to the fall.

To determine the effect of environmental factors on falls and fall injury events, we should consider categorizing potential hazard exposures into persistent and variable exposures (81). Persistent exposures are those that tend to be fixed into the building or unlikely to change frequently over time, thus making direct measurement easy. Cabinets, flooring, stairs, and the absence of grab bars in the bathroom are examples of persistent exposures. Variable exposures are those that change frequently and, thus, make direct measurement difficult. Lighting, for example, varies considerably during the day, throughout the year, and in different rooms. Lighting, glare, and other variable exposures can be best obtained through self-report. For both types of exposures, predetermined definitions should be established for variables, including "use areas," and staff should receive standardized training to evaluate the environment.

It is extremely difficult to compare homes of fallers and nonfallers, as there are many variations in room size and design. One useful approach is to develop a hazard index for an older person's living arrangements (67). This hazard index should be based on a valid, reliable instrument and on those factors shown to increase the risk of fall injury events. Public health practitioners could then use a standard hazard index form in a standard way during each visit to an older person's home.

Surveillance

Surveillance is a necessary activity to monitor health events on an ongoing basis (11). A surveillance system for falls should collect data that are representative of a defined population (11). Data from surveillance activities can then be used to determine the need for public health programs and to assess their effectiveness. Due to the geographic variation in the distribution of falls and resultant injuries, state and local injury surveillance systems are critical to set local public health priority areas (84).

Most falls do not result in injury or lead to medical care (35, 67, 87, 99). In addition, many falls and their resultant injuries may be forgotten by older persons, especially falls that resulted in minor or no injury (20, 87). It is clearly unrealistic for public health professionals to monitor all falls, regardless of outcome, or to develop surveillance systems based on definitions derived from the Kellogg International Work Group (45), which are more suitable for in-depth clinical investigations of falls.

A surveillance system based on the external causes of injury would lead to uniformity of data, thus allowing us to compare fall injury events by geographic area. Unfortunately, E-codes are not routinely collected in medical records, except on death certificates (94). Thus, reliable estimates of the incidence of fall injury events in a population-based setting are not readily available to the public health practitioner.

Currently, no national system of collecting data on the causes of nonfatal falls exists, although many states have hospital discharge data systems (94). Hospital discharge data systems contain many promising features of a useful surveillance system, including representativeness and specificity. E-coding of hospital discharge data has been recommended by the Council of State and Territorial Epidemiologists (16) and would fill the data gap between mortality and morbidity data (84, 94). Very few hospitals now use E-codes for injury information; however, in June 1991, the National Committee on Vital and Health Statistics unanimously passed the recommendation that E-codes be included soon in Uniform Hospital Discharge Datasets (65).

The use of E-codes to monitor falls and fall injury events has several shortcomings, all of which can be improved significantly (65, 84, 94). Specifically, the medical record often contains insufficient information to code the external cause and the place of injury. This problem is due to the previous lack of a national requirement for E-coding in hospitals and the exclusion of E-codes in the current reimbursement system for hospitals. Thus, hospitals have had no incentive to record comprehensive descriptive information on injuries. By including a description of the mechanism involved, a statement of the intent of the injury, and where the injury occurred, hospitals could markedly increase the ability of the system to provide useful information. This information could be included as an important component of quality improvement programs for hospitals that care for injured patients. Physician training to promote better reporting, both in death certificates and hospital discharge summaries, would greatly improve the system. Finally, the index for E-codes should be revised to clarify definitions for medical records personnel, and E-codes should be regularly refined and updated just as the other diseases in ICD-9-CM have been (65). Efforts to address all of these past problems associated with E-codes appear promising.

FUTURE PREVENTION EFFORTS

Although we have learned much over the last decade about the causes of falls, we still know little about the most effective ways of preventing their occurrence. We have many promising leads, however. For example, many current efforts to prevent chronic diseases through smoking cessation, exercise promotion, and alcohol reduction programs may also lead to the prevention of many falls and injuries.

Surveillance data should guide our prevention efforts. It can also help public health practitioners to describe the fall injury event problem in more detail, target high-risk individuals and high-risk areas, maximize use of limited resources, attract public attention to this problem, and monitor intervention strategies.

After identifying persons at high risk for a fall injury event, public health practitioners can use Haddon's matrix to conceptualize injury control options or minimize the consequences of injuries (Table 3). Haddon's matrix separates the injury event into three distinct phases: preevent, event, and postevent (37, 38). Each phase of the Haddon matrix can also include information on the potential impact of the host, agent, and environment. The preevent phase of injury might be affected by removing or altering energy sources that have the potential to increase a person's risk of falling, or by altering pathophysiologic conditions that would enable an older person to cope better. Proper stairway design and lighting, better control over multiple drug prescriptions, exercise programs designed for general muscle strengthening, and homes specifically designed for older persons are examples. Technological development of energy-absorbing flooring would be useful in managing the event phase of injury. Networks of emergency response call buttons or buddy systems could improve overall survival in older persons who fall, but cannot get help quickly.

It would also be useful for fall prevention efforts to be directed not only at older persons, but also at younger persons. For example, targeting young persons with smoking cessation, exercise promotion, and alcohol use reduction programs may reduce both chronic diseases and a potential outcome of these diseases—falls. Educating perimenopausal women about calcium intake, general nutrition, and the potential benefits and risks associated with estrogen use and teaching both middle-aged men and women about the need to maintain physical fitness and bone strength may reduce future injuries.

Prevention efforts must balance the need to reduce risks with the need to

Table 3 Possible elements of a public health program to prevent falls among the elderly based on the Haddon matrix

Phase	Elements
Preevent	Exercise promotion and physical conditioning
	Cessation of smoking and alcohol
	Nutrition education
	Reduction of psychotropic medication use
	Regular eye examinations
	Osteoporosis prevention
	Hazard evaluations and modifications of residential institutions
	Home hazard awareness
	Use of proper footwear
	Safe outdoor walk routes during all weather conditions
Event	Energy-absorbing flooring for high-risk areas[a]
	Hip protection devices for high-risk persons[a]
Postevent	Emergency response call systems or buddy systems
	Improvements in emergency communication systems
	Health promotion and hazard prevention (all elements listed under preevent)

[a] Currently under development.

maintain mobility, functional activities, personal autonomy, and quality of life. Reduction in activity and mobility after a fall cannot, by itself, eliminate the risk of falling. Fear of falling and excessive restrictions in activity may initially reduce a person's risk of falling, but may lead to increasing the risk over time by decreasing self-confidence and physical conditioning.

CONCLUSION

Public health practitioners must continue to rely on empirically derived interventions until effective prevention modalities are demonstrated for older persons (91). Clearly, more work is needed to determine which interventions can decrease the risk of a fall or fall injury event and how environmental factors interact with pathophysiologic processes, primary aging processes, and pharmacologic and behavioral factors in increasing or decreasing this risk. A need exists for better translation and dissemination by researchers of their findings to public health practitioners. Injury research must also include the principles of mechanics to investigate and explain the physical and physiologic responses to impact that result in fall injury events.

Understanding both the many components associated with the increased risk of falls and the ways to modify the injury event so that it does not lead to morbidity or disability requires a multidisciplinary approach (e.g. behavioral, medical, public health, and engineering disciplines). This understanding would provide the public health practitioner with the scientific base needed to institute effective fall intervention programs.

Literature Cited

1. Alderman, B. W., Weiss, N. S., Daling, J. R., Ure, C. L., Ballard, J. H. 1986. Reproductive history and postmenopausal risk of hip and forearm fracture. *Am. J. Epidemiol.* 124:262–67
2. Applegate, W. B., Miller, S. T., Elam, J. T. 1987. Impact of cataract surgery with lens implementation on vision and physical function in elderly patients. *J. Am. Med. Assoc.* 28:481–83
3. Archea, J. C. 1985. Environmental factors associated with stair accidents by the elderly. *Clin. Geriatr. Med.* 1:555–68
4. Bacon, W. E., Smith, G. S., Baker, S. P. 1989. Geographic variation in the occurrence of hip fractures among the elderly white US population. *Am. J. Public Health* 79:1556–58
5. Baker, S. P., O'Neil, B., Karpf, R. S. 1984. *The Injury Fact Book.* Lexington, Mass: Lexington Books
6. Brockelhurst, J. C., Exton-Smith, A. N., Lempert Barber, S. M., Hunt, L. P., Palmer, M. K. 1978. Fracture of the femur in old age: a two-centre study of associated clinical factors and the cause of the fall. *Age Aging* 7:2–15
7. Browner, W. S. 1986. Estimating the impact of risk factor modification programs. *Am. J. Epidemiol.* 123:143–53
8. Buchner, D. M., Larson, E. B. 1987. Falls and fractures in patients with Alzheimer-type dementia. *J. Am. Med. Assoc.* 257:1492–95
9. Campbell, A. J., Reinken, J., Allan, B. C., Martinez, G. S. 1981. Falls in old age: a study of frequencies and related clinical factors. *Age Aging* 10:264–70
10. Castle, O. M. 1950. Accidents in the home. *Lancet* 1:315–19
11. Cent. Dis. Control. 1988. Guidelines for evaluating surveillance systems. *Morbid Mortal. Wkly. Rep.* 37(Suppl. S-5):1–17
12. Cent. Dis. Control. 1983. *Training Resource Manual: Injury Control Surveys.* Atlanta: US Dep. Health Hum. Serv., Public Health Serv., Cent. Dis. Control, Cent. Environ. Health
13. Cohn, T. E., Lasley, D. J. 1985. Visual depth illusion and falls in the elderly. *Clin. Geriatr. Med.* 1:601–15
14. Comm. Trauma Res., Comm. Life Sci., Natl. Res. Counc., Inst. Med. 1985. *Injury in America.* Washington, DC: Natl. Acad. Press
15. Comm. Rev. Status Prog. Inj. Control Program, Cent. for Dis. Control. 1988. *Injury Control.* Washington, DC: Natl. Acad. Press
16. *CSTE Position Statement No. 7. 1988.*

Adopted by Counc. of State and Territ. Epidemiol.
17. Cummings, S. R. 1985. Are patients with hip fractures more osteoporotic? *Am. J. Med.* 78:487–94
18. Cummings, S. R., Black, D. 1986. Should perimenopausal women be screened for osteoporosis? *Ann. Intern. Med.* 104:817–23
19. Cummings, S. R., Kelsey, J. L., Nevitt, M. C., O'Dowd, K. J. 1985. Epidemiology of osteoporosis and osteoporotic fractures. *Epidemiol. Rev.* 7:178–208
20. Cummings, S. R., Nevitt, M. C., Kidd, S. 1989. Forgetting falls: the limited accuracy of recall of falls in the elderly. *J. Am. Geriatr. Soc.* 36:613–16
21. Droller, H. 1955. Falls among elderly people living at home. *Geriatrics* 10:239–44
22. Duthie, E. H. 1989. Falls. *Med. Clin. North Am.* 73:1321–36
23. Ettinger, B., Genant, H. K., Cann, C. E. 1985. Long-term estrogen replacement therapy prevents bone loss and fractures. *Ann. Intern. Med.* 102:319–24
24. Farmer, M. E., White, L. R., Brody, J. A., Bailey, K. R. 1984. Race and sex differences in hip fracture incidence. *Am. J. Public Health* 74:1374–80
25. Felson, D. T., Anderson, J. J., Hannan, M. T., Milton, R. C., Wilson, P. W. F., et al. 1989. Impaired vision and hip fracture: the Framingham Study. *J. Am. Geriatr. Soc.* 37:495–500
26. Felson, D. T., Kiel, D. P., Anderson, J. J., Kannel, W. B. 1988. Alcohol consumption and hip fractures: the Framingham Study. *Am. J. Epidemiol.* 128:1102–10
27. Felson, D. T., Sloutskis, D., Anderson, J. J., Anthony, J. M., Kiel, D. P. 1991. Thiazide diuretics and the risk of hip fracture: results from the Framingham Study. *J. Am. Med. Assoc.* 265:370–73
28. Fife, D. 1987. Injuries and deaths among elderly persons. *Am. J. Epidemiol.* 126:936–41
29. Fife, D., Barancik, J. I., Chatterjee, B. F. 1984. Northeastern Ohio Trauma Study. II. Incidence rates by age, sex, and cause. *Am. J. Public Health* 74:473–78
30. Flicker, L. 1991. The use of bone mass screening to prevent fractures. *Med. J. Aust.* 154:135–40
31. Folstein, M. F., Folstein, S. E. 1975. Mini-mental state: a practical method for grading the cognitive state of patients for the clinician. *J. Psychiatr. Res.* 12:189–98
32. Glynn, R. J., Seddon, J. M., Krug, J.

H., Sahagian, C. R., Chiavelli, M. E., et al. 1991. Falls in elderly patients with glaucoma. *Arch. Ophthalmol.* 109:205–10

32a. Goldman, L., Tosteson, A. N. A. 1991. Uncertainty about postmenopausal estrogen—time for action, not debate. *N. Engl. J. Med.* 325:800–2

33. Graitcer, P. L. 1987. The development of state and local injury surveillance systems. *J. Saf. Res.* 18:191–98

34. Grisso, J. A., Kelsey, J. L., Strom, B. L., Chiu, G. Y., Maislin, G., et al. 1991. Risk factors for falls as a cause of hip fracture in women. *N. Engl. J. Med.* 324:1326–31

35. Gryfe, C. I., Amies, A., Ashley, M. J. 1977. A longitudinal study of falls in the elderly population. I. Incidence and morbidity. *Age Aging* 6:201–10

36. Gurwitz, J. H., Avorn, J. 1991. The ambiguous relation between aging and adverse drug reactions. *Ann. Intern. Med.* 114:956–66

37. Haddon, W. Jr. 1970. On the escape of tigers: an ecologic note. *Tech. Rev.* 72:44–53

38. Haddon, W., Baker, S. P. 1981. Injury control. In *Preventive and Community Medicine*, ed. D. Clark, B. MacMahon, 8:109–40. Boston: Little Brown

39. Hingson, R., Howland, J. 1987. Alcohol as a risk factor for injury or death resulting from accidental falls: a review of the literature. *J. Stud. Alcohol* 48:212–19

40. Honkanen, R., Ertama, L., Kuosmanen, P., Linnoila, M., Alha, A., et al. 1983. The role of alcohol in accidental falls. *J. Stud. Alcohol* 44:231–45

41. Isaacs, B. 1985. Clinical and laboratory studies of falls in old people: prospects for prevention. *Clin. Geriatr. Med.* 1:513–25

42. Jacobsen, S. L., Goldberg, J., Miles, T. P., Brody, J. A., Stiers, W., et al. 1991. Seasonal variation in the incidence of hip fracture among white persons aged 65 years and older in the United States, 1984–1987. *Am. J. Epidemiol.* 133:996–1004

43. Johnston, C. C., Slemenda, C. W., Melton, L. J. 1991. Clinical use of bone densitometry. *N. Engl. J. Med.* 324:1105–9

44. Kapoor, W. N. 1987. Evaluation of syncope in the elderly. *J. Am. Geriatr. Soc.* 35:826–28

45. Kellogg Int. Work Group Prev. Falls by Elderly. 1987. The prevention of falls in later life. *Dan. Med. Bull.* 34(Suppl. 4):1–24

46. Kreiger, N., Kelsey, J. L., Holford, T.

R., O'Connor, T. 1982. An epidemiologic study of hip fracture in postmenopausal women. *Am. J. Epidemiol.* 116:141–46

47. Lach, H. W., Reed, A. T., Arfken, C. L., Miller, J. P., Paige, G. D., et al. 1991. Falls in the elderly: reliability of a classification system. *J. Am. Geriatr. Soc.* 39:197–202

47b. LaCroix, A. Z., Wienpahl, J., White, L. R., Wallace, R. B., Scherr, P. A., et al. 1990. Thiazide diuretic agents and the incidence of hip fractures. *N. Engl. J. Med.* 322:286–90

48. Lewis, D. J., Winsor, R. J. 1974. *Handle Yourself with Care—An Instructor's Guide for an Accident Prevention Course for Older Americans.* Washington, DC: US Dep. Health, Educ., Welf., Adm. Aging, Social, Rehabil. Serv.

49. Liebowitz, H. W., Shupert, C. L. 1985. Spatial orientation mechanisms and their implications for falls. *Clin. Geriatr. Med.* 1:571–80

50. Lindsay, R. 1988. Osteoporosis. *Clin. Geriatr. Med.* 4:411–30

51. Lipsitz, L. 1983. The drop attack: a common geriatric symptom. *J. Am. Geriatr. Soc.* 31:617–20

52. Lipsitz, L. 1983. Syncope in the elderly. *Ann. Intern. Med.* 99:92–105

53. Lotz, J. C., Hayes, W. C. 1990. The use of quantitative computed tomography to estimate the risk of fracture of the hip from falls. *J. Bone Joint Surg.* 72A:689–700

54. Lucht, U. 1971. A prospective study of accidental falls and resulting injuries in the home among elderly people. *Acta Socio-Med. Scand.* 2:105–20

55. MacDonald, J. B. 1985. The role of drugs in falls in the elderly. *Clin. Geriatr. Med.* 1:621–32

56. MacDonald, J. B., MacDonald, E. T. 1977. Nocturnal femoral fracture and continuing widespread use of barbiturate hypnotics. *Br. Med. J.* 2:483–85

57. McNutt, L. A., McAuliffe, T., Baird, S., Coles, B., Baron, R., et al. 1991. Impact of regulation on benzodiazepine use in a low-income, elderly population, New York State. *Epidemic Intell. Serv. 40th Annu. Conf., Atlanta, Ga, 1991,* p. 20. Atlanta: US Dep. Health Hum. Serv., Public Health Serv., Cent. Dis. Control

58. Meehan, P., Saltzman, L. E., Sattin, R. W. 1991. Suicides among older United States residents: epidemiologic characteristics and trends. *Am. J. Public Health* 81:1198–1200

59. Melton, L. J., Wahner, H. W., Richelson, L. S., O'Fallon, W. M., Riggs, B.

L. 1986. Osteoporosis and the risk of hip fracture. *Am. J. Epidemiol.* 124:254–61

60. Mendlein, J. M., Sattin, R. W., Waxweiler, R. J., Lui, K. J., McGee, D. L. 1990. Fall mortality and related medical conditions in the elderly: the association with pulmonary embolism. *J. Aging Health* 2:326–40

61. Meuleman, J. 1989. Osteoporosis and the elderly. *Med. Clin. North Am.* 73:1455–70

62. Morfitt, J. M. 1983. Falls in old people at home: intrinsic versus environmental factors in causation. *Public Health* 97:115–20

63. Naessen, T., Persson, I., Adami, H.-O., Bergstrom, R., Bergkvist, L. 1990. Hormone replacement therapy and the risk for first hip fracture: a prospective, population-based cohort study. *Ann. Intern. Med.* 113:95–103

64. Natl. Comm. Inj. Prev. Control. 1989. *Injury Prevention: Meeting the Challenge.* New York: Oxford Univ. Press

65. Natl. Comm. Vital Health Stat., Subcomm. Ambul. Hosp. Care Stat. 1991. *Report on the Need to Collect External Cause-of-Injury Codes in Hospital Discharge Data, June 1991.* Working Paper No. 38. Hyattsville, Md: Natl. Cent. Health Stat.

66. Natl. Saf. Counc. 1990. *Accident Facts.* Chicago: Natl. Saf. Counc.

67. Nevitt, M. C., Cummings, S. R., Kidd, S., Black, D. 1989. Risk factors for recurrent nonsyncopal falls: a prospective study. *J. Am. Med. Assoc.* 261:2663–68

68. Nickens, H. 1985. Intrinsic factors in falling among the elderly. *Arch. Intern. Med.* 145:1089–93

69. Deleted in proof

70. Owen, D. H. 1985. Maintaining posture and avoiding tripping: optical information for detecting and controlling orientation and locomotion. *Clin. Geriatr. Med.* 1:581–99

71. Paganini-Hill, A., Ross, R. K., Gerkins, V. R., Henderson, B. E., Arthur, M., et al. 1981. Menopausal estrogen therapy and hip fractures. *Ann. Intern. Med.* 95:28–31

72. Perrine, M. W. 1973. Alcohol influences on drinking-related behavior: a critical review of laboratory studies of neurophysiological, neuromuscular and sensory activity. *J. Saf. Res.* 5:165–84

73. Prudham, D., Evans, J. G. 1981. Factors associated with falls in the elderly: a community study. *Age Aging* 10:141–46

74. Radebaugh, T. S., Hadley, E., Suzman, R. 1985. Falls in the elderly: biologic and behavioral aspects. *Clin. Geriatr. Med.* 1:555–620

75. Rankin, J. G., Ashley, M. J. 1986. Alcohol-related health problems and their prevention. In *Maxcy-Rosenau Public Health and Preventive Medicine,* ed. J. M. Last, 27:1039–73. Norwalk, Conn: Appleton-Century-Crofts. 12th ed.

76. Ray, W. A., Blazer, D. G., Schaffner, W., Federspiel, C. F., Fink, R. 1986. Reducing long-term diazepan prescribing in office practice: a controlled trial of educational visits. *J. Am. Med. Assoc.* 256:2536–39

77. Ray, W. A., Griffin, M. R., Downey, W., Melton, L. J. 1989. Long-term use of thiazide diuretics and risk of hip fracture. *Lancet* 1:687–90

78. Ray, W. A., Griffin, M. R., Schaffner, W., Baugh, D. K., Melton, L. J. 1987. Psychotropic drug use and the risk of hip fracture. *N. Engl. J. Med.* 316:363–69

79. Rice, D. P., MacKenzie, E. J., Assoc. 1989. *Cost of Injury in the United States: a Report to Congress.* San Francisco: Inst. Health Aging, Univ. of Calif. Inj. Prev. Cent., Johns Hopkins Univ.

80. Ring, C., Nayak, U. S. L., Isaacs, B. 1988. Balance function in elderly people who have and who have not fallen. *Arch. Phys. Med. Rehabil.* 69:261–64

81. Rodriguez, J. G., Sattin, R. W., DeVito, C. A., Wingo, P. A. 1991. Developing an environmental hazards assessment instrument for falls among the elderly. In *Reducing Frailty and Falls in Older Persons,* ed. R. Weindruch, E. C. Hadley, M. Ory. Springfield, Mo: Thomas. In press

82. Rodriguez, J. G., Sattin, R. W., Waxweiler, R. J. 1989. Epidemiology of hip fractures, United States, 1970–1983. *Am. J. Prev. Med.* 5:175–81

83. Rodstein, M. 1964. Accidents among the aged: incidence, causes and prevention. *J. Chron. Dis.* 17:515–26

84. Rosenberg, M. L., Graitcer, P. L., Waxweiler, R. J. 1988. Introduction: moving from the 1990 injury control objectives to state and local surveillance systems. In *CDC Surveillance Summaries, February 1988, Morbid. Mortal. Wkly. Rep.,* 37(SS-1):1–4. Atlanta: US Dep. Health Hum. Serv., Public Health Serv., Cent. Dis. Control

85. Ross, P. D., Wasnich, R. D., Davis, J. W. 1990. Fracture prediction models for osteoporosis prevention. *Bone* 11:327–31

86. Rubenstein, L. Z., Robbins, A. S. 1984. Falls in the elderly: a clinical perspective. *Geriatrics* 39:67–78

87. Rubenstein, L. Z., Robbins, A. S., Schulman, B. L., Rosado, J., Osterweil, D., et al. 1988. Falls and instability in the elderly. *J. Am. Geriatr. Soc.* 36: 266–78

88. Sabin, T. 1982. Biologic aspects of falls and mobility limitations in the elderly. *J. Am. Geriatr. Soc.* 30:51–58

89. Sattin, R. W., Lambert Huber, D. A., DeVito, C. A., Rodriguez, J. G., Ros, A., et al. 1990. The incidence of fall injury events among the elderly in a defined population. *Am. J. Epidemiol.* 131:1028–37

90. Sattin, R. W., Nevitt, M. C. 1992. Injuries in later life: epidemiology and environmental aspects. In *The Oxford Textbook of Geriatric Medicine*, ed. T. F. Williams, J. G. Evans. Oxford: Oxford Univ. Press. In press

91. Sattin, R. W., Nevitt, M. C., Waller, P. F., Seiden, R. H. 1988. Injury prevention. In *Background Papers from the Surgeon General's Workshop on Health Promotion and Aging*, ed. F. G. Abdellah, S. R. Moore, D1–20. Washington, DC: US Public Health Serv.

92. Schelp, L., Svanstrom, L. 1986. One-year incidence of home accidents in a rural Swedish municipality. *Scand J. Soc. Med.* 14:75–82

93. Sheldon, J. H. 1960. On the natural history of falls in old age. *Br. Med. J.* 2:1685–90

94. Sniezek, J. E., Finklea, J. F., Graitcer, P. L. 1989. Injury coding and hospital discharge data. *J. Am. Med. Assoc.* 262:2270–72

95. States, J. D. 1985. Musculo-skeletal system impairment related to safety and comfort of drivers 55+. In *Drivers 55+: Needs and Problems of Older Drivers: Survey Results and Recommendations, Proc. of the Older Driver Colloquium, Orlando, Fla.*, ed. J. L. Malfetti, pp. 63–76. Falls Church, Va: AAA Found. Traffic Saf.

96. Tideiksaar, R. 1986. Preventing falls: home hazard checklists to help older patients protect themselves. *Geriatrics* 41:26–28

97. Tideiksaar, R. 1984. An assessment form for falls. *J. Am. Geriatr. Soc.* 32:538–39

98. Tinetti, M. E., Speechley, M. 1989. Prevention of falls among the elderly. *N. Engl. J. Med.* 320:1055–59

99. Tinetti, M. E., Speechley, M., Ginter, S. 1988. Risk factors for falls among elderly persons living in the community. *N. Engl. J. Med.* 319:1701–7

100. Tinetti, M. E., Williams, T. F., Mayewski, R. 1986. Fall risk index for elderly patients based on number of chronic disabilities. *Am. J. Med.* 80:429–34

101. US Consum. Prod. Saf. Comm. 1985. *Home Safety Checklist for Older Consumers*. Washington, DC: US Dep. Health Hum. Serv., Off. Hum. Dev. Serv., Adm. Aging

102. Viano, D. C., King, A. I., Melvin, J. W., Weber, K. 1989. Injury biomechanics research: an essential element in the prevention of trauma. *J. Biomech.* 22: 403–17

103. Waller, J. A. 1978. Falls among the elderly—human and environmental factors. *Accid. Anal. Prev.* 10:21–23

103b. Weintraub, M., Singh, S., Byrne, L., Maharaj, K., Guttmacher, L. 1991. Consequences of the 1989 New York State triplicate benzodiazepine prescription regulations. *J. Am. Med. Assoc.* 266:2392–97

104. Weiss, N. S., Ure, C. L., Ballard, J. H., Williams, A. R., Daling, J. R. 1980. Decreased risk of fractures of the hip and lower forearm with postmenopausal use of estrogen. *N. Engl. J. Med.* 303:1195–98

105. Wild, D., Nayak, U. S. L., Isaacs, B. 1981. Description, classification, and prevention of falls in old people at home. *Rheumatol. Rehab.* 20:153–59

Annu. Rev. Publ. Health. 1992. 13:509–28

NONFALL INJURIES IN OLDER ADULTS

Marsha E. Wolf[1,3] and Frederick P. Rivara[2,3]

Departments of [1]Epidemiology and [2]Pediatrics, University of Washington, and [3]the Harborview Injury Prevention and Research Center, Seattle, Washington 98104

KEY WORDS: trauma, motor vehicle crash, suicide, burns, assault

INTRODUCTION

In the United States, injuries are the most important cause of morbidity and mortality for persons between the ages of 1 and 44 years (59). Injuries are also an important cause of hospitalization and death in older adults, a problem often overlooked against the backdrop of cancer, cardiovascular disease, and stroke. This review outlines the epidemiology of nonfall trauma in older adults, including the incidence of the problem, special populations at risk, known risk factors, and proven and possible strategies for prevention.

Before examining patterns of injury in older adults, we should define injury and modern injury control. The term "injury" refers to damage resulting from acute exposure to physical or chemical agents (2). The term "accident" is purposely not used because it connotes randomness and fatalism, as in "accidents happen." The intent of the modern science of injury control is to reduce and control the damage from injuries, not to blame the victim or seek retribution for negligent or careless behavior (47).

It is important to distinguish events from the injuries themselves. The latter does not necessarily follow from the former. A motor vehicle crash (MVC) may occur, but injury can be prevented if the occupants are safely protected. Thus, one can examine the factors that predispose to the event (preevent) and those that follow the injury (postevent) from the injury itself. Combining this dimension of examining injuries with the classic epidemiology paradigm of

509

0163-7525/92/0501-0509$02.00

host, agent, and environment, Haddon created a matrix for examining the causes and prevention strategies for injuries. The matrix displays preevent, event, and postevent phases on one axis with host, vector, physical environment, and social environment on the other axis (2).

NONFALL INJURIES IN OLDER ADULTS

Overall Incidence

In the US in 1985, 2.1 million adults aged 65 and older had a nonfall injury (7346 per 100,000 persons) (Table 1). Contributing to this injury total were the estimated 1.9 million persons with medically treated injuries who did not require hospitalization, 141,000 with hospitalized injuries, and 21,500 with fatal injuries (59).

Injury rates vary with age and gender (Table 1). The most striking difference by gender is found among fatal injuries; men have rates 2.5 times greater than women in both the 65–74 and 75+ age groups. The rates and numbers of total injuries and nonhospitalized injuries are higher in the 65–74 age group than the 75+ age group. Although the actual number of persons hospitalized for injuries is larger for persons aged 65–74, the hospitalization and death rates for nonfall injuries are greater for those aged 75 and older.

Injuries as a cause of death in older adults may be underestimated, according to a study of multiple cause of death coding on death certificates (15). When an injury was listed on the death certificate as either a cause of death or a significant condition associated with death, the percentage with injury

Table 1   Nonfall injury rates in older adults by age and gender, 1985 (Rate per 100,000 persons)

Age and Gender	Total	Fatalities	Hospitalized	Nonhospitalized
Total	7346	75	494	6775
65–74	7793	60	419	5983
75+	6685	98	603	7312
Men				
65–74	6186	90	446	5652
75+	7259	168	669	6422
Women				
65–74	9033	36	398	8604
75+	6373	60	567	5744

Calculated from data in Ref. 59.

identified as the underlying cause of death was more than 90% for MVCs, assaults, and suicides. Hoewever, for other types of injuries listed on the death certificate, less than 70% identified the injury as the underlying cause of death for those aged 65–75, and less than 50% for those 85 and older.

Costs

An important aspect of the impact of injury is the economic cost. Rice, MacKenzie, and Associates (59) estimated the lifetime economic cost of injury, based on the direct cost for medical treatment and rehabilitation, and the indirect cost associated with life years lost, including the loss of earnings due to short- and long-term disability and premature death. The lifetime cost estimate for the 2.1 million older persons injured in the US in 1985 was $5.1 billion (Table 2). The direct expenditures for hospital care, physician services, nursing home care, drugs, and other medical and rehabilitation services account for $2.8 billion, 56% of the total lifetime costs. Indirect costs for morbidity and mortality are estimated as $1.8 billion and $441 million, respectively. In contrast to other ages, the economic burden of injury for older adults was greater for women than men. Mortality costs were similar in older men and women, but women had greater direct and morbidity costs.

Change in Lifestyle

Another very important measure of the impact of injury is changes in lifestyle as a result of trauma. Injuries in older adults may mean the difference between independent lives in private residences and dependent lives that require care in a nursing home. Adult children may force the older person to forgo driving after a motor vehicle crash. In Washington state, 20% of older adults who entered a hospital for a nonfall injury were discharged to a nursing home or intermediate care facility, rather than their own homes.

Table 2 Lifetime cost of nonfall injury for persons aged 65 and older, 1985

| | | Dollar Amount (millions) | | |
| | | | Indirect Cost | |
	Total	Direct	Morbidity	Mortality
Total	5054	2833	1780	441
Men	1841	1083	522	236
Women	3213	1751	1258	205

Calculated from data in Ref. 59.

CAUSE-SPECIFIC INJURIES

The major causes of nonfall injuries in older adults are MVCs (occupants and pedestrians), suicides, assaults, and burns; each is discussed below. Poisonings, drownings, and suffocations are less common in older adults and are not elaborated further.

Motor Vehicle Occupants

INCIDENCE   Motor vehicle crashes are the leading cause of injury death and the second leading cause (after falls) of medically treated injuries and hospitalizations (2). Although older adults appear to have low MVC rates compared with other ages, older adults drive about half as much as other age groups. Consequently, when the exposure of the number of miles driven is considered, drivers aged 65 and older have the second highest MVC rates after young adults. Drivers aged 85 and older have the highest crash rates per miles of travel (Figure 1) (8, 11, 24).

Older drivers have different crash patterns, which usually involve errors of omission, than do younger drivers (8, 11). Older drivers are more likely involved in intersection and turning crashes and head-on collisions in urban areas. They are also more likely to commit right-of-way and signal violations and to be charged with inattention. Some studies report they are more likely to be responsible for the MVC in which they are involved than are other ages (41). Conflicting results have been reported for overinvolvement in backing and parking related crashes. Conversely, older drivers are less likely to be involved in single vehicle crashes or to be cited for reckless driving, driving too fast, or drinking and driving (8, 11).

Older adults are more frequently admitted to the hospital and die from less severe injuries than younger persons. In one study, the proportions of hospital admissions that were for MVC trauma were 116 per 1000 emergency room visits for ages 65–74 and 248 per 1000 for age 75+, which are two and four times greater than the proportion of admissions for all other ages (3). Low severity injuries, as measured by injury severity scores (ISS), result in significant mortality for ages 70 and older, but are rarely fatal in younger persons (16). For example, 15% of MVC injury admissions with an ISS less than 20 died among those 70 and older, compared with less than 1% of individuals less than 50 years of age (2).

RISK FACTORS

Medical conditions   Conflicting results have been reported for associations between chronic medical conditions and MVCs. Drivers aged 60 and older with medical conditions of diabetes, epilepsy, cardiovascular disease,

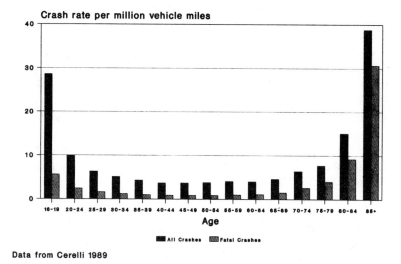

Data from Cerelli 1989

Figure 1   Motor vehicle crash rates per miles of travel by age.

alcoholism, and mental illness reported to the California Department of Licensing had twice as many crashes per 1 million miles of driving than drivers with no reported disease (72). Among persons with medical conditions reported to the Washington State Department of Licensing who had licensing and/or driving restrictions, such as special equipment, area or time of day restriction, or periodic reexamination, men older than 65 with reported epilepsy had increased risks of MVC. However, no increased risk of MVC or traffic violations was found for older adults with diabetes or heart disease license restrictions (13). These results among the small number of older adults conflict with the overall study findings of higher MVC rates for persons of all ages whose licenses were restricted as a result of diabetes, epilepsy, fainting, and other reported conditions. Slightly higher MVC rates that were not statistically significant were also found for drivers of all ages with heart disease restrictions. A recent study of diabetes and epilepsy in all ages, which attempted more complete ascertainment of persons with these medical conditions by identification from clinic and hospital records, found each condition had a relative risk of 1.3 for MVC, and both had a relative risk of 1.6 for MVCs causing injury (20).

A study comparing senile adults aged 60 and older to healthy 30–59-year-olds found that the older group had twofold greater MVC per miles driven; cardiovascular disease coupled with senility in the older adults increased MVCs fourfold (73).

Drugs   For persons of all ages, psychoactive drugs have been reported in several studies to be a risk factor for drivers involved in MVCs (25, 39, 63); one study found no increase (27). Although no published study has evaluated drugs and MVC risk in older drivers, Ray's study of Medicaid enrollees found current users of benzodiazepines, tricyclic antidepressants, or both agents had relative risks of 1.5, 2.2, and 2.1, respectively, for MVCs compared with nonusers (W. A. Ray 1991, unpublished observations). An increased risk was not found for current users of opioid analgesics or antihistamines.

Alcohol   Alcohol does not appear to be as major a risk factor for MVC in older adults as it is for younger persons. Of the approximately 6.6 million police-reported MVCs that occurred in the US in 1989, 1% of the crash-involved drivers aged 65 and older were reported by police as using alcohol, compared with 5% of drivers aged 21–24 and 25–34 (48). In fatal MVCs, 7% of drivers aged 65 and older had blood alcohol levels of 0.10 gm% of greater, compared with 35% of 20–24 year old drivers (46, 55). Of motor vehicle fatalities among persons aged 65 and older, 14% were alcohol related, compared with 52% of persons 20–24 (46).

In an 11-state survey conducted by the AAA Foundation for Traffic Safety and the Safety Research and Education Project at Columbia University, 42% of drivers aged 55 and older reported that they did not drink alcoholic beverages, compared with 17% of 30–45-year-old drivers (75). Only 0.4% of these older drivers and 1% of the younger drivers reported drinking more than one alcoholic beverage a day (75). The Alcohol Working Group of the Surgeon General's Workshop on Health Promotion and Aging stated that although it is not possible to determine the prevalence of alcohol abuse, reported drinking appears to decline as the population ages (57).

History of traffic infraction and MVC   Several studies report that drivers with a history of repeated traffic infractions and/or crashes may be at increased risk for subsequent MVC (34, 35), but the usefulness of driving history has been questioned, as the repeat offenders (violations and crashes) account for a small percentage of all crashes (33, 66). The role of either of these factors as a risk for MVC among older drivers is unknown.

PREVENTION   The strategies to prevent and reduce injury and death from MVC in older adults should be multifaceted. Control requires intervention at several levels, including federal, state, and local, and involves changes in the host, the agent, and the environment (47). Prevention approaches should include prevention of the occurrence of MVC, prevention of injury once MVC occurs, and prevention of adverse outcome when injury does occur. One of the tenets of modern injury control is that changes in the environment or products are more likely to result in a reduction of injuries than is a focus on behavior change (2, 47). Current prevention approaches include occupant protection, driver education, improved emergency medical and rehabilitation services, and license renewal changes.

Occupant protection The most effective interventions for motor vehicle occupants are seat restraints, including lap and shoulder belts and air bags. Studies have shown that seat belt restraints are 45% effective in preventing MVC fatalities and 50% effective in preventing moderate to critical MVC injuries (52). Not only do restraints reduce the risk of ejection, but they also prevent or mitigate the second collision of the occupant with the vehicle. New passenger cars are now required by federal vehicle safety standards to be equipped with shoulder/lap belts for front seat occupants and lap belts for rear seat occupants. Laws requiring front seat occupants and/or all passengers to use seat belts were enacted in 33 states and the District of Columbia by 1990 (46).

Overall usage of seat belt restraints has increased from less than 20% nationally in 1983 to the 49% estimated from observations of drivers in 19 cities in 1990 (49). Actual restraint use among older adults is unknown. In a 1989 seat belt observation study, seat belt use for drivers aged 50 or older was 45%, compared with 47% in drivers aged 25–49 (50). Older women drivers (53%) were more likely than men (41%) to buckle up (50).

Older adults report the main reasons for not using seat belts are difficulty of use and lack of comfort (75). The approaches to increasing restraint usage among older adults should include manufacturing changes for more easily reached, attached, and released belts and education/promotion of seat belt use. However, because passengers have failed to wear seat belts, air bags were developed and have been shown to be very effective in frontal collisions (47). Automatic seat belts and air bags in new automobiles will help reduce MVC injury.

Driver education In the late 1970s, the American Association of Retired Persons and the National Retired Teachers Association began sponsoring driver education courses for adults 55 and older. These refresher driver education courses, which attempt to update driving knowledge and refresh skills, are offered throughout the US by driving schools, automobile and safety organizations, and older adult organizations, usually in cooperation with state motor vehicle departments. Automobile insurance companies offer discount rates to older adults who complete the course. The effectiveness of these courses in improving driving is hard to assess, because of possible self-selection of better drivers who take the courses. Participants of California mature driver improvement courses had significantly lower rates of fatal or injury collisions and traffic convictions in the six months after the course than comparison drivers after adjusting for age, gender, license class, prior record, and area of residence (69).

Improved emergency medical and rehabilitation services   Interventions in the postevent phase are important in both reducing mortality and decreasing morbidity and disability among the survivors. Emergency medical service systems and regionalized trauma care have been effective in reducing the number of preventable deaths that occur in motor vehicle trauma and other types of serious injury (47). Rehabilitation care can enhance the degree of recovery attained by the trauma victim and, for the older adult trauma victim, may mean the difference between returning home to resume an active life or being discharged to a nursing home or other intermediate care facility.

License renewal changes   In the US, the frequency of state driver's license renewal varies from one to five years, and approximately 20% of the states do not require any vision screening with renewal (18, 29, 74). Approximately 20% of the states have increased, but varied, frequency of renewal regulations for older drivers (18). The varied policies for older drivers reflect inadequate scientific data on who is at high risk for MVC among older drivers. Studies are needed to assess whether such factors as medical conditions, drugs, sensory impairment, or driver history can help identify high risk drivers. Results from such studies would be useful for developing guidelines to screen drivers for more frequent and comprehensive license renewal. Such studies would also be helpful for clinicians and health educators so that they can better counsel and inform older adults about the safety of their driving.

Other prevention strategies   New prevention programs need to be developed, implemented, and evaluated. Long-term approaches might include license renewal changes, improved vehicular and roadway design, and improved public transportation alternatives.

Pedestrians

INCIDENCE   Since 1979, 14–17% of motor vehicle deaths in the US occurred to pedestrians, the second largest group of MVC after occupants. For persons aged 65 years and older, pedestrian injuries account for 22% of traffic-related deaths (26). Older adults have the highest pedestrian death rates of any age group, 4.7 per 100,000 persons in 1989. The rate for those aged 80 and older is more than twice as high as it is for persons aged 70–74 and younger persons. The pedestrian death rate for men is two to four times as high as for women in older ages, a pattern similar to the gender differences found at all ages.

Pedestrian-motor vehicle collisions (PMVCs) are qualitatively different from other types of motor vehicle-related trauma, as very few victims escape injury. Based on data from the National Highway Traffic Safety Administration, only 1.1% of pedestrians struck by a car are uninjured (51). In contrast, 94% of all MVCs involve no injury (52). The pedestrian injury rates in older adults are higher than those found in younger adults and second only to the rate in children when distance traveled, number of street crossings, and time spent as a pedestrian are considered (28, 70).

Two thirds of all pedestrian deaths occur in urban areas. For older adults, 33% of pedestrian fatalities and 50% of pedestrian injuries occurred at intersections, compared with 10–18% (fatalities) and 26–39% (injuries) for all other ages. Older pedestrian fatalities are more likely to occur during daylight (21). In contrast, pedestrians aged 26–64 are more likely to be fatally injured at night.

RISK FACTORS   There is a paucity of epidemiologic data on risk factors for pedestrian injuries and fatalities in older adults. In children, the other high-risk pedestrian group, male gender, low socioeconomic status, pedestrian action, and environmental factors have been identified as risk factors (44, 60). A case-control study of environmental factors found that children who lived in multifamily housing or in housing without yards had a more than fivefold increased risk of injury. Characteristics of the site that increased risk of injury were more than two lanes of traffic, high traffic volume, posted speed limits over 25 mph, and the presence of a marked crosswalk. The findings of an increased risk of injury for marked crosswalks has been shown in other studies (22).

Few studies of environmental factors have specifically been designed or evaluated for their effect on the risk of PMVC in older adults. The data for crosswalks, pedestrian signals, timing of signals, and right turn on a red light are reviewed below.

Crosswalks   Data regarding the safety benefits of crosswalks are conflicting. Herms reported a twofold increased risk of PMVC in marked crosswalks, controlling for differences in pedestrian volume (22). Older adults and children were found to have the greatest risks. However, this study did not address possible differences in age distribution of pedestrian volume, traffic volume, or other factors that may have contributed to the reason that the intersections were originally marked or signalized. Hauer (21) notes contrasting evidence, which uses a different outcome measure, comes from a study cited in the 1965 ITE handbook. This study found that painted crosswalks reduced pedestrian right-of-way violations. In addition, Tobey et al (70) reported that absence of crosswalk marking was a relatively hazardous intersection characteristic for pedestrians. Knoblauch et al (30) found that sites with marked crosswalks were safer than unmarked crosswalks. Marked crosswalks may provide pedestrians with a false sense of safety and may actually increase the risk of pedestrian injury.

Right turn on red   Allowing right turn on a red light has consistently been shown to increase the risk of pedestrian injury. In a study of the effect of right turn on red laws, adopted during 1974–1977, Zador (76) found the greatest increase for right turn PMVCs, 117%, was among adults aged 65 and older.

Pedestrian signals   Zegeer et al (77) reported intersections with standard pedestrian signals had more PMVCs than intersections without signals. However, these authors suggest that signalized crosswalks are most beneficial at low speed intersections with traffic signals. This study did not consider possible differences, such as pedestrian volume, age, or other reasons that intersection marking and signalization varied. In England, pedestrian crossings that had crosswalk markings and pedestrian activated traffic lights had half the risk of pedestrian injury, compared with crossings without such lights for the same levels of vehicle and pedestrian volume (71).

The assumed walking speed of 4 feet/second cited by the Manual on Uniform Traffic Control Device is the standard by which traffic engineers base the timing of pedestrian lights. From observations of adults aged 70 and older who were instructed to cross an intersection at a normal, comfortable speed, Dahlstedt found that almost 90% crossed at less than 4 feet/second (11). Lundgren-Lindquist et al (36) observed a comfortable walking speed mean of 3.4 and 3.0 feet/second for samples of 70-year-old men and women, respectively. Although older adults appear to have slower walking speed than current standards for timing of lights, the association between older adult PMVCs and timing of light has not been evaluated. A report from the Institute of Traffic Engineers recommends that a walk speed of 2.5 feet/second would provide adequate crossing time for 87% of older pedestrians (11).

Other environmental factors   Other factors that are relatively hazardous for pedestrians of all ages are major arterials, two or more traffic lanes, length of the block (250 feet or less), left turn channelization, no sidewalks or curbs, no street lighting or regularly spaced street lighting, residential and mixed use, and "T" intersection type (a street ending with outlets onto perpendicular street) (70).

PREVENTION   Pedestrian injuries, like MVC occupant injuries, are a complex problem for which multiple prevention approaches are necessary.

Environmental modifications   Research is necessary to identify and prioritize which environmental factors should be targeted for development of intervention programs for older adults. In the Queens Boulevard pedestrian prevention project, Retting et al (58) reported that the occurrence of fatal and near-fatal pedestrian injuries, especially among older adults, decreased by 43% and 86%, respectively, two years after implementation of interventions. These included stop light changes to increase pedestrian crossing time, modified roadway markings, pedestrian signals on median islands, tighter speed limit enforcement, and safety education presentations at senior centers. No adjustment was made for pedestrian volume in the study area. Citywide occurrence of fatal pedestrian injuries decreased by 4% over the same time period.

Vehicle design   The majority of injuries occurring in PMVCs are a result of the pedestrian being "run under" and thrown up onto the automobile, rather than being "run over" and having contact with the wheels or ground. Changes in motor vehicle design have been effective in decreasing the incidence and severity of motor vehicle occupant injuries. Research over the last decade indicates that similar design changes to the exterior of the vehicle (bumper, hood, and windshield) can potentially reduce by one-third the risk of serious injury to pedestrians who are struck (1, 38).

Legislation and enforcement   Legislation has been an effective component of many injury control programs, especially those related to motor vehicles. The extent to which laws and enforcement play significant roles in pedestrian safety, however, is a question that remains to be answered. Enforcement may be a key component. Lack of understanding of pedestrian laws and their enforcement may be a major reason for noncompliance by drivers in many areas of the country. Of 41 states surveyed, with the notable exception of California, enforcement of pedestrian safety laws receives little emphasis and is regarded as politically difficult (19).

In many states where laws are enforced, the emphasis traditionally has been on the pedestrian, rather than the driver. In Pennsylvania, changes in the code in 1977 resulted in virtually no change in driver behavior with regard to pedestrians, because the law went virtually unenforced (19). In Seattle, Washington, increased enforcement in the six months beginning September 1990 has resulted in 3625 tickets at $47 fine each, written against motorists who ignore persons in crosswalks, plus 1990 tickets at $19 fine each for jaywalkers. The effect of these measures is not yet known.

Pedestrian skill training program   Several promising reports on programs designed to improve children's pedestrian skills have appeared in the literature (47, 60). The literature is also replete with examples of programs that

have been ineffective. No similar programs for older adults have been undertaken. Such programs might be needed to help older adults change their
style of crossing as they age. Again, research is necessary to help illuminate
the focus of pedestrian skill training programs for older adults.

Suicide

INCIDENCE   When we hear of suicide, we often think of the adolescent
male. However, the highest rates of suicide are in men aged 65 and over;
those aged 85 or older have rates (67/100,000) two- to threefold greater than
those of adolescents and young adults (Figure 2) (45). Rates in older adult
men are four- to ninefold higher than in women, with highest rates among
whites, lowest rates among blacks. The rates among Asians and Hispanics are
intermediate between the two.

The number of nonfatal suicide attempts in older adults is not well known.
There appear to be fewer attempts compared with completed suicides in the
elderly than in persons younger than 40 years of age: 4 to 1 compared with 20
to 1 (4).

In a population-based survey in Washington state, completion rates for
suicide were age-dependent, ranging from 3.3% for teenage girls to 79% for
older men aged 65–74 (67).

RISK FACTORS

Marital status Durkeim first emphasized the association between widowhood and suicide 100 years ago; he described widowhood as "domestic
anomie." Married persons throughout life have the lowest rate of suicide (65).
Widowed and divorced older adult men and women have rates of suicide that

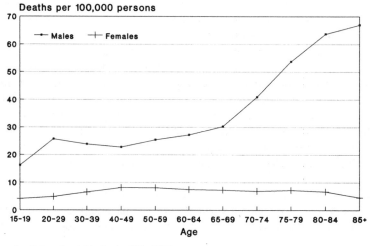

Figure 2 Rates of suicide in the US, 1987.

are two- to threefold greater than their married counterparts, which indicates the need for special intervention programs in these groups.

Physical illness   Chronic disabling illness may radically alter a person's sense of self-worth, as well as result in a loss of independence and increased isolation (23). Some studies suggest that older adult suicide victims have more physical disorders of metabolic, respiratory, and cardiovascular origin than older adults who do not attempt suicide (62).

Depression and mental illness   Depression is the most common mental health symptom in the over 65 age group and is considered a strong risk factor for suicide (23).

Availability of means   The availability of lethal means may convert an attempt into a successful suicide. Older adult men most commonly choose guns as their means, which may explain the high rate of completed suicides in this group. In a study in Arizona, more than one fourth of older adult suicide victims had obtained the firearm in the month before the suicide (43).

PREVENTION   Prevention of suicide among the high risk older population has been sorely neglected. Formal suicide prevention and psychological services are under-utilized by older adults, who generally represent only 1–2% of the caseloads of suicide prevention centers (40). Prevention of the problem must be multifaceted. Some potential strategies include the following:

Treatment of prior attempters   The single most important risk factor for suicide at any age is a history of a prior attempt. Treatment, ranging from outpatient therapy to inpatient hospitalization, is the primary intervention for those who attempt suicide (47).

Restrict availability of lethal means   This is a complex area for which definitive answers are not available. Elimination of carbon monoxide from gas for cooking and heating in Britain resulted in a reduction in the overall rates of suicide (32), whereas the same changes in Australia (5) and Bern, Switzerland (68), resulted in an offsetting increase in suicides by other means. Comparison of Seattle to Vancouver, BC, revealed equivalent rates of suicide among the elderly, despite more restrictive gun control laws in Vancouver (64).

Education of health professionals   Approximately 75% of older adults who kill themselves see a physician shortly before committing suicide (54). Many older adults do not see the physician with suicidal ideation as their chief complaint; instead, they present with somatic or depressive symptoms. Physicians need to be alert to such risks.

Services to decrease social isolation in the older adults   More global societal changes may be necessary to decrease suicide rates in this age group. Allowing individuals to work as long as they are able and making retirement a gradual process that involves counseling may decrease the sense of loss felt by many elderly at retirement (47). Programs to increase visitors for older adults, similar to those that have been developed for mothers at high risk of child abuse, may be necessary in a society in which economics and employment preclude older adults living with or even in the same city as their adult children.

Burns

INCIDENCE   Burns are the fourth leading cause of injury death in the US, accounting for approximately 5000 deaths each year (2). An additional 90,000 patients are hospitalized annually for the treatment of burns (2, 10, 59). The causes of deaths from burns are very different from those that result in hospitalizations, thus requiring different preventive strategies (2). In both situations, older adults and young children represent populations at increased risk.

Almost 90% of burn and fire deaths occur in residential fires (2). Residential fire deaths are highest in the South and lowest in the West (7). In all areas, residential fire deaths are much higher for adults over age 64 than they are for individuals aged 5–64 (Figure 3). These rate differences are most pronounced in the South.

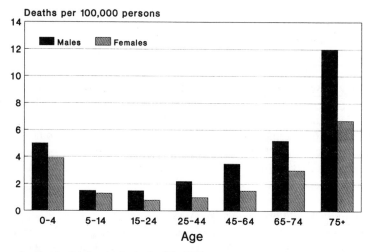

Figure 3   Residential fire deaths in the US, 1985.

In contrast to fatal burn injuries, nonfatal injuries do not occur most frequently in the older adults. The incidence of hospitalization in Massachusetts for flame/flash burns, scalds, and other burns was lower in those aged 55 and older than in children under the age of 5 and those aged 5–54 (61). The same age trends were found for all burns that required emergency room care (10) and all burns that required medical care (37).

These differences in relative incidence of fatal and nonfatal burn injuries reflect not only the difference in the etiology of these two major categories of burns, but also the increased case-fatality rate among older adults. Young children and older adults have far higher fatality rates than older children and adults for the same degree and extent of burn (9).

Scald burns, usually caused by a hot food or drink, were the most common category of nonfatal burns in older adults (10). A subset of scald burns are those caused by hot tap water, accounting for approximately 10% of scald burns in this age group. Nonfatal flame burns often involve clothing ignition and/or flammable substances. One third of fabric ignitions among older adults happen in the kitchen, nearly always associated with cooking. Rossignol et al (61) noted that 62% of nonhouse fire burns among older adults involved clothing ignition, compared with 30% for all younger persons.

RISK FACTORS   Risk factors for burn injuries in older adults are likely to be the same as those in other age groups. Poverty is clearly one of the strongest risk factors for fatalities from residential fires. Mierley & Baker (42) reported a strong correlation between economic conditions and house-fire deaths for both blacks and whites.

Cigarettes are estimated to cause 45% of all fires and 22–56% of residential fire deaths (47). Most cigarettes made in this country contain additives that cause the cigarette to burn for as long as 28 minutes, even if left unattended. Many of the individuals who smoke also consume alcohol, a known risk factor for house fires and deaths.

PREVENTION   Prevention strategies for burn injuries have been successful and can make a large impact on morbidity and mortality.

Smoke detectors are perhaps the most inexpensive injury prevention strategy that one can implement (47). The majority of fire deaths do not involve burns, but rather smoke inhalation. Evaluation of smoke detectors reveals that they reduce the potential of death in 86% of fires and the risk of severe injuries in 88% (14). The effectiveness of smoke detectors is increased if a sprinkler system is also used, thereby markedly reducing the spread of a fire. Building regulations could be changed to require that all new housing is equipped with relatively inexpensive sprinkler systems.

The technology exists to manufacture a self-extinguishing, fire-safe cigarette. The benefits of producing fire-safe cigarettes would far outweigh the costs to the tobacco industry. If only fire-safe cigarettes were smoked in this country, nearly 2000 deaths and more than 6000 burn injuries would be prevented annually (47, 59).

One success story in injury control has been that of efforts to reduce tap water temperatures. Lowering the water-heater setting to 125° F can prevent most tap water-related scald burns (2). The appliance manufacturers have tentatively agreed to voluntarily preset all new heaters at the lower temperature. Many utilities offer free home services to adjust water heater settings.

Assault

SCOPE OF PROBLEM   In 1987, 1330 persons aged 65 and older died from assault (45). However, these figures far underestimate the true nature of the problem. Just as the 1960s brought to light the problem of child abuse and neglect, the 1980s taught us that domestic violence against older adults was a common and tragic problem.

There are no national studies on the extent of this problem. Data are limited and come from small prevalence surveys. In the Major Trauma Outcome Study of patients admitted to 111 US and Canadian hospitals for the care of trauma, stab and gunshot wounds accounted for 8.1% of admissions in those aged 65 and older (9). These injuries had very high case-fatality rates: 17.3% and 52.1%, respectively, of those assaulted died from their injuries. Men and women were equally represented.

In a community-based survey of older adults in Boston, 2% reported they had been physically abused, the most common form of maltreatment suffered in this age group (56). Only a small fraction of this abuse appears to come to public attention. In Massachusetts, only one of 14 cases was reported (56). Thus, official estimates of older adult abuse and assault far underestimate the extent of the problem.

The abuser is a relative in 86% of cases and lives with the older adult in 75% of cases (12). Approximately 50% of older adult abusers are children or grandchildren of the victim, and about 40% are spouses.

RISK FACTORS   Few analytical studies of assaults to older adults have been conducted; knowledge of risk factors comes nearly entirely from case series. In the Boston survey, men were three times more likely to be physically abused than women, and those in poor health were fourfold more likely to be abused than those in excellent health (56). Many other studies have found women to be a greater risk than men. However, women appear to be more seriously abused than older adult men, and thus are more likely to come to official attention. Other studies have also reported an association of older adult abuse with physical and mental impairment (17).

Dependency on others appears to place the older adult at risk of abuse (12). Although dependency may not be the sole explanation, it may act as a trigger by creating stress on a caretaker who is poorly equipped to adapt and cope with this burden.

It is unclear whether socioeconomic status is a risk factor, as older adult abuse appears to exist at all levels of household income (12).

In some studies (31), advanced age appears to be a risk factor for abuse. In other studies (56), the risk of abuse was similar in those over age 75 compared with the 65–75 age group.

Alcohol appears to be a risk factor for all domestic violence, including that involving older adults (31). Alcohol abuse may affect the victim, the perpetrator, or both.

PREVENTION   Prevention of older adult abuse and assault has only recently been attempted. In 1985, states spent an average of $22 per child for prevention and care of child abuse. However, only $2.90 is spent per elderly person for the prevention of abuse in this age group (6). No interventions have yet been evaluated; thus, none should be implemented without a research component (47).

Risk assessment   Because health providers are often the only professionals who interact with abuse victims, risk assessment tools for use by these groups may be useful in early detection and treatment. This can take the form of an informal assessment with knowledge of the common presentations of older adult abuse (53) or the use of more formal standardized screening instruments (47). Key elements are the history, physical findings, observation of the patient and/or individual accompanying patient, and whether the severity or nature of the injury match the explanation of events. None of these methods, however, has been tested in a prospective fashion with attempts to identify false-positives and false-negatives.

Community education campaigns   Several communities have launched public education campaigns designed to increase community awareness of the problem of older adult abuse; however, none have been evaluated to date. Given the past performance of many community education campaigns, none should be widely implemented until proved to be effective (47).

Community projects   Many communities have developed programs to decrease the isolation of older adults and help prevent abuse. These include programs in churches, businesses, and public and private agencies. Adult day care and respite care programs are examples of the concrete services provided by these community-based projects. Outcomes from these programs should be monitored for their effects on reducing the rates of older adult assaults in the community.

SUMMARY

Nonfall injuries are an important cause of morbidity and mortality in older adults. In addition to the loss of life and human suffering, the economic costs and the changes in lifestyle are important aspects of the consequences of trauma. Rates of injury as a result of MVCs (occupant and pedestrian), suicide, and residential fire are higher in the younger and older segments of the population, as indicated by J-shaped or U-shaped curves. Domestic violence against older adults is a recognized, but not well investigated, problem. Although risk factors have been identified for some of the cause specific injuries, the continuation of epidemiologic research is important to elucidate risk factors, especially those for which interventions can be developed. The development, implementation, and evaluation of the intervention programs are necessary for a multifaceted approach to injury control in older adults.

Literature Cited

1. Ashton, S. I. 1982. Vehicle design and pedestrian injuries. In *Pedestrian Accidents,* ed. A. J. Chapman, H. C. Foot, F. M. Wade, pp. 169–202. Chichester, England: Wiley
2. Baker, S. P., O'Neill, B., Karpf, R. S. 1984. *The Injury Fact Book.* Lexington, Mass: Lexington
3. Barancik, J. I., Chatterjee, B. F., Greene-Craden, Y. C., Michenzi, E. M., Kramer, C. F., et al. 1986. Motor vehicle trauma in Northeastern Ohio. I: Incidence and outcome by age, sex, and road-use category. *Am. J. Epidemiol.* 123:846–61
4. Blazer, D. G., Bachar, J. R., Manton, K. G. 1986. Suicide in later life. Review and commentary. *J. Am. Geriatr. Soc.* 34:519–25
5. Burvill, P. W. 1980. Changing patterns of suicide in Australia, 1910–1977. *Acta Psychiatr. Scand.* 62:258–68
6. Callahan, J. J. 1988. Elder abuse: some questions for policymakers. *Gerontologist* 28:453–58
7. Cent. Dis. Control. 1987. Regional distribution of deaths from residential fires—United States, 1978–84. *Morbid. Mortal. Wkly. Rep.* 36:645–48
8. Cerelli, E. 1989. *Older Drivers, the Age Factor in Traffic Safety.* Natl. Highway Traffic Safe. Adm. Dep. Transp. DOT HS 807 402
9. Champion, H. R., Copes, W. S., Buyer, D., Flanagan, M. E., Bain, L., Sacco, W. J. 1989. Major trauma in Geriatric patients. *Am. J. Public Health* 79:1278–82
10. Chatterjee, B. F., Barancik, J. I., Fratianne, R. B., Waltz, R. C., Fife, D. 1986. Northeastern Ohio Trauma Study: V. Burn Injury. *J. Trauma* 26:844–47
11. Comm. for the Study on Improving Mobility and Safe. for Older Persons. 1988. Special Rep. 218, Transp. in an Aging Soc., Vol. 1, Washington, DC: Transp. Res. Board, Natl. Res. Counc.
12. Counc. on Sci. Aff. 1987. Elder abuse and neglect. *J. Am. Med. Assoc.* 257:966–71
13. Crancer, A., McMurray, L. 1968. Accident and violation rates of Washington's medically restricted drivers. *J. Am. Med. Assoc.* 205:74–78
14. Fed. Emerg. Manage. Agency. 1980. An evaluation of residential smoke detector performance under actual field conditions: final report. Washington, DC: Fed. Emerg. Manage. Agency
15. Fife, D. 1987. Injuries and deaths among elderly persons. *Am. J. Public Health* 126:936–41

16. Fife, D., Barancik, J. I., Chatterjee, B. F. 1984. Northeastern Ohio trauma study: II. Injury rates by age, sex, and cause. *Am. J. Public Health* 74:473–78

17. Godkin, M. A., Wolf, R. S., Pillemer, K. A. 1989. A case-comparison analysis of elder abuse and neglect. *Int. J. Aging Hum. Dev.* 28:207–25

18. Graca, J. L. 1986. Driving and aging. *Clin. Geriatr. Med.* 2:577–89

19. Haight, F. A., Olsen, R. A. 1981. Pedestrian safety in the United States: some recent trends. *Accident Anal. Prev.* 13:43–55

20. Hansotia, P., Boste, S. K. 1991. The effect of epilepsy or diabetes mellitus on the risk of automobile accidents. *N. Engl. J. Med.* 324:22–26

21. Hauer, E. 1988. The safety of older persons at intersections. See Ref. 11, pp. 194–252

22. Herms, B. F. 1973. Pedestrian crosswalk study: accidents in painted and unpainted crosswalks. Highway Res. Rec. No. 406:1

23. Hirst, S. P., Brockington, W., Sheesley, L. 1985. Suicide among the aged: concern for caregivers. *Dimensions* Dec:25–27

24. Hogue, C. C. 1982. Injury in late life: Part I. Epidemiology. *J. Am. Geriatr. Soc.* 30:183–89

25. Honkanen, R., Ertama, L., Linnoila, M., Alha, A., Lukkari, I., et al. 1980. Role of drugs in traffic accidents. *Br. Med. J.* 281:1309–12

26. Insurance Inst. for Highway Safe. 1990. *Fatality Facts*. Arlington, Va: IIHS

27. Jick, H., Hunter, J. R., Dinan, B. J., Madsen, S., Stergachis, A. 1981. Sedating drugs and automobile accidents leading to hospitalization. *Am. J. Public Health* 71:1399–1400

28. Jonah, B. A. 1983. Measuring the relative risk of pedestrian accidents. *Accident Anal. Prev.* 15:163

29. Keltner, J. L., Johnson, C. A. 1987. Visual function, driving safety, and the elderly. *Opthamology* 94:1180–88

30. Knoblauch, R. L., Justin, B. H., Smith, S. A., Pietrucha, M. J. 1988. *Investigation of Exposure Based Pedestrian Accident Areas: Crosswalks, Sidewalks, Local Streets, and Major Arterials*. McLean, Va: Fed. Highway Adm.

31. Kosberg, J. I. 1988. Preventing elder abuse: identification of high risk factors prior to placement decisions. *Gerontologist* 28:43–50

32. Kreitman, N. 1976. The coal gas story: United Kingdom suicide rates, 1960–1971. *Br. J. Prev. Soc. Med.* 30:86–93

33. Liddell, F. D. K. 1982. Motor vehicle accidents (1973–76) in a cohort of Montreal drivers. *J. Epidemiol. Community Health* 36:140–45

34. Lui, K. J., Marchbanks, P. A. 1990. A study of the time between previous traffic infractions and fatal automobile crashes, 1984–1986. *J. Safe. Res.* 21:45–51

35. Lund, A. 1984. *Driver Records and Crash Protection*. Insur. Inst. for Highway Safe. Res. Note No. 106. Washington, DC

36. Lundgren-Lindquist, B., Aniansson, A., Rundren, A. 1983. Functional studies in 79-years-old. *Scand. J. Rehab. Med.* 15:125

37. Mackay, A., Halpern, J., McLoughlin, E., Locke, J., Crawford, J. D. 1979. A comparison of age-specific burn injury rates in five Massachusetts communities. *Am. J. Public Health* 69:1146–50

38. Mackay, M. 1988. Crash protection for older persons. See Ref. 11, pp. 158–93

39. MacPherson, R. D., Perl, J., Starmer, G. A., Homel, R. 1984. Self-reported drug usage and crash incidence in breathalyzed drivers. *Accident Anal. Prev.* 16:139–48

40. McIntosh, J. L. 1985. Suicide among the elderly: levels and trends. *Am. J. Orthopsychiatr.* 5:288–93

41. McKnight, A. J. 1988. Driver and pedestrian training. See Ref. 11, pp. 101–33

42. Mierley, M., Baker, S. P. 1983. Fatal house fires in an urban population. *J. Am. Med. Assoc.* 249:1466–68

43. Miller, M. 1978. Geriatric suicide: The Arizona study. *Gerontologist* 18:488–95

44. Mueller, B. A., Rivara, F. P., Lii, S. M., Weiss, N. S. 1990. Environmental factors and the risk for childhood pedestrian-motor vehicle collision occurrence. *Am. J. Epidemiol.* 132:550–60

45. Natl. Cent. for Health Stat. 1990. *Vital Statistics of the United States, Vol. 2: Part B Mortality*. Hyattsville, Md: DHHS, PHS

46. Natl. Cent. for Stat. Anal. 1989. *Fatal Accident Reporting System 1989: A Review of Information on Fatal Traffic Crashes in the United States in 1989*. Washington, DC: Natl. Highway Traffic Safe. Adm. Dep. Transp. DOT HS 807 693

47. Natl. Comm. for Injury Prev. and Control. 1989. *Injury Prevention: Meeting the Challenge*. New York: Oxford Univ. Press

48. Natl. Highway Traffic Safe. Adm. 1990. *General Estimates System 1989—A Review of Information on Police-Reported Traffic Crashes in the United*

States. Washington, DC: Dep. Transp. DOT HS 807 665

49. Natl. Highway Traffic Safe. Adm. 1990. *Occupant Protection Trends in 19 Cities*. Oct. 1990. Washington, DC: Dep. Transp.

50. Natl. Highway Traffic Safe. Adm. 1990. *Restraint System Use in 19 Cities 1989 Annual Report*. Washington, DC: Dep. Transp. DOT HS 807 595

51. Natl. Highway Traffic Safe. Adm. 1981. *Pedestrian Injury Causation Parameters—Phase II*. Washington, DC: Dep. Transp. DOT HS 806 148

52. Natl. Safe. Counc. 1990. *Accident Facts*. Chicago: Natl. Safe. Counc.

53. O'Malley, T. A., Everitt, D. E., O'Malley, H. C., Campion, W. 1983. Identifying and preventing family-mediated abuse and neglect of elderly persons. *Ann. Int. Med.* 98:998–1005

54. Osgood, N. J. 1982. Suicide in the elderly. *Postgrad. Med.* 72:123–30

55. Perrine, M. W., Peck, R. C., Fell, J. C. 1989. Epidemiology and data management. In *Surgeon General's Workshop on Drunk Driving: Background Papers*, pp. 35–76. Rockville, Md: US Dep. of Health and Hum. Serv. PHS Off. of the Surgeon General

56. Pillemer, K., Finkelhor, D. 1988. The prevalence of elder abuse: a random sample survey. *Gerontologist* 28:51–57

57. Public Health Serv. 1989. Surgeon general's workshop on health promotion and aging: summary recommendations of the alcohol working group. *Morbid. Mortal. Wkly, Rep.* 38:285–88

58. Retting, R., Schwartz, S. I., Kulewicz, M., Buhrmeister, D. 1989. Queens boulevard pedestrian safety project—New York City. *Morbid. Mortal. Wkly. Rep.* 38:61

59. Rice, D. P., MacKenzie, E. J., and Assoc. 1989. *Cost of Injury in the United States: A Report to Congress*. San Francisco, Calif: Inst. Health & Aging, Univ. of Calif. and Injury Prev. Cent., Johns Hopkins Univ.

60. Rivara, F. P. 1990. Child pedestrian injuries in the United States: Current status of the problem, potential intervention, and future research needs. *Am. J. Dis. Child.* 144:692–96

61. Rossignol, A. M., Boyle, C. M., Locke, J. A., Burke, J. F. 1986. Hospitalized burn injuries in Massachusetts: an assessment of incidence and product involvement. *Am. J. Public Health* 76:1341–43

62. Sendbuehler, J. M. 1977. Suicide and attempted suicide among the aged. *Can. Med. Assoc. J.* 117:418–19

63. Skegg, D. C. G., Richards, S. M., Doll, R. 1979. Minor tranquilizers and road accidents. *Br. Med. J.* 1:917–19

64. Sloan, J. H., Rivara, F. P., Reay, D. T., Ferris, J. A. J., Kellermann, A. L. 1990. Firearm regulations and rates of suicide. A comparison of two metropolitan areas. *N. Engl. J. Med.* 322:369–73

65. Smith, J. C., Mercy, J. A., Conn, M. 1988. Marital status and the risk of suicide. *Am. J. Public Health* 78:78–80

66. Solomon, D. 1985. The older driver and highway design. See Ref. 75, pp. 55–62

67. Starzyk, P. 1989. *Suicide Attempts and Deaths in Washington State, 1985–1987*. Olympia, Wa: Dep. Soc. Health Serv.

68. Stengel, S. 1964. *Suicide and Attempted Suicide*, pp. 34–35. Baltimore: Penguin

69. Stylos, L., Janke, M. K. 1989. *Annual Tabulations of Mature Driver Program Driving Record Comparisons—1989*. State Calif. Dep. Motor Vehicles. CAL-DMV-RSS-89-119

70. Tobey, H. N., Shunamen, E. M., Knoblauch, R. L. 1983. *Pedestrian Trip Making Characteristics and Exposure Measures*. Washington, DC: Fed. Highway Adm. Off. of Safe. Traffic Oper.

71. Wade, R. M., Foot, H. C., Chapman, A. J. 1982. Accidents and the physical environment. See Ref. 1, pp. 237–64

72. Waller, J. A. 1967. Cardiovascular disease, aging and traffic accidents. *J. Chron. Dis.* 20:615–20

73. Waller, J. A. 1965. Chronic medical conditions and traffic safety. *N. Engl. J. Med.* 273:1413–20

74. Waller, P. F. 1988. Renewal licensing of older adults. See Ref. 11, pp. 72–100

75. Yee, D. 1985. A survey of the traffic safety needs and problems of drivers age 55 and over. In *Drivers 55+: Needs and Problems of Older Drivers: Survey Results and Recommendations*, ed. J. L. Malfetti, pp. 96–128. Falls Church, Va: AAA Found. Traffic Safe.

76. Zador, P. 1982. Adoption of right turn on red: effects on crashes at signalized intersections. *Accident. Anal. Prev.* 14:219

77. Zeeger, C. V., Opiela, K. S., Cynecki, M. J. 1985. *Pedestrian Signalization Alternatives*. Washington, DC: US Dep. Transp.

SUBJECT INDEX

A

Acquired immunodeficiency syndrome (AIDS)
children and, 1–23
clinical management in children of, 19–22
college students and, 260
diagnosis in children of, 16–19
heterosexual transmission of, 1–6
mortality from
African American, 3
Hispanic American, 3
women and, 1–4
prevention of, 22–23
prognosis in children with, 22
sub-Saharan Africa and, 1–2
women and, 1–23
(See also Human immunodeficiency virus (HIV) infection)
Acute confusional states
drug-related, 411–27
elderly and, 411–27
anticholinergic drugs and, 418–21
polypharmacy and, 411–27
prevention of, 426–27
Adolescent health, 253–66
(See also Adolescents, College students)
Adolescents
depression among, 325–28, 330–31
smoking among, 294–96
restrictions on access to tobacco and, 302–3
Teenage Attitudes and Practices Survey (TAPS) and, 294–95
Youth Risk Behavior Survey and, 294–95
Adult Use of Tobacco Survey, 289, 292
Adverse drug reactions
elderly and, 415–27
Aerobic capacity
age-related decline in, 471
exercise and, 101–21, 471
physical activity and, 457, 470–71
Aerobic power (See Aerobic capacity)
Affective disorders (See Depression, Mood disorders)

African Americans
AIDS mortality among, 3
Age-period-cohort studies
mood disorders and, 325–27
Agency for Health Care Policy and Research, 365, 378–81
Medical Treatment Effectiveness Program of, 378
practice guidelines and, 365, 379–80
Aging, 411–526
Alzheimer's disease and, 418, 431–45
bone density and, 452, 457–58
dementia and, 431–45
disease prevention and, 411–13
health promotion and, 411–13
Healthy People 2000 goals for, 411–12
injury and
falls and, 489–504
nonfall, 509–26
physical activity and
effects of, 451–84
polypharmacy and, 415–27
AIDS (See Acquired immunodeficiency syndrome)
Alameda Population Laboratory, 459
Alaskan natives (See American Indians)
Alcohol abuse
dementia and, 433
Alcohol use
college students and, 260
elderly and
falls among, 499
Aluminum exposure
Alzheimer's disease and, 433, 439–40
Alz-50 antibody, 444
Alzheimer's disease, 418, 431–35
dementia and, 431–45
Down syndrome and, 443–44
epidemiology of, 437–41
aluminum exposure and, 439–40
family history and, 437–38
head trauma and, 438–39
viruses and, 440–41
incidence of, 436–37
pathogenesis of, 441–44
Alz-50 antibody and, 444
β-amyloid and, 442–44

amyloid percursor protein and, 442–44
chromosome 21 and, 442–44
neurofibrillary tangles and, 443
prevalence of, 434–35
American College of Sports Medicine (ACSM)
exercise prescriptions of, 102–3
American Indians, 269–83
infant mortality among, 269–83
Americans with Disabilities Act of 1990, 24
Amitriptyline, 420
β-Amyloid
Alzheimer's disease and, 442–44
Amyloid precursor protein
Alzheimer's disease and, 442–44
Anticholinergic drugs
acute confusional states in elderly and, 418–21
Appropriateness
unnecessary surgery and, 363–81
(See also Surgery)
Arrythmia
reduced risk for lethal ventricular exercise and, 104
Assault
elderly and injuries from, 509, 524–26
Association of State and Territorial Health Officials (ASTHO)
tobacco prevention and control network of, 304–5
tobacco use control and, 289, 294–96, 304–5, 308–9
Audience analysis
social marketing and, 341–60
Azidothymidine, 19
AZT, 19

B

B-cell dysfunction
HIV-infected children and, 14
Behavior
health-seeking
immunization and, 385–88
Behavioral Risk Factor Surveillance System

529

smoking and, 290–92, 299
Behavioral risks
smoking and, 287–315
Benzodiazepines, 420, 498–99
cognitive impairment in elderly and, 420
falls among elderly and, 498–99
Biological Effects of Ionizing Radiation (BEIR) Committee, 134–35
Bipolar disorder, 320–21, 328–36
genetics of, 328
Body fat distribution
excercise and, 106–7
Bone density, 452, 457–58, 478–79
exercise and, 478–79
physical activity and, 452, 457–58
Burns
elderly and, 509, 522–24

C

Cancer
breast
exercise and, 107, 109, 112
colon
exercise and, 107, 109
lung
firefighters and, 160–61
radiation-induced, 127–28, 130–46
breast, 134–44
colon, 134
esophagus, 134
leukemia, 128, 134, 138–42, 144
lung, 134, 136–37, 142
multiple myeloma, 134, 139, 142
ovary, 134
stomach, 134
thyroid, 134, 144
urinary tract, 134
reproductive
exercise and, 107, 109
Cancer Prevention Research Program
Fred Hutchinson Cancer Research Center, 38–39
Cancer risk
extremely-low-frequency magnetic fields and, 184–88, 191
Carcinogenesis, 127–28, 130–46
heritable mutations and, 132–33, 137
mechanisms of irradiation injury and, 130–31

radiation exposure and, 127–28, 130–31
radon and, 127, 129–30, 136–37, 145–46
threshold hypothesis for abandonment of, 127–28, 145–46
Cardiac pacemakers
effects of extremely-low-frequency magnetic fields on, 189
Cardiovascular disease
diabetes mellitus and exercise and, 106
firefighters and, 163–65
physical activity and older adults and, 459–64
physical fitness and, 100–1, 103–11
Centers for Disease Control Behavioral Risk Factor Survey, 38–39
Cesarian section, 365–66, 373
Chernobyl, 143–44
Children
AIDS in
clinical management of, 19–22
clinical presentation of, 12–16
incubation period of, 12–13
prognosis for, 22
cyclothymia among, 331
depression among, 325–28, 330–31
global immunization for, 223–37, 239–50
Children's Vaccine Initiative and, 234
Declaration on the Survival, Protection, and Development of Children and, 227
diptheria and, 223
hepatitis B vaccine and, 234
measles and, 223–24, 229, 231–33, 240
neonatal tetanus and, 223–24, 232, 240, 248
poliomyelitis and, 223, 233–34, 239–50
tuberculosis and, 223, 240
World Summit for Children, 227
HIV infection in, 1–23
clinical management of, 19–22
clinical presentation of, 12–16
incubation period of, 12–13
maternal factors affecting, 9–10

prevention of, 22–23
prognosis of, 22
transmission of, 1–12
low preschool immunization coverage in US of, 385–95
universal immunization among, 234
Children's Vaccine Initiative, 234
Chlamydia trachomatis
increased risk of HIV infection and, 6
Cholesterol
high density lipoprotein exercise and, 104–5
Chromosome 21
Alzheimer's disease and, 442–44
Down syndrome and, 443–44
Civil liberties
worksite drug testing and, 199, 203–5, 218
Coagulation
exercise and favorable effect on blood, 104
Cognition
exercise and, 456–57, 478
Cognitive disfunction
elderly and
motor vehicle crashes and, 512–14
polypharmacy and, 415–27
Cognitive therapy, 334–35
College health services, 256–66
future of, 264–66
health care structure and, 262–66
health promotion and, 257–58
history of, 256–57
medical care and, 257
psychological care and, 257–58
student health centers and, 257
College students
health problems of, 253–66
acute, 259
AIDS and, 260
chronic, 259–60
disabled, 254–55
health professions, 255
injuries and, 259
international, 255
nontraditional, 255–56
sexually transmitted diseases and, 259–60
unwanted pregnancy, 261
vaccine-preventable, 259
Combustion gases
health hazards of firefighters and, 151–67

Community-based health promotion and disease prevention, 31–54
Community education, 341
social marketing and, 341–60
developing countries and, 48–53
Congenital abnormalities
natural background radiation and, 132
Consensus panels, 363, 376–78
National Institutes of Health Consensus Conferences and, 376
unnecessary surgery and, 363, 376–78
Coronary artery bypass graft surgery, 366, 374
Coronary heart disease risk
firefighters', 163–65
physical activity in older adults and, 459–60
physical fitness and, 100–1, 103–11
Cost containment, 399–410
Medicaid and, 399–400
drug formularies and, 400–10
Current Population Survey, 290–94
Cutter polio vaccine incident, 393–94
Cyclothymia, 321–22, 331
Cytomegalovirus
HIV-infected children and, 14, 21

D

Delirium
polypharmacy and
elderly and, 415–27
Dementia, 431–45
alcohol abuse and, 433
Alzheimer's disease and, 431–45
brain damage and, 433, 438–39
causes of, 432–34
depression and, 433
drug toxicity and, 433
Huntington disease and, 433
incidence of, 436–37
metabolic disorders and, 433
multiinfarct, 433–34
neurotoxins and, 433
normal pressure hydrocephalus and, 433
Parkinson's disease and, 433
Pick's disease and, 433
prevalence of, 434–35
progressive supranuclear palsy and, 433

Dementia pugilistica, 438
Depression
age-period cohort studies of, 325–27
changing rates of, 325–27
children and, 325–28, 330–31
dementia and, 433
dysthemia, 321–22, 323, 325
epidemiology of, 319–28
exercise and, 103
genetics of, 328–30
inactivity and, 458–59
major, 321, 323–27
quality of life and, 331–32
treatment of, 332–36
pharmacologic, 332–33
psychotherapy for, 334
Depression Awareness, Recognition, and Treatment Program (DART), 335–36
Developing countries
immunization in, 223–37
social marketing in, 48–60
Diabetes mellitus, 99, 106, 112–13
cardiovascular disease and, 106
exercise and, 99, 106
Diarrhea
HIV-infected children and, 14
Dideoxydytidine (ddC), 19
Dideoxyinosine (ddI), 19
Dietary behavior
self-reporting of, 48–49
Digoxin, 421
Diptheria
vaccine against, 229, 240, 248
Diptheria-pertussis-tetanus vaccine, 240, 248
Disability
inactivity and, 452–64
Disease prevention
community-based interventions for, 31–54
evaluation of, 31–54
exercise
older adults and, 454, 470–84
falls among elderly and, 503–4
health objectives and, 59–76
health status indicators and, 66–71
physical activity
older adults and, 451–84
targets and priorities for, 59, 73–75
US national health goals for, 59–76
Down syndrome
Alzheimer's disease and, 443–44

Drug abuse
national trends in, 205–6
worksite drug testing and, 197–218
Drug expenditures, 399–410
Medicaid drug formulary and, 402–10
Medicaid reibursement for drugs and, 399–410
new legislation regarding, 408–10
Drug formulary
Medicaid, 400–10
drug expenditures and, 402–5
lag access to new drugs and, 406–7, 409
Drug-free Workplace Act of 1988, 202–3
Drug-induced disease
elderly and, 415–27
prevention of, 426–27
Drug pricing, 409–10
Drug reactions
adverse
elderly and, 415–27
Drugs
public perception of, 206
urine screening for, 197–218
use among workers of, 206
worksite drug testing and, 197–218
public attitudes toward, 206–7
Drug therapy
multiple
delirium among elderly and, 415–27
Drug toxicity
dementia and, 433
Drug use
elderly and
falls among, 498–99
motor vehicle crashes and, 514
Dysthymia, 321–23, 325, 330–36

E

Edmonston-Zagreb strain of measles vaccine, 229, 231
Elderly
acute confusional states among
drug-related, 417–27
epidemiology of, 416–17
polypharmacy and, 415–27
falls among, 489–504
chronic diseases and, 496
environmental risk factors for, 500–1

gait and balance
    abnormalities and,
    496–97
  medication use and, 198
  mental status and, 497
  osteoporosis and, 495–96
  vision and, 497
frail, 469
health status of
  effects of physical activity
    on, 451–84
  inactivity among, 452–64
  depression and, 458–59
  disability and, 451–64
  nonfall injuries among
    motor vehicle crash and,
      509, 512–16
    risk factors for, 512
  physical fitness and, 470–84
    bone density and, 452,
      457–58, 478–79
    cognition and, 456–57, 478
Electric blankets
  ELF magnetic fields and,
    183–84
Employee assistance programs,
    198–99
  worksite drug testing and,
    198–99
Encephalopathy
  progressive
    HIV-infected children and,
      13
  static
    HIV-infected children and,
      13
Ergonomics
  firefighters' health concerns
    and, 152–53, 165–66
Evaluation methods
  health promotion and disease
    prevention and, 31–54
Executive Order 12564
  federal worksite drug testing
    regulations and, 201–2
Exercise
  aerobic capacity and, 101–21,
    470–71
  American College of Sports
    Medicine recommenda-
    tions for, 102–3
  clinical studies of, 101–7
  cognition and, 478
  definition of, 101
  dose response relationship to
    health of, 115–18
  duration of, 102, 105
  frequency of, 102–3
  gait, balance, and physical
    function and, 473–79
  intensity of, 102, 105
  intervention studies of older
    adults and, 473–84

older adults and, 454, 470–
    84
  osteoporosis and, 478–79
  physical fitness and, 99–121,
    470–84
  older adults and, 470–84
  physiologic effects of, 103–
    7
Exercise science
  development of, 100
Expanded Programme on Im-
    munization, 223–37, 240–
    50, 349–52
  achieving full coverage and,
    228–30
  disease surveillance and, 230
  global immunization plan of,
    223–37
  goals of, 226–27
  hepatitis B vaccine and, 234
  measles reduction and, 231–
    32
  neonatal tetanus elimination
    and, 223–24, 232
  poliomyelitis eradication and,
    223, 233–34
  social marketing and, 349,
    351–52
Extremely-low-frequency (ELF)
    magnetic fields, 173–91
  biological effects of, 179–82
    cardiac fibrillation and, 181
    magnetophosphenes and,
      179–82, 190
    visually evoked potentials
      and, 180
  cardiac pacemakers and, 189
  effects of combined static
    and, 178–79
    calcium ion uptake, 178
    fibroblast proliferation,
      178
    ion movements through
      membrane channels,
      178–79
  exposure guidelines for, 189–
    90
  health effects of, 173–91
  human health studies of, 182–
    89
    cancer risk and, 184–88
    electric blankets and, 183–
      84
    video display terminals
      and, 184
  interaction with tissue and,
    176–78, 191
    ligand-receptor interactions
      and, 177, 191
    RNA transcriptase patterns
      and, 177
  measurement of, 174
  sources of, 175

F

Factor 1000, 216–17
Failure to thrive
  HIV-infected children and,
    13–14
Falls
  definitions of, 490–92
  elderly morbidity and mortal-
    ity from, 489–504
  epidemiology of, 490–500
  incidence of, 492–94
  prevention of, 490–503
  risk factors for, 494–501
    age and sex, 494
    chronic diseases, 496
    environmental, 500–1
    gait and balance
      abnormalities, 496–97
    medication use, 498
    mental status and, 497
    osteoporosis, 495–96
    vision and, 497
Fetal alcohol syndrome
  American Indian infant
    mortality from, 279–80
Firefighters, 151–67
  health hazards of
    chemical, 153–57
    ergonomic, 152–53, 165–66
    psychological, 157–58
    thermal, 152–53
  occupational health effects of,
    158–67
Fluoxetine, 333
Fourth Amendment
  worksite drug testing and,
    203
Framingham Heart Study, 106,
    109
Functional status
  exercise and
    older adults and, 473–79

G

Genetic epidemiology
  mood disorders and, 319,
    328–36
Geographic variations
  unnecessary surgery and, 364,
    367–70
Geriatrics (See Aging, Elderly)

H

Hantaan virus, 80–84, 90
  vaccine for, 90
Hantaviruses, 79–94
  diagnosis of, 89–90
  Hantaan, 80–84
  Leakey, 80, 88–89
  molecular biology of, 89–90

Prospect Hill, 80, 87–88
Puumula, 79–80, 84–85
Seoul, 79–81, 85–87
transmission of, 80–81
vaccine for, 89–90
virus isolation of, 89–90
in US, 90–93
Health
definition of, 101
physical fitness and, 101,
456–64
Health Care Financing Administration (HCFA), 363, 371
Health care services
overuse of
unnecessary surgery and,
363–81
Health communication
social marketing and, 341–60
developing countries and,
348–53
Health departments
Association of State and Territorial Health Officials
(ASTHO), 289, 294–96,
304–5, 308–9
state, 287–89, 294–96, 304–
15
Institute of Medicine report
on The Future of
Public Health and,
288
tobacco use prevention and,
288
Health maintenance organizations (HMOs), 364, 368,
370
Health objectives, 59–76
individual, 63–64
statistical issues in setting,
61–66
statistical models for small
areas and, 72–73
targets for, 73–75
Health promotion
community-based in-
terventions for, 31–54
evaluation of, 31–54
elderly and
prevention of falls among,
503–4
prevention of nonfall injuries among, 514–16,
518–26
health objectives and, 59–76
health status indicators and,
66–71
Indian Health Service and,
281–83
older adults and
exercise and, 454, 470–84
physical activity and, 451–
84

social marketing and, 341–60
developing countries and,
348–53
targets for, 59, 73–75
US national health goals and,
59–76
Health seeking behavior, 385–88
health belief model of, 386–
87
socioeconomic status and,
387–95
Health services, 385–95
Aid for Dependent Children
(AFDC) and, 391, 394
consumer demand for im-
munization and, 386–88
immunization and, 389–95
socioeconomic status and,
387–95
Women, Infants and Children
(WIC) program and,
391, 394
Health status indicators, 59, 66–
71
criteria for, 66–71
statistical models for small
areas and, 72–73
composite estimation, 73
regression estimation, 72–
73
structure-preserving estimation, 73
synthetic estimation, 72
Hematologic abnormalities
HIV-infected children and, 14
Hemorrhagic fever
Korean, 81–84
Hantaan virus and, 81–84
Healthy People 2000
American Indian health care
and, 282
college student health, 264
health objectives and, 59–76
implementation of, 75–76
statistical issues in setting,
61–66
targets and priorities for,
73–75
health status indicators and,
66–71
tobacco use and, 288–94,
296, 299
Hemorrhagic fever with renal
syndrome (HFRS), 79–94
diagnosis of, 89–90
hantaviruses and, 79–94
laboratory-rat-associated, 87
ribavirin and, 84, 93
in US, 90–93
vaccine for, 89–90
Hepatitis B vaccine, 234
Hepatosplenomegaly
HIV-infected children and, 13

Herpes simplex virus type II
increased risk of HIV infec-
tion and, 6
High blood pressure
exercise and reduced, 105–
6
High density lipoprotein
cholesterol
effect of exercise on, 104–5
Higher education
health services in, 253–66
Hispanic Americans
AIDS-related mortality
among, 3
Hispanic Health and Nutrition
Examination Survey
(HHANES), 290–92
HIV (See Human im-
munodeficiency virus)
Homicide
American Indian infant
mortality and, 281
Honolulu Heart Program, 459–
60
Human immunodeficiency virus
(HIV) infection, 1–23
children and, 1–23
clinical management of, 19–
22
diagnosis in children of, 16–
19
epidemiology of, 2–7
sexually transmitted dis-
eases and, 6, 8
incidence of
CDC estimates of, 1–3
WHO estimates worldwide
of, 1–2
IV drug use and, 1–3, 8
pregnancy and, 7–8
prevention of, 22–23
prognosis in children of, 22
transmission of
heterosexual, 1–6
intrapartum, 11–12
intrauterine, 10–11
maternal factors and, 9–10
parenteral, 6–7
postnatal, 12
vertical, 8–12
women and, 1–23
(See also Acquired im-
munodeficiency syn-
drome)
Huntington disease
dementia and, 433
Hyergammaglobulinemia
HIV-infected children and, 14
Hypertension
exercise and, 105–8
hantaviruses and, 79, 81, 93
Hypotension
iatrogenic-induced, 421

I

Immunization
barriers to, 389–93
disease surveillance and, 230
Expanded Programme on,
223–37, 240–50, 349–52
follow-up systems for, 392–
93
global, 223–37, 239–50
hepatitis B vaccine and, 234
measles reduction and, 231–
32
missed opportunities for, 390–
92
neonatal tetanus elimination
and, 223–24, 232
polio
Brazil and, 243–45
Cuba and, 243–44
Pan American Health
Organization (PAHO)
and, 240–50
US and, 244–45
poliomyelitis eradication and,
223, 233–34, 239–50
Western hemisphere, 239–
50
research and development
and, 235–36
socioeconomic status and,
387–95
vaccines
new and improved, 234
Immunization compliance, 385–
95
barriers to, 389–93
health insurance
availability of, 387–95
health-seeking behavior and,
385–95
Immunization programs, 385–95
Aid for Dependent Children
(ADFC) and, 391, 394
barriers to utilization of, 389–
93
missed opportunities in, 390–
92
Women, Infants and Children
(WIC) program and,
391, 394
Immunologic function
exercise and enhanced, 107
Impramine, 420
Inactivity
coronary heart disease and,
452
depression and, 452
disability and, 452–64
disuse hypothesis and, 453
fractures and, 452
frailty and, 452

mortality and, 452, 461–64
Indian Health Care Improvement
Act, 282
Indian Health Care Service,
269–83
death and disease rates and
calculating Indian, 270
Healthy People 2000 and,
282
infant mortality rates by area,
274–76
maternal and child health program of, 281–83
Induced currents, 173–91
(See also Extremely-low-
frequency (ELF) magnet-
ic fields)
Infant mortality, 269–83
American Indian, 269–83
congenital abnormalities
and, 279–80
factors contributing to,
276–81
homicide and, 281
injuries and, 274–76, 281
low birthweight and, 278–
79
meningitis and, 274–76
pneumonia and influenza
and, 274–76
sudden infant death syn-
drome and, 274–76,
280–81
Influenza
American Indian infant
mortality from, 274–
76
Injuries
American Indian infant
mortality and, 274–76,
281
elderly and
assault and, 524–26
burns and, 522–24
costs of, 511
disease model of, 490
falls and, 489–504
incidence of, 510–12
lifestyle changes and, 511
motor vehicle crashes and,
509, 512–16
pedestrian injuries and,
516–20
suicide and, 520–22
firefighting and, 159
Institute of Medicine report on
*The Future of Public
Health,* 288
Insulin sensitivity
exercise and, 106
Interpersonal psychotherapy,
334–35

Interventions
community-based, 31–54
evaluation of, 31–54
physical activity and health of
older adults, 469–84

K

Henry J. Kaiser Family Founda-
tion
Community Health Promotion
Grants Program of, 34–
35, 38–39, 53
Kaiser Health Promotion
Evaluation Project, 41
Kellog International Work
Group, 490
Korean Hemorrhagic fever, 81–
84

L

Leakey virus, 80, 88–89
Left ventrical function
exercise and, 103–4
Linear energy transfer, 130–31,
135
low-level irradiation injury
and, 130–31
Lipoprotein levels
exercise and, 104–5
Lymphadenopathy
HIV infections in children
and, 13
Lymphocytic infiltration
diffuse
HIV-infected children and,
13
focal
HIV-infected children and,
13
Lymphoid interstitial pneumonitis
HIV-infected children and, 13

M

Magnetophosphenes, 173, 179–
82, 190
cardiac fibrillation and, 181
retina and, 180
visually evoked potentials
and, 180
Managed care
unnecessary surgery and, 364,
368, 370
Measles, 223–24, 229, 231–32,
240
Edmonston-Zagreb vaccine
for, 229, 231
recommended immunization
schedule for, 229

Measles eradication, 231–32, 240
Mechanisms of interaction
extremely-low-frequency magnetic fields and, 173–91
Medicaid
cost containment and, 399–410
new drugs and
lag in access to, 406–7, 409
pharmaceutical reimbursements for
new legislation regarding, 408–10
restrictions in, 400–10
Membrane interactions
extremely-low-frequency magnetic fields and, 173, 176–82, 191
Meningitis
American Indian infant mortality from, 274–76
Methyldopa, 421
Mood disorders, 319–36
bipolar disorder, 320–21, 323–24
depressive disorders, 319–22
changing rates of, 325–27
dysthymia, 321–22, 323, 325, 330
major, 321, 323–27
genetics of, 328–30
quality of life and, 331–32
treatment of, 332–36
pharmacologic, 332–33
psychotherapy, 334
Motor vehicle crashes
elderly and, 509, 512–16
MRFIT Study, 44
Multiinfarct dementia, 433–34
Muscle strength
older adults and
age-related decline in, 471
physical activity and, 457
physical fitness and, 471–72
physical function and, 473–78
Musculoskeletal system, 99, 114–15
physical fitness and, 114–15
Mutation
heritable, 132–33, 137
mechanisms of injury by irradiation and, 130–31
radiation exposure and, 127–28, 130–46
threshold hypothesis for abandonment of, 127–28, 145–46

Myocardial hypertrophy
exercise and, 102–3
Myocardial oxygen supply and demand
exercise and, 103

N

National Cancer Institute
COMMIT intervention trial to reduce cancer mortality rate, 305–7, 311, 313
National Health and Nutrition Survey (NHANES), 290
National Health Interview Survey (HIS)
tobacco use and, 289
National Institute on Aging Established Populations for Epidemiologic Studies of the Elderly, 460
National Institute on Drug Abuse (NIDA), 290, 294
Native Americans
(See American Indians)
Neonatal tetanus elimination, 223–24, 232
Nephropathia epidemica, 79, 84–85
Puumala virus and, 84–85
Nephropathy
HIV-infected children and, 14
Neurofibrillary tangles, 443
Normal pressure hydrocephalus
dementia and, 433
Norway rats
Seoul virus and, 80–81, 85–87
Nutrition
college students and, 262

O

Obesity
exercise and, 106–7
Occupational health
cancer risk and
extremely-low-frequency magnetic fields and, 187–88
firefighting exposures and, 151–67
radiation exposure and, 139–42
worksite drug testing and, 197–218
Omnibus Budget Reconciliation Act, 400
Oral rehydration solution
social marketing and, 347, 350

Oral rehydration therapy
social marketing and, 350
Osteoarthritis
running and risk of, 113
Osteoporosis
exercise and, 478–79
falls among elderly and, 495–96
physical fitness and, 114

P

Pan American Health Organization (PAHO)
polio eradication and, 240–50
initiative for, 241
program strategies for, 241–47
Paralysis
acute flaccid
poliomyelitis vaccine-associated, 243
Parkinson's disease
dementia and, 433
Pediatrics
HIV and AIDS and, 1–23
Peer Review Organization (PRO)
unnecessary surgery and, 365, 372
Pertussis, 223–24, 240, 248
Pharmaceuticals
Medicaid drug formularies and, 400–10
lag in access to new drugs and, 406–7, 409
Medicaid reimbursements for, 399, 410
new legislation regarding, 408–10
restrictions on access to Medicaid and, 399–410
Physical activity, 99–121, 262
college students and, 262
definition of, 101
dose-response relationship to health of, 115–18
epidemiologic studies of, 107–20
older adults and, 451–84
bone density and, 457–58
coronary heart disease risk and, 459–60
depression and, 458–59
disability and, 451–64
health and, 456–64
intervention studies on, 469–84
metabolism and, 458
mortality and, 461–64
muscle strength and, 457, 471–72

neurological function and, 456–57
observational studies on, 451–64
public health recommendations for, 115–18
Physical fitness
cancer risk and, 107, 109, 112
cardiovascular diseases and, 100–1, 103–11
definition of, 101
diabetes and, 106, 112–13
epidemiologic studies of, 107–20
exercise and, 99–121
physiologic effects of, 102–8
older adults and
aerobic capacity and, 470–71
cognitive status and, 473
physical status and, 472–73
skeletal muscle strength and, 471–72
osteoarthritis risk and, 113
osteoporosis and, 114
public health recommendations for, 115–18
Physical function
exercise and
older adults and, 473–79
Pick's disease
dementia and, 433
Pneumocystis carinii infections
HIV-infected children and, 13, 15–16, 20
Pneumonia
American Indian infant mortality from, 274–76
Pneumocystis carinii
HIV-infected children and, 13, 15–16, 20
Poliomyelitis, 223, 233–34, 239–50
Cutter poliomyelitis vaccine incident and, 393–94
eradication in Western Hemisphere of, 239–50
trivalent oral poliomyelitis vaccine for, 233–34
vaccine for, 239–50
Poliomyelitis eradication, 223, 233–34, 239–50
Pan American Health Organization (PAHO) and, 240–50
progress of, 248–50
Polypharmacy in elderly
acute confusional states and, 415–27
anticholinergic drugs and, 418–21

prevention of, 426–27
Practice guidelines, 363, 365, 379–81
Agency for Health Care Policy and Research (AHCPR) and, 365, 378–81
Peer Review Organizations (PROs) and, 365, 372
Pregnancy
HIV transmission and, 7–12
smoking and, 292
tetanus immunization during, 224, 232
unwanted
college students and, 261
Preschool immunization
causes of low rates in US of, 385–95
Privacy
worksite drug testing and, 199, 203–5
Prospect Hill virus, 80, 87–88, 90
Prudent Purchasing Act of 1990, 408
Psychiatric diagnosis
mood disorders and, 319–22
Psychiatric epidemiology, 319–28
Pulmonary disease, 13
acute and chronic
HIV-infected children and, 13
firefighters and, 161–63
Puumala virus, 79–80, 84–85
nephropathia epidemica and, 84–85

Q

Quality-adjusted life years, 71

R

Radiation
carcinogenesis and, 127–28, 130–33
exposure limits of, 127–28, 145–46
low-level ionizing, 127–46
medical, 143–44
mutation and, 127–28, 130–33
natural background, 128–30, 132–33
radon, 127, 129–30, 136–37
occupational, 139–42
sources of environmental, 128–30
cosmic rays, 129–30

external gamma radiation, 129–30
internal radiation, 129–30
man-made, 130, 142–44
teratogenic effect of, 136
Radiation accidents, 142–43
Chernobyl, 143–44
Three Mile Island, 143
Radionuclide, 127
Radon, 127, 129–30, 136–37, 145–46
exposure limits to, 146
RAND Health Insurance Experiment, 38–39
RAND Health Services Utilization Study, 369
RAND Medical Outcomes Study, 70–71
Randomization, 40–41
Rape
college students and, 259
Rehabilitation Act of 1973, 204
Renal disease
chronic
hanta viruses and, 79–94
nephropathia epidemica, 84–85
Puumala virus and, 84–85
Resonance interactions, 173–91
(See also Extremely-low-frequency magnetic fields)
Respiratory disorders
firefighting and, 159–60
Ribavirin
treatment of hemorrhagic fever with renal syndrome with, 84, 93
Rocky Mountain Tobacco-Free Challenge, 304, 313
Rodent-borne zoonoses, 79–94
hantaviruses, 79–94
Seoul virus, 79–81, 85–87

S

School health
college-level, 253–66
(See also College students, College health services)
Scopolamine, 418–19
Self-contained breathing apparatus (SCBA)
firefighting and, 152, 157–58
Self-reported health characteristics, 46–49
dietary behavior and, 48–49
smoking behavior and, 47–49
Seniors
activity patterns among, 454–55

exercise and, 454, 470–84
  cognition and, 456–57
health status of
  effects of physical activity
    on, 452–84
  inactivity among, 452–64
  depression among, 458–
    59
  disability among, 451–84
  physical fitness and, 470–84
    bone density and, 452,
      457–58, 478–79
  (See also Aging, Elderly,
    Physical activity,
    Physical Fitness)
Seoul virus, 79–81, 85–87, 91
Sexually transmitted diseases
  college students and, 259–
    60
  HIV epidemiology and, 6, 8
Smoke inhalation
  firefighting and, 151–57
Smoking
  health department and com-
    munity-based programs
    to prevent, 304–15
  cessation programs, 307
  high risk groups and, 307–
    8
  NCI COMMIT intervention
    trial, 305–7, 311, 313
  legislation and policies
    against, 299–304
  clean-indoor-air, 300–2
  restrictions on access, 302–
    3
  restrictions on advertising,
    303
  tax increases, 303–4
  preventing, 287–315
  public information campaigns,
    308–9
  social marketing and, 308–
    9
  surveillance of, 289–98
  Year 2000 Objectives for the
    Nation on Tobacco and
    Health, 314–15
Smoking behavior, 38–39
  biochemical validation of, 47–
    49
  community-level measures of,
    51–53
  self-reporting of, 47–49
Social and Economic Accounts
  System (SEAS), 51
Social marketing, 48–60, 308,
  341–60
  antismoking campaigns and,
    308–9
  developing countries and, 48–
    60
  ethical issues of, 346–48

Stanford Three-Community
  Hear Disease Study and,
    353–54
Socioeconomic status
  health insurance and
    availability of, 387–95
  immunization and, 387–95
  health-seeking behavior
    and, 387–88
Stanford Five-City Project, 44
Stanford Three-Community
  Heart Disease Study
  social marketing and, 353–54
Statistical rates
  standardization of
    methods of, 65–66
Stress
  college students and, 260–62
  firefighters and, 151, 157–58
Stroke, 108–11
  physical fitness and, 108–11
Student health
  college, 253–66
    (See also College students)
Sudden infant death syndrome
  American Indians and, 274–
    76, 280–81
Suicide
  college students and, 261–62
  elderly and, 509, 520–22
Surgery
  unnecessary, 363–81
    definition of, 365–67
    geographic variations and,
      363–64
    methods of payment and,
      370
    outcomes research and,
      378–79
    policy implications of,
      380–81
    practice guidelines and,
      363, 365, 379–80
    precertification programs
      and, 372–73
    reasons for, 374–78
    second surgical opinion
      programs, 363, 370–72
Surgical second opinion program, 363, 370–72
Surveillance
  Expanded Programme on Im-
    munization and, 230
  falls among elderly and, 501–
    3
  health objectives and, 59–76
  health status indicators and,
    66–71
  Pan American Health Organ-
    ization program to eradi-
    cate polio and, 245
  tobacco use prevention and
    control and, 289–98

Adult Use of Tobacco Sur-
  vey, 289, 292
Behavioral Risk Factor Sur-
  veillance System, 290–
  92
Current Population Surveys,
  290–94
excise tax data and tobacco
  consumption, 297
Hispanic Health and Nutri-
  tion Examination Sur-
  vey, 290–92
National Health Interview
  Survey, 289
National Health and Nutri-
  tion Examination Sur-
  vey, 290
National Institute on Drug
  Abuse National House-
  hold Surveys on Drug
  Abuse, 290, 294
public opinion polls, 296
Smoking Attributable
  Mortality, Morbidity,
  and Economic Costs
  (SAMMEC and SAM-
  MEC II), 299
Teenage Attitudes and
  Practices Survey
  (TAPS), 294–95
Syphilis
  increased risk of HIV infec-
    tion and, 6

T

Teenage Attitudes and Practices
  Survey (TAPS), 294–95
Tetanus, 223–24, 232, 240, 248
  neonatal, 224, 232
Third World
  immunization in, 223–37,
    239–50
Three Mile Island, 143
Threshold hypothesis
  radiation exposure and, 127–
    28, 145–46
Tobacco use
  Adult Use of Tobacco Sur-
    vey, 289, 292
  smokeless, 306
  Year 2000 Objectives for the
    Nation on Tobacco and
    Health, 314–15
  (See also Smoking)
Trauma
  college students and, 259
  elderly and
    assault and, 509, 524–26
    burns among, 509, 522–24
    falls among, 489–504
    motor vehicle crashes
      among, 509, 512–16

pedestrian injuries and,
516–20
suicide among, 509, 520–
22
Trihexyphenidyl, 419–20
Trivalent oral poliomyelitis vaccine, 229, 233–34, 240–50
Tuberculosis, 223, 229, 240
vaccine against, 229, 240

U

United Nations Children's Fund
(UNICEF)
Child Survival and Development Initiative, 359–60
global immunization and,
224, 234
social marketing and, 349,
351–52, 358–60
United Nations Scientific Committee on the Effects of
Atomic Radiation (UN-
SCEAR), 133, 135
US national health goals, 59–76
health status indicators and,
66–71
Healthy People 2000, 59–76
statistical issues in setting,
61–66
targets and priorities for, 59,
73–75

V

Vaccination
Brazil and, 243–45
Cuba and, 243–44
Expanded Programme on Im-
munization and global,
223–37, 240
low rates of US preschool immunization and, 385–95

Pan American Health Organization (PAHO) initiative
and, 240–50
polio, 239–50
US rates of, 244–45
Vaccine
diptheria-pertussis-tetanus vaccine, 223, 229, 240, 248
hantavirus, 89–90
measles, 229, 231, 240
Edmonston-Zagreb strain
of, 229, 231
polio
delivery of, 243–45
inactivated, 239–40
live oral, 240–50
oral, 239–50
trivalent oral, 229, 233–34,
240–50
tuberculosis, 223, 229
Video display terminals
ELF magnetic fields and, 184

W

Washington State Cancer-
Related Behavioral Risk
Factor Survey, 39–39
Women
HIV infection in, 1–23
Worksite drug testing, 197–218
costs and benefits of, 216–17
detection from, 211–12
effectiveness of, 209–10, 213,
218
federal regulations for, 202
federal regulatory initiatives
for, 201
Fourth Amendment and, 203
job performance and, 213–16
US corporations and, 200–1
US military and, 200–1

World Health Assembly
(WHA), 223–37, 250
Expanded Programme on Im-
munization and, 223–37,
250
goals of, 226–27
World Health Organization
(WHO)
Expanded Programme on Im-
munization of, 223–37,
250
goals of, 226–27
expert committee on new
approaches to health
education, 357–60
HIV infection estimates worldwide of, 1–2
social marketing and, 349,
351–52, 357–60

X

X-ray irradiation, 127–28, 130,
142–46
carcinogenesis and mutagenesis and, 127–28, 130,
142–46

Y

Year 2000 Objectives for the
Nation on Tobacco and
Health, 314–15
Youth Risk Behavior Survey,
294–95, 312

Z

Zidovudine, 19, 22
Zoonoses
rodent-borne, 79

CUMULATIVE INDEXES

CONTRIBUTING AUTHORS, VOLUMES 1–13

A

Alcalay, R., 3:179–99
Allan-Andrilla, C. H., 13:31–57
Allen, D., 9:503–26
Altman, S. H., 2:117–43
Andrus, J. K., 13:239–52
Archer, J., 3:445–68
Ashford, N. A., 6:383–401
Ashley, M. J., 9:233–71
Auffrey, C., 10:281–97
Autry, J. H., 7:535–43
Axelson, O., 12:235–55
Axnick, N., 11:251–66

B

Baker, D. B., 6:367–81
Baker, E. L., 9:223–32
Banton, J., 12:17–40
Barer, M. L., 12:481–518
Barnes, B., 1:277–95
Battista, R. N., 9:21–45
Beauchamp, D. E., 1:121–36
Beck, J. C., 3:55–83
Bellinger, D., 12:111–41
Bender, T. R., 11:251–66
Benfari, R. C., 2:431–71;
  3:101–28
Beresford, S. A. A., 13:469–88
Berger, B. B., 3:359–92
Bergner, M., 8:191–210;
  11:165–83
Bergthold, L., 12:157–75
Berkman, L., 4:69–90;
  5:413–32
Bernier, R. H., 13:385–98
Best, J. A., 9:161–201
Bice, T. W., 1:137–61
Bigoness, W. J., 3:201–24
Bingham, E., 11:419–34
Blair, S. N., 9:403–25;
  13:99–126
Blount, J. H., 6:85–106
Bor, D. H., 10:363–83
Bosworth, K., 8:387–415
Brenneman, G., 13:269–85
Breslow, L., 3:129–51;
  8:289–307; 11:1–28

Breslow, N., 3:29–54;
  5:385–411
Brock, D. B., 8:211–34
Brody, J. A., 8:211–34
Brown, B. W. Jr., 5:267–92
Brown, C., 8:441–67
Brown, E. R., 11:377–400
Brown, J. L., 9:503–26
Brown, K. S., 9:161–201
Brown, S. L., 6:247–67
Brown, S. T., 11:251–66
Brownell, K. D., 7:521–33
Bruce-Chwatt, L. J., 8:75–110
Buchner, D. M., 13:451–68,
  469–88
Bunker, J. P., 1:277–95;
  7:391–409
Burby, R. J., 4:47–67

C

Calabrese, E. J., 6:131–46
Caldart, C. C., 6:383–401
Callas, P., 7:441–71
Canada, A. T., 6:131–46
Capron, A. M., 7:59–75
Caskey, C. T., 10:27–48
Casper, R., 7:535–43
Caspersen, C. J., 8:253–87
Castleman, B. I., 8:1–19
Cayten, C. G., 12:401–24
Chaffin, D. B., 7:77–104
Chang, S.-L., 3:393–418
Cheadle, A. C., 13:31–57
Cherkin, D., 12:141–56
Chewning, B., 8:387–415
Chiang, C. L., 12:281–307
Childs, J. E., 13:79–98
Chin, J., 11:127–42
Clarkson, T. W., 4:375–80
Clever, L. H., 9:273–303
Clough, V. M., 13:151–71
Colsher, P. L., 10:203–19
Conn, J. M., 8:417–40
Connell, F. A., 8:51–74
Conrad, D., 12:141–56
Conroy, C., 5:163–92
Cook, N. R., 4:1–23
Cousins, N., 2:93–99

Crowley, J., 5:385–411
Crump, K. S., 3:339–57
Curran, A. S., 12:85–109
Cushner, I. M., 2:201–18
Cutts, F. T., 13:385–98

D

Dallek, G., 11:377–400
Damasio, A. R., 10:115–40
Damasio, H., 10:115–40
Davidson, L. E., 8:417–40
Davis, D. L., 6:195–221
Davis, K., 2:159–82
Davis, R. M., 13:287–318
DeFriese, G. H., 11:401–18
de Macedo, C. G., 13:239–52
de Quadros, C. A., 13:239–52
DesJardins, R. B., 3:201–24
de Tornyay, R., 1:83–94
Dey, L. J., 13:31–57
Deyo, R. A., 12:141–56
Diehr, P., 8:51–74
Diehr, P. H., 13:31–57
Dowling, W. L., 1:95–119
Drury, T. F., 5:83–106
Dworkin, R. B., 6:107–30
Dwyer, J. T., 12:309–34

E

Eaker, E., 2:431–71
Edwards, J., 9:427–50
Ehrenberg, R., 4:397–402
Eisenstadt, E., 4:391–95
Eissa, M., 12:519–41
Elinson, L., 13:197–221
Elston, M. A., 8:111–35
English, C. W., 6:269–94
Ennever, F. K., 11:69–87
Enterline, P. E., 12:459–80
Eriksen, M. P., 9:47–70
Eskenazi, B., 7:441–71
Evans, R. G., 12:481–518

F

Faden, R. R., 12:335–60
Farewell, V. T., 7:35–58

Farfel, M. R., 2:219–51; 6:333–60
Farquhar, J. W., 6:147–93
Feldman, J. J., 1:1–36
Ferris, B. G. Jr., 4:385–90
Fielding, J. E., 4:91–130; 5:237–65; 11:401–18; 12:209–34
Fine, L. J., 11:89–103
Fineberg, H. V., 3:225–48; 6:1–20
Fingerhut, L. A., 1:1–36
Flora, J. A., 10:181–201
Foege, W. H., 11:251–66
Franklin, B. A. K., 13:341–62
Fraumeni, J. F. Jr., 3:85–100
Frazier, T. M., 6:419–32
Freed, J. R., 2:71–92
Frerichs, R. R., 12:257–80
Freund, D. A., 8:137–63
Friberg, L., 4:367–73
Fried, L. P., 10:319–32

G

Gearon, S. A. N., 13:341–62
German, P. S., 10:319–32
Gerr, F., 12:543–66
Gershey, E. L., 10:299–317
Gibbs, R. A., 10:27–48
Gillings, D. B., 1:163–225
Glass, G. E., 13:79–98
Gold, M., 2:159–82
Gordon, N. F., 13:99–126
Gordon, N. P., 7:127–49
Gostin, L., 13:197–221
Grace, T. W., 13:253–68
Green, L. W., 3:321–38; 5:215–36; 11:319–34
Greenberg, R. S., 6:223–45
Greenblatt, M., 4:131–54
Greenough, W. B. III, 10:221–44
Greenwald, P., 7:267–91
Grosse, R. N., 10:281–97
Grover, S. A., 9:21–45
Gruenberg, E. M., 3:445–68
Grumbach, K., 11:297–318
Guess, H. A., 3:339–57
Guidotti, T. L., 13:151–71
Gusman, S., 7:293–312
Gustafson, D. H., 8:387–415

H

Hale, W. E., 13:415–30
Hall, J. A., 10:163–80
Halperin, W. E., 6:419–32
Handler, A., 13:269–85
Handsfield, H. H., 6:85–106
Hanis, C. L., 11:105–25
Hanley, J. A., 4:155–80
Hanley, R. J., 12:67–84

Harley, N. H., 13:127–50
Harris, R. H., 6:269–94
Harris, R. L., 3:201–24
Harrison, R., 7:441–71
Hart, L. G., 8:51–74
Harter, P. J., 7:293–312
Hawkins, R. P., 8:387–415
Henderson, D. A., 11:335–58; 13:239–52
Hertzman, C., 12:481–518
Herzstein, J., 7:217–35
Higashi, G. I., 9:483–501
Highland, J. H., 6:269–94
Hochberg, M. C., 9:379–401
Hogan, M. D., 8:355–85
Holford, T. R., 12:425–57
Holmes, K. K., 6:85–106
Holtzman, N. A., 2:219–51; 7:237–66
Hopps, H. E., 9:203–21
Hornbrook, M. C., 6:295–324
Hubert, H. B., 7:493–502
Huff, J. E., 8:355–85
Hughes, J. M., 7:171–92
Hunt, A. T., 6:325–32
Hurley, R. E., 8:137–63
Hyman, B. T., 10:115–40

I

Idler, E. L., 4:181–201
Interagency Regulatory Liaison Group, 1:345–93
Iverson, D. C., 3:321–38

J

Jacob, R. G., 4:285–310
Jameson, W. J., 11:297–318
Jamison, D. T., 11:335–58
Jelliffe, D. B., 2:145–58
Jelliffe, E. F. P., 2:145–58
Jernigan, D. H., 10:245–79
Jordan, P., 4:311–34

K

Kane, R. A., 1:227–53
Kane, R. L., 1:227–53
Kaplan, N. M., 7:503–19
Kasl, S. V., 4:69–90; 5:319–41
Kass, N. E., 12:335–60
Katzman, R. L., 13:431–49
Kellermann, A. L., 12:17–40
Kelsey, J. L., 9:379–401
Kendrick, J. S., 8:253–87
Keyserling, W. M., 7:77–104
Khoury, M. J., 7:237–66
Kim-Farley, R., 13:223–37
King, M.-C., 5:1–52
Klein, R. C., 10:299–317
Kleinbaum, D. G., 6:223–45
Kleinman, J. C., 10:423–40

Kleinstein, R. N., 5:369–84
Klerman, G. L., 13:319–39
Kneip, T., 10:1–25
Koch, G. G., 1:163–225; 9:123–60
Koepsell, T. D., 13:31–57
Kogevinas, M., 8:111–35
Kohl, M. H. W., 13:99–126
Köhler, L., 12:177–93
Koplan, J. P., 11:267–96
Koskela, K., 6:147–93
Kottke, T. E., 6:147–93
Kramer, P. S., 9:333–59
Kraus, J. F., 5:163–92; 6:403–18; 9:99–121
Kreuter, M. W., 11:319–34
Kristal, A. R., 13:31–57
Kukull, W. A., 13:431–49
Kuller, L., 3:153–78
Kunins, H., 12:361–82
Kuritz, S. J., 9:123–60

L

Labarthe, D. R., 7:193–215; 12:519–41
LaCroix, A. Z., 13:451–68, 469–88
Landis, J. R., 9:123–60
Landrigan, P. J., 2:277–98; 7:337–56; 11:359–75; 12:543–66
Larson, E. B., 8:165–90; 13:431–49, 451–68, 469–88
Lave, J. R., 5:193–213; 10:141–61
Lave, L. B., 1:255–76; 2:183–200; 5:193–213; 11:69–87
Lawrence, R. S., 10:363–83
Leaf, A., 7:411–39
Leaning, J., 7:411–39
Leape, L. L., 13:363–83
Lebowitz, M. D., 4:203–21
LeDuc, J. W., 13:79–98
Lee, G. M., 5:1–52
Lee, P. R., 7:217–35; 11:297–318
Lee, R. K., 12:17–40
LeMaistre, C. A., 9:47–70
Leonard, C. O., 2:219–51
Letz, R., 12:543–66
Levin, L. S., 4:181–201
Levy, R. I., 2:49–70
Lewis, C. E., 4:259–83
Lewis, M. A., 4:259–83
Lindheim, R., 2:1–29; 4:335–59
Lindsteadt, J. F., 13:341–62
Ling, J. C., 13:341–62
Lioy, P. J., 10:69–84
Lippmann, M., 10:49–67
Lomas, J., 12:41–65
Louis, T. A., 4:25–46; 6:1–20
Lovato, C. Y., 13:253–68

Luthy, D. A., 8:165–90
Lyle, J., 13:269–85
Lynch, B. S., 7:267–91
Lyons, B., 9:427–50

M

Maccoby, N., 6:147–93;
    10:181–201
Mahler, H., 9:71–97
Maibach, E. W., 10:181–201
Makuc, D., 2:159–82
Mallino, D. L., 11:359–75
Mandula, B., 6:195–221
Mann, J. M., 11:127–42
Marmot, M. G., 2:253–76;
    8:111–35
Marsland, D., 7:357–89
Martin, D. C., 13:31–57
Mayo, F., 7:357–89
McAlister, A., 6:147–93
McGinnis, J. M., 8:441–67;
    11:231–49
McIntyre, K. M., 3:101–28
McNeil, B. J., 5:135–61
Meade, M. S., 7:313–35
Meader, W. V., 11:419–34
Mechanic, D., 12:1–15
Meilahn, E., 3:153–78
Meisels, S. J., 9:527–50
Mendeloff, J. M., 12:401–24
Mercy, J. A., 12:17–40
Meredith, C. N., 12:309–33
Mills, S. L., 13:287–318
Modlin, J., 13:1–30
Moolgavkar, S. H., 7:151–69
Morrison, P. R., 6:325–32
Moses, L. E., 5:267–92;
    8:309–53
Mosher, J. F., 10:245–79
Mosley, W. H., 11:335–58
Mosteller, F., 6:1–20
Muir, C. S., 11:143–63
Mullen, P. D., 9:305–32
Murnaghan, J. H., 2:299–361
Murt, H. A., 5:107–33

N

Navarro, V., 8:1–19; 10:85–94
Needleman, H. L., 2:277–98;
    12:111–14
Nelkin, D., 10:95–113
Nelson, N., 4:363–65; 11:29–37
Nersesian, W. S., 9:361–77
Newell, G. R., 9:47–70
Newhouse, J. P., 11:207–30
Nissinen, A., 6:147–93
Norman, M., 4:131–54
Novotny, T. E., 13:287–318

O

Ockene, J. K., 3:101–28
O'Hara, N. M., 9:403–25
Okun, D. A., 4:47–67
Olive, J. M., 13:239–52
Omenn, G. S., 6:107–30;
    9:273–303
Ongerth, H. J., 3:419–44
Ongerth, J. E., 3:419–44
Orenstein, W. A., 13:385–98
Osborn, J. E., 9:551–83
Osterman-Golkar, S., 4:397–402
Ouslander, J. G., 3:55–83

P

Paffenbarger, R. S. Jr., 13:99–
    126
Pagano, M., 6:325–32
Parcel, G. S., 9:403–25
Pardes H., 10:403–22
Parkman, P. D., 9:203–21
Party, E., 10:299–317
Pate, R. R., 9:403–25
Patrick, D. L., 11:165–83;
    13:31–57
Patrick, K., 13:253–68
Pauker, S. G., 5:135–61
Pearlman, L. A., 3:225–48
Pels, R. J., 10:363–83
Perine, P. L., 6:85–106
Perrin, E. B., 13:31–57
Pickett, G., 1:297–321
Pierce, J. P., 12:383–400
Pollack, S. H., 11:359–75
Porter, I. H., 3:277–319
Powell, K. E., 8:253–87
Prentice, R. L., 7:35–58
Puska, P., 6:147–93

Q

Quinn, T. C., 13:1–30

R

Rall, D. P., 8:355–85
Rankin, J. G., 9:233–71
Rao, K. S., 3:1–27
Reatig, N., 7:535–43
Reisine, S. T., 9:1–19
Renner, C., 10:85–94
Rhoades, E. R., 13:269–85
Richardson, W. C., 1:95–119
Richmond, J. B., 11:185–205
Rivara, F. P., 13:509–28
Robbins, F. C., 7:105–25
Robbins, J. B., 7:105–25
Robertson, L. S., 7:13–34
Rogan, W. J., 4:381–84
Romano, R. A., 13:287–318
Room, R., 5:293–317

S

Rosenberg, M. L., 8:417–40
Rosenfield, A., 10:385–401;
    12:361–82
Rosenfield, P. L., 4:311–34
Rosenstock, L., 7:337–56
Roter, D. L., 10:163–80
Rothenberg, R. B., 11:267–96
Rothman, M. L., 8:191–210
Rowland, D., 9:427–50
Russ, A., 13:1–30

S

Sacco, C., 6:131–46
Salonen, J. T., 6:147–93
Sanazaro, P. J., 1:37–68
Santi, S. M., 9:161–201
Sasco, A. J., 11:143–63
Sattin, R. W., 13:489–508
Schaffarzick, R. W., 7:391–409
Schoen, M. H., 2:71–92
Schull, W. J., 11:105–25
Schweitzer, S. O., 13:399–410
Schwetz, B. A., 3:1–27;
    8:355–85
Scitovsky, A. A., 7:59–75
Scrimshaw, N. S., 11:53–68
Shapiro, A. P., 4:285–310
Shapiro, S. H., 4:25–46
Sharp, D. S., 7:441–71
Shiota, S. R., 13:399–410
Shonick, W., 5:53–81
Shopland, D., 8:441–67
Shore, R. E., 13:127–50
Shy, K. K., 8:165–90
Siegel, J. M., 5:343–67
Sigal, L. H., 12:85–109
Silverman, M. M., 10:403–22
Simons-Morton, B. G., 9:403–
    25
Simopoulos, A. P., 7:475–79,
    481–92
Smith, A. H., 7:441–71
Smith, E. A., 9:161–201
Smith, G. S., 9:99–121
Smith, J. C., 8:417–40
Socholitzky, E., 2:117–43
Sondik, E., 7:267–91
Sorensen, G., 8:235–51
Sorsa, M., 4:403–7
Spinner, N. B., 5:1–52
Stallones, R. A., 1:69–82
Starfield, B., 6:21–40
Stason, W. B., 6:41–63
Stewart, R. B., 13:415–30
Stokes, M. E., 1:163–225
Stoll, J. G., 2:431–71
Stoto, M., 13:59–78
Stover, E. S., 7:535–43
Sullivan, J., 3:249–76
Syme, S. L., 3:179–99; 4:335–
    59

T

Taylor, C. E., 10:221–44
Tenforde, T. S., 13:173–96
Tennant, R. W., 8:355–85
Terris, M., 1:323–44; 11:39–51
Thomas, D. C., 9:451–82
Thompson, P. D., 8:253–87
Thomson, G., 5:1–52
Thomson, S. J., 9:161–201
Toniolo, P., 10:1–25
Torrens, P. R., 6:65–83
Townsend, M., 3:153–78
Tuomilehto, J., 6:147–93
Tyler, C. W. Jr., 4:223–58

U

Upton, A. C., 10:1–25; 13:127–50

V

Vainio, H., 4:403–7
Vanderpool, N. A., 11:185–205

Van Hoesen, G. W., 10:115–40
Varas, C., 12:519–41
Verbrugge, L. M., 8:235–51; 10:333–61
Vladeck, B. C., 9:333–59
Vogt, T. M., 2:31–47
Volinn, E., 12:141–56

W

Wagner, E. H., 13:31–57, 451–68, 469–88
Wallace, R. B., 10:203–19
Waller, J. A., 8:21–49
Walsh, D. C., 7:127–49; 13:197–221
Ware, J. H., 4:1–23
Warner, K. E., 5:107–33
Warren, K. S., 2:101–15
Watts, C. A., 1:95–119
Weeks, J. L., 12:195–207
Wegman, D. H., 6:363–65; 11:89–103
Wehrle, P. F., 2:363–95

Weill, H., 7:171–92
Weinberg, G., 3:153–78
Weinstein, I. B., 4:409–13
Weinstein, M. C., 6:41–63
Weissman, M. M., 13:319–39
Wennberg, J. E., 1:277–95
West, A., 10:403–22
Whittemore, A. S., 2:397–429
Wiener, J. M., 12:67–84
Wilkerson, A., 10:299–317
Wilkins, J., 2:363–95
Williams, T. F., 8:211–34
Wilson, R. W., 1:1–36; 5:83–106
Wingard, D. L., 5:433–58
Winkelstein, W. Jr., 2:253–76
Wolf, M. E., 13:509–28
Wolman, A., 7:1–12
Wood, M., 7:357–89
Woolson, R. F., 10:423–40
Wrensch, M. R., 5:1–52

Y

Yankauer, A., 3:249–76

CHAPTER TITLES, VOLUMES 1–13

AGE AND DISEASE SPECIFIC

Long-Term Care: Can Our Society Meet the
  Needs of its Elderly?   R. L. Kane, R. A. Kane   1:227–53
The Decline in Cardiovascular Disease
  Mortality   R. I. Levy   2:49–70
Prevention of Dental Disease: Caries and
  Periodontal Disease   M. H. Schoen, J. R. Freed   2:71–92
The Control of Helminths: Nonreplicating
  Infectious Agents of Man   K. S. Warren   2:101–15
Recent Trends in Infant Feeding   D. B. Jelliffe, E. F. P. Jelliffe   2:145–58
Maternal Behavior and Perinatal Risks:
  Alcohol, Smoking, and Drugs   I. M. Cushner   2:201–18
Issues in Antenatal and Neonatal Screening
  and Surveillance for Hereditary and
  Congenital Disorders   N. A. Holtzman, C. O. Leonard,
                     M. R. Farfel   2:219–51
Primary Prevention of Ischemic Heart
  Disease: Evaluation of Community
  Interventions   W. Winkelstein Jr., M. Marmot   2:253–76
Immunizing Agents: Potential for Controlling
  or Eradicating Infectious Diseases   P. F. Wehrle, J. Wilkins   2:363–95
Defining the Health Problems of the Elderly   J. G. Ouslander, J. C. Beck   3:55–83
Control of Hereditary Disorders   I. H. Porter   3:277–319
The Chronically Medically Disabled and
  "Deinstitutionalization"   J. Archer, E. M. Gruenberg   3:445–68
Health Consequences of the Experience of
  Migration   S. V. Kasl, L. Berkman   4:69–90
Deinstitutionalization: Health Consequences
  for the Mentally Ill   M. Greenblatt, M. Norman   4:131–54
Schistosomiasis Control: Past, Present, and
  Future   P. Jordan, P. L. Rosenfield   4:311–34
Mortality and Morbidity from Injuries in
  Sports and Recreation   J. F. Kraus, C. Conroy   5:163–92
Alcohol Control and Public Health   R. Room   5:293–317
Vision Disorders in Public Health   R. N. Kleinstein   5:369–84
Postneonatal Mortality   B. Starfield   6:21–40
Epidemiology of the Sexually Transmitted
  Diseases   P. L. Perine, H. H. Handsfield,
                     K. K. Holmes, J. H. Blount   6:85–106
Legal Aspects of Human Genetics   R. B. Dworkin, G. S. Omenn   6:107–30
Medical Care at the End of Life: The
  Interaction of Economics and Ethics   A. A. Scitovsky, A. M. Capron   7:59–75
Monitoring for Congenital Malformations   N. A. Holtzman, M. J. Khoury   7:237–66
Diet and Chemoprevention in NCI's Research
  Strategy to Achieve National Cancer
  Control Objectives   P. Greenwald, E. Sondik,
                     B. S. Lynch   7:267–91
Public Health Aspects of Nuclear War   J. Leaning, A. Leaf   7:411–39

Symposium on Nutrition
  Introduction   A. P. Simopoulos   7:475–79
  Obesity and Body Weight Standards   A. P. Simopoulos   7:481–92

The Importance of Obesity in the
  Development of Coronary Risk Factors and
  Disease   H. B. Hubert   7:493–502
Dietary Aspects of the Treatment of
  Hypertension   N. M. Kaplan   7:503–19
Public Health Approaches to Obesity and Its
  Management   K. D. Brownell   7:521–33
Anorexia Nervosa and Bulimia   J. H. Autry, E. S. Stover,
                                            N. Reatig, R. Casper   7:535–43
Malaria and Its Control: Present Situation and
  Future Prospects   L. J. Bruce-Chwatt   8:75–110
Evaluating a New Technology: The
  Effectiveness of Electronic Fetal Heart Rate
  Monitoring   K. K. Shy, E. B. Larson,
                                            D. A. Luthy   8:165–90
Trends in the Health of the Elderly
  Population   J. A. Brody, D. B. Brock,
                                            T. F. Williams   8:211–34
The Impact of Dental Conditions on Social
  Functioning and the Quality of Life   S. T. Reisine   9:1–19
Early Detection of Cancer: An Overview   R. N. Battista, S. A. Grover   9:21–45
A Public Health Approach to the Prevention
  of Alcohol-Related Health Problems   M. J. Ashley, J. G. Rankin   9:233–71
Infant Mortality in Socially Vulnerable
  Populations   W. S. Nersesian   9:361–77
Vaccines for Parasitic Diseases   G. I. Higashi   9:483–501
Hunger in America   J. L . Brown, D. Allen   9:503–26
The AIDS Epidemic: Six Years   J. E. Osborn   9:551–83
Alzheimer's Disease   B. T. Hyman, H. Damasio, A. R.
                                            Damasio, G. W. Van Hoesen   10:115–40
Prevention and the Elderly: Public Health
  Issues and Strategies   P. S. German, L. P. Fried   10:319–32
HIV Infections and AIDS in the 1990s   J. Chin, J. M. Mann   11:127–42
Prospects for Cancer Control in the 1990s C. S. Muir, A. J. Sasco   11:143–63
Child Health in the United States: Prospects
  for the 1990s   N. A. Vanderpool, J. B. Richmond 11:185–205
Injury Prevention and Control: Prospects for
  the 1990s   S. T. Brown, W. H. Foege,
                                            T. R. Bender, N. Axnick   11:251–66
Symposium on Selected Clinical Syndromes Associated with Aging
  Acute Confusional States in Older Adults and
    the Role of Polypharmacy   W. E. Hale, R. B. Stewart   13:415–30
  Cognitive Impairment: Dementia and
    Alzeimer's Disease   E. Larson, W. A. Kukull,
                                            R. L. Katzman   13:431–49
  Effects of Physical Activity on Health Status
    in Older Adults I: Observational Studies E. Wagner, M.D., M.P.H.   13:451–68
  Effects of Physical Activity on Health Status
    in Older Adults II: Intervention Studies D. M. Buchner, S. A. A.
                                            Beresford, E. B. Larson,
                                            A. Z. LaCroix, E. H. Wagner   13:469–88
  Falls Among Older Persons: A Public Health
    Perspective   R. W. Sattin   13:489–508
  NonFalls Injuries in Older Adults   M. E. Wolf, F. P. Rivara   13:509–28
BEHAVIORAL ASPECTS OF HEALTH
  Public Health and Individual Liberty   D. E. Beauchamp   1:121–36
  Behavioral Interventions and Compliance to
    Treatment Regimes   R. C. Benfari, E. Eaker, J. G. Stoll 2:431–71
  Control of Cigarette Smoking from a
    Psychological Perspective   R. C. Benfari, J. K. Ockene,
                                            K. M. McIntyre   3:101–28

Control of Cigarette Smoking from a Public
Policy Perspective — L. Breslow — 3:129–51
Control of Cigarette Smoking from a Medical
Perspective — S. L. Syme, R. Alcalay — 3:179–99
School Health Education — L. W. Green, D. C. Iverson — 3:321–38
Improving the Health of Children: Must the
Children Be Involved? — C. E. Lewis, M. A. Lewis — 4:259–83
Nonpharmacologic Approaches to the
Treatment of Hypertension — A. P. Shapiro, R. G. Jacob — 4:285–310
Economic Incentives for Health — K. E. Warner, H. A. Murt — 5:107–33
Modifying and Developing Health Behavior — L. W. Green — 5:215–36
The Community-Based Strategy to Prevent
Coronary Heart Disease: Conclusions from
the Ten Years of the North Karelia Project — P. Puska, A. Nissinen,
J. Tuomilehto, J. T. Salonen,
K. Koskela, A. McAlister,
T. E. Kottke, N. Maccoby,
J. W. Farquhar — 6:147–93

Behavioral and Environmental Interventions
for Reducing Motor Vehicle Trauma — L. S. Robertson — 7:13–34
Legal Approaches to Smoking Deterrence — D. C. Walsh, N. P. Gordon — 7:127–49
Social/Economic Status and Disease — M. G. Marmot, M. Kogevinas,
M. A. Elston — 8:111–35
Women, Work, and Health — G. Sorensen, L. M. Verbrugge — 8:235–51
Computer-Based Health Promotion:
Combining Technological Advances with
Problem-Solving Techniques to Effect
Successful Health Behavior Changes, — D. H. Gustafson, K. Bosworth,
B. Chewning, R. P. Hawkins — 8:387–415
The Emergence of Youth Suicide: An
Epidemiologic Analysis and Public Health
Perspective — M. L. Rosenberg, J. C. Smith,
L. E. Davidson, J. M. Conn — 8:417–40
Tobacco and Health: Trends in Smoking and
Smokeless Tobacco Consumption in the
United States — J. M. McGinnis, D. Shopland,
C. Brown — 8:441–67
Preventing Cigarette Smoking Among School
Children — J. A. Best, S. J. Thomson, S. M.
Santi, E. A. Smith, K. S. Brown — 9:161–201
Health Promotion and Patient Education
Benefits for Employees — P. D. Mullen — 9:305–32
Communicating Technological Risk: The
Social Construction of Risk Perception — D. Nelkin — 10:95–113
The Role of Media Across Four Levels of
Health Promotion Intervention — J. A. Flora, E. W. Maibach,
N. Maccoby — 10:181–201
New Directions in Alcohol Policy — J. F. Mosher, D. H. Jernigan — 10:245–79
Literacy and Health Status in Developing
Countries — R. N. Grosse, C. Auffrey — 10:281–97
Health Promotion as a Public Health Strategy
for the 1990s — L. W. Green, M. W. Kreuter — 11:319–34
Health Risk Appraisal in the 1990s:
Opportunities, Challenges, and Expectations — G. H. DeFriese, J. E. Fielding — 11:401–18
Nutrition and Exercise: Effects on Adolescent
Health — C. N. Meredith, J. T. Dwyer — 12:309–33
Bioethics and Public Health in the 1980s:
Resource Allocation and AIDS — R. R. Faden, N. E. Kass — 12:335–60
The 20-Year Experiment: Accounting for,
Explaining, and Evaluating Health Care
Cost Containment in Canada and the
United States — R. G. Evans, M. L. Barer,
C. Hertzman — 12:481–518

Depression: Current Understanding and
  Changing Trends   M. M. Weissman, G. L. Klerman   13:319–39
Social Marketing: Its Place in Public Health   J. C. Ling, B. A. K. Franklin,
                                                J. F. Lindsteadt, S. A. N. Gearon   13:341–62

ENVIRONMENTAL HEALTH
Economic Evaluation of Public Health
  Programs   L. B. Lave   1:255–76
Scientific Bases for Identification of Potential
  Carcinogens and Estimation of Risks   Interagency Regulatory Liaison
                                                  Group, Work Group on Risk
                                                  Assessment, J. V. Rodricks, chm.   1:345–93
Balancing Economics and Health in Setting
  Environmental Standards   L. B. Lave   2:183–200
The Health Effects of Low Level Exposure to
  Lead   H. L. Needleman, P. J. Landrigan   2:277–98
Air Pollution and Respiratory Disease   A. S. Whittemore   2:397–429
Reproductive Toxicity of Environmental
  Agents   K. S. Rao, B. A. Schwetz   3:1–27
Labor-Management Aspects of Occupational
  Risk   R. B. DesJardins, W. J. Bigoness,
                                                  R. L. Harris   3:201–24
Drinking Water and Cancer: Review of
  Recent Epidemiological Findings and
  Assessment of Risks   K. S. Crump, H. A. Guess   3:339–57
Water and Wastewater Quality Control and
  the Public Health   B. B. Berger   3:359–92
The Safety of Water Disinfection   S.-L. Chang   3:393–418
Health Consequences of Wastewater Reuse   H. J. Ongerth, J. E. Ongerth   3:419–44
Land Use Planning and Health   R. J. Burby, D. A. Okun   4:47–67
Health Effects of Indoor Pollutants   M. D. Lebowitz   4:203–21
Environments, People, and Health   R. Lindheim, S. L. Syme   4:335–59

Special Section: Some Recent Events in Biological Monitoring
Introduction   N. Nelson   4:363–65
Cadmium   L. Friberg   4:367–73
Mercury   T. W. Clarkson   4:375–80
Persistent Pesticides and Polychlorinated
  Biphenyls   W. J. Rogan   4:381–84
Respiratory Assessments—Expired Air
  Ventilatory Performance   B. B. Ferris, Jr.   4:385–90
Biological Assays for Mutagens in Human
  Samples   E. Eisenstadt   4:391–95
Dosimetry of Electrophilic Compounds by
  Means of Hemoglobin Alkylation   S. Osterman-Golkar, L. Ehrenberg   4:397–402
Application of Cytogenetic Methods for
  Biological Monitoring   H. Vainio, M. Sorsa   4:403–7
The Monitoring of DNA Adducts as an
  Approach to Carcinogen Detection   I. B. Weinstein   4:409–13
Trace Elements and Public Health   E. J. Calabrese, A. T. Canada,
                                                  C. Sacco   6:131–46
Airborne Asbestos and Public Health   D. L. Davis, B. Mandula   6:195–221
Quantitative Risk Assessment of
  Environmental Hazards   S. L. Brown   6:247–67
Hazardous Waste Disposal: Emerging
  Technologies and Public Policies to Reduce
  Public Health Risks   R. H. Harris, C. W. English,
                                                  J. H. Highland   6:269–94
Reducing Lead Exposure in Children   M. R. Farfel   6:333–60

Symposium on Occupational Health
Introduction   D. H. Wegman   6:363–65
The Study of Stress at Work   D. B. Baker   6:367–81

The "Right to Know": Toxics Information
Transfer in the Workplace N. A. Ashford, C. C. Caldart 6:383–401
Fatal and Nonfatal Injuries in Occupational
Settings: A Review J. F. Kraus 6:403–18
Surveillance for the Effects of Workplace
Exposure W. E. Halperin, T. M. Frazier 6:419–32
Occupational Ergonomics - Methods to
Evaluate Physical Stress on the Job W. M. Keyserling, D. B. Chaffin 7:77–104
Asbestos as a Public Health Risk: Disease
and Policy H. Weill, J. M. Hughes 7:171–92
Mediating Solutions to Environmental Risks S. Gusman, P. J. Harter 7:293–312
Occupational Health: The Intersection
Between Clinical Medicine and Public
Health L. Rosenstock, P. J. Landrigan 7:337–56
Delayed Health Hazards of Pesticide
Exposure D. S. Sharp, B. Eskenazi,
R. Harrison, P. Callas,
A. H. Smith 7:441–71

International Mobility of Hazardous Products,
Industries, and Wastes B. I. Castleman, V. Navarro 8:1–19
Injury: Conceptual Shifts and Preventive
Implications J. A. Waller 8:21–49
Alternatives to Using Human Experience in
Assessing Health Risks D. P. Rall, M. D. Hogan,
J. E. Huff, B. A. Schwetz,
R. W. Tennant 8:355–85
Health Hazards of Passive Smoking M. P. Eriksen, C. A. LeMaistre,
G. R. Newell 9:47–70
Organic Solvent Neurotoxicity E. L. Baker 9:223–32
Hazards for Health Care Workers L. H. Clever, G. S. Omenn 9:273–303
Public Health Aspects of Toxic Chemical
Disposal Sites A. C. Upton, T. Kneip, P. Toniolo 10:1–25
Effects of Ozone on Respiratory Function and
Structure M. Lippmann 10:49–67
Exposure Assessment of Oxidant Gases and
Acidic Aerosols P. J. Lioy 10:69–84
Low-Level Radioactive Waste from U. S.
Biomedical and Academic Institutions:
Policies, Strategies, and Solutions A. Wilkerson, R. C. Klein,
E. Party, E. L. Gershey 10:299–317
Toxics and Public Health in the 1990s N. Nelson 11:29–37
Toxic Substances Control in the 1990s: Are
We Poisoning Ourselves with Low-level
Exposures? L. B. Lave, F. K. Ennever 11:69–87
Occupational Health in the 1990s D. H. Wegman, L. J. Fine 11:89–103
Child Labor in 1990: Prevalence and Health
Hazards S. H. Pollack, P. J. Landrigan,
D. L. Mallino 11:359–75
Governmental Regulation of Environmental
Hazards in the 1990s E. Bingham, W. V. Meader 11:419–34
The Health Effects of Low Level Exposure to
Lead H. L. Needleman, D. Bellinger 12:111–40
Occupational Health and Safety Regulation in
the Coal Mining Industry: Public Health at
the Workplace J. L. Weeks 12:195–207
Smoking Control at the Workplace J. E. Fielding 12:209–34
Occupational and Environmental Exposures to
Radon and Cancer Risks O. Axelson 12:235–55
Trauma Systems and Public Policy J. M. Mendeloff, C. G. Cayten 12:401–24
Carcinogenic Effects of Man-Made Vitreous
Fibers P. E. Enterline 12:459–80
Upper-Extremity Musculoskeletal Disorders of
Occupational Origin F. Gerr, R. Letz, P. J. Landrigan 12:543–66

The Health Effects of Low-Level Ionizing
  Radiation   A. C. Upton, R. E. Shore,
                                              N. H. Harley   13:127–50
Occupational Health Concerns of Firefighting T. L. Guidotti, V. M. Clough   13:151–71
Biological Interactions and Potential Health
  Effects of Extremely-Low-Frequency
  Magnetic Fields from Power Lines and
  Other Common Sources   T. S. Tenforde   13:173–96
Worksite Drug Testing   D. C. Walsh, L. Elinson, L. Gostin 13:197–221

EPIDEMIOLOGY/BIOSTATISTICS
Health and Disease in the United States   L. A. Fingerhut, R. W. Wilson,
                                              J. J. Feldman   1:1–36
To Advance Epidemiology   R. A. Stallones   1:69–82
Biostatistical Implications of Design,
  Sampling, and Measurement to Health
  Science Data Analysis   G. G. Koch, D. B. Gillings,
                                              M. E. Stokes   1:163–225
Epidemiology as a Guide to Health Policy   M. Terris   1:323–44
Health Indicators and Information System for
  the Year 2000   J. H. Murnaghan   2:299–361
Design and Analysis of Case-Control Studies N. Breslow   3:29–54
Epidemiologic Approaches to Cancer
  Etiology   J. F. Fraumeni, Jr.   3:85–100
Design and Analysis Methods for
  Longitudinal Research   N. R. Cook, J. H. Ware   4:1–23
Critical Issues in the Conduct and
  Interpretation of Clinical Trials   T. A. Louis, S. H. Shapiro   4:25–46
Appropriate Uses of Multivariate Analysis   J. A. Hanley   4:155–80
Genetic Epidemiology   M.-C. King, G. M. Lee,
                                              N. B. Spinner, G. Thomson,
                                              M. R. Wrensch   5:1–52
Interpreting Trends in Illness and Disability:
  Health Statistics and Health Status   R. W. Wilson, T. F. Drury   5:83–106
Decision Analysis for Public Health:
  Principles and Illustrations   B. J. McNeil, S. G. Pauker   5:135–61
Stress and Health   S. V. Kasl   5:319–41
Type A Behavior: Epidemiologic Foundations
  and Public Health Implications   J. M. Siegel   5:343–67
Statistical Analysis of Survival Data   J. Crowley, N. Breslow   5:385–411
Assessing the Physical Health Effects of
  Social Networks and Social Support   L. F. Berkman   5:413–32
The Sex Differential in Morbidity, Mortality,
  and Lifestyle   D. L. Wingard   5:433–58
Findings for Public Health from
  Meta-Analyses   T. A. Louis, H. V. Fineberg,
                                              F. Mosteller   6:1–20
Mathematical Modeling Strategies for the
  Analysis of Epidemiologic Research   R. S. Greenberg, D. G. Kleinbaum 6:223–45
The Effects of Computer Science
  Advancements on Public Health Research   A. T. Hunt, P. R. Morrison,
                                              M. Pagano   6:325–32
Relative Risk and Odds Ratio Regression   R. L. Prentice, V. T. Farewell 7:35–58
Carcinogenesis Modeling: From Molecular
  Biology to Epidemiology   S. H. Moolgavkar   7:151–69
Geographic Analysis of Disease and Care   M. S. Meade   7:313–35
Practice-Based Recording as an
  Epidemiological Tool   M. Wood, F. Mayo, D. Marsland   7:357–89
The Use of Large Data Bases in Health Care
  Studies   F. A. Connell, P. Diehr, L. G. Hart 8:51–74
Health Status Measures: An Overview and
  Guide for Selection   M. Bergner, M. L. Rothman   8:191–210

Physical Activity and the Incidence of
Coronary Heart Disease | K. E. Powell, P. D. Thompson,
| C. J. Caspersen, J. S. Kendrick | 8:253–87
Setting Objectives for Public Health | L. Breslow | 8:289–307
Graphical Methods in Statistical Analysis | L. E. Moses | 8:309–53
Alcohol and Residential, Recreational, and
Occupational Injuries: A Review of the
Epidemiologic Evidence | G. S. Smith, J. F. Kraus | 9:99–121
A General Overview of Mantel-Haenszel
Methods: Applications and Recent
Developments | S. J. Kuritz, J. R. Landis,
| G. G. Koch | 9:123–60
Epidemiology of Chronic Musculoskeletal
Disorders | J. L. Kelsey, M. C. Hochberg | 9:379–401
Health-Related Physical Fitness in Childhood:
Status and Recommendations | B. G. Simons-Morton, G. S. Parcel,
| N. M. O'Hara, S. N. Blair,
| R. R. Pate | 9:403–25
Models for Exposure-Time-Response
Relationships with Applications to Cancer
Epidemiology | D. C. Thomas | 9:451–82
The Application of Recombinant DNA
Technology for Genetic Probing in
Epidemiology | R. A. Gibbs, C. T. Caskey | 10:27–48
Is Modest Alcohol Consumption Better than
None at All? An Epidemiologic Assessment | P. L. Colsher, R. B. Wallace | 10:203–19
Control of Diarrheal Diseases | C. E. Taylor, W. B. Greenough, III | 10:221–44
Recent, Present, and Future Health of
American Adults | L. M. Verbrugge | 10:333–61
Perspectives on Statistical Significance
Testing | R. F. Woolson, J. C. Kleinman | 10:423–40
The Future of Public Health: Prospects in the
United States for the 1990s | L. Breslow | 11:1–28
Nutrition: Prospects for the 1990s | N. S. Scrimshaw | 11:53–68
Genetics and Public Health in the 1990s | W. J. Schull, C. L. Hanis | 11:105–25
Measurement of Health Status in the 1990s | D. L. Patrick, M. Bergner | 11:165–83
Setting Objectives for Public Health in the
1990s: Experience and Prospects | J. M. McGinnis | 11:231–49
The Epidemiological Basis for the Prevention
of Firearm Injuries | A. L. Kellermann, R. K. Lee,
| J. A. Mercy, J. Banton | 12:17–40
Epidemiologic Surveillance in Developing
Countries | R. R. Frerichs | 12:257–80
Competing Risks in Mortality Analysis | C. L. Chiang | 12:281–307
Progress and Problems in International Public
Health Efforts to Reduce Tobacco Usage | J. P. Pierce | 12:383–400
Understanding the Effects of Age, Period,
and Cohort on Incidence and Mortality
Rates | T. R. Holford | 12:425–57
HIV Infection and AIDS in Children | T. C. Quinn, A. Ruff, J. Modlin | 13:1–30
Selected Methodological Issues in Evaluating
Community-Based Health Promotion and
Disease Prevention Programs | T. D. Koepsell, E. H. Wagner,
| A. C. Cheadle, D. L. Patrick,
| D. C. Martin, P. H. Diehr,
| E. B. Perrin, A. R. Kristal,
| C. H. Allan-Andrilla, L. J. Dey | 13:31–57
Public Health Assessment in the 1990s | M. A. Stoto | 13:59–78
The Hantaviruses, Etiologic Agents of
Hemorrhagic Fever with Renal Syndrome:
A Possible Cause of Hypertension and
Chronic Renal Disease | J. W. LeDuc, J. E. Childs,
| G. E. Glass | 13:79–98

How Much Physical Activity Is Good for
Health?   S. N. Blair, H. W. Kohl, N. F.
                                         Gordon, R. S. Paffenbarger, Jr.   13:99–126

PUBLIC HEALTH PRACTICE
Recent Developments in Mental Health:
Perspectives and Services   D. Mechanic   12:1–15
Lyme Disease: A Multifocal Worldwide
Epidemic   L. H. Sigal, A. S. Curran   12:85–109
Cost, Controversy, Crisis: Low Back Pain
and the Health of the Public   R. A. Deyo, D. Cherkin,
                                         D. Conrad, E. Volinn   12:141–56
Infant Mortality: The Swedish Experience L. Köhler   12:177–93
Abortion: A Legal and Public Health
Perspective   H. Kunins, A. Rosenfield   12:361–82
Childhood Precursors of High Blood Pressure
and Elevated Cholesterol   D. R. Labarthe, M. Eissa, C. Varas 12:519–41
Global Immunization   R. Kim-Farley, Expanded
                                         Programme on Immunization
                                         Team   13:223–37
Polio Eradication from the Western
Hemisphere   C. de Quadros, J. K. Andrus,
                                         J. Olive, C. G. de Macedo,
                                         D. A. Henderson   13:239–52
Health Issues for College Students   K. Patrick, T. W. Grace,
                                         C. Y. Lovato   13:253–68
Mortality of American Indian and Alaska
Native Infants   E. R. Rhoades, G. Brenneman,
                                         J. Lyle, A. Handler   13:269–85
The Public Health Practice of Tobacco
Control: Lessons Learned and Directions
for the States in the 1990s   T. E. Novotny, R. A. Romano,
                                         R. M. Davis, S. L. Mills   13:287–318

HEALTH SERVICES
Quality Assessment and Quality Assurance in
Medical Care   P. J. Sanazaro   1:37–68
Public Health Nursing: The Nurse's Role in
Community-Based Practice   R. de Tornyay   1:83–94
Strategies for the Reimbursement of
Short-term Hospitals   C. A. Watts, W. L. Dowling,
                                         W. C. Richardson   1:95–119
Health Planning and Regulation Effects on
Hospital Costs   T. W. Bice   1:137–61
The Need for Assessing the Outcome of
Common Medical Practices   J. E. Wennberg, J. P. Bunker,
                                         B. Barnes   1:277–95
The Future of Health Departments: The
Governmental Presence   G. Pickett   1:297–321
Birthing Centers and Hospices: Reclaiming
Birth and Death   R. Lindheim   2:1–29
Risk Assessment and Health Hazard Appraisal T. M. Vogt   2:31–47
Laymen and Medical Technology   N. Cousins   2:93–99
The Cost of Ambulatory Care in Alternative
Settings: A Review of Major Research
Findings   S. H. Altman, E. Socholitzky   2:117–43
Access to Health Care for the Poor: Does the
Gap Remain?   K. Davis, M. Gold, D. Makuc   2:159–82
Low-Cost Medical Practices   H. V. Fineberg, L. A. Pearlman   3:225–48
The New Health Professionals: Three
Examples   A. Yankauer, J. Sullivan   3:249–76
Lessons from Health Care Regulation   J. E. Fielding   4:91–130
Self-Care in Health   L. S. Levin, E. L. Idler   4:181–201

The Public Health Implications of Abortion   C. W. Tyler, Jr.   4:223–58
Early Developments and Recent Trends in the
  Evolution of the Local Public Hospital   W. Shonick   5:53–81
Hospital Cost Functions   J. R. Lave, L. B. Lave   5:193–213
Health Promotion and Disease Prevention at
  the Worksite   J. E. Fielding   5:237–65
Experiences with Evaluating the Safety and
  Efficacy of MedicalTechnologies   L. E. Moses, B. W. Brown, Jr.   5:267–92
Cost-Effectiveness of Interventions to Prevent
  orTreat Coronary Heart Disease   M. C. Weinstein, W. B. Stason   6:41–63
Hospice Care: What Have We Learned?   P. R. Torrens   6:65–83
Techniques for Assessing Hospital Case Mix   M. C. Hornbrook   6:295–324
Medical Care at the End of Life: The
  Interaction of Economics and Ethics   A. A. Scitovsky, A. M. Capron   7:59–75
Current Status and Prospects for Some
  Improved and New Bacterial Vaccines   F. C. Robbins, J. B. Robbins   7:105–25
Mild Hypertension: The Question of
  Treatment   D. R. Labarthe   7:193–215
International Drug Regulation   P. R. Lee, J. Herzstein   7:217–35
Reimbursement Incentives for Hospital Care   J. P. Bunker, R. W. Schaffarzick   7:391–409
Managed Care in Medicaid: Selected Issues in
  Program Origins, Design, and Research   D. A. Freund, R. E. Hurley   8:137–63
Setting Objectives for Public Health   L. Breslow   8:289–307
Present Status of WHO's Initiative, "Health
  for All by the Year 2000"   H. Mahler   9:71–97
Viral Vaccines and Antivirals: Current Use
  and Future Prospects   P. D. Parkman, H. E. Hopps   9:203–21
Case-Mix Measures: DRGs and Alternatives   B. C. Vladeck, P. S. Kramer   9:333–59
Medicaid: Health Care for the Poor in the
  Reagan Era   D. Rowland, B. Lyons, J. Edwards   9:427–50
Developmental Screening in Early Childhood:
  The Interaction of Research and Social
  Policy   S. J. Meisels   9:527–50
Why is Our Population of Uninsured and
  Underinsured Persons Growing? The
  Consequences of the "Deindustrialization"
  of America   C. Renner, V. Navarro   10:85–94
The Effect of the Medicare Prospective
  Payment System   J. R. Lave   10:141–61
Studies of Doctor-Patient Interaction   D. L. Roter, J. A. Hall   10:163–80
Decision Making for Introducing Clinical
  Preventive Services   R. J. Pels, D. H. Bor,
                          R. S. Lawrence   10:363–83
Modern Contraception: A 1989 Update   A. Rosenfield   10:385–401
Prevention and the Field of Mental Health: A
  Psychiatric Perspective   H. Pardes, M. M. Silverman,
                            A. West   10:403–22
Public Health Policy for the 1990s   M. Terris   11:39–51
Geographic Access to Physician Services   J. P. Newhouse   11:207–30
Chronic Disease in the 1990s   R. B. Rothenberg, J. P. Koplan   11:267–96
Physician Payment in the 1990s: Factors that
  Will Shape the Future   P. R. Lee, K. Grumbach,
                           W. J. Jameson   11:297–318
The Health Sector in Developing Countries:
  Problems for the 1990s and Beyond   W. H. Mosley, D. T. Jamison,
                                       D. A. Henderson   11:335–58
State Approaches to Financing Health Care
  for the Poor   E. R. Brown, G. Dallek   11:377–400
Words Without Action? The Production,
  Dissemination, and Impact of Consensus
  Recommendations   J. Lomas   12:41–65
Long-Term Care Financing: Problems and
  Progress   J. M. Wiener, R. J. Hanley   12:67–84

The Fat Kid on the Seesaw: American
Business and Health Care Cost
Containment, 1970-1990   L. Bergthold   12:157–75
Unnecessary Surgery   L. L. Leape   13:363–83
Causes of Low Preschool Immunization
Coverage in the United States   F. T. Cutts, W. A. Orenstein,
                                      R. H. Bernier   13:385–98

Access and Cost Implications of State
Limitations on Medicaid Reimbursement for
Pharmaceuticals   S. O. Schweitzer, Ph.D.,
                                      S. R. Shiota, M.P.H.   13:399–410

PREFATORY CHAPTER
Is There a Public Health Function?   A. Wolman   7:1–12

ANNUAL REVIEWS INC.

a nonprofit scientific publisher
4139 El Camino Way
P. O. Box 10139
Palo Alto, CA 94303-0897   •   USA

Annual Reviews Inc. publications may be ordered directly from our office; through booksellers and subscription agents, worldwide; and through participating professional societies.

Prices are subject to change without notice.   ARI Federal I.D. #94-1156476

- **Individuals:** Prepayment required on new accounts by check or money order (in U.S. dollars, check drawn on U.S. bank) or charge to MasterCard, VISA, or American Express.

- **Institutional Buyers:** Please include purchase order.

- **Students: $10.00 discount** from retail price, per volume. Prepayment required. Proof of student status must be provided. (Photocopy of Student I.D. is acceptable.) Student must be a degree candidate at an accredited institution. Order direct from Annual Reviews. Orders received through bookstores and institutions requesting student rates will be returned.

- **Professional Society Members:** Societies who have a contractual arrangement with Annual Reviews offer our books at reduced rates to members. Contact your society for information.

- **California orders** must add applicable sales tax.

- **CANADIAN ORDERS:** We must now collect 7% General Sales Tax on orders shipped to Canada. Canadian orders will not be accepted unless this tax has been added. Tax Registration # R 121 449-029. **Note:** Effective 1-1-92 Canadian prices increase from USA level to "other countries" level. See below.

- **Telephone orders,** paid by credit card, welcomed. Call Toll Free **1-800-523-8635** (except in California). California customers use 1-415-493-4400 (not toll free). M-F, 8:00 am - 4:00 pm, Pacific Time. Students ordering by telephone must supply (by FAX or mail) proof of student status if proof from current academic year is not on file at Annual Reviews. Purchase orders from universities require written confirmation before shipment.

- **FAX: 415-855-9815   Telex: 910-290-0275**

- **Postage paid by Annual Reviews** (4th class bookrate). UPS domestic ground service (except to AK and HI) available at $2.00 extra per book. UPS air service or Airmail also available at cost. UPS requires street address. P.O. Box, APO, FPO, not acceptable.

- **Regular Orders:** Please list below the volumes you wish to order by volume number.

- **Standing Orders:** New volume in the series will be sent to you automatically each year upon publication. Cancellation may be made at any time. Please indicate volume number to begin standing order.

- **Prepublication Orders:** Volumes not yet published will be shipped in month and year indicated.

- **We do not ship on approval.**

ANNUAL REVIEWS SERIES *Volumes not listed are no longer in print*	Prices, postpaid, per volume		Regular Order Please send Volume(s):	Standing Order Begin with Volume:
	Until 12-31-91 USA & Canada / elsewhere	After 1-1-92 USA / other countries (incl. Canada)		
Annual Review of ANTHROPOLOGY				
Vols. 1-16 (1972-1987)........................	$33.00/$38.00 ⎫			
Vols. 17-18 (1988-1989)........................	$37.00/$42.00 ⎬ $41.00/$46.00			
Vols. 19-20 (1990-1991)........................	$41.00/$46.00 ⎭			
Vol. 21 (avail. Oct. 1992)...............	$44.00/$49.00	$44.00/$49.00	Vol(s)._____	Vol.____
Annual Review of ASTRONOMY AND ASTROPHYSICS				
Vols. 1, 5-14, (1963, 1967-1976)				
16-20 (1978-1982)........................	$33.00/$38.00 ⎫			
Vols. 21-27 (1983-1989)........................	$49.00/$54.00 ⎬ $53.00/$58.00			
Vols. 28-29 (1990-1991)........................	$53.00/$58.00 ⎭			
Vol. 30 (avail. Sept. 1992).............	$57.00/$62.00	$57.00/$62.00	Vol(s)._____	Vol.____
Annual Review of BIOCHEMISTRY				
Vols. 30-34, 36-56 (1961-1965, 1967-1987) ...	$35.00/$40.00 ⎫			
Vols. 57-58 (1988-1989)........................	$37.00/$42.00 ⎬ $41.00/$47.00			
Vols. 59-60 (1990-1991)........................	$41.00/$47.00 ⎭			
Vol. 61 (avail. July 1992)	$46.00/$52.00	$46.00/$52.00	Vol(s)._____	Vol.____

ANNUAL REVIEWS SERIES	Prices, postpaid, per volume		Regular Order	Standing Order
Volumes not listed are no longer in print	Until 12-31-91 USA & Canada / elsewhere	After 1-1-92 USA / other countries (incl. Canada)	Please send Volume(s):	Begin with Volume:

Annual Review of BIOPHYSICS AND BIOMOLECULAR STRUCTURE

Vols. 1-11	(1972-1982)	$33.00/$38.00			
Vols. 12-18	(1983-1989)	$51.00/$56.00	$55.00/$60.00		
Vols. 19-20	(1990-1991)	$55.00/$60.00			
Vol. 21	(avail. June 1992)	$59.00/$64.00	$59.00/$64.00	Vol(s)._____	Vol.____

Annual Review of CELL BIOLOGY

Vols. 1-3	(1985-1987)	$33.00/$38.00			
Vols. 4-5	(1988-1989)	$37.00/$42.00	$41.00/$46.00		
Vols. 6-7	(1990-1991)	$41.00/$46.00			
Vol. 8	(avail. Nov. 1992)	$46.00/$51.00	$46.00/$51.00	Vol(s)._____	Vol.____

Annual Review of COMPUTER SCIENCE

Vols. 1-2	(1986-1987)	$41.00/$46.00	$41.00/$46.00		
Vols. 3-4	(1988, 1989-1990)	$47.00/$52.00	$47.00/$52.00	Vol(s)._____	Vol.____

Series suspended until further notice. Volumes 1-4 are still available at the special promotional price of $100.00 USA /$115.00 other countries, when all 4 volumes are purchased at one time. Orders at the special price must be prepaid.

Annual Review of EARTH AND PLANETARY SCIENCES

Vols. 1-10	(1973-1982)	$33.00/$38.00			
Vols. 11-17	(1983-1989)	$51.00/$56.00	$55.00/$60.00		
Vols. 18-19	(1990-1991)	$55.00/$60.00			
Vol. 20	(avail. May 1992)	$59.00/$64.00	$59.00/$64.00	Vol(s)._____	Vol.____

Annual Review of ECOLOGY AND SYSTEMATICS

Vols. 2-18	(1971-1987)	$33.00/$38.00			
Vols. 19-20	(1988-1989)	$36.00/$41.00	$40.00/$45.00		
Vols. 21-22	(1990-1991)	$40.00/$45.00			
Vol. 23	(avail. Nov. 1992)	$44.00/$49.00	$44.00/$49.00	Vol(s)._____	Vol.____

Annual Review of ENERGY AND THE ENVIRONMENT

Vols. 1-7	(1976-1982)	$33.00/$38.00			
Vols. 8-14	(1983-1989)	$60.00/$65.00	$64.00/$69.00		
Vols. 15-16	(1990-1991)	$64.00/$69.00			
Vol. 17	(avail. Oct. 1992)	$68.00/$73.00	$68.00/$73.00	Vol(s)._____	Vol.____

Annual Review of ENTOMOLOGY

Vols. 10-16, 18	(1965-1971, 1973)				
20-32	(1975-1987)	$33.00/$38.00			
Vols. 33-34	(1988-1989)	$36.00/$41.00	$40.00/$45.00		
Vols. 35-36	(1990-1991)	$40.00/$45.00			
Vol. 37	(avail. Jan. 1992)	$44.00/$49.00	$44.00/$49.00	Vol(s)._____	Vol.____

Annual Review of FLUID MECHANICS

Vols. 2-4, 7	(1970-1972, 1975)				
9-19	(1977-1987)	$34.00/$39.00			
Vols. 20-21	(1988-1989)	$36.00/$41.00	$40.00/$45.00		
Vols. 22-23	(1990-1991)	$40.00/$45.00			
Vol. 24	(avail. Jan. 1992)	$44.00/$49.00	$44.00/$49.00	Vol(s)._____	Vol.____

Annual Review of GENETICS

Vols. 1-12, 14-21	(1967-1978, 1980-1987)	$33.00/$38.00			
Vols. 22-23	(1988-1989)	$36.00/$41.00	$40.00/$45.00		
Vols. 24-25	(1990-1991)	$40.00/$45.00			
Vol. 26	(avail. Dec. 1992)	$44.00/$49.00	$44.00/$49.00	Vol(s)._____	Vol.____

Annual Review of IMMUNOLOGY

Vols. 1-5	(1983-1987)	$33.00/$38.00			
Vols. 6-7	(1988-1989)	$36.00/$41.00	$41.00/$46.00		
Vol. 8	(1990)	$40.00/$45.00			
Vol. 9	(1991)	$41.00/$46.00	$41.00/$46.00		
Vol. 10	(avail. April 1992)	$45.00/$50.00	$45.00/$50.00	Vol(s)._____	Vol.____